Received 5/94 $65

D0077066

1993
YEAR BOOK OF
DIAGNOSTIC
RADIOLOGY®

Statement of Purpose

The YEAR BOOK Service

The YEAR BOOK series was devised in 1901 by practicing health professionals who observed that the literature of medicine and related disciplines had become so voluminous that no one individual could read and place in perspective every potential advance in a major specialty. In the final decade of the 20th century, this recognition is more acutely true than it was in 1901.

More than merely a series of books, YEAR BOOK volumes are the tangible results of a unique service designed to accomplish the following:

- to *survey* a wide range of journals of proven value
- to *select* from those journals papers representing significant advances and statements of important clinical principles
- to provide *abstracts* of those articles that are readable, convenient summaries of their key points
- to provide *commentary* about those articles to place them in perspective

These publications grow out of a unique process that calls on the talents of outstanding authorities in clinical and fundamental disciplines, trained literature specialists, and professional writers, all supported by the resources of Mosby, the world's preeminent publisher for the health professions.

THE LITERATURE BASE

Mosby subscribes to nearly 1,000 journals published worldwide, covering the full range of the health professions. On an annual basis, the publisher examines usage patterns and polls its expert authorities to add new journals to the literature base and to delete journals that are no longer useful as potential YEAR BOOK sources.

The Literature Survey

The publisher's team of literature specialists, all of whom are trained and experienced health professionals, examines every original, peer-reviewed article in each journal issue. More than 250,000 articles per year are scanned systematically, including title, text, illustrations, tables, and references. Each scan is compared, article by article, to the search strategies that the publisher has developed in consultation with the 270 outside experts who form the pool of YEAR BOOK editors. A given article may be reviewed by any number of editors, from one to a dozen or more, regardless of the discipline for which the paper was originally published. In turn, each editor who receives the article reviews it to determine whether or not the article should be included in the YEAR BOOK. This decision is based on the article's inherent quality, its probable usefulness to readers of that YEAR BOOK, and the editor's goal to represent a balanced picture of a given field in each volume of the YEAR BOOK. In addition, the editor indicates when to include figures and tables from the article to help the YEAR BOOK reader better understand the information.

Of the quarter million articles scanned each year, only 5% are selected for detailed analysis within the YEAR BOOK series, thereby assuring readers of the high value of every selection.

THE ABSTRACT

The publisher's abstracting staff is headed by a physician-writer and includes individuals with training in the life sciences, medicine, and other areas, plus extensive experience in writing for the health professions and related industries. Each selected article is assigned to a specific writer on this abstracting staff. The abstracter, guided in many cases by notations supplied by the expert editor, writes a structured, condensed summary designed so that the reader can rapidly acquire the essential information contained in the article.

THE COMMENTARY

The YEAR BOOK editorial boards, sometimes assisted by guest commentators, write comments that place each article in perspective for the reader. This provides the reader with the equivalent of a personal consultation with a leading international authority—an opportunity to better understand the value of the article and to benefit from the authority's thought processes in assessing the article.

ADDITIONAL EDITORIAL FEATURES

The editorial boards of each YEAR BOOK organize the abstracts and comments to provide a logical and satisfying sequence of information. To enhance the organization, editors also provide introductions to sections or individual chapters, comments linking a number of abstracts, citations to additional literature, and other features.

The published YEAR BOOK contains enhanced bibliographic citations for each selected article, including extended listings of multiple authors and identification of author affilliations. Each YEAR BOOK contains a Table of Contents specific to that year's volume. From year to year, the Table of Contents for a given YEAR BOOK will vary depending on developments within the field.

Every YEAR BOOK contains a list of the journals from which papers have been selected. This list represents a subset of the nearly 1,000 journals surveyed by the publisher, and occasionally reflects a particularly pertinent article from a journal that is not surveyed on a routine basis.

Finally, each volume contains a comprehensive subject index and an index to authors of each selected paper.

The 1993 Year Book Series

Year Book of Anesthesia and Pain Management: Drs. Miller, Abram, Kirby, Ostheimer, Roizen, and Stoelting

Year Book of Cardiology®: Drs. Schlant, Collins, Engle, Gersh, Kaplan, and Waldo

Year Book of Chiropractic: Drs. Phillips and Adams

Year Book of Critical Care Medicine®: Drs. Rogers and Parrillo

Year Book of Dentistry®: Drs. Meskin, Currier, Kennedy, Leinfelder, Berry, Roser, and Zakariasen

Year Book of Dermatologic Surgery: Drs. Swanson, Salasche, and Glogau

Year Book of Dermatology®: Drs. Sober and Fitzpatrick

Year Book of Diagnostic Radiology®: Drs. Federle, Clark, Gross, Madewell, Maynard, Sackett, and Young

Year Book of Digestive Diseases®: Drs. Greenberger and Moody

Year Book of Drug Therapy®: Drs. Lasagna and Weintraub

Year Book of Emergency Medicine®: Drs. Wagner, Burdick, Davidson, Roberts, and Spivey

Year Book of Endocrinology®: Drs. Bagdade, Braverman, Horton, Kannan, Landsberg, Molitch, Morley, Odell, Rogol, Ryan, and Sherwin

Year Book of Family Practice®: Drs. Berg, Bowman, Davidson, Dietrich, and Scherger

Year Book of Geriatrics and Gerontology®: Drs. Beck, Reuben, Burton, Small, Whitehouse, and Goldstein

Year Book of Hand Surgery®: Drs. Amadio and Hentz

Year Book of Health Care Management: Drs. Heyssel, Brock, Moses, and Steinberg, Ms. Avakian, and Messrs. Berman, Kues, and Rosenberg

Year Book of Hematology®: Drs. Spivak, Bell, Ness, Quesenberry, and Wiernik

Year Book of Infectious Diseases®: Drs. Wolff, Barza, Keusch, Klempner, and Snydman

Year Book of Infertility: Drs. Mishell, Paulsen, and Lobo

Year Book of Medicine®: Drs. Rogers, Bone, Cline, O'Rourke, Greenberger, Utiger, Epstein, and Malawista

Year Book of Neonatal and Perinatal Medicine®: Drs. Klaus and Fanaroff

Year Book of Nephrology: Drs. Coe, Favus, Henderson, Kashgarian, Luke, Myers, and Curtis

Year Book of Neurology and Neurosurgery®: Drs. Bradley and Crowell

Year Book of Neuroradiology: Drs. Osborn, Eskridge, Harnsberger, and Grossman

Year Book of Nuclear Medicine®: Drs. Hoffer, Gore, Gottschalk, Zaret, and Zubal

Year Book of Obstetrics and Gynecology®: Drs. Mishell, Kirschbaum, and Morrow

Year Book of Occupational and Environmental Medicine: Drs. Emmett, Brooks, Frank, and Hammad

Year Book of Oncology®: Drs. Young, Longo, Ozols, Simone, Steele, and Glatstein

Year Book of Ophthalmology®: Drs. Laibson, Adams, Augsburger, Benson, Cohen, Eagle, Flanagan, Nelson, Rapuano, Reinecke, Sergott, and Wilson

Year Book of Orthopedics®: Drs. Sledge, Poss, Cofield, Frymoyer, Griffin, Hansen, Johnson, Simmons, and Springfield

Year Book of Otolaryngology–Head and Neck Surgery®: Drs. Holt and Paparella

Year Book of Pathology and Clinical Pathology®: Drs. Gardner, Bennett, Cousar, Garvin, and Worsham

Year Book of Pediatrics®: Dr. Stockman

Year Book of Plastic, Reconstructive, and Aesthetic Surgery: Drs. Miller, Cohen, McKinney, Robson, Ruberg, and Whitaker

Year Book of Podiatric Medicine and Surgery®: Dr. Kominsky

Year Book of Psychiatry and Applied Mental Health®: Drs. Talbott, Frances, Freedman, Meltzer, Perry, Schowalter, and Yudofsky

Year Book of Pulmonary Disease®: Drs. Bone and Petty

Year Book of Sports Medicine®: Drs. Shephard, Eichner, Sutton, and Torg, Col. Anderson, and Mr. George

Year Book of Surgery®: Drs. Copeland, Deitch, Eberlein, Howard, Ritchie, Robson, Souba, and Sugarbaker

Year Book of Transplantation®: Drs. Ascher, Hansen, and Strom

Year Book of Ultrasound: Drs. Merritt, Mittelstaedt, Carroll, Babcock, and Goldstein

Year Book of Urology®: Drs. Gillenwater and Howards

Year Book of Vascular Surgery®: Dr. Porter

Roundsmanship® '93–'94: A Student's Survival Guide to Clinical Medicine Using Current Literature: Drs. Dan, Feigin, Quilligan, Schrock, Stein, and Talbott

Editors

Michael P. Federle, M.D.

Professor, Department of Radiology, University of Pittsburgh, Pittsburgh, Pennsylvania

Robert A. Clark, M.D.

Department of Radiology, Moffitt Cancer Center, University of South Florida, Tampa, Florida

Barry H. Gross, M.D.

Professor of Radiology, University of Michigan Medical Center, Ann Arbor, Michigan

John E. Madewell, M.D.

Professor and Chairman, Department of Radiology, Pennsylvania State University, Hershey, Pennsylvania

C. Douglas Maynard, M.D.

Professor and Chairman, Department of Radiology, Bowman Gray School of Medicine, Wake Forest University, Winston-Salem, North Carolina

Joseph F. Sackett, M.D.

Professor and Chairman, Department of Radiology, University of Wisconsin Hospital and Clinics, Madison, Wisconsin

Lionel W. Young, M.D.

Director of Pediatric Radiology, Loma Linda University Children's Hospital, Loma Linda, California

1993

The Year Book of
DIAGNOSTIC
RADIOLOGY®

Editors

Michael P. Federle, M.D.
Robert A. Clark, M.D.
Barry H. Gross, M.D.
John E. Madewell, M.D.
C. Douglas Maynard, M.D.
Joseph F. Sackett, M.D.
Lionel W. Young, M.D.

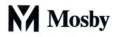 Mosby

St. Louis Baltimore Boston Chicago London Philadelphia Sydney Toronto

Editor-in-Chief, Year Book Publishing: Kenneth H. Killion
Associate Acquisitions Editor: Gretchen C. Templeton
Sponsoring Editor: Bernadette Buchholz
Manager, Literature Services: Edith M. Podrazik
Senior Information Specialist: Terri Santo
Senior Medical Writer: David A. Cramer, M.D.
Assistant Director, Manuscript Services: Frances M. Perveiler
Assistant Managing Editor, Year Book Editing Services: Tamara L. Smith
Senior Production/Desktop Publishing Manager: Max F. Perez
Proofroom Manager: Barbara M. Kelly

Editorial Office:
Mosby, Inc.
200 North LaSalle St.
Chicago, IL 60601

International Standard Serial Number: 0098-1672
International Standard Book Number: 0-8151-1127-4

Table of Contents

Journals Represented

Mosby subscribes to and surveys nearly 1,000 U.S. and foreign medical and allied health journals. From these journals, the Editors select the articles to be abstracted. Journals represented in this YEAR BOOK are listed below.

Acta Radiologica
American Heart Journal
American Journal of Gastroenterology
American Journal of Medicine
American Journal of Neuroradiology
American Journal of Otolaryngology
American Journal of Roentgenology
American Journal of Surgery
American Journal of Surgical Pathology
American Surgeon
Annals of Emergency Medicine
Annals of Surgery
Annals of Thoracic Surgery
Annals of Vascular Surgery
Archives of Disease in Childhood
Archives of Emergency Medicine
Archives of Internal Medicine
Archives of Neurology
Archives of Orthopaedic and Trauma Surgery
Archives of Otolaryngology-Head and Neck Surgery
Archives of Physical Medicine and Rehabilitation
Archives of Surgery
Arthritis and Rheumatism
Australasian Radiology
British Heart Journal
British Journal of Industrial Medicine
British Journal of Obstetrics and Gynaecology
British Journal of Radiology
British Journal of Surgery
British Medical Journal
Canadian Association of Radiologists Journal
Canadian Journal of Neurological Sciences
Cancer
Cardiovascular and Interventional Radiology
Chest
Childs Nervous System
Circulation
Clinical Genetics
Clinical Imaging
Clinical Nuclear Medicine
Clinical Orthopaedics and Related Research
Clinical Radiology
Critical Care Medicine
Diseases of the Colon and Rectum
Epilepsia
European Journal of Nuclear Medicine
Gastroenterology
Gastrointestinal Radiology
Hepatology
International Orthopaedics

Investigative Radiology
Italian Journal of Orthopaedics and Traumatology
Journal of Bone and Joint Surgery (American Volume)
Journal of Clinical Ultrasound
Journal of Computer Assisted Tomography
Journal of Hand Surgery (British)
Journal of Laryngology and Otology
Journal of Medical Ethics
Journal of Medical Genetics
Journal of Neurology, Neurosurgery and Psychiatry
Journal of Neurosurgery
Journal of Nuclear Medicine
Journal of Pediatric Gastroenterology and Nutrition
Journal of Pediatric Orthopedics
Journal of Pediatric Surgery
Journal of Pediatrics
Journal of Rheumatology
Journal of Thoracic and Cardiovascular Surgery
Journal of Trauma
Journal of Ultrasound in Medicine
Journal of Urology
Journal of Vascular Surgery
Journal of the American College of Cardiology
Journal of the American Medical Association
Journal of the Neurological Sciences
Kidney International
Lancet
Magnetic Resonance Imaging
Magnetic Resonance in Medicine
Medical Physics
Neuroradiology
Neurosurgery
New England Journal of Medicine
Nuclear Medicine and Biology–Part B
Obstetrics and Gynecology
Ophthalmology
Orthopedics
Pediatric Cardiology
Pediatric Infectious Disease Journal
Pediatric Radiology
Radiology
Respiratory Medicine
Seminars in Oncology
Skeletal Radiology
Southern Medical Journal
Spine
Stroke
Surgical Neurology
Urologic Radiology
Urology
Zeitschrift fur Kinderchirurgie

STANDARD ABBREVIATIONS

The following terms are abbreviated in this edition: acquired immunodeficiency syndrome (AIDS), central nervous system (CNS), cerebrospinal fluid (CSF), computed tomography (CT), diethylenetriaminepentaacetic acid (DTPA), electrocardiography (ECG), gadolinium (Gd), human immunodeficiency virus (HIV), and magnetic resonance (MR) or MR imaging (MRI), positron emission tomography (PET), and single-photon emission computed tomography (SPECT).

1 Thorax

Introduction

Although it was a great pleasure to contribute to the 1992 YEAR BOOK OF DIAGNOSTIC RADIOLOGY, it is an even greater pleasure to get to do it again in 1993—even after they've seen my work! I am certain that this is in no small part a reflection on Murray Rebner's excellent comments on mammography. I thank him for helping to keep me on the team and for his even larger contribution this year. Murray's articles on breast cancer and breast imaging follow his introductory comments and constitute the first section of this chapter.

I have subdivided the remainder of the chapter under almost exactly the same headings as were used in the 1992 YEAR BOOK. The first section is topics in CT. I especially call your attention to Swensen's article on CT of the solitary pulmonary nodule. It may change our practices as profoundly as the Hopkins work in the mid-1980s on thin-section CT evaluation of diffuse calcification of pulmonary nodules.

The next section is lung cancer. Several articles discuss missed radiographic findings in lung cancer patients, and several others deal with new imaging agents for lung cancer. The key article in this section is by McLoud. This is a reassessment of the accuracy of mediastinal staging by CT in lung cancer patients. As with Swensen's article, the potential impact on the role of CT in real life is profound.

A new section for me is ultrasound. Although I (and my American chest radiology colleagues) don't do much with thoracic ultrasound, there are many interesting applications that have been pursued by our Asian and European counterparts. It may be time to expand the role of ultrasound in chest radiology; if so, the articles presented here may be a good place for us to start.

Under the heading of new applications in diagnosis and therapy, I expected a flood of articles on digital chest radiography, because more departments are using this new technology. The flood didn't materialize; I actually saw more ultrasound articles this year. Nevertheless, 2 excellent articles on digital chest radiography lead off the section and provide a good model for future investigations. Other applications in this section include MR evaluation of lung parenchyma, complications of newer therapies (e.g., bone marrow and lung transplantation), and new surgical tools.

Utilization review was probably my major theme in the 1992 YEAR BOOK. There is a smaller section on this subject in 1993. It is no less important than it was previously, and there is again some nice work on the proper role of chest radiography in diverse conditions such as acute asthma, febrile neutropenic patients, and breast cancer. Next year I hope to find good articles that discuss the appropriate use of chest CT.

The final section in this chapter is a potpourri of general topics. There is no overriding theme. Several articles (1 on meningioma and 1 on thymolipoma) question what is generally regarded as common knowledge. Other articles (e.g., the article on searching for lung nodules) are nice treatments of subjects that don't comfortably reside in other sections. As usual, my special favorites are 2 very cute case reports. I hope you get as much pleasure from their images as I did.

Barry H. Gross, M.D.

Breast Cancer and Breast Imaging

Nonpalpable Breast Lesions: Findings of Stereotaxic Needle-Core Biopsy and Fine-Needle Aspiration Cytology
Dowlatshahi K, Yaremko ML, Kluskens LF, Jokich PM (Rush-Presbyterian-St Luke's Med Ctr, Chicago)
Radiology 181:745–750, 1991   1–1

Background.—Although there have been advances in the technique of mammography, it is still difficult to predict accurately the benign or malignant nature of mammographically detected breast lesions. The findings of stereotaxic needle-core biopsy and fine-needle aspiration (FNA) cytology in cases of nonpalpable breast lesions were reviewed.

Methods.—A total of 250 mammographically detected nonpalpable lesions suspicious for malignancy were localized stereotaxically. These lesions were found in women undergoing routine screening mammography. In each case, FNA cytologic specimens and needle-core biopsy specimens were obtained before open biopsy.

Findings.—Of the lesions, 76 (30.4%) were malignant and 83% were 1 cm long or smaller. Needle-core biopsy alone conclusively diagnosed 41% of these cancers. Fine-needle aspiration cytologic study alone was diagnostic in 32%. There were no false positive results in either test. The same diagnosis was reached in 54% when the results of both tests were combined. When the 2 needle tests were applied to 125 mammographically defined low-suspicion lesions, 68% were found to be benign by either 1 or both needle tests. There was 1 lobular carcinoma in situ. When the algorithm was applied, 34% of patients with abnormal mammograms, or one third of those recommended for open biopsy, may have avoided surgery.

Conclusion.—It appears that stereotaxic needle biopsy of nonpalpable breast lesions will play an important role in the future diagnosis and management of breast cancer. It will decrease the number of unnecessary breast biopsies and the associated cost, and more women will be encouraged to participate in screening mammographic surveillance for early detection of breast cancer.

▶ With the increased use of the stereotactic localization device, the accuracy of FNA cytology has improved, and stereotactic-guided needle-core biopsy has also started to assume importance in the management of nonpalpable breast lesions. The authors note a sensitivity rate of 86% for FNA cytology vs. 71% for fine-needle core biopsy. Specificity for fine-needle core biopsy was 96%, greater than the 72% for FNA cytology.

Both techniques can help to minimize unnecessary surgery for benign lesions, and they can potentially allow 1-stage diagnosis and staging for malignant lesions. It is important to note the poorest results with FNA cytology and fine-needle core biopsy occurred with calcifications. A biopsy of these lesions is still needed if they are mammographically suspicious, despite a negative cytology result. A good cytologist and pathologist are required for both procedures. Optimal needle size and what procedure (FNA cytology or fine-needle core biopsy) is best for a specific type of lesion still may need to be determined with additional comparative studies.—Murray Rebner, M.D.

Nonpalpable Breast Lesions: Stereotactic Automated Large-Core Biopsies
Parker SH, Lovin JD, Jobe WE, Burke BJ, Hopper KD, Yakes WF (Radiology Imaging Assoc, Englewood, Colo; Fitzsimons Army Med Ctr, Aurora, Colo; Pennsylvania State Univ, Hershey, Pa)
Radiology 180:403–407, 1991   1–2

Objective.—If needle biopsy of the breast could be made accurate and dependable, it would probably replace surgical excisional biopsy. Surgical excisional biopsy of the breast was compared with automated stereotactic gun biopsy (using 14-gauge cutting needles exclusively) in 102 patients with mammographically suspicious nonpalpable lesions.

Observations.—The results of gun biopsy and surgical excisional biopsy agreed histologically in 98 cases, including 22 of 23 carcinomas. Two cases that were missed at surgical biopsy were correctly diagnosed with gun biopsy. Two cases missed by gun biopsy were correctly diagnosed by surgical biopsy.

Conclusion.—Stereotactic gun biopsy can be an acceptable alternative to surgical biopsy in women with mammographically suspicious lesions, particularly if a 14-gauge needle is used.

▶ This paper is one of the first to describe stereotactic-guided large-core biopsy of nonpalpable breast lesions. The authors demonstrated that the technique, when correctly applied, has a high degree of accuracy (96% agreement with histologic diagnosis). The procedure offers an alternative to surgical biopsy if a negative result is obtained. The authors' pioneering work with this modality will hopefully reap benefits for many years to come.

One question that arises is whether a 14-gauge needle is required. Other authors have shown equally impressive results and perhaps less morbidity with the use of 18-gauge needles. It will be interesting to see if bigger is, in fact, better for needle size.—M. Rebner, M.D.

Stereotaxic Localization for Fine-Needle Aspiration Breast Biopsy: Initial Experience With 300 Patients
Mitnick JS, Vazquez MF, Roses DF, Harris MN, Gianutsos R, Waisman J (New York Univ Med Ctr, New York)
Arch Surg 126:1137–1140, 1991   1–3

Background.—Research has shown that aspiration biopsy is a valuable method for diagnosing palpable masses. Recently, it has been applied to the diagnosis of nonpalpable masses as well. However, the accuracy varies widely when ultrasound or radiography has been used for guiding the needle, probably because of an inability to verify its location. Stereotaxic localization may permit greater accuracy in aspiration biopsy for nonpalpable lesions.

Methods and Findings.—A group of 300 consecutive patients with nonpalpable mammographic lesions was studied. Sixty-eight (23%) had suspicious or malignant aspirates on stereotaxic aspiration biopsy. All were later proved malignant by assessment of operative specimens. Among the 216 patients with benign aspirates, 65 were confirmed at surgery; 151 had subsequent mammography at 6- and 12-month intervals with no demonstrable changes. In 10 cases, the aspirates were atypical, and in 6, they were nondiagnostic. In all 16 cases, biopsy specimens were obtained and were malignant in 8. Stereotaxic breast aspiration for diagnosing cancer had a sensitivity of 96% and a specificity of 100%.

Conclusion.—Stereotaxic aspiration permitted precise localization of nonpalpable lesions for cytologic assessment in this series. It proved highly reliable for identifying lesions that required surgery. In the current series, all the nonpalpable breast lesions that yielded suspicious or malignant aspirates proved to be malignant by subsequent resection. No lesion that was benign by aspiration proved malignant.

▶ This paper by Mitnick et al. shows that the use of stereotactic guided fine-needle aspiration cytology, the predecessor of core biopsy, is still an accurate tool in the diagnosis of nonpalpable breast lesions. The authors note a high correlation between either a negative or positive cytology result and subsequent histologic diagnosis. A small number of cases (6 of 300) were not diagnostic. What was surprising was that no lesion that was benign by aspiration proved malignant. Other series have noted that sampling errors (e.g., obtaining cells from the desmoplastic reactive tissue of a cancer and not from the tumor itself) do occur. Kudos to the authors for their excellent needle work. This technique, along with stereotactic-guided core biopsy, will continue to help reduce the number of breast biopsies for benign lesions. Having this article published in the *Archives of Surgery* hopefully will enhance the credibility of stereotactic-guided fine-needle aspiration cytology for breast surgeons.—M. Rebner, M.D.

Application of Estrogen Receptor Immunocytochemical Assay to Aspirates From Mammographically Guided Fine Needle Biopsy of Nonpalpable Breast Lesions

Masood S, Frykberg ER, McLellan GL, Bullard JB (Univ of Florida, Jacksonville, Fla)
South Med J 84:857–861, 1991   1–4

Background.—Hormone receptors have played an important role in managing and determining the prognosis of breast cancer. However, they are difficult to apply to the growing numbers of very small breast cancers being detected. The feasibility of applying the estrogen receptor immunocytochemical assay (ER-ICA) to ctyologic specimens was studied.

Methods.—One hundred patients who were undergoing fine-needle aspiration (FNA) biopsy of mammographically detected nonpalpable breast lesions were studied. In all cases, these lesions were surgically excised just after cytologic aspiration. Ultimately, 20 malignancies were diagnosed histologically; 17 had been diagnosed cytologically. Specific monoclonal antibody for ER was used in applying ER-ICA to cytologic preparation of 15 malignant neoplasms with enough cellular material for the assay.

Results.—Immunostaining was positive in 9 cases. There was no expression of ER in 6. When an immunocytochemical assay was done on frozen tissue of the corresponding surgically removed tumors, there was an 86.6% concordance between the 2 results.

Conclusion.—The combination of mammographically guided FNA biopsy and ER-ICA on the cytologic specimens appears to be a safe, reliable, and cost-effective alternative to open surgical biopsy and biochemical ER assay in the diagnosis and management of nonpalpable breast lesions. Estrogen receptor immunocytochemical assay offers many advantages and should be the method of choice for hormone receptor assay of breast malignances.

▶ The authors describe an ICA technique used on fine-needle aspirates of nonpalpable breast lesions to measure ERs. The advantage of this method, which uses anti-ER antibodies instead of the traditional biochemical assays, is that it can be used with smaller volumes of tissue. There is a high degree of correlation between ER-ICA and conventional biochemical assays. In addition, the method permits a precise determination of tumor heterogeneity. It is tumor heterogeneity that correlates with prognosis and responsiveness to hormonal manipulation.

Thanks to this new assay, it now appears that mammographically guided FNA biopsy can aid not only in diagnosis, but also in choice of treatment of nonpalpable breast cancer. It will be interesting to see whether this method supplants the traditional biochemical assay for ERs in the future.—M. Rebner, M.D.

Gadopentetate Dimeglumine-Enhanced Chemical-Shift MR Imaging of the Breast
Rubens D, Totterman S, Chacko AK, Kothari K, Logan-Young W, Szumowski J, Simon JH, Zachariah E (Univ of Rochester, Ridgewood Diagnostic Imaging, Breast Clinic of Rochester, Rochester, NY; Honolulu)
AJR 157:267–270, 1991   1–5

Background.—Because of the high background signal from fat in the breast, standard T_1-weighted MR images enhanced with gadopentetate dimeglumine only minimally enhance breast lesions. Lesions that are strongly enhanced may become isointense compared with the fat signal, and they also may become invisible or indistinct after contrast administration. In other areas of the body where a strong lipid signal is present, fat-suppressed chemical-shift imaging (CSI), combined with administration of gadopentetate dimeglumine, improves lesion detection and characterization. Therefore, this technique was assessed in the breast.

Methods.—Twenty patients with mammographic lesions were studied with standard unenhanced T_1- and T_2-weighted images and enhanced T_1-weighted images. Chemical-shift imaging was also performed before and after gadopentetate dimeglumine was administered. The patients were independently ranked for border and matrix characteristics. The borders were assessed for smooth, irregular, or spiculated margins, and the matrix or internal substance was assessed for visibility and enhancement type, homogeneous or inhomogeneous.

Results.—The enhanced CSI images depicted border and matrix characteristics better than the other images. A corresponding mass was detected on MRI in 14 of the 20 patients. In 2 of those 14, only the enhanced CSI images demonstrated the lesion. In several cases, chemical-shift artifacts on enhanced T_1-weighted images obscured border detail.

Conclusion.—Compared with conventional MRI with or without enhancement, enhanced CSI improves visualization of breast lesions. Enhanced CSI produces differential enhancement between glandular tissue and lesions whereas suppressing the fat signal. As a result, the visualization of border and matrix characteristics is improved, and lesions are depicted that may otherwise be obscured.

▶ This study notes the value of Gd-enhanced chemical-shift MRI of the breast. When the high background signal from fat in the breast is suppressed, lesion detection and characterization may improve. The authors noted better border definitions and matrix characteristics than on standard conventional Gd-enhanced T_1-weighted images.

However, we should be aware of the method's limitations. As the authors note, 6 of the 20 lesions were not imaged with this technique. Further studies are needed to determine whether sensitivity and specificity for breast lesions will be improved with Gd-enhanced CSI. It is likely that MRI will remain a complementary tool to mammography in the workup of nonpalpable breast lesions.—M. Rebner, M.D.

Three-Dimensional Gadolinium-Enhanced MR Imaging of the Breast: Pulse Sequence With Fat Suppression and Magnetization Transfer Contrast: Work in Progress
Pierce WB, Harms SE, Flamig DP, Griffey RH, Evans WP, Hagans JE (Baylor Univ, Dallas)
Radiology 181:757–763, 1991   1–6

Background.—The results of breast screening studies have demonstrated that early detection of breast carcinoma can significantly reduce mortality. Even when breast MRI is enhanced with gadopentetate dimeglumine, the tumor is often isointense with fat on T_1-weighted images and may be obscured by the hyperintense surrounding fat. A steady-state pulse sequence with fat suppression, called magnetization transfer with fast adiabatic trajectory in the steady state (MT-FATS), can produce high-resolution 3-dimensional images of the breast in rapid imaging time.

Method.—Fourteen women were evaluated with MRI before and after infusion of gadopentetate dimeglumine. In the MT-FATS technique, a special preparation pulse is applied off resonance, before the main sequence, to produce magnetization transfer contrast, which attenuates signal from normal fibroglandular tissue and improves lesion conspicuity after administration of gadopentetate dimeglumine. Twelve of the women participating had clinical or mammographic findings (or both) suspicious for malignancy, and 2 were healthy volunteers (1 with silicone implants). The imaging time was approximately 7 minutes for each set of 128 sections. All carcinomas were enhanced on postcontrast images.

Findings.—Multifocal and inflammatory carcinoma could be clearly visualized. In 2 patients with fat necrosis or scar, enhancement was not clear, but in 1 patient with fibrocystic changes, the areas were visible as increased signal intensity on preinfusion images.

Conclusion.—Fat-suppressed 3-dimensional imaging with this pulse sequence provides improved resolution and image contrast in diagnosing breast cancer compared with conventional breast MRI. Although the high cost of MRI will preclude its use as a screening method, it may be helpful in problematic clinical cases that cannot be resolved with conventional diagnostic imaging methods.

▶ Like the report summarized in Abstract 1–5, this work notes a new MRI technique for the breast. The authors use a combination of fat suppression, Gd enhancement, and a special preparation pulse (MT-FATS) applied off resonance to attenuate signals from normal glandular elements. This method has shown promise not only in detecting mammographically suspicious carcinomas, but also in finding occult multifocal breast cancer. Fat necrosis and scarring older than 6 months did not enhance and were able to be differentiated from carcinoma. Further studies are needed to determine whether other benign entities, such as fibroadenomas and fibrocystic change, can be characterized accurately with this procedure. If future study results continue to show progress, we are likely to see improved, dedicated breast coils for MRI become more readily accessible to breast imagers.—M. Rebner, M.D.

Radiologic Recommendation for Breast Biopsy on Screening Mammography Reports

Geelhoed GW, Barr HM, Curtis DJ, Olmsted WW (George Washington Univ Med Ctr, Washington DC)
Am Surg 57:419–424, 1991   1–7

Background.—Screening programs for breast cancer have been introduced among asymptomatic women, especially those with identified risk factors, to facilitate diagnosis. Although the recommendation for biopsy of nonpalpable lesions is a conservative policy, it is unsettling for patients. Noncancer of the breast can usually be diagnosed on the basis of clinical and mammographic findings instead of subjecting patients to invasive diagnostic procedures.

Methods and Findings.—Eighty-four patients were referred for needle localization of nonpalpable mammographically detected lesions thought to be suspicious on screening. In 15 patients, or 21%, new radiographic reports reinterpreting the findings without biopsy were written on the original mammogram. Needle localization was done in 69 patients. Cancer was found in 28% compared with the national average of 14%. The patients who did not undergo biopsies were then reviewed. In the log of patients undergoing needle localization, the prereading by the mammographer doing the needle localization was recorded before biopsy confirmation, with a specificity of 94% and a sensitivity of 96%. Of the cancers detected, 39% were proved in patients older than 50 years of age.

Conclusion.—Benign breast conditions imaged in screening of patients without clinical findings can be diagnosed with confidence. Radiologically directed biopsy recommendation should be reserved for patients with mammographically suspicious lesions. This policy can safely

double the positive biopsy rate on needle localization of mammographically detected findings.

▶ This paper addresses the issue of decreasing the number of breast biopsies for benign conditions. In today's tense medicolegal climate, it is refreshing to read an article in a surgery journal that advocates additional radiologic
workup for lesions that are not definitely malignant. It is also noteworthy that
our surgical colleagues do not want the national radiology flower to be the
"hedge." The authors state that it is inappropriate for a mammography report to read "mammographic findings indeterminate: recommend biopsy."
Additional mammography views or other imaging modalities can often better
characterize an abnormality. Hopefully, more radiologists will use these techniques and also will use the same mammographic lexicon as advocated by
Dr. Kopans and the American College of Radiology to standaridize reports.
Surgeons too, not only radiologists, want to increase their positive biopsy
rate.—M. Rebner, M.D.

**Breast Cancer Screening in a Biracial Community: The Charleston
Tricounty Experience**
Lackland DT, Dunbar JB, Keil JE, Knapp RG, O'Brien PH (Med Univ of South
Carolina, Charleston, SC)
South Med J 84:862–866, 1991   1–8

Introduction.—Breast cancer remains a major cause of death among
American women. In South Carolina alone, breast cancer accounts for
more than 450 deaths per year. Although mammography, breast self-ex-
amination (BSE), and clinical breast examination are effective methods
for early detection of breast cancer, women's use of these procedures
remains relatively low. Knowledge of breast screening methods was surveyed among women living in a tricounty area in South Carolina.

Methods.—A total of 503 women between the ages of 18 and 91 years
was interviewed by telephone. Sample selection was by random telephone dialing. The respondents were asked whether they ever had a
mammogram and, if so, when the most recent mammogram was done.
Additional questions pertained to the frequency of BSE, the frequency of
clinical breast examination, estrogen usage, family history of cancer, and
demographics.

Results.—Most women (92%) reported that they knew how to do
BSE, and 57% reported doing BSE at least once each month. However,
13% of black women and 6% of white women did not know how to perform BSE. More than 90% of the women reported ever having had a
clinical breast examination, and 69% had had such an examination
within the past year. Mammography use varied significantly by age, income, and race, but overall, only 40% of the women reported ever having had a mammogram and only 22% of them had had a mammogram
within the past year. A total of 5% of the white women and 18% of the

black women interviewed had never heard of a mammogram. Whereas 40% of the women could not give any reason for never having had a mammogram, only 3% of the women gave as the reason that they could not afford it. Thus, the women surveyed for this report appeared to be reasonably compliant with clinical breast examinations and BSE, but compliance with mammography screening at the recommended frequencies was much lower.

Conclusion.—Educational interventions to familiarize health care professionals, as well as the public in general, with the importance of regular mammography screening for breast cancer are needed.

▶ Despite advances in the quality of mammography and the ability to detect breast cancer at an earlier phase in its development, this paper by Lackland et al. points out the important fact that many women are not participating in breast cancer screening. In the Charleston, South Carolina tricounty area, only 40% of surveyed women reported ever having had a mammogram. This is in contrast to 92% who reported they knew how to do BSE. Younger women were more knowledgeable about mammography recommendations. Black women were more likely than white women to report never having heard of mammography (blacks, 18%; whites, 5%). This study noted that the major obstacles to mammography were a belief that a woman does not need regular mammography and physicians' failure to recommend it.

It seems unfortunate that the use of a beneficial system, breast screening, has not kept pace with the technical improvements in the system itself. Hopefully, with increased education and low-cost screening mammography, this trend will not continue to prevail.—M. Rebner, M.D.

The American College of Radiology Mammography Accreditation Program
McLelland R, Hendrick RE, Zinninger MD, Wilcox PA (Univ of North Carolina, Chapel Hill, NC; Univ of Colorado Health Sciences Ctr, Denver; American College of Radiology, Reston, Va)
AJR 157:473–479, 1991   1–9

Background.—In the early to mid-1980s, when dedicated mammographic equipment became readily available and widely used, many radiologists believed that the use of this equipment was all that was needed to ensure optimal image quality at low radiation dose. Later in the decade, several findings raised doubts about the validity of that assumption. Those findings served as an impetus for the American College of Radiology (ACR) Mammography Accreditation Program.

Program Results.—Since the start of the program in August 1987, application rates have increased steadily. Nearly half the mammographic units in the United States have applied for accreditation voluntarily, and approximately one fourth are now accredited. Surprisingly, the failure rate among first-time applicants has remained consistently high, at 28% to 30%. Failure rates, resulting from phantom and/or clinical image assessments, were highest for mobile units, at 24%. The failure rates were 15% for hospitals, 13% for multispecialty clinics, 12% for private offices, and 10% for multiple settings. Although there is no clear association between quality and the practice setting of a radiology-based mammographic practice, there is a clear connection between quality and the number of mammograms obtained at a mammographic site in a given time.

Conclusion.—The success of the ACR Mammography Accreditation Program is encouraging. However, the task of improving the quality of mammography is still not complete. Radiologists must implement meaningful quality assurance procedures and devote the necessary personnel, time, and attention to assessing and improving quality on an ongoing basis.

▶ This paper discusses the background, goals, criteria, current results, impact, and future directions of the ACR mammography accreditation program. As the authors note, the goals of the program are to establish standards of quality for mammography, to provide a mechanism for radiologists to compare voluntarily their own performance with national standards, to collect and disseminate data on the current practice of mammography, to encourage quality assurance practices in mammography, and to ensure high-quality images at low-radiation dose to the patients. Approximately half the mammography units in the United States have applied for accreditation, and roughly 25% of the units are accredited.

No other radiologic subspecialty has evoked such high standards for equipment, performance, and professional criteria. It is interesting that some states have adopted this program into legislation, whereas others have made certain standards even tougher for those who do not comply with ACR's guidelines. It will not be surprising to see other imaging subspecialties invoke similar standards of quality assurance and continuing medical education. After talking to many mammographers, I have heard only 1 negative comment about the program, and that involves the time it takes to go through the accreditation process. This program will continue to help improve the quality of mammography practiced across the country.—M. Rebner, M.D.

Periodic Mammographic Follow-Up of Probably Benign Lesions: Results in 3,184 Consecutive Cases
Sickles EA (Univ of California, San Francisco)
Radiology 179:463–468, 1991   1–10

Objective.—Routine mammography frequently reveals nonpalpable lesions with a very low probability of malignancy. To avoid the expense and morbidity associated with biopsy, such lesions can be followed up with mammographic surveillance. Periodic mammographic surveillance among 3,184 consecutive cases of nonpalpable, probably benign breast lesions was evaluated.

Methods and Criteria.—There were 2 major categories of probably benign findings: localized and generalized. The former was characterized by a focal distribution in 1 segment of 1 breast. A generalized distribution consisted of multiple similar lesions randomly distributed in both breasts. Four follow-up mammographic examinations were scheduled during a 3- or 3.5-year period. Repeat mammography of the ipsilateral breast was first performed at 6 months.

Findings.—Tiny calcifications accounted for 58.2% of the cases, well-defined nodules for 26.4%, and focal asymmetric areas of fibroglandular density for 14.1%. During follow-up, 161 biopsies were performed, with most being prompted by mammographic demonstration of interval change. Fifteen of the 17 malignancies in this study population were detected in biopsy specimens after mammography demonstrated interval change. The results of biopsies performed without evidence of such change were all negative. All 17 tumors were either stage 0 or stage 1. At a median follow-up of 60 months, none of the women with malignancy showed evidence of tumor recurrence.

Discussion.—Under certain conditions, mammographic surveillance can successfully replace biopsy of probably benign lesions. The lesions must be nonpalpable, and supplementary magnification mammograms in orthogonal projections must be acquired and evaluated.

▶ This paper by Ed Sickles points out the value of mammographic follow-up in the management of probably benign breast lesions. These lesions must be nonpalpable, and the benign characteristics of the lesion must be demonstrated in 2 orthogonal views. The significant decrease in expense and morbidity associated with fewer surgical biopsies is obvious. It is encouraging that, of the 131 biopsies performed because of mammographic demonstration of interval change, only 15 cancers were found. All of the carcinomas found were either stage 0 or I tumors. Hopefully, the results of this study will make periodic mammographic follow-up of probably benign lesions more acceptable to both radiologists and clinicians and will also help make mammographic screening more cost-effective.—M. Rebner, M.D.

A New Coaxial Needle for Pre-Operative Localization of Breast Abnormalities

Schoenberger SG, Bamber JC, Rank W, Sutherland CM, Nichols RL (Tulane Univ, New Orleans; Royal Marsden Hospital, Sutton, England)
Br J Radiol 64:699–707, 1991   1–11

Background.—The increase in the number of women who have mammography for the detection of asymptomatic nonpalpable breast cancer has resulted in an increase in the number of preoperative breast localizations for suspicious lesions. A new coaxial needle has been developed for mammographic and sonographic localization of such breast abnormalities before surgery.

Methods.—Both in vitro experiments and clinical studies were done. The new needle contains a retractable anchoring wire with a helical tip, which provides the needle with a number of potential advantages over other localization needles currently available.

Observations.—Quantitative and qualitative data from the in vitro comparisons of the new needle with other needles suggested that the new needle can be expected to have improved anchoring ability, be deflected less by tough fibrous tissue interfaces, and be more visible in sonography. The anchoring wire can be retracted and repositioned. The preliminary clinical studies with the needle supported these expectations.

Conclusion.—Because of its design characteristics, this new breast localization needle is called the "double helix" needle. The distal helix at the tip of the anchoring wire may be screwed into the target breast tissue in a manner identical to the visible proximal helix. The overall improved anchoring ability is important because it may reduce the chance of a position change during the time between localization and excision.

▶ The authors describe a new coaxial needle for mammographic and sonographic localization of nonpalpable breast masses. The new needle contains a retractable anchoring wire with a helical tip. The potential advantages of this system include improved anchoring ability, increased visibility under sonography, better penetration through tough fibrous breast tissue, and the ability of the wire to be retracted and repositioned.

To me, the most attractive feature of this needle is its anchoring capability. This can be advantageous in a fatty breast, in which changes in the position of the wire after localization are not that uncommon. Hopefully, once this double-helix needle become commercially available, it will be comparably priced with other localizing needles.—M. Rebner, M.D.

Occult Breast Masses: Use of a Mammographic Localizing Grid for US Evaluation
Conway WF, Hayes CW, Brewer WH (Med College of Virginia, Richmond)
Radiology 181:143–146, 1991   1–12

Introduction.—Ultrasonography (US) is useful for the characterization of mammographically detected, nonpalpable breast masses. It may, however, be difficult for the examiner to positively determine whether a mass seen with US is the same mass seen on the mammogram when there is more than 1 mass in the breast. Many areas of varying echogenicity may be found, and some normal breast parenchyma may mimic solid masses. A fenestrated mammographic compression grid was used to stabilize the breast and guide the ultrasound examination.

Methods.—Fifty mammographically distinct masses in 47 patients scheduled to undergo needle localization were identified. Six masses were localized in an area of the breast that contained other opacities, which could have interfered with identification. Freehand US results were compared with results when a fenestrated mammographic compression guide was used. Needle localization was performed while the breast was still in the grid.

Findings.—Five of 50 masses (10%) detected by freehand US and thought to be the mammographically detected masses were found to represent different areas of the breast when US was performed with the compression grid. There is a potential for misidentification of masses with freehand US.

Conclusion.—Because of the small number of patients studied, grid-directed US of the breast is not universally recommended. It is recommended when there are adjacent mammographic masses, when the mass is in dense tissue, or when there is a significant size difference between the mammographic and ultrasonographic depictions of the mass.

▶ Dr. Conway and his colleagues describe the use of a mammographic localizing compression grid to aid in the sonographic evaluation of nonpalpable breast masses. Of the 50 masses included in their study, 5 (10%) were misidentified with free-hand US. This method may help reduce the possibility of characterizing a malignant lesion as benign by ensuring that the mammographic and sonographic abnormality are the same lesion.

Although this technique requires a transducer small enough to fit into the localizing grid, it does offer the opportunity to reduce diagnostic error when there are adjacent mammographic masses that could be confused, and there is a significant size difference between a mass seen at mammography and at sonography. The authors are to be commended for taking a standard mammographic localizing grid and using it in a different fashion with sonography.—M. Rebner, M.D.

Lobular Carcinoma In Situ of the Breast: Clinical, Pathologic, and Mammographic Features
Beute B, Kalisher L, Hutter RVP (St Barnabas Med Ctr, Livingston, NJ)
AJR 157:257–265, 1991   1–13

Introduction.—Lobular carcinoma in situ (LCIS) is a rare lesion of the lobule of the breast that is difficult to diagnose by mammography. In an effort to identify mammographic features or predictors of LCIS, 165 breasts diagnosed as having LCIS were examined.

Pathologic Findings.—In younger women, LCIS was more common than other breast cancers. Multifocal disease was detected in 70% of the cases. When both breasts were examined, bilateral foci were detected in

50% of the cases. In 37% of the breasts, simultaneous invasive cancers occurred within the breast.

Mammographic Correlation.—Results of mammography were normal in 44% of breasts with LCIS. It was rare in an N1 breast or in a breast with less than 25% of its parenchymal area occupied by fibroglandular density. Compared with an age-matched control group, breasts with LCIS had more than 50% fibroglandular density and a significantly higher frequency of the DY pattern. In postmenopausal women, these 2 prognostic factors were seen at nearly double the rate detected in the control group.

Implications.—In postmenopausal women, mammographically dense breasts are a marker for increased cancer risk. In the premenopausal age group, this marker is too nonspecific to be useful diagnostically. Mammography does not appear to be useful in the specific detection of LCIS.

▶ This study shows that LCIS of the breast has no distinct mammographic correlation. Microcalcifications were a nonspecific finding at mammography. They were often found in tissues *adjacent* to foci of LCIS and not directly within it. Of the breasts with LCIS, 37% had simultaneously occurring invasive carcinomas in the same breast. The authors also note that patients with LCIS have a higher rate of fibroglandular and parenchymal density, as well as a higher rate of the DY pattern. They believe that dense breasts are a marker for increased cancer risk in the postmenopausal age group.

As radiologists, we need to be aware that patients with LCIS have a 2% chance per year for the rest of their lives of invasive ductal or lobular carcinoma developing in either breast. Given the increased relative risk of breast cancer and dense postmenopausal breasts, we may wish to become more aggressive in the workup and management of lesions in this population.—M. Rebner, M.D.

Lobular Carcinoma In Situ: Mammographic-Pathologic Correlation of Results of Needle-Directed Biopsy

Sonnenfeld MR, Frenna TH, Weidner N, Meyer JE (Harvard Med School, Boston)
Radiology 181:363–367, 1991   1–14

Background.—Lobular carcinoma in situ (LCIS) appears to be a marker for increased risk of subsequent invasive breast carcinoma. The correlation between the mammographic finding that prompts the performance of needle-directed biopsy and the histologic finding of areas of LCIS was studied.

Methods.—During a 3½-year period, 41 patients with isolated LCIS were studied. This group was drawn from 437 malignancies detected during the same period. Preoperative and localization mammograms and pathologic slides were reviewed for each patient. The median age was 50 years, and 19 patients were 40–49 years of age.

Results.—The indication for biopsy was clustered microcalcifications in 31 patients; in 24 of these, calcifications were found in areas with benign breast disease, and LCIS appeared as a separate process. When microcalcifications appeared in association with LCIS, as they did in a few patients, more similar calcifications were noted in adjacent areas of benign disease. Benign foci were found when biopsy was done for soft tissue abnormalities, except in 1 patient who had LCIS in and adjacent to a fibroadenoma.

Conclusion.—There appear to be no characteristic mammographic features of LCIS. This tumor is found incidentally at breast biopsy in patients whose mammographic abnormality represents a benign condition.

▶ This abstract, like the previous one, notes that LCIS of the breast is a marker for increased risk of subsequent invasive breast carcinoma. Microcalcifications were a nonspecific finding. As in the previous paper, they were more often found in adjacent areas of benign disease and were not found directly in areas of LCIS. There were no characteristic mammographic features of LCIS.

I have included both papers on LCIS for 2 reasons. First, they are both well-done scientific studies. Second, the fact that they both reach a similar conclusion should not detract from their merit. A study on a topic does not have to find something new or different to be published. Corroborating the results of a prior study is important to enhance the validity of the data to the readers of the journal.—M. Rebner, M.D.

Atypical Hyperplasia of the Breast: Mammographic Appearance and Histologic Correlation
Helvie MA, Hessler C, Frank TS, Ikeda DM (Univ of Michigan, Ann Arbor)
Radiology 179:759–764, 1991   1–15

Background.—Little is known about the mammographic features of atypical hyperplasia (AH), despite extensive pathologic and epidemiologic data. The mammographic characteristics of AH were determined retrospectively and were correlated with histologic findings.

Methods and Findings.—Of 58 cases of AH of the breast, there was a direct correlation between mammographic and histologic findings in 41%, a near correlation in 26%, and a remote correlation in 33%. The most common mammographic abnormality that directly correlated with AH at histologic assessment was clustered microcalcifications. Atypical ductal hyperplasia was much more often associated with a direct correlation than was atypical lobular hyperplasia, those percentages being 48% and 9%, respectively.

Conclusion.—Although no pathognomonic appearance for AH was found in this series, mammographic abnormalities similar to those of small cancers were concluded to be directly correlated with histologic results in 41% of the cases. Because AH has been associated with five-fold to tenfold increase in the risk of subsequent invasive carcinoma, frequent clinical follow-up and mammography at least once yearly should be done after AH is discovered.

▶ The authors describe 58 cases of AH of the breast. There was a direct correlation between mammographic and histologic findings in 41% of the cases and a near correlation in 26%. No distinct appearance was found for AH. Clustered calcifications were the mammographic abnormality that directly correlated most often with AH.

This paper is noteworthy because it describes features of a borderline, possibly premalignant condition. Epidemiologic data has shown a fivefold to tenfold relative risk increase of subsequent invasive carcinoma for patients with AH. When surgical pathology results reveal AH, we should not treat this result as simply another benign diagnosis. Rather, we should recommend close clinical follow-up and mammography at least every year.—M. Rebner, M.D.

Topics in CT

Solitary Pulmonary Nodule: CT Evaluation of Enhancement With Iodinated Contrast Material. A Preliminary Report

Swensen SJ, Morin RL, Schueler BA, Brown LR, Cortese DA, Pairolero PC, Brutinel WM (Mayo Clinic and Found, Rochester, Minn; Mayo Clinic, Jacksonville, Fla)
Radiology 182:343–347, 1992   1–16

Background.—The investigation of a solitary pulmonary nodule (SPN) aims to expedite resection of potentially curable cancer and to minimize the number of benign nodules that are removed at thoracotomy. Even with current analytic methods, approximately one fourth to one third of resected SPNs are benign. In searching for a radiologic technique that could allow better distinction between benign and malignant nodules, it was hypothesized that the degree of contrast material enhancement of a pulmonary nodule seen at CT may indicate the likelihood of malignancy.

Methods.—A total of 52 patients with uncalcified SPNs measuring 6–30 mm was studied to evaluate SPN attenuation before and after intravenous administration of iodinated contrast material. Five single serial thin-section CT scans were obtained at 1-minute intervals after injection of 100 mL of nonionic contrast material. Twenty-two nodules were excluded because of a technically inadequate examination or an inadequate observation period.

Findings.—Of 30 nodules in 30 patients, 23 were neoplastic, 22 being malignant and 1 a benign fibrous mesothelioma. Seven nodules were benign. In the first 2 minutes after injection, all the malignant nodules and

TABLE 1.—Maximum Enhancement of Malignant Nodules During First 2 Minutes
After Injection of Contrast Material

Patient	Enhancement (HU)*	Diagnosis	Nodule Characteristics Diameter (mm)	Edge
A	25	Non–small cell carcinoma	25	L, I
C	30	Metastasis, adenocarcinoma	27	L, S
D	57	Large cell carcinoma	8	S
E	20	Metastasis, adenocarcinoma	15	L, S
F	31	Spindle cell carcinoma	8	S
H	33	Adenocarcinoma	25	L, I
J	32	Adenocarcinoma	12	S, L
K	35	Adenocarcinoma	14	S, L
M	22	Squamous cell carcinoma	27	L, I
O	38	Metastasis, squamous cell carcinoma	22	S
1	52	Squamous cell carcinoma	15	L, S
3	61	Adenocarcinoma	20	S
9	58	Squamous cell carcinoma	30	L, I
10	30	Large cell carcinoma	12	S
12	56	Metastasis, adenocarcinoma	12	S
14	24	Adenocarcinoma	10	S
15	48	Squamous cell carcinoma	10	L, S
16	32	Fibrous mesothelioma	12	L, S
19	36	Bronchial carcinoid	20	S
22	28	Adenocarcinoma	18	L, S
25	38	Adenocarcinoma	12	S
30	26	Adenocarcinoma	10	L, S
37	36	Squamous cell carcinoma	20	L, S

Abbreviations: I, infiltrating; *L,* lobulated; *S,* smooth.
* Values represent maximum change in attenuation value between precontrast and postcontrast images; mean value ± standard deviation = 37 HU ± 12.
(Courtesy of Swensen SJ, Morin RL, Schueler BA, et al: *Radiology* 182:343–347, 1992.)

1 benign nodule had enhanced by 20 HU or more (Tables 1 and 2; Fig 1–1).

Conclusion.—The degree of enhancement of SPNs measured with CT may be helpful in differentiating uncalcified malignant nodules from benign pulmonary nodules. Malignant nodules usually enhanced significantly more than did benign nodules. The measurements made within the first 2 minutes after injection of contrast material appear to be diagnostically important in indicating the likelihood of malignancy.

▶ This could represent a second great leap forward in noninvasive characterization of SPNs. The first leap was made with the work of Siegelman and others (1, 2), who used thin-section CT and later added a chest phantom to decide whether a nodule is diffusely calcified. Because we all know that calcification alone does not make a lesion benign, it will be very useful to have a completely different criterion for benign vs. malignant SPNs.

TABLE 2.—Maximum Enhancement of Benign Nodules During First 2 Minutes
After Injection of Contrast Material

Patient	Enhancement (HU)*	Diagnosis	Nodule Characteristics Diameter (mm)	Edge
G	18	Granuloma‡	6	S†
L	8	Granuloma‡	25	S
7	9	Granuloma‡	25	L, S
18	42	Granuloma‡	8	L, S
21	19	Granuloma‡	12	L, S
24	12	Granuloma‡	12	S†
33	18	Granuloma‡	20	L, S

Abbreviations: L, lobulated; *S,* smooth.
* Values represent maximum change in attenuation value between precontrast and postcontrast images;
mean value ± standard deviation = 18 HU ± 12.
† High probability of benignity, as indicated with CT reference phantom.
‡ Presumptive diagnosis because of nodule stability during follow-up of 2-years or more.
(Courtesy of Swensen SJ, Morin RL, Schueler BA, et al: *Radiology* 182:343–347, 1992.)

Obviously, the problem thus far is the small number of cases. At this point, it looks as though enhancement by 20 HU is both sensitive and specific regarding malignant SPNs. With more experience, we can sacrifice some specificity as long as we maintain very high sensitivity; in other words, whatever enhancement criterion we use, we are willing to resect some benign lesions if we are certain to get all (or very nearly all) of the malignant ones.

Another article on SPNs applied spiral volumetric CT to their evaluation (3). With a 12-second breath hold (requiring some patient selection), 4 addi-

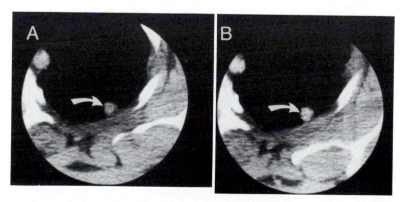

Fig 1–1.—A, a 2-mm CT section through an uncalcified, 8-mm–diameter SPN (*arrow*). Scanning was performed without intravenously administered contrast material. The mean attenuation value was 2 HU. **B,** a 2-mm CT section through the same nodule as in **A** (*arrow*), obtained 1 minute after the start of injection of contrast material. The mean attenuation value was 55 HU. At 1 minute, enhancement of 53 HU was measured manually by area indentification. The nodule proved to be a large cell bronchogenic carcinoma. (Courtesy of Swensen SJ, Morin RL, Schueler BA, et al: *Radiology* 182:343–347, 1992.)

tional nodules were detected in 20 patients. There is 1 problem: when it comes to small additional nodules, I'm not certain whether I want to find them, because I certainly won't know what to do with them.—B.H. Gross, M.D.

References

1. Siegelman SS, et al: *Radiology* 160:307, 1986.
2. Zerhouni EA, et al: *Radiology* 160:319, 1986.
3. Costello P, et al: *Radiology* 179:875, 1991.

The Role of Computed Tomography (CT) in the Investigation of Unexplained Haemoptysis
Millar AB, Boothroyd AE, Edwards D, Hetzel MR (University College and Middlesex Hospital, London, England)
Respir Med 86:39–44, 1992   1–17

Objective.—As many as 50% of patients referred for evaluation of hemoptysis may remain without a diagnosis despite clinical history and examination, conventional chest radiographs, and fiberoptic bronchoscopy. The role of CT in the evaluation of these patients was studied prospectively.

Patients.—Computed tomography, with or without contrast, was performed in 40 patients who had unexplained hemoptysis with normal chest radiographs apart from evidence of chronic airflow limitation and normal fiberoptic bronchoscopy (or blood alone in the bronchial tree).

Findings.—Abnormalities were seen in 20 CT scans (50%), such as diffuse cystic changes in a patient with histiocytosis X; bronchiectasis in 7 patients, including 1 with probably malignant mass; abnormal masses in 4 (2 tuberculous and 2 malignant); areas of alveolar consolidation in 4; abnormal vessels in contrast-enhanced CT in 3 patients, including 2 with arteriovenous malformations; and multiple nodules in 1 patient. In 93 control patients undergoing CT for preoperative assessment of bronchogenic carcinoma, 6 (6%) patients had abnormalities in the contralateral lung. This control group included older patients and more smokers who were expected to have increased pulmonary abnormalities. Compared with control patients, the relative risk ratio for patients with unexplained hemoptysis having abnormal CT scans was 7.75.

Conclusion.—Computed tomography is a valuable tool in the evaluation of patients with unexplained hemoptysis.

▶ It always bothers me when someone scientifically disproves what I innately (and *very* unscientifically) know to be true. Hemoptysis that is unexplained by conventional radiographs and fiberoptic bronchoscopy *must* be a poor indication for CT and, in my limited anecdotal experience, it has been.

The authors strongly suggest the opposite, and for the time being I will be less of an obstructionist in this setting.—B.H. Gross, M.D.

Low-Dose High-Resolution CT of Lung Parenchyma
Zwirewich CV, Mayo JR, Müller NL (University of British Columbia, Vancouver General Hospital, Vancouver, BC, Canada)
Radiology 180:413–417, 1991   1–18

Background.—High-resolution CT is now widely accepted for the assessment of patients with known or suspected diffuse lung disease. The efficacy of low-dose, high-resolution CT was tested in the assessment of lung parenchyma.

Methods.—A total of 31 patients underwent 1.5-mm collimation, 2-second, 120-kVp scans at 20 and 200 mamp at selected identical levels in the chest. Three observers assessed the visualization of normal pulmonary anatomy, various parenchymal abnormalities and their distribution, and artifacts.

Findings.—Low-dose and conventional scans were equivalent in assessment of vessels, lobar and segmental bronchi, and anatomy of secondary pulmonary lobules. They were also comparable in characterizing the extent and distribution of reticulation, honeycomb cysts, and thickened interlobular septa. The low-dose method did not show groundglass opacity in 2 of 10 cases and emphysema in 1 of 9. Those findings were evident, although subtle, on the high-dose scans. The differences were not significant statistically. Linear streak artifact was more pronounced on images obtained with the low-dose method, but the 2 techniques were considered to be equally diagnostic in 97% (Figs 1–2 and 1–3).

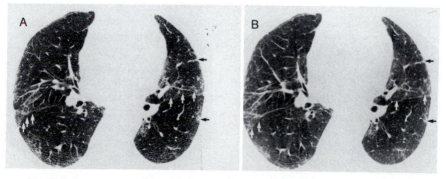

Fig 1–2.—Demonstration of ground-glass opacities and mild reticulation in a patient with early changes of usual interstitial pneumonia. Ground-glass opacities (*white arrows*) and reticulation (*black arrows*) are visualized on both the 20-mamp (**A**) and 200-mamp (**B**) scans, as is the peripheral, predominantly subpleural distribution of the infiltrates. Ground-glass opacities are slightly better visualized on the 200-mamp scan. Equivalent demonstration of subsegmental bronchi and vessels is seen in the right upper lobe. (Courtesy of Zwirewich CV, Mayo JR, Müller NL: *Radiology* 180:413–417, 1991.)

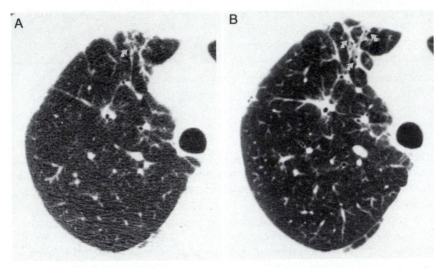

Fig 1–3.—High-resolution CT scans demonstrate mild cylindric bronchiectasis peripherally in the right upper lobe. Dilated bronchi (*arrows*) in the anterior segment can be identified on both the 20-mamp **(A)** and 200-mamp **(B)** scans, but they are much better seen on the high-dose scan. (Courtesy of Zwirewich CV, Mayo JR, Müller NL: *Radiology* 180:413–417, 1991.)

Conclusion.—High-resolution CT images acquired at 20 mamp yield anatomical data equivalent to that acquired with 200-mamp scans in most patients. There is no significant loss of spatial resolution or image degradation from linear streak artifact.

▶ I'm not yet sold on the clinical usefulness of high-resolution CT of the lung parenchyma. I have seen beautiful examples at various meetings, but I always wonder whether the actual patient (not his or her disembodied slides) benefited from the CT scan. For example, I've been shown quite convincingly that CT can diagnose invasive pulmonary aspergillosis in patients with leukemia earlier than chest radiographs can. But what febrile leukemic patient isn't already receiving antifungal drug therapy?

The authors highlight an undiscussed problem of high-resolution CT. Skin doses of 12–14 rad for each scan are not trivial. The trade-off suggested in this article is dose for diagnosis; low-dose scans failed to diagnose ground-glass opacity in 2 of 10 patients and emphysema in 1 of 9. Although these differences were not statistically significant, they would sure bother me if I believed in this technique. I'm afraid you'll have to judge for yourselves. To help, I am referencing additional recent articles on high-resolution CT of the lung parenchyma (1–3).—B.H. Gross, M.D.

References

1. Leung AN, et al: *AJR* 157:693, 1991.
2. Remy-Jardin M, et al: *Radiology* 181:157, 1991.
3. Muller N: *AJR* 157:1163, 1991.

Complications After CT-Guided Needle Biopsy Through Aerated Versus Nonaerated Lung

Haramati LB, Austin JHM (Columbia-Presbyterian Med Ctr, New York)
Radiology 181:778, 1991
1–19

Background.—Complication rates as high as 60% have been reported for patients undergoing percutaneous needle biopsy of the lungs. The relationship between complication rate and the traversal of aerated versus nonaerated lung was investigated.

Methods.—During a 6-year period, 131 CT-guided percutaneous needle biopsies of the lung were performed in 123 patients. Ninety-six percent were done with a 21- or 22-gauge needle. The CT images were examined to ascertain whether the needle traversed aerated lung. For each

Complications After Percutaneous
CT-Guided Needle Biopsy of the Lung
$(n = 131)$

Complication	Traversal of Aerated Lung	
	Yes $(n = 79)$	No $(n = 52)$
Major	8 (10)	0 (0)
Pneumothorax requiring chest tube	6	0
Hemoptysis (estimated 150 mL)	1	0
Ventricular tachycardia	1	0
Moderate	15 (19)	0 (0)
Pneumothorax ≥5% not requiring chest tube	15	0
Minor	18 (23)	1 (2)
Pneumothorax		
<5%	15	0
Focal*	12	0
Nonfocal†	3	0
Hemoptysis ≤5 mL	3	1
None	39 (49)‡	51 (98)‡

Note: The numbers in parentheses are percentages, which may not equal 100% because of rounding.
* Focal pneumothorax is defined as loculated at the biopsy site.
† Nonfocal pneumothorax is defined as extending over the apex of the lung.
‡ $P < .0001$ (χ^2 analysis).
(Courtesy of Haramati LB, Austin JHM: *Radiology* 181:778, 1991.)

patient, CT sections of the sampled region were assessed for the presence of pneumothorax.

Results.—Aerated lung was not traversed in 52 biopsies; in 34 cases, the needle passed through the pleura directly into a cancer. None of these patients had pneumothorax develop, and only 1 had minor hemoptysis develop. However, of 79 biopsies in which the aerated lung was traversed, pneumothorax developed in 46%. Other complications were more common as well (table).

Conclusion.—Pneumothorax and other complications are unlikely to occur in percutaneous CT-guided lung biopsy when the needle does not traverse aerated lung. Analyses of the complication rate of this procedure should consider patients who do and do not have traversal of aerated lung as separate risk populations.

▶ To balance a previous article, here is a scientific investigation with a conclusion that agrees with that of our intuition.—B.H. Gross, M.D.

Diagnosis and Localization of Laceration of the Thoracic Duct: Usefulness of Lymphangiography and CT
Sachs PB, Zelch MG, Rice TW, Geisinger MA, Risius B, Lammert GK (Cleveland Clinic Found, Cleveland, Ohio)
AJR 157:703–705, 1991   1–20

Objective.—The relative value of lymphangiography and CT in detecting and localizing lacerations of the thoracic duct was examined in 12 patients who were seen 3 days–9 months after having had thoracic or abdominal surgery with chylothorax or chylous ascites.

Methods.—Bipedal lymphangiography was carried out in all patients using ethiodized oil and saline. The last 4 patients also had CT scanning of the chest without oral or intravenous contrast medium, immediately after lymphangiography was completed.

Findings.—A leak from the thoracic duct was seen on lymphangiography in 5 patients. One other patient had a lymphocele, and 1 had evidence of lymphatic obstruction but no evident leakage. There were no complications from the study. Exploration confirmed the lymphangiographic findings in all 4 patients who underwent thoracic duct ligation. Chylothorax resolved spontaneously after lymphangiography in the remaining patient. Computed tomography confirmed a leak in 1 patient, and confirmed negative lymphangiographic findings in 3 others.

Conclusion.—Lymphangiography still is the preferred means of diagnosing and localizing lacerations of the thoracic duct. Computed tomography is of little added diagnostic value.

▶ I like this approach. Take a focused question comparing the utility of an old diagnostic tool that is moderately invasive with a newer tool that is relatively noninvasive. Use surgical proof as the gold standard. Whether the new modality measures up or not, the result is important. In this case, the message is clear: "Laceration of the thoracic duct was accurately diagnosed and localized with lymphangiography. CT was of little additional value."—B.H. Gross, M.D.

Lung Cancer

Radiographically Occult Endobronchial Obstruction in Bronchogenic Carcinoma
Shure D (VA Med Ctr, San Diego)
Am J Med 91:19–22, 1991   1–21

Background.—Central endobronchial tumors may become detectable radiographically when they cause significant endobronchial obstruction. However, the incidence of radiographically undetectable obstruction is unknown. The incidence of radiographically undetectable completely obstructing lesions encountered during routine diagnostic bronchoscopy was studied prospectively in 77 patients.

Methods.—The patients were referred to 1 center for bronchoscopy because of suspected bronchogenic carcinoma on the basis of chest radiographic abnormalities or clinical symptoms. Chest radiographs were routinely interpreted 24 hours before bronchoscopy.

Results.—Eighty-one completely obstructing lesions were detected in the 77 patients. Thirty-six completely obstructing endobronchial lesions, or 44%, gave no radiographic signs of obstruction. Cell type did not affect the rate of radiographically occult tumors. Segmental bronchial obstruction was more likely to be undetectable than that of more proximal airways. In 13, or 16%, chest radiographs were normal. All 13 had risk factors for bronchogenic carcinoma and symptoms that were suggestive of the disease (Fig 1–4).

Conclusion.—Complete endobronchial obstruction from bronchogenic carcinoma can frequently occur in patients at risk for lung cancer. The significant incidence of radiographically undetectable complete obstruction has implications for diagnosing, staging, and assessing treatment.

▶ This is the kind of manuscript that almost has to be written by a pulmonologist. A radiologist wouldn't want to write about lesions prospectively missed on conventional chest radiographs, because it might say more about the radiologist than about the entity. Chest radiologists might add that a random series of abnormalities missed on conventional chest radiographs is unimportant if the radiographs weren't interpreted by experienced chest radiologists.

Balderdash! At Ford Hospital, we have 6 radiologists whose interests, training, and skills merit the designation "chest radiologist." Nevertheless, a large number of daily chest radiographs is interpreted by others without that desig-

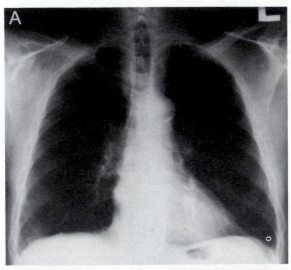

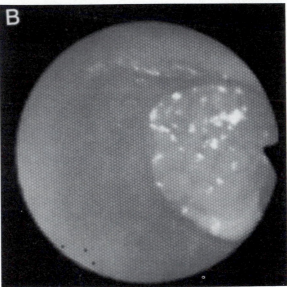

Fig 1–4.—**A,** normal, chest radiograph; **B,** mass occluding left upper lobe bronchus in the same patient. (Courtesy of Shure D: *Am J Med* 91:19–22, 1991.)

nation. If that's how it works at your hospital, the routine prospective interpretations are fair game for a study. However, the results of this study are not as shocking as they first seem. Although it is prominently proclaimed that 44% of completely obstructing endobronchial lesions showed no radiographic signs of obstruction, only 16% had normal chest radiographs. The remainder of this group included 11 patients with a solitary pulmonary nodule, 8 with a hilar mass, 3 with peripheral infiltrate without volume loss, and 1 with bilateral interstitial infiltrates. In other words, most of these patients were bound for further investigation, regardless of whether there was radiographic evidence of obstruction.

The message to take away is that 16% of patients with complete bronchial obstruction had normal chest radiography. Liberal usage of bronchoscopy in the presence of appropriate symptoms or in the right patient population seems advisable.—B.H. Gross, M.D.

Missed Bronchogenic Carcinoma: Radiographic Findings in 27 Patients With a Potentially Resectable Lesion Evident in Retrospect

Austin JHM, Romney BM, Goldsmith LS (Columbia-Presbyterian Med Ctr, Goldsmith, Tabak and Richman, PC, New York)
Radiology 182:115–122, 1992   1–22

Introduction.—Failure of a radiologist to detect bronchogenic carcinoma seen retrospectively on a chest radiograph is common and occurs in a minimum of 12% to 30% of the cases. The clinical and radiologic findings were studied in 27 patients with potentially resectable bronchogenic carcinomas revealed retrospectively on serial chest radiographs.

Data Analysis.—Eighteen radiologists failed to detect the missed bronchogenic carcinoma in 27 patients. Women (67%) were more affected than men (33%). The mean diameter of the lesions was 1.6 cm,

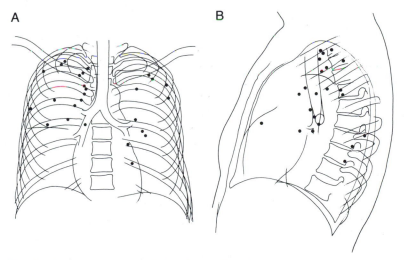

Fig 1–5.—Graphic representation of sites of missed bronchogenic carcinoma as evident retrospectively on **(A)** posteroanterior radiographs (26 patients) and **(B)** lateral radiographs (23 patients). Most (81% [*n* = 22]) of the lesions were in an upper lobe, especially the right upper lobe (56% [*n* = 15]). On lateral-projection chest x-ray films, the major sites of missed lesions were the pulmonary apices (30% [*n* = 7]) and over the spine (30% [*n* = 7]). (Courtesy of Austin JHM, Romney BM, Goldsmith LS: *Radiology* 182:115–122, 1992.)

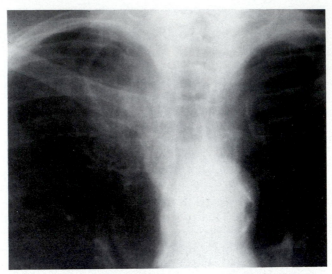

Fig 1–6.—Chest x-ray film shows the medial aspect of the right clavicle partially obscuring a poorly marginated primary adenocarcinoma of the lung in a woman, aged 71 years. This lesion, which was estimated to be 3.4 cm in diameter, was the largest missed cancer in this series. At later evaluation, 1 of 6 radiologists failed to identify it, despite knowing that a lung cancer had been missed in this patient. (Courtesy of Austin JHM, Romney BM, Goldsmith LS: *Radiology* 182:115–122, 1992.)

and 81% of the cancers involved the upper lobe, especially the right upper lobe (Fig 1–5). A well-defined margin was evident in only 7% of the patients, whereas slight levels of opacity occurred in 59%. Two or 3 overlapping bones obscured the missed lesion in 64% of patients with an upper lobe cancer (Figs 1–6 and 1–7). A lateral radiograph revealed the missed carcinoma better than a posteroanterior chest radiograph in 17% of the patients (Fig 1–8). The single most frequently identified cause of missed diagnoses was failure of the radiologist to evaluate the current chest radiographs in relation to previous chest radiographs. The delay in radiologic diagnosis affected prognosis in 18 of 27. Twenty-two cancers were evaluated by 6 consultants who were biased by knowledge that cases were of missed bronchogenic carcinoma. Each consultant missed a mean of 26% of the lesions, and at least 1 consultant missed the lesion in 73% of the cases.

Conclusion.—Difficulty of radiographic detection, female gender, and location of the lesion in an upper lobe, especially on the right side, contribute primarily to radiographically missed but potentially curable bronchogenic carcinomas.

▶ As a companion piece for Abstract 1–21, here are radiologists writing about missed lung cancer. We have a choice here. We can retreat into the "Mayo Clinic Defense," a defense against malpractice that I advocate based on the experience from the Mayo Clinic lung cancer screening project (1). In that study, even experts at the Mayo Clinic (who were looking specifically for

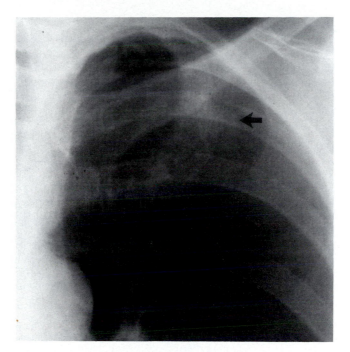

Fig 1–7.—Chest x-ray film shows the ribs obscuring a lightly radiopaque adenocarcinoma (*arrow*) in the apical-posterior segment of the left upper lobe in a woman, aged 56 years. Initially undetected, this lesion was also not identified by 1 of 6 radiologists at later evaluation, despite knowledge that a lung cancer had been missed in this patient. The missed cancer was estimated to be 1.4 cm in diameter. (From Austin JHM, Romney BM, Goldsmith LS: *Radiology* 182:115–122, 1992. Courtesy of Romney BM, Austin JHM: *Semin Roentgenol* 25:45–63, 1990.)

lung cancers in a high-risk population) initially missed a large number of lesions (that kind of statement sounds *so* good to lay juries!).

Better yet, we can learn where problems lie. The authors point out that failure to compare the current study with older radiographs was the single most frequently identified cause of missed diagnoses. They also suggest that lesions in female patients and upper lobe lesions (especially right upper lobe) are more commonly missed. Let's apply this to our daily work in an effort to make this kind of case collection more difficult.—B.H. Gross, M.D.

Reference

1. Muhm JR, et al: *Radiology* 148:609, 1983.

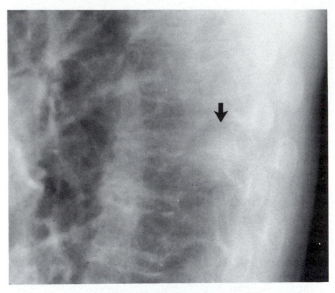

Fig 1-8.—Ribs and posterior elements of the spine obscure an undifferentiated carcinoma (*arrow*) in the superior segment of the left lower lobe of a woman, aged 76 years. This lesion was evident retrospectively only on a lateral-projection chest x-ray film. All 6 consultant radiologists failed to identify this lesion, despite their knowing that a lung cancer had been missed in this patient. (Courtesy of Austin JHM, Romney BM, Goldsmith LS: *Radiology* 182:115-122, 1992.)

Radioiodinated Somatostatin Analog Scintigraphy in Small-Cell Lung Cancer
Kwekkeboom DJ, Krenning EP, Bakker WH, Oei HY, Splinter TAW, Kho GS, Lamberts SWJ (University Hospital Dijkzigt, Rotterdam, The Netherlands)
J Nucl Med 32:1845-1848, 1991   1-23

Background.—Small cell lung cancer (SCLC), which account for nearly 25% of all lung cancers, is characterized by neuroendocrine properties. The staging procedures to differentiate between limited and extensive disease are complex, and the disease has a poor 2-year survival rate despite chemotherapy and irradiation. Somatostatin receptors have been characterized on SCLC biopsy specimens and on cultured human SCLC cells. The in vitro visualization of somatostatin receptor–positive tumors after injection of iodine 123-Tyr-3-octreotide, a radiolabeled somatostatin analog has been described. The in vivo visualization of SCLC was done using ^{123}I-Tyr-3-octreotide scintigraphy.

Methods.—The somatostatin analogue ^{123}I-Tyr-3-octreotide was used in imaging 11 patients with histologically confirmed lung cancer.

Findings.—Tumor deposits were demonstrated in 5 of 8 patients with SCLC, and unexpected metastases were found in 2 patients (Figs 1-9 and 1-10). In 3 patients with SCLC and 1 patient with a squamous cell carcinoma and a bronchial adenoma, the tumors were not visualized. In 1 pa-

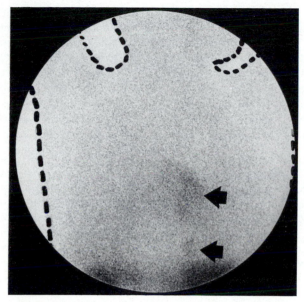

Fig 1–9.—Posterior chest image of a patient 2 hours after injection of ^{123}I-Tyr-3-octreotide. The *arrows* indicate tumor sites. (Courtesy of Kwekkeboom DJ, Krenning EP, Bakker WH, et al: *J Nucl Med* 32:1845–1848, 1991.)

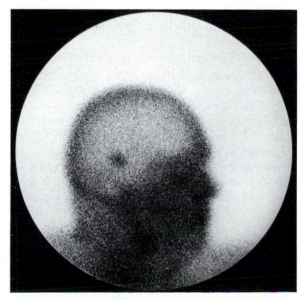

Fig 1–10.—Right lateral image of the skull of another patient 2 hours after injection of ^{123}I-Tyr-3-octreotide. (Courtesy of Kwekkeboom DJ, Krenning EP, Bakker WH, et al: *J Nucl Med* 32:1845–1848, 1991.)

tient with SCLC, this may have been explained by tumor necrosis and recent radiotherapy. The neoplasm was visualized in 1 of 2 patients with malignant small-cell tumors as described by Askin. The somatostatin receptor status of these tumors has not yet been investigated, but this finding should prompt an investigation.

Conclusion.—In the majority of patients with SCLC, the tumor and metastases can be visualized with ^{123}I-Tyr-3-octreotide scintigraphy. The scintigraphy may be useful in determining somatostatin receptor–positive tumors, but its specificity and sensitivity should be tested further.

▶ Biochemically specific imaging and therapy are becoming realities with the advent of monoclonal antibodies. Small cell lung cancer is a particularly appealing candidate because its intrathoracic morphology is usually far from subtle, rendering cross-sectional imaging less important, and because it has a significant predilection for distant spread. Radioiodinated somatostatin analogue scintigraphy detected SCLC in only 5 of 8 affected patients. Nevertheless, the promise of the technique lies in the concurrent detection of metastases in 2 of the 5 patients with positive scintigraphy.—B.H. Gross, M.D.

Technetium-99m Monoclonal Antibody Fragment (FAb) Scintigraphy in the Evaluation of Small Cell Lung Cancer: A Preliminary Report
Morris JF, Krishnamurthy S, Antonovic R, Duncan C, Turner FE, Krishnamurthy GT (VA Med Ctr and Oregon Health Sciences Univ, Portland, Ore)
Nucl Med Biol 18:613–620, 1991   1–24

Introduction.—A wide range of measures is needed to determine the extent of small cell lung cancer, which grows rapidly and metastasizes early. In a preliminary study, scintigraphy using monoclonal antibody labeled with technetium-99m was evaluated in 5 untreated patients with histologically proved small cell lung cancers.

Method.—Scintigraphy was carried out using a digital gamma camera after the injection of the monoclonal antibody NR-LU-10 (NeoRx Corporation, Seattle) labeled with 25–30 mCi of ^{99m}Tc. Tomographic data also were acquired using a large-field digital dyna camera fitted with a LEAP collimator.

Findings.—Fifteen lesions were found in the chest, 6 in bone, and 1 in the head. Scintigraphy detected all but 1 of the chest lesions and missed a 2-cm brain lesion. Four of the 6 bone lesions were detected scintigraphically, whereas 2 rib lesions failed to concentrate ^{99m}Tc-monoclonal antibody. All 3 positive spinal lesions were confirmed as metastases by MRI. Two adrenal lesions detected by CT failed to concentrate technetium activity. Planar imaging detected all the SPECT-positive lesions, but SPECT images better demonstrated the actual size of lesions.

Conclusion.—This limited experience indicates that monoclonal antibody labeled with ^{99m}Tc can be a useful scintigraphic imaging agent for detecting and staging small cell lung cancers.

▶ Perhaps more promising than somatostatin analogue is monoclonal antibody fragment scintigraphy. This is a better study, as well, using only untreated patients who had histologically proved small cell lung cancer. The greater promise is demonstrated by the multiplicity of metastases detected and by the fact that all 5 patients had detectable chest disease. The authors are too hard on themselves. They note that 2 adrenal masses detected by CT failed to concentrate monoclonal antibody fragment. In the absence of biopsy proof, I am unwilling to conclude that these are scintigraphic false negatives; they may be CT false positives, because nonhyperfunctioning adrenal adenomas are so common. Obviously, this must be evaluated in more than 5 patients, but it appears to be a great start.—B.H. Gross, M.D.

Thallium-201 SPECT Depicts Radiologically Occult Lung Cancer
Tonami N, Yokoyama K, Taki J, Hisada K, Watanabe Y, Takashima T, Nonomura A (Kanazawa University, Kanazawa, Japan)
J Nucl Med 32:2284–2285, 1991   1–25

Background.—Thallium 201 chloride administered intravenously accumulates in lung neoplasms and can be detected by SPECT. A male patient had positive sputum cytology results for lung cancer, but no abnormal mass was seen on chest radiographs or CT (Fig 1–11). Thallium 201 SPECT delineated the involved area of lung cancer.

Method.—A man, 66, had a positive sputum cytology for lung cancer. Although chest radiography did not show any abnormal findings, trans-

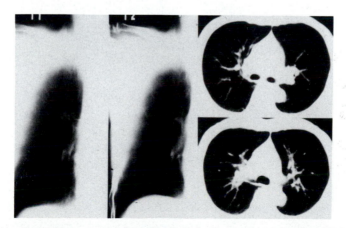

Fig 1–11.—Computed tomograms of the right chest showing no abnormal findings. No abnormal mass other than the irregularity of the right main bronchus was found. (Courtesy of Tonami N, Yokoyama K, Taki J, et al: *J Nucl Med* 32:2284–2285, 1991.)

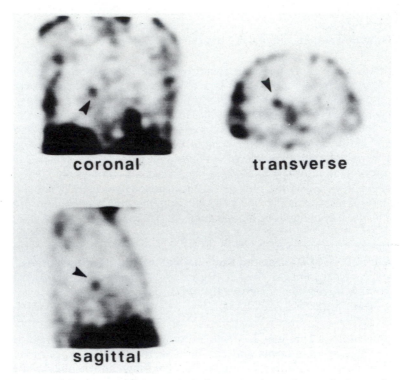

coronal   transverse

sagittal

Fig 1–12.—Thallium-201–delayed scans clearly demonstrate abnormal accumulation near the right hilum (*arrowhead*). (Courtesy of Tonami N, Yokoyama K, Taki J, et al: *J Nucl Med* 32:2284-2285, 1991.)

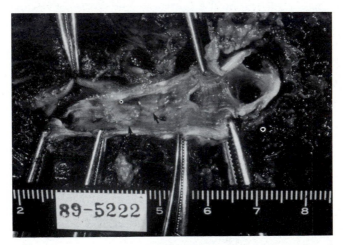

Fig 1–13.—Surgical specimen of the right bronchus showing the area of irregularly surfaced mucosa extending about 15 mm in the right bronchus 3b (*arrows*) and across to the bifurcation of the right bronchus 3a. (Courtesy of Tonami N, Yokoyama K, Taki J, et al: *J Nucl Med* 32:2284-2285, 1991.)

bronchial fiberoscopy revealed a tumor-like lesion at the right bronchus 3, and biopsy results suggested squamous cell carcinoma. Thallium 201 SPECT of the chest was performed to locate the primary lesion and to assess mediastinal lymph node involvement (Fig 1–12).

Findings.—The delayed ratio of SPECT was not high, but the high retention index suggested a malignant lesion. Since surgery, during which a well-differentiated squamous cell carcinoma was removed, the patient has been free of recurrence for 16 months (Fig 1–13).

Conclusion.—It is difficult to detect small lung cancers radiologically. Transbronchial fiberoscopy, biopsy, and aspiration cytology are used, but they may not always be successful. The use of SPECT after intravenous administration of ^{201}Tl-chloride has been successful in visualizing small lesions, despite its limited spatial resolution. The lesion described had enough tumor volume and ^{201}Tl radioactivity to be visualized even though the mass lesion was not evident on radiologic examination.

▶ A more limited application of lung cancer scintigraphy is described in this abstract. Thallium 201 SPECT was *not* important in making the diagnosis in this patient; bronchoscopy detected the primary neoplasm. However, if ^{201}Tl SPECT was positive in this case, it might also be positive in a patient with positive sputum cytology results and negative chest radiography, CT, *and* bronchoscopy. It is another tool to keep in mind.—B.H. Gross, M.D.

Bronchogenic Carcinoma: Analysis of Staging in the Mediastinum With CT by Correlative Lymph Node Mapping and Sampling

McLoud TC, Bourgouin PM, Greenberg RW, Kosiuk JP, Templeton PA, Shepard J-AO, Moore EH, Wain JC, Mathisen DJ, Grillo HC (Massachusetts Gen Hosp, Boston)
Radiology 182:319–323, 1992   1–26

Introduction.—Computed tomography enables noninvasive assessment of mediastinal nodes in bronchogenic carcinoma, but recent studies have suggested significant limitations of the technology. The accuracy of CT in the assessment of mediastinal lymph node metastases was evaluated.

Methods.—In a prospective study, 143 patients with bronchogenic carcinoma were studied with CT. Mediastinal lymph nodes were localized according to the lymph node mapping scheme of the American Thoracic Society and were considered abnormal if they exceeded 1 cm in short-axis diameter. The patients also underwent surgical staging by either mediastinoscopy alone or mediastinoscopy and thoracotomy. All accessible nodes were either removed or sampled.

Results.—Forty-two patients had nodal metastases confirmed at either mediastinoscopy or thoracotomy, for a prevalence of 29%. The sensitiv-

TABLE 1.—Accuracy of CT in N Staging

| | Sensitivity | | Specificity | | No. of Lymph Nodes | |
| | N2 and N3 | N1 | N2 and N3 | N1 | | |
Variable	(%)	(%)	(%)	(%)	N2 and N3	N1
All patients (per-patient basis) (*n* = 143 patients)	64	63	62	58	401	42
All nodal stations	44	23	85	79	401	42
Obstructive pneumonitis and atelectasis (*n* = 40 patients)	70	50	43	54	110	21
T1 (all nodal stations) (*n* = 36 patients)	59	50	90	90	123	13

(Courtesy of McLoud TC, Bourgouin PM, Greenberg RW, et al: *Radiology* 182:319-323, 1992.)

ity of CT for mediastinal nodes on a per-patient basis was 64%, and the specificity was 62% (Table 1). The sensitivity of CT for individual nodal stations involved with tumor was only 44% (Table 2). The specificity of CT was reduced to 43% when obstructive pneumonia was present, but the sensitivity was not appreciably altered. Although the likelihood of metastases increased with lymph node size, 37% of the lymph nodes that were 2–4 cm in diameter were hyperplastic and did not contain metastases (Table 3).

Conclusion.—Early investigations of CT reported a sensitivity in the staging of mediastinal disease as high as 88% to 94%. The sensitivity of CT for mediastinal nodes on a per-patient basis appears to be 64%; the specificity, 62%. The relative insensitivity of CT may make formal nodal

TABLE 2.—Accuracy of CT in N
Staging of Individual Nodal Stations

Node Group	Sensitivity (%)	Specificity (%)	No. of Lymph Nodes
2R	...	...	10
2L	...	...	7
4R	78	79	104
4L	33	86	70
5	83	83	30
7	25	91	108
10R	30	72	42
10L	27	94	29
11R	29	73	22
11L	17	86	20
8R	...	...	1
8L	...	...	0

(Courtesy of McLoud TC, Bourgouin PM, Greenberg RW, et al: *Radiology* 182:319-323, 1992.)

TABLE 3.—Prevalence of Metastases
Related to Size of Nodes on CT Scan

No. of Lymph Nodes	Size (cm)	Metastases (%)
336	<1	13
57	1.0–1.9	25
13	2.0–2.9	62
6	3.0–3.9	67
2	>4	100

(Courtesy of McLoud TC, Bourgouin PM, Greenberg RW, et al: *Radiology* 182:319–323, 1992.)

sampling at mediastinoscopy or thoracotomy essential to detect lymph node metastases.

▶ I was having a pretty good year until this article was published. It raises serious questions about multiple prior studies that showed CT's sensitivity for mediastinal staging to be 90%, with a specificity in the 65% range. We had the specificity right, but in this prospective study of 143 patients, the sensitivity was only 64%. A decrease of 26% may not seem earthshaking, but if it is correct, it indicates a radical revision of CT's role in patients with lung cancer. The primary goal of CT staging is to prevent unnecessary "exploratory thoracotomies." False positives can be accommodated for by invasive confirmation of abnormal CT findings, but false negatives (which result in unnecessary surgery) need to be avoided. If CT's sensitivity is only 64%, false negatives will occur in significant numbers.

I have a great deal of respect for the authors of this study, and I am certain that this is a careful and important piece of work. Nevertheless, I am not yet ready to throw in the towel. There are many studies, not just those to which I have contributed, that have arrived at a CT sensitivity of 85% to 90%. Furthermore, most thoracic surgeons use preoperative CT as a guide to appropriate therapy, and we haven't yet heard of a rash of unnecessary thoracotomies. How this ultimately plays out as further studies are published will have major economic implications for us as radiologists and for society as a whole.

If we stop doing staging CT in patients with lung cancer, perhaps we can still use chest CT to answer other questions pertaining to lung cancer (1, 2).—B.H. Gross, M.D.

References

1. Yokoi K, et al: *Radiology* 181:147, 1991.
2. Gaeta M, et al: *AJR* 157:1181, 1991.

Ultrasound

Ultrasound-Guided Aspiration Biopsy of Small Peripheral Pulmonary Nodules

Yuan A, Yang P-C, Chang D-B, Yu C-J, Lee Y-C, Kuo S-H, Luh K-T (National Taiwan University Hospital, Taipei, Taiwan)
Chest 101:926–930, 1992   1–27

Background.—The etiologic diagnosis of small peripheral pulmonary nodules is difficult because of their size and location. Roentgenographic features are helpful for differential diagnosis, but they are not conclusive. Ultrasound-guided aspiration biopsy has good sensitivity and specificity in the transthoracic biopsy of peripheral lung lesions and mediastinal tumors. The diagnostic value of ultrasound-guided aspiration biopsy was assessed in patients with peripheral pulmonary nodules.

Method.—The diagnostic yields of ultrasound-guided transthoracic aspiration biopsy, sputum cytology, fiberoptic bronchoscopy, and biopsy in 30 patients with peripheral pulmonary nodules were compared. Four nodules were less than 1 cm in diameter, 12 were between 1.1 and 2 cm, and 14 were between 2.1 and 3 cm. Confirmed final diagnoses revealed 24 malignant lesions and 6 benign lesions.

Results.—The size of the lesions did not affect the diagnostic yield and complication rate. Confirmative diagnoses were made in 27 of the 30 patients who underwent ultrasound-guided transthoracic fine-needle aspiration biopsy (Fig 1–14). Diagnosis was made by cytologic and microbiologic examinations in 22 of 24 patients with malignant nodules and 5

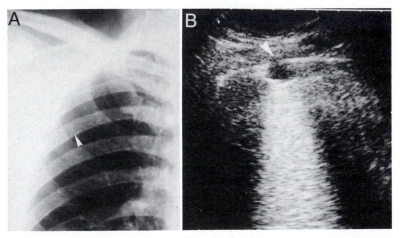

Fig 1–14.—**A,** chest radiograph of a man, 41, showing multiple small nodules in the right lung. The *arrowhead* indicates a minute .5 × .5-cm nodule in the right upper lobe. **B,** transverse scan at the right 2nd intercostal space reveals a hypoechoic subpleural nodule with smooth margin. The pleural line was interrupted (*arrowhead*). (Courtesy of Yuan A, Yang P-C, Chang D-B, et al: *Chest* 101:926–930, 1992.)

of 6 patients with benign lesions. Two patients had fiberoptic bronchoscopy diagnosed at biopsy, and none received a diagnosis by sputum cytology.

Conclusion.—The overall diagnostic yield by ultrasound-guided transthoracic needle aspiration in 30 patients with pulmonary nodules was 90% for all small peripheral pulmonary nodules, 92% for malignant nodules, and 83% for benign lesions. Sputum cytology and fiberoptic bronchoscopic biopsy had a very low diagnostic yield in this patient group. Ultrasound-guided transthoracic needle aspiration biopsy is a simple, safe, and accurate diagnostic approach for peripheral pulmonary nodules, even when the nodules are smaller than 3 cm in diameter.

▶ This is a new section for me. Although I did 6 months of ultrasonography during my fellowship, I have never used it as a chest radiologist. Interestingly, most of the authors in this section are working outside the United States. In American chest radiology, we seem to have bypassed ultrasound for more expensive technologies. The expense may ultimately catch up with us, and perhaps we will look more seriously at ultrasound as an alternative diagnostic modality. Whether ultrasound is the right answer or not, this is the kind of trend that deserves encouragement. For example, we would probably be practicing better radiology if we spent more time analyzing conventional radiographs, used more oblique views, and performed more chest fluoroscopy. Then again, our clinical colleagues could similarly improve their style of practice by performing more careful physical examinations and pondering their lists of differential diagnosis more carefully.

In any event, in this study of biopsies performed using ultrasound guidance, 27 of 30 peripheral lung nodules were successful. Most nodules were in the 1- to 3-cm size range. Only 1 patient had a complication, and that was a small pneumothorax. The authors correctly note that small lesions are sometimes difficult to biopsy using CT or fluoroscopy; they may not be well visualized at fluoroscopy, and patient motion and breathing may render them inaccessible (or at least difficult to biopsy) at CT. The cost, speed, lack of radiation, and real-time image monitoring of ultrasound are advantages that may be worth pursuing.—B.H. Gross, M.D.

Diagnosis of Pneumothorax by Ultrasound Immediately After Ultrasonically Guided Aspiration Biopsy
Targhetta R, Bourgeois J-M, Chavagneux R, Balmes P (Montpellier-Nimes University Hospital, Nimes, France)
Chest 101:855–856, 1992   1–28

Introduction.—Chest radiography or CT is generally used to diagnose pneumothorax after thoracic puncture. Although peripheral pulmonary tumors are most often punctured during ultrasonically guided aspiration biopsy (UGAB), no reports have suggested the use of ultrasound to diagnose pneumothorax after pulmonary puncture.

Case.—Man, 55, was admitted for diagnostic evaluation of a peripheral lesion of the upper left lobe of the lung. Previous diagnostic studies had failed to establish a diagnosis. The patient underwent UGAB using a linear scanner with a central guide channel to introduce a fine needle. A hypoechoic tumor with no tapered edges was seen on an ultrasonogram with the real-time image showing movement of the tumor and respiratory excursions of the visceral pleura. Immediately after puncture, ultrasound examination detected pneumothorax, which was confirmed by chest radiography. With the development of penumothorax, the tumor and pleural respiratory excursions were no longer visible.

Conclusion.—Ultrasound can be used to diagnose pneumothorax occurring immediately after UGAB. The technique is simple and is especially suitable in emergencies and when radiographic equipment is unavailable.

▶ If you are going to do UGABs, it will be important to be able to diagnose pneumothoraces with ultrasound. The simple sign described here is the ultrasound disappearance of the nodule on which a biopsy was being performed because of interposed pleural air. The same authors also report several sonographic signs for diagnosing hydropneumothorax (1).—B.H. Gross, M.D.

Reference

1. Targhetta R, et al: *Chest* 101:931, 1992.

Factors Affecting the Development of Pneumothorax Associated With Thoracentesis
Raptopoulos V, Davis LM, Lee G, Umali C, Lew R, Irwin RS (Univ of Massachusetts Med Ctr, Worcester, Mass)
AJR 156:917–920, 1991   1–29

Objective.—Grogan et al. recently showed that sonographically guided thoracentesis produces fewer complications, including pneumothoraces. An attempt was made to see whether this applies to a broader range of patients by reviewing 342 thoracenteses done in 30 months, 154 conventionally and 188 with sonographic guidance.

Findings.—Pneumothorax complicated 18% of conventional thoracenteses and 3% of sonographically guided procedures. The need for chest tube placement also differed significantly (7% vs. 2%). Regression analysis showed that the method of thoracentesis was the dominant factor in whether pneumothorax developed. Excluding the method used, the type of tap (diagnostic or therapeutic) and needle size were factors, but the size of the effusion was not.

Conclusion.—Sonography makes thoracentesis a safer procedure without substantially increasing its cost. Sonographically guided thoracentesis should at least be used in critically ill patients, those with severe lung disease, and those requiring respiratory assistance.

▶ I put this in the ultrasound section because more than half the thoracenteses in this series were done with sonographic guidance. There was a statistically significant difference in the complication rate between the 2 groups. With ultrasound guidance, pneumothorax developed in only 3% of patients (vs. 18% with conventional thoracentesis), and the need for chest tube placement was also statistically significantly different. I have always told clinicians to attempt thoracentesis first, using only lateral decubitus views and percussion. Based on their findings, the authors of this study suggest that sonographic guidance should be extended at least to critically ill patients, those with severe lung disease, and those requiring respiratory assistance. Another study of pneumothorax, this time as a complication of percutaneous lung aspiration biopsy, concludes that when patients are positioned with the puncture site down after the procedure, they are much less likely to need a chest tube (1).—B.H. Gross, M.D.

Reference

1. Moore EH, et al: *Radiology* 181:385, 1991.

Lung Abscesses: US Examination and US-Guided Transthoracic Aspiration
Yang P-C, Luh K-T, Lee Y-C, Chang D-B, Yu C-J, Wu H-D, Lee L-N, Kuo S-H
(National Taiwan University Hospital No 1, Taipei, Taiwan)
Radiolgoy 180:171–175, 1991   1–30

Introduction.—Transthoracic needle aspiration is the most reliable method for obtaining specimens from lung abscesses for microbiological diagnosis. Ultrasound (US)–guided transthoracic needle aspiration is used to diagnose pleural diseases and mediastinal tumors, but transthoracic needle aspiration of lung abscesses with US guidance has not previously been reported.

Patients.—During a 5-year study period, 35 patients aged 1–70 years had a diagnosis of lung abscess based on clinical history and chest radiography. Twenty-three patients had been treated with parenteral antibiotics for at least 3 days before undergoing needle aspiration. Fiberoptic bronchoscopy was performed in 25 patients, 15 of whom also had bronchoalveolar lavage. In 3 patients, a malignant tumor was diagnosed.

Results.—On US, a lung abscess was usually depicted as an ovoid-shaped hypoechoic lesion with irregular outer margins. The central cavity appeared inhomogeneously hypoechoic and an abscess cavity appeared as a hyperechoic ring. Abscess walls were of irregular thickness (Fig 1–15). Two patients had abscess lesions that were not in contact with the pleura, and neither lesion was depicted with US. The other 33 le-

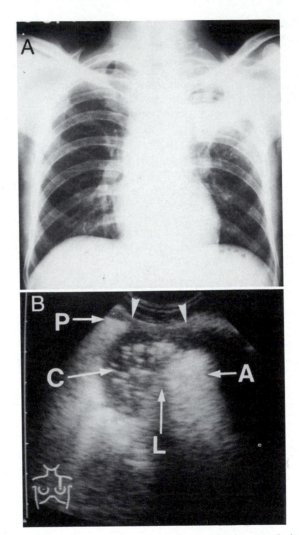

Fig 1–15.—A, radiograph of the chest of a man, 45, shows a lung abscess in the left upper lobe; B, longitudinal ultrasound examination of the chest, obtained with the use of a convex scanner, reveals a hypoechoic lesion with a central hyperechoic cavity (C). Hyperechoic air (A) is present in the upper part, and inhomogeneous abscess fluid is present in the lower half, with a sharp demarcation line of air-fluid level (L). The visceral-pleural echo (P) was interrupted at the pleural contact area. The *arrowheads* indicate the lesion-pleura symphysis. (Courtesy of Yang P-C, Luh K-T, Lee Y-C, et al: *Radiology* 180:171–175, 1991.)

sions were depicted, and all showed areas of visceral or pleural involvement and the presence of a cavity (Fig 1–16). Twenty-five abscesses (71%) had local adhesion to parietal pleura. Ultrasound-guided transthoracic needle aspiration of fluid from the abscess cavity was successful in 31 of 33 patients (94%) in whom the abscess was depicted. Sixty-five or-

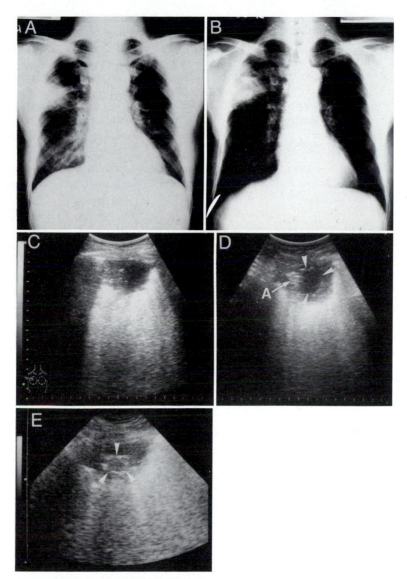

Fig 1–16.—A, posteroanterior radiograph of chest of a man, 62, shows segmental pneumonia in the right upper lobe at the time of admission; **B,** abscess cavity with air-fluid level developed 1 week later; **C,** ultrasound examination of the chest shows segmental consolidation at the time of admission; **D,** a follow-up US scan of the chest 3 days after admission shows a hypoechoic cystic lesion that developed in the consolidated lung (*arrowheads*). A = air echogenicity. Chest radiograph at this time did not demonstrate the abscess cavity. Lung aspirates from the cystic lesion grew *Peptostreptocccus* species, *B intermedius,* and unidentified gram-negative bacilli. **E,** an ultrasound scan of the chest 1 week later shows a hyperechoic, ringlike abscess cavity more clearly (*arrowheads*). (Courtesy of Yang P-C, Luh K-T, Lee Y-C, et al: *Radiology* 180:171–175, 1991.)

ganisms were isolated from the 31 aspirates, including 41 anaerobes and 24 aerobes, even though 23 patients had previously been treated with antibiotics. All 65 organisms were considered to be significant pathogens. Only 2 pathogens (3%) were recovered from blood culture, 7 (11%) from sputum culture, and 2 (3%) from bronchoalveolar lavage. On the basis of the culture results, the antibiotic regimen was changed in 10 patients, 7 of whom improved after the change in regimen. Thirty abscess cavities closed within 4–6 weeks. Three patients died of underlying disease. Two patients were operated on when the cavity had not closed after more than 6 weeks.

Conclusion.—Ultrasound-guided transthoracic aspiration of a lung abscess is a safe and useful diagnostic modality for collecting specimens for culture.

▶ I have a hard time relating this study to my daily work. We see far fewer lung abscesses than the 35 seen in this series in a 5-year period. Most of our lung abscesses resolve with percussion and postural drainage supplementing antibiotic therapy. We are very reluctant to transgress uninfected pleura to needle an abscess, but 33 of the 35 abscesses in this study involved the pleura. Most importantly, aspiration led to a change in antibiotic therapy in 10 patients. For patients with lung abscesses not responding to therapy, percutaneous aspiration (perhaps using US guidance) may be helpful. Another recent application of thoracic US is the detection of thymic involvement in Hodgkin's disease (1), and again, the authors work outside the United States.—B.H. Gross, M.D.

Reference

1. Wernecke K, et al: *Radiology* 181:375, 1991.

New Applications in Diagnosis and Therapy

Efficacy of Digital Radiography for the Detection of Pneumothorax: Comparison With Conventional Chest Radiography
Elam EA, Rehm K, Hillman BJ, Maloney K, Fajardo LL, McNeill K (Univ of Arizona, Tucson)
AJR 158:509–514, 1992   1–31

Background.—Exploratory studies of digital radiography continue to define its many possible advantages over conventional techniques. A comparative study of radiologists' abilities to detect pneumothorax using different digital radiographic formats was performed.

Methods.—Five experienced radiologists reviewed 23 frontal chest radiographs showing pneumothorax and 22 other chest radiographs showing normal findings or other abnormalities. Images were reviewed in each of 4 formats: conventional chest radiographs, small- and large-format computed radiographs, and digital images viewed on an electronic work station.

Findings.—No significant differences were noted in mean areas under the receiver-operating-characteristic curves, which ranged from .869 for the electronic work station to .915 for film-screen images. Neither was there any difference in specificities, which ranged from .90 for large-format computed radiographs to .96 for the electronic work station. However, sensitivity was .65 for the work station compared with .82 for film-screen images; small-format computed images also increased sensitivity.

Conclusion.—Pneumothorax can be detected equally well on conventional radiographs and digital images printed on film. Use of an electronic viewing console appears to decrease detection of pneumothorax. More development and evaluations of the usefulness of these work stations are needed.

▶ With the comparatively new technology of digital chest radiography, this is the right question to ask. We have purchased 1 such unit, and we use it for all portable intensive care unit films. Its advantages include cost, radiation dose, and consistency of the resultant computed radiograph; the latter is its key advantage in patients who have daily films looking for minor changes. An additional (probably undiscussed) advantage is that I can read these smaller radiographs more quickly. I hope it's not at the cost of missed diagnoses, although the images I've seen are clearly inferior for evaluating subtle lung parenchymal abnormality. However, I believe that the authors are correct in stating that there is no statistically significant difference between conventional radiographs and computed radiographs in detecting pneumothorax. An important point in this study is that viewing images at an electronic work station *does* reduce the sensitivity for detecting pneumothorax in a meaningful way.—B.H. Gross, M.D.

Plain and Computed Radiography for Detecting Experimentally Induced Pneumothorax in Cadavers: Implications for Detection in Patients
Carr JJ, Reed JC, Choplin RH, Pope TL, Case LD (Wake Forest Univ, Winston-Salem, NC)
Radiology 183:193–199, 1992   1–32

Background.—Detecting pneumothorax, especially in critically ill patients, is extremely important to avoid serious consequences and to ensure patient recovery. The incidence of pulmonary barotrauma as a complication of continuous positive-pressure breathing is estimated at 5% to 15%. Pneumothorax is usually documented on chest radiograph in an erect inspiratory frontal view position, but other positions have been recommended to improve detection. Cadavers with induced pneumothorax were used to determine the effects of patient positioning and imaging modality on radiographic findings.

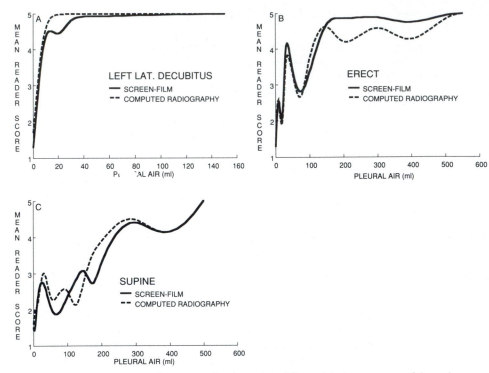

Fig 1–17.—A–C, mean reader score vs. pleural air volume. The y axis is the mean score of the readers (1–5 scale with 5 indicating a definite presence of pneumothorax), and the x axis is the volume of air (in millimeters) in the pleural space. Smooth spline curves were used to interpolate between the estimated mean scores at each volume of air for screen-film (*solid line*) and computed (*dashed line*) radiography. **A,** graph for diagnosis of pneumothorax with LLD view. Readers became confident of the diagnosis of pneumothorax (average score > 4) at air volumes of 10–20 mL. **B,** graph for cadavers in the erect position demonstrates variation in the scoring until 100–150 mL of air was present. With more air than this, readers were able to make a confident and reliable diagnosis of pneumothorax. **C,** for the supine position, a confident diagnosis was not made by the readers until more than 200 mL of air was present. (Courtesy of Carr JJ, Reed JC, Choplin RH, et al: *Radiology* 183:193–199, 1992.)

Method.—Chest radiography with conventional screen-film and computed radiography was performed with 3 fresh, unembalmed cadavers in the supine frontal, erect frontal, and left lateral decubitus (LLD) positions. Radiography was performed at baseline and after injection of incremental quantities of air into the pleural space. The radiographs were independently interpreted by 5 radiologists who rated each on a 1 to 5 scoring system, with 5 equal to definite presence of pneumothorax.

Findings.—The ability of the radiologists to diagnose pneumothorax varied by the cadaver position and depended on volume of air (Fig 1–17). The LLD position had 88% sensitivity for diagnosis of pneumothorax, followed by 59% for the erect position and 37% for the supine position. Conventional screen-film radiography and computed radiography performed similarly with no statistically significant difference in diagnostic proficiency.

Conclusion.—The LLD view was the most sensitive for diagnosis of pneumothorax, followed by the erect and supine views.

▶ Without intending to slight this excellent article, it made an even better radiographic display. I saw it at the 1991 Roentgen Ray meeting and was pleased to see it win the Gold Medal. You honestly could not ask for a more compact, elegant, and scientific example of the medium.

This study concurs with the previous study's conclusion that there is no difference in pneumothorax detection between conventional and computed radiographs. Additional information found in this study is that lateral decubitus radiography is the most sensitive technique for detecting pneumothorax and is capable of detecting amounts of pleural air as small as 5 mL. At 20 mL or more, all readers in the study confidently diagnosed pneumothorax. The erect position was less sensitive, and pneumothorax paradoxically became less detectable as the volume of pleural air increased in the 5 to 200-mL range. In the supine position, even 400 mL of air did not lead to consensus among the readers that pneumothorax was present.

A number of critical questions are raised, and then answered. What more can we ask?—B.H. Gross, M.D.

Intrathoracic Complications Following Allogeneic Bone Marrow Transplantation: CT Findings
Graham NJ, Müller NL, Miller RR, Shepherd JD (University of British Columbia, Vancouver, BC, Canada)
Radiology 181:153–156, 1991   1–33

Introduction.—Pulmonary problems and complications often accompany allogeneic bone marrow transplantation (BMT). Computed tomographic scans of patients with intrathoracic complications after undergoing BMT were compared with radiographic and pathologic studies of the same patients.

Methods.—Eighteen patients who received BMT had 21 intrathoracic complications. There were 7 women and 11 men, with a mean age of 32 years. The chest radiographs were performed on the initial indication of a pulmonary problem; the CT scans were taken after the patient had had a major lung symptom that could not be defined by a radiograph. All 18 patients had pathologic or microbiologic diagnosis (or both) of the lung difficulty. With lung complications occurring 1–30 months after the BMT, 13 of the 21 complications related to an infection. Two patients had pulmonary graft-vs.-host disease (GVHD) 9 and 11 months after BMT.

Results.—The chest CT scans showed significant findings not found on the radiograph in 12 of the 18 patients with pulmonary complications. Twenty radiographs demonstrated some abnormality, but in 1 patient with Hodgkin's disease no radiographic abnormality was present.

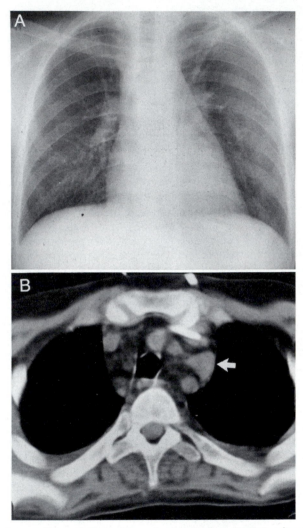

Fig 1–18.—Images of 20-year-old man 12 months after allogeneic BMT. **A,** radiograph showing no evidence of lymphadenopathy; **B,** conventional CT scan (10-mm collimation) demonstrating an enlarged left superior paratracheal lymph node (region 2L) (*arrow*), which at anterior mediastinotomy demonstrated recurrent Hodgkin's disease. (Courtesy of Graham NJ, Müller NL, Miller RR, et al: *Radiology* 181:153–156, 1991.)

The CT scan demonstrated the pathologic condition (Fig 1–18), which occurred 12 months after BMT. When acute abnormalities did not appear on radiographs, the CT scans of the same individual and area clearly demonstrated the lesion (Fig 1–19). The CT scan revealed a peripheral distribution in 1 patient with bronchiolitis obliterans organizing pneumonia and 1 with an eosinophilic drug reaction (Fig 1–20). Al-

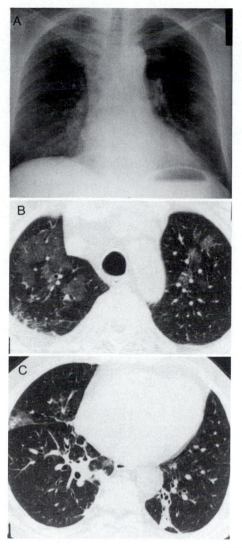

Fig 1–19.—Images of a man, 49, who had fever and cough 2 years after BMT. **A,** radiograph is abnormal, showing bilateral areas of scarring, particularly in the middle and lower lung zones. Those radiographic findings had not changed over the previous 3 months. **B,** high-resolution CT scan (1.5-mm collimation with use of high-spatial-frequency reconstruction algorithm) obtained at the level of aortic arch shows a bilateral ground-glass pattern. Mild parenchymal scarring can be seen in the posterior aspect of the right upper lobe. **C,** high-resolution CT scan through the lung bases shows more extensive scarring and cylindrical bronchiectasis, but only minimal ground-glass pattern. On the basis of the CT findings, bronchoalveolar lavage was performed in the right upper lobe and demonstrated the presence of *Pseudomonas aeruginosa* pneumonia. (Courtesy of Graham NJ, Müller NL, Miller RR, et al: *Radiology* 181:153–156, 1991.)

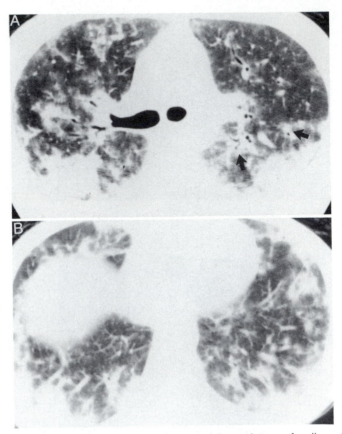

Fig 1–20.—Images of a man, 22, with severe dyspnea and dry cough 1 year after allogeneic BMT. **A,** high-resolution CT scan obtained at the level of the right upper lobe bronchus shows peribronchial (*arrows*) and subpleural consolidation. **B,** 10-mm collimation CT scan shows peripheral distribution at the lung bases. Open lung biopsy demonstrated graft-vs.-host disease. (Courtesy of Graham NJ, Müller NL, Miller RR, et al: *Radiology* 181:153–156, 1991.)

though the CT scan revealed the abnormalities in those patients, it gave no significant additional data in 9 patients.

Conclusion.—The CT scan can provide useful additional information in the diagnosis of intrathoracic complications associated with allogeneic BMT. The CT scan gives much better information about the presence and extent of lesions than does the conventional radiograph in these patients.

▶ In this select patient population, negative chest radiographs may necessitate chest CT. The potential advantages include earlier detection of disease and better localization of a site for lavage or biopsy; Figure 1–19 is especially impressive. A disadvantage of CT is the overlap of different diseases with the same CT pattern. I'm also not clear why it was helpful to find cystic changes at CT in a patient with *Pneumocystis carinii* pneumonia who had groundglass abnormality on the chest radiograph; the cystic changes would only have confused me regarding the diagnosis.—B.H. Gross, M.D.

Pulmonary Metastases: MR Imaging With Surgical Correlation—A Prospective Study

Feuerstein IM, Jicha DL, Pass HI, Chow CK, Chang R, Ling A, Hill SC, Dwyer AJ, Travis WD, Horowitz ME, Steinberg SM, Frank JA, Doppman JL (Dept of Diagnostic Radiology, Natl Insts of Health, Natl Cancer Inst, Bethesda, Md; Georgetown Univ)

Radiology 182:123–129, 1992   1–34

Purpose.—The sensitivity of MRI for detection of pulmonary metastases was evaluated in a prospective, controlled study.

Patients.—Eleven patients scheduled for thoracotomy and curative resection of metastases were studied. In a blinded fashion, findings on MRI using .5 tesla were compared with those of CT, chest radiography, and thoracotomy in 12 cases (1 patient had 2 separate occurrences of pulmonary metastases).

Findings.—The combination of all MR sequences correctly identified all 12 (100%) cases of pulmonary metastases. By design, CT identified at least 1 lung nodule in all 12 cases (100%), whereas chest radiography identified only 64%. For detection of individual pulmonary nodules, MRI allowed more detection of nodules than CT, although the difference was not significant; MR was significantly more sensitive than chest radiography. Compared with unenhanced T_1-weighted images, gadopentetate dimeglumine–enhanced T_1-weighted images improved detection of 35% of the lung nodules, including potentially useful morphologic data, (e.g., central necrosis and homogenous enhancement in 2 cases. However, Gd-enhanced T_1-weighted images also provided the most false positive findings. Short inversion time inversion-recovery (STIR) images were the most sensitive MR sequence (82%) and allowed detection of paracardiac pulmonary metastases that were not visible on CT. All modalities missed the diagnosis in 2 metastases less than 5 mm in diameter. One nodule, 25 mm in diameter located adjacent to the aorta, was missed on MRI and identified as a flow artifact.

Conclusion.—Magnetic resonance imaging is equally effective as CT for the detection of pulmonary metastases greater than 5 mm in diameter. Because STIR is as sensitive as all MR sequences taken together, detection of pulmonary metastases can be accomplished with a reduced number of sequences, possibly even with a single STIR sequence.

▶ It is probably not good enough for MRI to equal CT in the detection of pulmonary metastases, as it did in this study. Because of CT's advantages in length of examination and availability, MRI must do better than CT and must do so in a clinically meaningful way to replace CT. It is not clinically meaningful to detect 13 metastases in a patient if CT detects 9; it is meaningful to detect some lesions when CT detects none and to detect more than 1 lesion when CT detects only 1, although we get back to the earlier troubling question of what to do with multiple very small nodules. Technical issues in the development of MRI of the lung parenchyma have recently been addressed by the Stanford group (1, 2).—B.H. Gross, M.D.

References

1. Bergin CJ, et al: *Radiology* 179:777, 1991.
2. Bergin CJ, et al: *Radiology* 180:845, 1991.

Imaged Thoracoscopic Surgery: A New Thoracic Technique for Resection of Mediastinal Cysts

Lewis RJ, Caccavale RJ, Sisler GE (Univ of Medicine and Dentistry of New Jersey, New Brunswick)
Ann Thorac Surg 53:318–320, 1992   1–35

Background.—Until recently, the only 2 approaches to the intrathoracic organs were through thoracoscopy and thoracotomy. Recently, imaged thoracoscopic surgery, using video optics and projection of images on a screen, has been used successfully in patients with mediastinal cysts.

Case 1.—Man, 40, underwent thoracoscopic surgery for the removal of a small mediastinal mass. The soft, pliable cyst was found in the posterior medias-

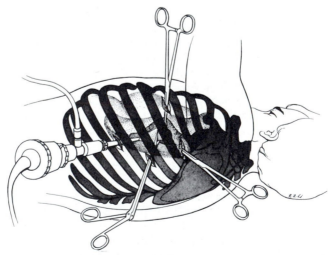

Fig 1–21.—With a clamp holding the lung and the camera in place, the cyst is excised. (Courtesy of Lewis RJ, Caccavale RJ, Sisler GE: *Ann Thorac Surg* 53:318–320, 1992.)

tinum. It was opened, drained, cultured, and excised to its base. It was diagnosed as a benign bronchogenic cyst. The patient's recovery was uneventful.

Case 2.—Man, 31, had a cyst drained, cultured, and excised to its base with imaged thoracoscopic surgery. The cyst was ablated with a coagulator, and the patient returned to normal activity within 10 days.

Discussion.—The main patient benefit of imaged thoracoscopic surgery is the avoidance of the thoracotomy incision with its inherent pain and morbidity. Both patients required only 4 incisions: a 2-cm midaxillary line incision in the sixth intercostal space, a 1.5-cm incision in the anterior axillary line in the fifth intercostal space, and 2 1.5-cm incisions in the posterior axillary line at the fourth and sixth intercostal spaces (Fig 1–21). Imaged thoracoscopic surgical techniques allow full participation of all members of the operating team and excellent visualization of the thorax and its contents. The ribs need not be spread, because the work is performed through the intercostal spaces. Both patients experienced minimal pain postoperatively and made a quick recovery.

Conclusion.—Imaged thoracoscopic surgery is more difficult and tedious than traditional thoracotomy, but the patients benefit from an apparent shortened recovery time. Procedures such as lung biopsy and resection of tumors, recurrent pneumothorax, and pericardial cysts have been successfully performed with the new technique.

▶ To the uninformed eye of this layman, imaged thoracoscopic surgery is to thoracotomy what arthroscopic surgery is to arthrotomy. My brother had open surgery for a knee injury 20 years ago. When he subsequently injured the contralateral knee, painful experience had taught him to opt for conservative therapy. He is now a physiatrist. Five years ago I had arthroscopic knee surgery for a similar injury, and if need be I'll do it again. I suspect patients would gladly opt for a procedure that doesn't necessitate thoracotomy or spreading of the ribs.—B.H. Gross, M.D.

The Prevalence and Management of Bronchial Anastomotic Complications in Lung Transplantation
Schafers H-J, Haydock DA, Cooper JD (Washington Univ, St Louis, Mo; University of Toronto, Toronto, Ont, Canada)
J Thorac Cardiovasc Surg 101:1044–1052, 1991   1–36

Objective.—Disruption of the bronchial anastomosis and formation of a bronchopleural or bronchovascular fistula were the common causes of death in patients who survived the first 2 weeks after lung transplantation. The prevalence and management of bronchial anastomotic complications in 53 patients undergoing lung transplantation between 1963 and 1978 were studied.

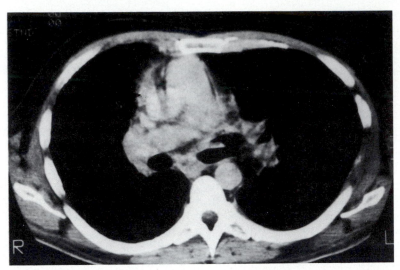

Fig 1–22.—A CT scan of the chest taken 34 days after left lung transplantation. A defect in the left main bronchus can be seen. (Courtesy of Schafers H-J, Haydock DA, Cooper JD: *J Thorac Cardiovasc Surg* 101:1044–1052, 1991.)

Patients.—Fifty patients survived more than 2 weeks after lung transplantation and were considered to be at risk for bronchial complications. Bronchial omentopexy was performed in all but 1 patient, and all received immunosuppression consisting of cyclosporine, azathioprine,

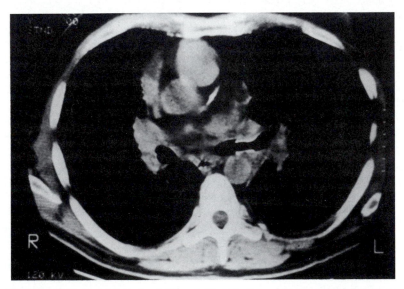

Fig 1–23.—A CT scan of the patient in Figure 1-22, with silicone rubber stent in place. (Courtesy of Schafers H-J, Haydock DA, Cooper JD: *J Thorac Cardiovasc Surg* 101:1044–1052, 1991.)

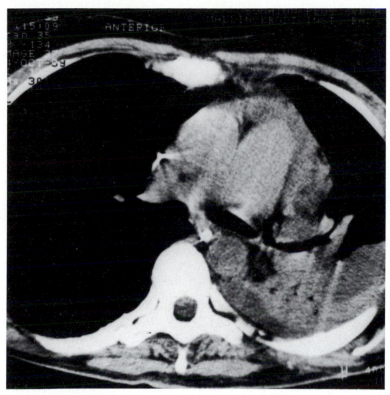

Fig 1–24.—A CT scan demonstrating an air pocket outside the airway anastomosis with a cartilaginous flap obstructing the airway. There is a considerable amount of consolidation in the lower lobe of the transplanted lung. (Courtesy of Schafers H-J, Haydock DA, Cooper JD: *J Thorac Cardiovasc Surg* 101:1044–1052, 1991.)

and horse antilymphocyte globulin. Orally administered prednisolone was started 2–3 weeks after transplantation.

Findings.—Seven (14%) patients had significant bronchial complications, for a prevalence of 11.6% per anastomosis. Three patients died, but only 1 (2%) died as a direct result of the airway complication, for a prevalence of 1.7% per anastomosis. Four long-term survivor patients required airway stenting. The bronchial dehiscence was well contained by the omentum in 3 patients (Fig 1–22). Healing occurred by secondary intention, followed by stenosis of the left main bronchus in 3 patients. The stenosis was managed by dilation and, ultimately, stenting of the bronchus with adequate airway (Fig 1–23). One patient who had airway breakdown on the cartilaginous portion of the anastomosis showed an air pocket outside the airway on CT, with considerable collapse and consolidation of the left lower lobe (Fig 1–24). The patient improved with stenting (Fig 1–25).

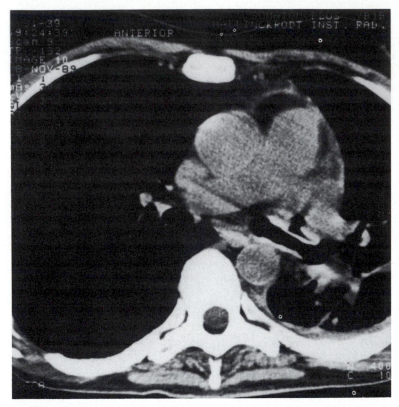

Fig 1–25.—A CT scan after stent placement. The stent bridges the defect and holds back the flap obstruction of the airway. There has been considerable clearing of the lower lobe of the transplanted lung. (Courtesy of Schafers H-J, Haydock DA, Cooper JD: *J Thorac Cardiovasc Surg* 101:1044–1052, 1991.)

Conclusion.—With bronchial omentopexy and current immunosuppressive protocols, airway healing after lung transplantation is normal in most patients. Airway complications as a cause of death are not common, and they are usually amenable to bronchoscopic management with good long-term results.

▶ In the past, bronchial anastomotic complications were a common cause of late death after lung transplantation. This article examines more recent experience that incorporates advances such as bronchial omentopexy and improved immunosuppression regimens. These advances and the improved bronchoscopic management of bronchial stenosis have virtually eliminated airway complications as a cause of death. Another complication of lung transplantation is bronchiolitis obliterans, occurring in 10% of patients in a recently published series (1). Chest radiographic and high-resolution CT findings are illustrated.—B.H. Gross, M.D.

Reference

1. Morrish WF, et al: *Radiology* 179:487, 1991.

Thoracoscopic Neodymium: Yttrium-Aluminum Garnet Laser-Assisted Pulmonary Resection

Landreneau RJ, Herlan DB, Johnson JA, Boley TM, Nawarawong W, Ferson PF (Univ of Pittsburgh, Pittsburgh; Univ of Missouri, Columbia, Mo)
Ann Thorac Surg 52:1176–1178, 1991   1–37

Introduction.—A renewed interest in therapeutic thoracoscopy and pressures to perform less invasive surgery have combined to promote laser-assisted resection of pulmonary disease by this approach. In the present case, the neodymium:yttrium-aluminum-garnet (Nd:YAG) laser was used to remove a 2.5-cm adenocarcinoma from the left lower lobe of an elderly patient who had a synchronous squamous carcinoma of the larynx and serious chronic obstructive lung disease.

Case Report.—Man, 74, had an uncalcified lung nodule identified on chest radiography during staging of a (stage I) laryngeal carcinoma. Computed tomography demonstrated an isolated lesion in the periphery of an emphysematous

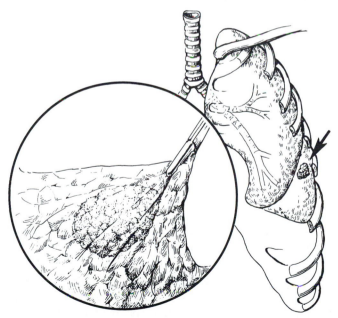

Fig 1–26.—Endoscopic forceps grasping the lung over the lesion to facilitate demarcation of the lesion from the collapsed normal lung. (Courtesy of Landrendeau RJ, Herlan DB, Johnson JA, et al: *Ann Thorac Surg* 52:1176–1178, 1991.)

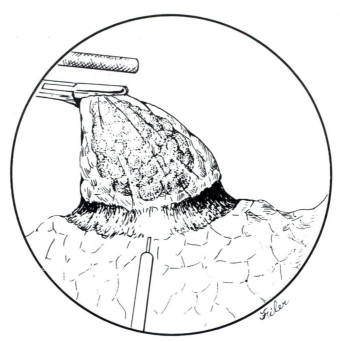

Fig 1–27.—The margin of Nd:YAG laser resection established beneath the lesion. A laser crater is formed as coagulation and vaporization of the surrounding lung tissue occurs. (Courtesy of Landreneau RJ, Herlan DB, Johnson JA, et al: *Ann Thorac Surg* 52:1176–1178, 1991.)

lower lobe. The patient was a long-time smoker and had a forced expiratory volume in 1 second (FEV_1) of 1.4 L. After bronchoscopy, endoscopic forceps were introduced via the operating laparoscope and served to isolate the lesion (Fig 1–26). Laser resection then was performed, with a 1.5-cm margin of normal lung tissue (Fig 1–27). The lesion was a well-differentiated adenocarcinoma. The procedure ended with the placement of underwater seal drainage. Air leakage was minimal.

Conclusion.—Limited experience suggests that thoracoscopic pulmonary resection using the Nd:YAG laser may be a valuable approach to selected peripheral lung lesions. At present, it is proposed only for limited-stage primary pulmonary malignancies in patients with severely impaired lung function or with other problems that seriously increase the risk of conventional resection. Tumors less than 3 cm that are in the outer third of the lung are most suitable.

▶ This is a new approach to limited-stage lung cancers in patients with severe lung function abnormality or other risk factors that preclude thoracotomy. The competitive procedure is radiation therapy, and they should be compared in a double-blind fashion for complications and for survival times.—B.H. Gross, M.D.

Utilization Review

Acute Asthma: Admission Chest Radiography in Hospitalized Adult Patients

White CS, Cole RP, Lubetsky HW, Austin JHM (Columbia-Presbyterian Med Ctr, New York)
Chest 100:14–16, 1991   1–38

Background.—The clinical usefulness of a chest x-ray (CXR) examination obtained in adult patients hospitalized with acute asthma has been controversial. Results from several studies have showed that the results of the CXR study influence treatment in only 1% to 5% of patients. The effect of the admission CXR examination on immediate management decisions after unsuccessful therapy for acute asthma in the emergency ward was evaluated.

Patients.—Fifty-eight consecutive admissions of 54 adult patients with acute asthma were prospectively reviewed. The patients were admitted after a 12-hour course of bronchodilator therapy in the emergency ward failed.

TABLE 1.—Admission Chest Radiographic Abnormalities in
Acute Asthma

Abnormalities	No. (%)
Major	
Focal parenchymal opacity	7 (12)*
IIM	6 (10)
Enlarged cardiac silhouette	5 (8)
Pulmonary vascular congestion	3 (5)
New pulmonary nodule	1 (2)
Pneumothorax	1 (2)
TOTAL	23†
Minor	
Hyperinflation	13 (22)
Pleural thickening	8 (14)
Elevated hemidiaphragm	3 (5)
Calcified granuloma	2 (3)
Scoliosis	2 (3)
TOTAL	28‡

* Percentage based on 58 admissions.
† Twenty admissions (34% of total series).
‡ Twenty-four admissions (41% of total series).
(Courtesy of White CS, Cole RP, Lubetsky HW, et al: *Chest* 100:14–16, 1991.)

TABLE 2.—Antibiotic Use in Patients With Radiographic Focal Opacities or Increased Interstitial Markings

	Antibiotics Used*	Antibiotics not Used*
Focal opacity or IIM	11	2
No focal opacity or IIM	19	26

* Fisher exact test, P = .0073.
(Courtesy of White CS, Cole RP, Lubetsky HW, et al: *Chest* 100:14–16, 1991.)

Findings.—Major radiographic abnormalities were found on 20 of 58 (34%) chest radiographs. The major abnormalities were focal parenchymal opacity, increased interstitial markings (IIM), enlarged cardiac silhouette, pulmonary vascular congestion, new pulmonary nodule, or pneumothorax (Table 1). Antibiotic treatment was instituted significantly more frequently in the 22% of patients with admission CXR studies demonstrating a focal pulmonary opacity or IIM than in patients without these radiographic findings (Table 2). Immediate management and antibiotic use was affected even in afebrile patients when focal opacity or IIM were present (Table 3). Antibiotic use was not correlated with elevated blood leukocyte count.

Conclusion.—The most common abnormalities found on CXR studies were significantly associated with antibiotic use. Because the CXR studies had a significant effect on immediate management of 22% of the patients with radiographic abnormalities independent of elevated blood leukocyte count and body temperature, it is recommended that chest radiographs be obtained for all adult patients admitted because of acute asthma.

▶ This a good utilization review study. My experience with patients with asthma admitted to the hospital is that most have normal radiographs or hyperinflation. I don't believe that 22% of our patients with asthma have chest radiographic abnormalities that affect immediate management. Now it's up to me (or to one of you) to study this issue further. One article is a good start, but it needn't be the final answer.—B.H. Gross, M.D.

TABLE 3.—Antibiotic Use in Afebrile Patients With Focal Opacities or Increased Interstitial Markings

	Antibiotics Used*	Antibiotics not Used*
Focal opacity or IIM	8	2
No focal opacity or IIM	16	26

* Fisher exact test, P = .020.
(Courtesy of White CS, Cole RP, Lubetsky HW, et al: *Chest* 100:14–16, 1991.)

Comparison of Physician Judgment and Decision Aids for Ordering Chest Radiographs for Pneumonia in Outpatients

Emerman CL, Dawson N, Speroff T, Siciliano C, Effron D, Rashad F, Shaw Z, Bellon EL (MetroHealth Med Ctr, Case Western Reserve Univ, Cleveland)
Ann Emerg Med 20:1215–1219, 1991   1–39

Background.—The symptoms of respiratory tract infection, such as cough, fever, or sputum production, can indicate a range of problems from minor to significant. Chest radiographs are used for a differential diagnosis of pneumonia, but studies have indicated that physicians have difficulty in predicting pneumonia in outpatients and are found to over-estimate pneumonia. Physicians' clinical judgments were compared with published decision aids for ordering chest radiographs in the evaluation of outpatients with symptoms of respiratory infection.

Methods.—The prospective observational study included 290 adult patients with a recent history of acute cough or exacerbation of chronic

Diehr et al Score[9] — Add Points for Each Variable Present

Variable	Point
Rhinorrhea	−2
Sore throat	−1
Night sweats	1
Myalgias	1
Sputum all day	1
Respirations of more than 25	2
Temperature of more than 37.7 C	2

Heckerling et al Score[10] — Add 1 Point for Each Variable Present

Variable

Temperature of more than 37.8 C
Pulse of more than 100
Rales
Decreased breath sounds
Absence of asthma

Gennis et al Rule[11] — Order Chest Radiograph if Any Variable Present

Variable

Temperature of more than 37.8 C
Pulse of more than 100
Respirations of more than 20

Singal et al Score[8] — Calculate Probability of Pneumonia

Probability $= 1/(1 + E^{-Y})$
where $Y = -3.095 + 1.214$ (cough) $+ 1.007$ (fever) $+ 0.823$ (crackles); each variable is
0 if absent and 1 if present.

Fig 1–28.—(Courtesy of Emerman CL, Dawson N, Speroff T, et al: *Ann Emerg Med* 20:1215–1219, 1991.)

TABLE 1.—Comparison of Physician Judgment and Decisions Aids in Ordering Chest Radiographs to Diagnose Pneumonia Decision Aids

	Physician Judgment	Decision Aids			
		Gennis et al[11]	Diehr et al[9]	Heckerling et al[10]	Singal et al[8]
Sensitivity	.86 (18/21)	.62 (13/21)	.67 (14/21)	.71 (15/21)	.76 (16/21)
Specificity	.58 (155/269)	.76 (205/269)†	.67 (180/269)*	.67 (181/269)*	.55 (148/269)
Positive predictive value	.14 (18/132)	.17 (13/77)	.14 (14/103)	.15 (15/103)	.12 (16/137)
Negative predictive value	.98 (155/158)	.96 (205/213)	.96 (180/187)	.97 (181/187)	.97 (148/153)
Accuracy	.60 (173/290)	.76 (218/290)†	.67 (194/290)	.68 (196/290)*	.54 (164/290)

* P < .012 compared with physician judgment.
† P < .001 compared with physician judgment.
Notes: true positive, radiograph ordered demonstrating pneumonia; true negative, no radiograph ordered in patients without pneumonia; sensitivity, true positives/all with pneumonia; specificity, true negatives/all without pneumonia; positive predictive value, true positives/all patients with radiographs ordered; negative predictive value, true negatives/all patients with radiographs not ordered; accuracy, true positives plus true negatives/all patients.
(Courtesy of Emerman CL, Dawson N, Speroff T, et al: *Ann Emerg Med* 20:1215–1219, 1991.)

cough plus either fever, sputum production, or hemoptysis. Physician intent to order chest radiographs was surveyed. Thirty-nine physicians, including 15 attending physicians and 24 medical housestaff, participated. Four previously published decision aids by Diehr, Singal, Heckerling, and Gennis were applied retrospectively to the patient population (Fig 1–28).

Findings.—Of the 290 patients, 7% had pneumonia. The sensitivity of physician judgment exceeded that of all 4 decision aids. The specificity of the Diehr, Heckerling, and Gennis rules exceeded that of physician judgment, and the accuracy of the Gennis and Heckerling rules ex-

TABLE 2.—Comparison of Attending and Housestaff Judgment

	Attending	Housestaff
Sensitivity	.83 (10/12)	.89 (8/9)
Specificity	.57 (119/207)	.58 (36/62)
Positive predictive value	.10 (10/98)	.24 (8/34)
Negative predictive value	.98 (119/121)	.97 (36/37)
Accuracy	.59 (129/219)	.62 (44/71)

(Courtesy of Emerman CL, Dawson N, Speroff T, et al: *Ann Emerg Med* 20:1215–1219, 1991.)

ceeded physician accuracy (Table 1). The differing level of experience among the attending and housestaff physicians did not influence judgment (Table 2).

Conclusion.—The physicians' decisions for ordering chest radiographs to diagnose pneumonia had high sensitivity and lower specificity but were reasonably accurate. Two of the published decision rules, Gennis and Heckerling, had a higher specificity and accuracy than physician judgment, which would make them useful in patient evaluation.

▶ I think most physicians hate practice guidelines, decision aids, and the like. It makes them feel like automatons, stinting their individual creativity. Like them or not, they're coming soon to a hospital near you. Large managed care organizations require more uniformity than the typical anarchic practice spawns. I don't know with whom to agree. I hate the idiosyncratic ordering patterns of some of our clinicians, but I don't want someone codifying and quantifying the radiographic signs that should result in a diagnosis of congestive heart failure. So here's where it stands: practice guidelines are good for them but not for us.—B.H. Gross, M.D.

The Role of the Chest Roentgenogram in Febrile Neutropenic Patients

Donowitz GR, Harman C, Pope T, Stewart FM (Univ of Virginia, Charlottesville, Va)
Arch Intern Med 151:701–704, 1991   1–40

Background.—The immunocompromised patient with fever and neutropenia may experience pneumonia or certain types of bacteremia (Ta-

TABLE 1.—Infections

	Initial	Persistent	Recurrent
Pneumonia	13	5	1
Sepsis	31	1	1
Urinary tract infections	6	0	0
Local*	12	2	5
Noninfectious (tumor, drug fever)	6	1	6
Presumed fungal† infection	1	4	3
Fever of unknown origin‡	77	9	11

* Local infections include skin and soft tissue infections, sinusitis, stomatitis, and gastroenteritis.
† Amphotericin-B-responsive fever without focal findings.
‡ Fever of unknown origin is defined as fever not associated with an identifiable pathogen or site of infection, and that is unassociated with noninfectious causes of fever (administration of blood products, chemotherapy, or underlying disease).
(Courtesy of Donowitz GR, Harman C, Pope T, et al: *Arch Intern Med* 151:701–704, 1991.)

TABLE 2.—Roentgenographic Findings During
Febrile Episodes

Febrile Episodes

	Initial	Persistent	Recurrent
No. of episodes	146	22	27
Abnormal chest roentgenograms, No. (%)	28 (19)	8 (36)*	5 (19)†
Findings on chest roentgenograms			
Pneumonia	13	5	1
Pleural effusion	5	1	1
Congestive failure	1	1	1
Indeterminate‡	9	1	2

* Seven of 8 patients had chest roentgenographic abnormalities (including 5 pneumonias) within 5 days of an initial normal film. One patient had worsening of a previously abnormal film.
† Four of 5 patients had chest roentgenographic abnormalities (including 1 pneumonia) after an initial normal film.
‡ This includes atelectasis and/or nonspecific parenchymal infiltrates believed not to represent pneumonia, congestive failure, or tumor.
(Courtesy of Donowitz GR, Harman C, Pope T, et al: *Arch Intern Med* 151:701-704, 1991.)

ble 1). These patients routinely have chest roentogenograms to evaluate their conditions. The role of chest roentgenograms in the clinical management of this patient population was investigated through a retrospective review of the medical records.

Methods.—The records of all patients with both neutropenia and fever (> 38.3°C) admitted from September 1982 to July 1987 were reviewed. The febrile episodes were defined as initial, persistent, or recurrent. All patients received an aminoglycoside and either an anti-*Pseudomonas* species penicillin or a third-generation cephalosporin. Those with persistent or recurrent fevers had chest roentgenograms.

Results.—Most of the 127 identified patients had acute leukemia, lymphoma, or solid tumors. The 127 patients had 146 febrile episodes, with 22 of the 146 fevers persisting after the initiation of antibiotic therapy. An overall total of 195 febrile episodes was evaluated, and 187 chest roentogenograms were obtained. Of the 146 initial fevers, 19% were accompanied by abnormal chest roentgenograms, with penumonia diagnosed in 13 patients. Eighteen of the 22 patients with persistent fevers received chest roentgenograms, which showed abnormalities in 8. Five of these 8 patients had pneumonia. In 27 of the 146 initial episodes of fever, fever recurred after starting antibiotics; 5 of 23 chest roentgenograms showed abnormalities, with 1 patient having pneumonia (Table 2). Overall, 17% of the patients had chest roentgenographic abnormalities, even though they had no other signs or symptoms of pulmonary disease (Table 3). During persistent or recurrent febrile episodes, chest roentgenogram results promoted an alteration of therapy in 8 of 13 episodes (61%), with 6 patients (40%) improving.

TABLE 3.—Clinical Findings: Correlation With Findings on Chest Roentgenograms

No. (%)

	Normal Chest Roentgenogram, n = 146	Abnormal Chest Roentgenogram, n = 41	*P**
Symptoms			
New cough	22 (15)	16 (39)	.0012
Chest pain	2 (1.4)	4 (9.8)	.027
Dyspnea	11 (7.5)	12 (29)	.004
Absence of symptoms	117 (80)	17 (41.5)	<.0001
Physical findings			
Tachypnea	4 (2.7)	6 (14.6)	.009
Rales	24 (16.4)	24 (58.5)	<.0001
Decreased breath sounds	7 (4.8)	9 (21.9)	.0021
Rhonchi	5 (3.4)	1 (2.4)	1.0
Absence of abnormalities on examination	113 (77)	13 (31.7)	<.0001
Absence of both symptoms and abnormalities on examination	102 (70)	7 (17)	.0002

* Two-tailed Fisher's Exact Test.
(Courtesy of Donowitz GR, Harman C, Pope T, et al: *Arch Intern Med* 151:701–704, 1991.)

Implications.—The signs and symptoms of pulmonary disease are significantly related to abnormalities on chest roentgenograms, although 30% of the febrile episodes showed similar signs and symptoms with normal chest roentgenograms. Chest roentgenograms serve as an important diagnostic tool in evaluating persistent or recurrent fever in these patients.

▶ The conclusion of this abstract is important. ("Chest roentgenograms serve as an important diagnostic tool in evaluating persistent or recurrent fever in these [febrile neutropenic] patients.") Just as important is the additional clause in the abstract: "but [are] of little use during initial febrile episodes." The latter conclusion is fully supported by the fact that the chest radiographic findings did not lead to changes in therapy for the initial febrile episodes. The number of studies in each category is striking: 146 were for initial episodes (and thus useless), whereas only 18 were for persistent fevers, and only 23 were for recurrent fevers. In other words, lots of money was wasted.

There was a number of interesting recent articles on immunocompromised patients (1–5), highlighting interesting radiographic appearances, new associations between entities, and invasive diagnostic procedures.—B.H. Gross, M.D.

References

1. Ganti S, et al: *NY State J Med* 91:265, 1991.
2. Scott WW Jr, et al: *Radiology* 180:419, 1991.
3. Groskin SA, et al: *Radiology* 180:423, 1991.
4. Boisserie-Lacroix M, et al: *J Radiol* 72:243, 1991.
5. Carson PJ, et al: *Chest* 100:675, 1991.

Chest Pain in the Accident and Emergency Department: Is Chest Radiography Worthwhile?
Templeton PA, McCallion WA, McKinney LA, Wilson HK (The Ulster Hospital, Dundonald, Belfast, Northern Ireland)
Arch Emerg Med 8:97–101, 1991   1–41

Purpose.—Chest radiography is often performed routinely in the evaluation of patients admitted to the Accident and Emergency Department (A & E) with chest pain, but the efficacy of this approach is conflicting. The role of routine chest radiography in the evaluation of these patients and the accuracy by which casualty officers in the A & E interpret the chest x-ray films were evaluated in a prospective, double-blind study.

Data Analysis.—During a 2-month period, 327 of 7,738 (4%) patients attending the A & E complained of chest pain. Of these, 297 had chest radiographs, including 131 (44%) with abnormalities. Overall, 23% of the chest x-ray films showed abnormalities influencing patient management; this increased to 40% in patients admitted to the cardiac unit. Although 29% of chest x-ray films were misinterpreted by casualty officers, mismanagement occurred in only 6 (3.3%) patients (table). The regular audit of A & E chest radiographs within 24 hours by the consultant radiologist averted potentially serious errors.

False Positive Errors Made in Chest Radiograph Interpretation and Their Significance

CXR 'abnormality' misdiagnosed by Casualty Officer	Number of CXRs with this false positive error	False positive errors resulting in mismanagement
Acute inflammation	6	2
Chronic inflammation	5	0
Pulmonary vascular congestion	3	0
Atelectasis	1	0
Cardiomegally	1	0
Total	16	2

(Courtesy of Templeton PA, McCallion WA, McKinney LA, et al: *Arch Emerg Med* 8:97–101, 1991.)

Conclusion.—These data indicate that 96.7% of the patients seen in the A & E with chest pain are managed correctly. Chest x-ray films remain a useful investigation, but early audit of all A & E chest radiographs by a radiologist and continuing education of casualty officers will further reduce patient mismanagement.

▶ Articles in utilization review more commonly study chest radiographs than CT. This probably reflects the complex influence of CT on patient management, with multiple organs evaluated. It seems easier to ask and answer a simple question with chest radiographs. The simple answer here is that chest radiography is worthwhile for patients in the emergency department with chest pain. The interesting footnote is that 29% of chest radiographs were misinterpreted by the clinicians before audit by the consultant radiologist. And they want their own ultrasound machine?—B.H. Gross, M.D.

Chest Radiography in the Management of Breast Cancer
Moskovic E, Parsons C, Baum M (Royal Marsden Hospital, London, England)
Br J Radiol 65:30–32, 1992   1–42

Introduction.—There is little evidence to suggest that detection of clinically occult metastatic disease on follow-up chest radiographs confers any survival benefits for patients with early breast cancer. To evaluate further, a retrospective analysis was conducted of the medical records and chest radiographs of 141 patients with a diagnosis of early breast cancer. Primary treatment included mastectomy and local excision with axillary clearance. Results of every chest radiograph were correlated with subsequent therapeutic decision making.

Data Analysis.—There were 1,161 chest radiographs performed on 141 patients. Of these, 174 (15%) were requested for direct clinical reasons and 987 (85%) were performed either as part of "routine" follow-up procedures, or for unknown reasons not resulting in management change. Asymptomatic pulmonary metastases were identified on routine chest radiographs in only 4 patients, representing less than 3% of the total number of patients examined and less than .4% of the total number of routine chest radiographs performed. Chest radiographs were performed for a clinical reason in 2.2% of the requests among 91 patients with no recurrence or metastasis, compared with 33% in 43 patients who had distant metastases.

Implications.—Routine chest radiography should not be performed in asymptomatic patients being followed after treatment for primary breast cancer. It should be used to address specific clinical problems relating to the thorax, whereas the cessation of all other chest radiography in asymptomatic patients during follow-up should result in significant budgetary implications.

▶ Music to my ears! So few asymptomatic metastases were detected in breast cancer patients that the authors flat out say, "Routine CXRs are not performed on patients being followed up after treatment for primary breast cancer at this institution . . . resulting in inevitable savings of both valuable budgetary resources and unnecessary radiation to both patients and staff." Bravo!—B.H. Gross, M.D.

Pulmonary: General Topics

Milk of Calcium Pericardial Effusion: Case Report
Sarosi MG, Crummy AB, McDermott JC, Kroncke GM (Univ of Wisconsin, Madison, Wis)
Cardiovasc Intervent Radiol 14:314–315, 1991   1–43

Setting.—Milk of calcium (MOC) pericardial effusion developed in a patient previously treated with radiotherapy to the mediastinum for Hodgkin's disease. During evaluation for massive hemoptysis, a chest x-ray film showed pleural and pulmonary fibrosis, calcified lymph nodes, and pericardial calcification. On fluoroscopy, calcification along the posteroinferior portions of the pericardium moved like a liquid. This was confirmed at CT with demonstration of a fluid-MOC level and density measurements. Dense pericardial fibrosis, thin calcified pericardial plaques, and MOC effusion were observed on pericardiectomy.

Discussion.—Pericardial effusion is the most common pericardial manifestation of radiotherapy-related cardiotoxicity, but MOC pericardial effusion has not been previously studied. The pericardial sac appears to be an ideal location for the development of MOC caused by the presence of inflammation, effusion, and stasis—prerequisites of MOC elsewhere in the body.

▶ This is 1 of my 2 favorite cases this year (the other is the last case in this chapter). I especially like this case, because it really doesn't belong here. When an occasional cardiovascular paper accidentally finds its way to me, I usually send it back posthaste (and postage due). My repayment for the (admittedly minimal) energy I've wasted is this splendid chest radiograph and CT.—B.H. Gross, M.D.

Coaxial Transthoracic Fine-Needle Biopsy in Patients With a History of Malignant Lymphoma
Wittich GR, Nowels KW, Korn RL, Walter RM, Lucas DE, Dake MD, Jeffrey RB (Stanford Univ Med Ctr, Stanford, Calif)
Radiology 183:175–178, 1992   1–44

Background.—Diagnosis and classification of malignant lymphoma has traditionally been made on the basis of histologic evaluation. Large cutting needle biopsy has been utilized in some cases. Recently, the role of fine-needle biopsy and cytologic examination has been proved. The safety and efficacy of percutaneous fine-needle biopsy of thoracic lesions was evaluated when combined with cytologic, immunocytochemical, and microbiologic evaluation of tissue in patients with a history of malignant lymphoma and new chest lesions.

Method.—A group of 54 patients with a history of biopsy-proved malignant lymphoma was included. In the standard biopsy technique with a coaxial approach, a 22-gauge needle with a removable hub was inserted into the lesion, and an 18-gauge cannula was advanced coaxially to the edge of the lesion. Multiple samples were then obtained through the cannula by using 22-gauge Chiba and 21-gauge cutting needles.

Findings.—Twenty-one patients had recurrent lymphoma. Correct diagnosis was achieved with 1 biopsy in 17 of 21, for a sensitivity of 81%. The sensitivity increased to 95% with a repeat needle biopsy in 3 patients. Immunophenotyping was essential for establishing a definitive diagnosis of lymphoma in 3 patients. Nonlymphomatous malignancies were correctly diagnosed in 14 patients.

Conclusion.—The use of coaxial transthoracic fine-needle biopsy had a sensitivity of 81% in patients with lymphoma, which increased to 95% with repeat biopsy. Biopsy also correctly identified all nonlymphomatous malignancies. Transthoracic fine-needle biopsy is a safe and accurate first-line diagnostic method in patients with suspected relapse of lymphoma. The use of large cutting needles or surgical biopsy can be restricted to patients with negative findings at fine-needle biopsy and patients in whom transformation of malignant lymphoma is suspected.

▶ I have no argument with fine-needle biopsy in suspected recurrent lymphoma, particularly if pathologic slides from the original presentation are available for review. With the addition of immunocytochemical studies, diagnosis rests on solid ground. Things become murky when we consider biopsy of new anterior mediastinal masses (1), in other words, no history of lymphoma. A recent study showed only 42% sensitivity for diagnosing lymphoma, 20% sensitivity for Hodgkin's disease, and 71% for thymoma. The authors conclude that transthoracic needle biopsy is useful in metastatic disease and germ cell tumors; however, because we rarely know the diagnosis before the biopsy, I still don't consider a new anterior mediastinal mass to be a good target for fine-needle aspiration.—B.H. Gross, M.D.

Reference

1. Herman SJ, et al: *Radiology* 180:167, 1991.

Cigarette Smoking and Small Irregular Opacities

Weiss W (Hahnemann Univ, Philadelphia)
Br J Ind Med 48:841–844, 1991   1–45

Background.—Cigarette smoke leads to pathologic evidence of chronic inflammation, structural damage, and interstitial fibrosis in the lungs. It is unclear whether diffuse pulmonary fibrosis caused by smoking can be detected radiographically. In a controlled study, workers exposed to acrylic dust were compared with unexposed workers. The study was designed to determine whether exposure to acrylic dust, cigarette smoking, or both, was associated with radiographic findings of diffuse abnormalities suggestive of pneumoconiosis.

Method.—The International Labour Office (ILO) classification of radiographs for pneumoconiosis was done using standard films for comparison. Workers with exposure to asbestos were excluded from the study. Chest x-ray films from 100 workers exposed to acrylic dust were compared with 81 unexposed workers who were matched by age, year hired, and smoking habit. The radiograph readers were blind to smoking history and dust exposure of the subjects. Profusions of 0/1 and 1/0 are classified as "suspect" pneumoconiosis according to the ILO guidelines.

Findings.—There was no relation between dust exposure and prevalence of abnormalities. In 181 radiographs read, 23 radiographs were 0/1, 3 were 1/0, and 2 were 1/1. One nonsmoker (2.2%) and 20% of the smokers were classified 0/1 or greater, a statistically significant difference. The 5 films with a profusion of 1/0 or 1/1 occurred among smokers. Prevalence was 10% among former smokers, 5.3% in those who currently smoked less than 1 pack per day, 31.3% in heavier cigarette smokers, and 52.9% in 17 heavy cigarette smokers aged 50–64. The prevalence rate increased steadily with increasing age among smokers to a maximum of 32% for those aged 50–64 years.

Conclusion.—The diffuse abnormalities seen on x-ray studies that were similar to small irregular opacities found in some smokers may be interpreted as pneumoconiosis. This abnormality occurs in low profusion with a prevalence that is dose related to cigarette smoking. Small irregular opacities are directly related to age and smoking habits among workers not exposed to hazardous dust.

▶ Several years ago we tried to do a somewhat similar study that also incorporated pulmonary function test data. We never finished it, but I believed then (and believe more strongly after reading this article) that there is such a thing as the "dirty chest" of cigarette smokers. Radiographic diagnosis of chronic obstructive pulmonary disease is a tricky and contentious subject, with greatest success reported for emphysema. A recent study concluded that expiratory chest CT is particularly effective for diagnosing emphysema (1).—B.H. Gross, M.D.

Reference

1. Knudson RJ, et al: *Chest* 99:1357, 1991.

Intracranial Meningioma With Pulmonary Metastases: Diagnosis by Percutaneous Fine-Needle Aspiration Biopsy and Electron Microscopy
Jha RC, Weisbrod GL, Dardick I, Herman SJ, Chamberlain D (University of Manitoba, Winnipeg, Man, Canada; Toronto General Hospital, Toronto, Ont, Canada)
Can Assoc Radiol J 42:287–290, 1991   1–46

Introduction.—Metastatic menangioma is rare and has usually been diagnosed at autopsy or thoracotomy. Meningioma metastatic to the lung was diagnosed in 1 patient from a specimen obtained by percutaneous fine-needle aspiration biopsy.

Case Report.—Woman, 37, underwent a right frontal craniotomy for removal of a large tumor found to be a benign meningioma. At 5 and 14 years after the initial operation (1977 and 1986), recurrent meningiomas with no histologic features of malignancy were removed. In February 1990, the woman had increasing pain and trismus in the right temporomandibular joint. Computed tomography revealed extensive tumor along the right cavernous sinus and the infratemporal fossa down to the right hemimandible and the right orbit. A preoperative chest radiograph (Fig 1–29) and CT (Fig 1–30) showed 2 lung nodules. The specimen obtained at biopsy was examined by light and electron microscopy and confirmed as metastatic meningioma.

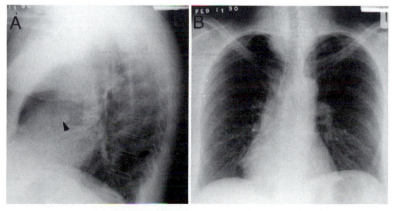

Fig 1–29.—Lateral (**A**) and posterior (**B**) chest radiographs of a patient with recurrent intracranial menengioma show nodules in the right apex and lingula (*arrowhead* in **A**). (Courtesy of Jha RC, Weisbrod GL, Dardick I, et al: *Can Assoc Radiol J* 42:287–290, 1991.)

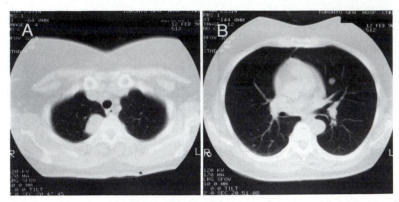

Fig 1–30.—Computed tomography scans show right apical and lingular nodules. (Courtesy of Jha RC, Weisbrod GL, Dardick I, et al: *Can Assoc Radiol J* 42:287–290, 1991.)

Implications.—It is suggested that radiologists and pathologists should consider metastatic disease as part of the differential diagnosis of a pulmonary nodule in patients with intracranial meningiomas. In this case, extracranial spread may have resulted from repeated craniotomy, although the 4 resected tumor specimens did not have accepted characteristics of malignancy. Electron microscopy can reveal the ultrastructural features specific to metastatic meningioma.

▶ I've always taught that you don't see pulmonary metastases from CNS primaries. What am I going to do now? (The exception that proves the rule?) (What does that mean, anyway?)—B.H. Gross, M.D.

Searching for Lung Nodules: The Guidance of Visual Scanning
Kundel HL, Nodine CF, Toto L (Univ of Pennsylvania, Philadelphia)
Invest Radiol 26:777–781, 1991   1–47

Introduction.—An eye position-interactive display has been developed that uses data on eye position to determine whether to display a nodule. In this way, the display may be limited to a part of the visual field without otherwise disturbing the appearance of the chest image.

Objective and Methods.—This display technology was used to determine the optimal size of the scanning field for lung nodules. The image of the nodule was restricted in a stepwise manner to the central visual field. Digitally synthesized nodules were placed at various sites in the lungs of test images. Eye position was recorded by a limbus reflecting technique. Three radiologists and a psychologist experienced in detecting nodules viewed the display at a distance of 70 cm.

Findings.—The time needed to scan the image and fixate a nodule was least for nodules that were accessible to the peripheral vision. Progressive reduction in the size of the peripheral field that could access the nodules influenced search performance only when the field was less than 5 degrees.

Implications.—This study supports a model of visual search in which the first step is global analysis of the image to identify conspicuous targets and major landmarks. Identified targets are checked by central vision, and discovery scanning then begins. Scanning can be interrupted by input from the peripheral visual field.

▶ I'm fascinated by Dr. Kundel's work. It is very difficult to set up this kind of study. For most of us, it's hard to even figure out what *needs* to be studied. It is also important to go the next step and use the information gained to improve our approach to the radiograph.—B.H. Gross, M.D.

Thymolipoma in Association With Myasthenia Gravis

Le Marc'hadour F, Pinel N, Pasquier B, Dieny A, Stoebner P, Couderc P (Hospital Albert Michallon, Grenoble, France)

Am J Surg Pathol 15:802–809, 1991   1–48

Introduction.—Nine cases of thymolipoma associated with myasthenia gravis have been reported. This rare, benign tumor consists of thymic tissue and mature adipose tissue elements.

Case Report.—Man, 52, had progresssive weakness and fatigue on mastication, and electromyography confirmed the presence of myasthenia gravis. The patient improved without treatment, but he became generally weak 2 years later, and a thymoma was discovered (Fig 1–31). Antistriated muscle antibody was present in a titer of 1:100. A large tumor was removed and found to consist of

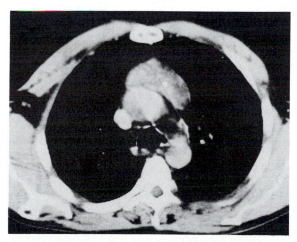

Fig 1–31.—A CT scan shows a mass in the anterior mediastinum (*small white square*). (Courtesy of Le Marc'hadour F, Pinel N, Pasquier B, et al: *Am J Surg Pathol* 15:802–809, 1991.)

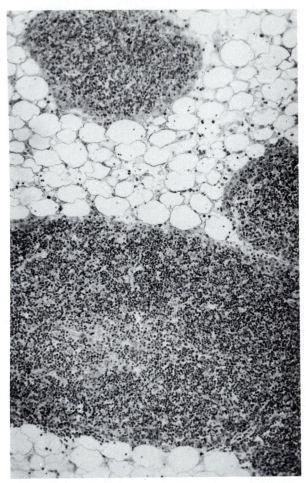

Fig 1–32.—The tumor shows cords and nests of thymic tissue enbedded in mature adipose elements. (Courtesy of Le Marc'hadour F, Pinel N, Pasquier B, et al: *Am J Surg Pathol* 15:802–809, 1991.)

large lobules of mature fat tissue and thymic tissue (Fig 1–32). The latter included mostly cortical areas, in which the thymocytes stained immunohistochemically like cortical cells. Electron microscopy affirmed predominantly cortical differentiation of the thymic component.

Discussion.—Many of the previous patients with thymolipoma have been asymptomatic. The average age is more than 50 years. The authors believe that thymolipoma may be a true thymoma that is so well differentiated as to remain encapsulated and undergo adipose involution. The coexistence of thymolipoma with immune or neoplastic disorders often associated with thymoma, such as hyperthyroidism and Hodgkin's disease, supports this hypothesis.

▶ Although thymoma and thymolipoma are clearly different, histologically and at CT, the authors present compelling evidence that they may be the same tumor.—B.H. Gross, M.D.

Elevated Right Hemidiaphragm With Yellow Sputum Production
Cammarata SK, Dircks J, Grambau G, Hyzy R (Henry Ford Hosp, Detroit; Michigan State Univ, Kalamazoo, Mich)
Chest 99:1463–1465, 1991   1–49

Background.—The authors encountered a woman, 40, with newly diagnosed acute lymphocytic leukemia, who had lymphadenopathy and was febrile when seen for induction chemotherapy. She was granulocytopenic; fever resolved on antibiotic treatment but recurred after a rapid response to chemotherapy. The right hemidiaphragm was elevated, and a gas-containing soft tissue density was present in the subdiaphragmatic hepatic cavity (Fig 1–33). Thoracic ultrasonography showed no pleural fluid. Liver function was abnormal, and a technetium 99m hepatoiminodiacetic acid scan showed a bronchobiliary fistula (Fig 1–34). Labeled bile entered the bronchial tree within 45 minutes of nuclide injection. Specimens of the right lower lung lobe, right hemidiaphragm, and medial part of the liver revealed mucormycosis. The patient did well after 2 thoracoabdominal operations for debridement and omental packing of the diaphragmatic defect.

Discussion.—This patient had a bronchobiliary fistula secondary to mucormycosis of the liver. Pulmonary mucormycosis can lead to erosion of bronchi with hemoptysis. The presence of bile in the sputum (bilioptysis) is pathognomonic for bronchobiliary fistula. Nuclide scanning clearly demonstrated the fistula in this case. Neither the gallbladder nor the duodenum was seen, indicating biliary tract obstruction, but a patent biliary system was seen on endoscopic retrograde cholangiopancreatography.

▶ Great images! I love the nuclear scan most of all!—B.H. Gross, M.D.

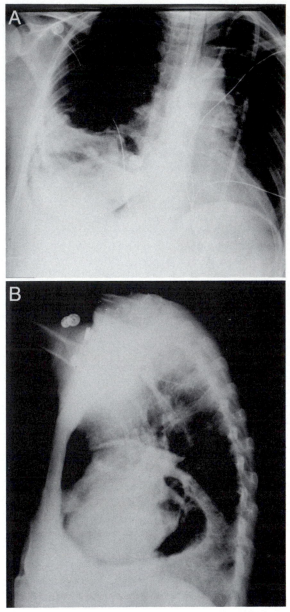

Fig 1–33.—Chest roentgenogram showing an elevated right hemidiaphragm with a gas-containing soft tissue density in the subdiaphragmatic hepatic cavity. (Courtesy of Cammarata SK, Dircks J, Grambau G, et al: *Chest* 99:1463–1465, 1991.)

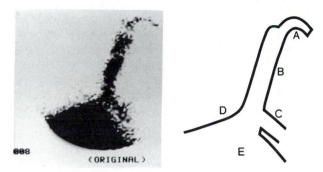

(ORIGINAL)

Fig 1–34.—A ^{99m}-Tc-HIDA scan (anterior projection) performed 60 minutes after injection of radionuclide, with illustration of *A,* oropharynx; *B,* trachea; *C,* left mainstream bronchus; *D,* right mainstream bronchus; *E,* elevated dome of the liver. (Courtesy of Cammarata SK, Dircks J, Grambau G, et al: *Chest* 99:1463–1465, 1991.)

2 Cardiovascular and Interventional Radiology

Introduction

This has been an exciting and innovative year for cardiovascular and interventional radiology. The abstracts in this section represent the wide diversity of cardiovascular imaging and intervention literature. No other area of radiology incorporates so many anatomical areas, imaging modalities, and technical procedures. The diversity carries the mixed blessing of continual stimulation, challenge, and change. All who manage to master this area of radiology have my deepest respect.

Magnetic resonance imaging of the heart has progressed this year, with the clinical research focus on myocardial infarction and coronary artery disease. Magnetic resonance angiography has progressed into clinical trials with comparisons to other vascular imaging modalities. Trials for evaluation of angioscopy and intravascular sonography have begun, although few centers have yet to use these new technologies.

There have been continued investigations into methods of arterial revascularization, including research on costs and utilization, as well as efficacy. There also have been fewer reports of new lasers, atherectomy devices, and drills, and more studies evaluating the use of arterial stents. Balloon angioplasty remains the standard for revascularization, although studies this year evaluated its efficacy when combined with laser recanalization and when monitored by laser spectroscopy or intravascular untrasound.

There were far fewer investigations of embolization therapy this year, and reports of nonvascular interventions in the gastrointestinal tract continue to outnumber those in the genitourinary system.

Interest in the portal venous system—specifically portal hypertension, was renewed this year for 2 reasons. First, the evolving maturity of color-flow Doppler ultrasound and MR angiography make efficacy studies timely. Second, the introduction of a new intervention for the management of portal hypertension, transjugular intrahepatic portal-systemic shunting, has renewed interest in the noninvasive diagnosis and follow-up of this condition.

The more things change, however, the more some things stay the same. Despite the change in content or focus of articles as noted earlier, the format of the titles of this year's abstracts is unchanged from last year. I looked at 5 parameters of title style and compared this year's titles to last year's (table). There is no significant difference between the rates of the style parameters in the 2 years. This lack of change represents either constancy of editing style by the reviewed journals, monotony of style among authors, or an inherent bias in the type of articles that I choose for inclusion in the YEAR BOOK. At any rate, in both years there was an obvious absence of any title that contained an exclamation mark! I keep searching for such an article, such as "Atherosclerosis is cured!" or "Gallstones don't matter anymore!" However, I have waited in vain, because of either subject deficiencies or author modesty. (Hint to authors: although an exclamation mark in the title won't automatically get your article abstracted in YEAR BOOK, it will most assuredly get it read closely by this reader and most others. Chutzpah alone counts for something!)

Although the articles abstracted in this section are free of exclamation marks, they represent the breadth and quality of work in cardiovascular and interventional radiology this year. As always, I apologize to the authors of all the excellent articles that could not be included because of space limitations. I hope these selections are useful to all radiologists practicing in this dynamic specialty.

Robert A. Clark, M.D.

Analysis of Titles of Abstracted Articles

	1993		1992	
	No.	%	No.	%
Articles abstracted	47	100	50	100
Title in form of a question	4	9	3	6
Title contains an abbreviation	7	15	11	22
Title contains a clause or statement following a colon	22	47	23	46
Title contains a hyphenated term	18	38	13	26
Title includes the word "percutaneous"	14	30	14	28

Cardiovascular Imaging

Acute, Subacute, and Chronic Myocardial Infarction: Quantitative Analysis of Gadolinium-Enhanced MR Images
van Dijkman PRM, van der Wall EE, de Roos A, Matheijssen NAA, van Rossum AC, Doornbos J, van der Laarse A, van Voorthuisen AE, Bruschke AVG (University Hospital, Leiden, The Netherlands; Free University Hosp, Amsterdam, The Netherlands; Interuniversity Cardiology Inst of The Netherlands,

Utrecht, The Netherlands)
Radiology 180:147–151, 1991   2–1

Background.—Magnetic resonance imaging depicts good natural contrast between ventricular walls and cavities. It can determine left ventricular wall thickness, mass, and ejection fraction and enables characterization of myocardial tissue with use of T_1 and T_2 relaxation times. Because of the overlap between characteristics of normal and infarcted myocardium, exact delineation of acute myocardial infarction (AMI) with MRI may be improved by the use of paramagnetic contrast agents. The value of gadopentetate dimeglumine in depicting the infarcted myocardium during MR was assessed in 84 patients after AMI.

Methods.—Eighty-four patients with AMI and 5 normal controls underwent MRI before and 20 minutes after administration of gadopentetate dimeglumine. The 111 MRI examinations were divided into 4 groups. In group 1, MRI examinations were obtained within 1 week after AMI (Fig 2–1). In group 2, 26 MRI examinations were obtained 1–3 weeks after AMI. In group 3, 12 MRI examinations were obtained 3–6 weeks after AMI. In group 4, 8 MRI examinations were done more than 6 weeks after AMI (Fig 2–2).

Results.—In groups 1, 2, and 3, the mean intensity ratio after administration of gadopentetate was significantly higher than it was before Gd enhancement. In group 4, no significant difference was observed. The intensity ratio after Gd enhancement was abnormally increased in 82% of the MRI examinations in group 1, in 62% of group 2, in 58% in group 3, and in 12% of group 4.

Conclusion.—The paramagnetic contrast agent gadopentetate dimeglumine improved visualization of AMI at MRI as long as 6 weeks after the onset of symptoms. Use of Gd within 1 week of the onset of symptoms allowed the maximal effect.

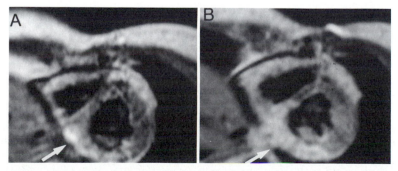

Fig 2–1.—Magnetic resonance images of a short-axis, midventricular section of a patient with transmural inferior wall infarction obtained 1 week after AMI, before (**A**) and 20 minutes after (**B**) administration of intravenous gadopentetate dimeglumine. Increased signal intensity of the inferior wall is visible after Gd-enhancement (*arrows*). (Courtesy of van Dijkman PRM, van der Wall EE, de Roos A, et al: *Radiology* 180:147–151, 1991.)

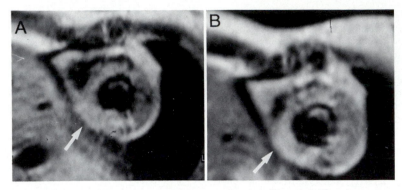

Fig 2–2.—Magnetic resonance images of the same patient as in Figure 2–1. These images were obtained 2 months after AMI, before (**A**) and 20 minutes after (**B**) administration of intravenous gadopentetate dimeglumine. Only mirror enhancement of the signal intensity of the inferior wall is observed after Gd-enhancement (*arrows*). (Courtesy of van Dijkman PRM, van der Wall EE, de Roos A, et al: *Radiology* 180:147–151, 1991.)

▶ This study confirms that MRI can accurately assess the extent of AMI. The addition of Gd enhancement improved visualization of infarction 1–2 weeks after the acute event. Given the limitations of cardiac monitoring and handling of ill inpatients by many MRI units in this country, it is unlikely that most MIs will be routinely assessed in this manner. Nevertheless, this is a good, reproducible method to estimate myocardial damage by facilities that can handle the management of such patients in their scanners.—R.A. Clark, M.D.

First-Pass Nuclear Magnetic Resonance Imaging Studies Using Gadolinium-DTPA in Patients With Coronary Artery Disease
Manning WJ, Atkinson DJ, Grossman W, Paulin S, Edelman RR (Beth Israel Hosp, Harvard Med School, Boston; Siemens Med Systems, Inc, Iselin, NJ)
J Am Coll Cardiol 18:959–965, 1991   2–2

Background.—Nuclear MRI accurately portrays cardiac anatomy and function. Recently, ultrafast imaging sequences, coupled with administration of a nuclear MR contrast agent and acquisition first-pass images through the heart, have been used to assess regional myocardial perfusion. This technique was used to evaluate patients with chest pain and angiographically documented normal and diseased coronary arteries.

Methods.—Ultrafast nuclear MRI was used in conjunction with a T_1 (longitudinal relaxation time) contrast agent to evaluate 17 patients with chest pain who had undergone cardiac catheterization. Twelve patients had significant coronary artery stenoses, and 4 underwent repeat nuclear MR study after myocardial revascularization. Cardiac images at rest were obtained during a rapid bolus injection of Gd-DTPA. The ultrafast images were all electrocardiograph gated with successive images acquired every 3 to 4 seconds.

Findings.—After injection of the contrast agent, there was pronounced signal enhancement in the right ventricular cavity, followed by enhancement in the left ventricular cavity and myocardium (Fig 2–3). The regional myocardium that was perfused by coronary arteries with stenosis had a lower peak signal intensity and a lower rate of signal increase compared with myocardium perfused by coronary arteries without stenosis (Fig 2–4). After revascularization, the repeat nuclear MR study showed an increase in peak signal intensity.

Conclusion.—Ultrafast nuclear MRI and dynamic Gd-DTPA–enhanced nuclear MRI were useful in obtaining clinical cardiac images for the assessment of coronary stenosis in patients with chest pain. Combining dynamic first-pass Gd-DTPA studies with nuclear MRI may be useful for noninvasive evaluation of patients with suspected coronary artery disease.

▶ Abstract 2–1 described the assessment of myocardial damage after infarction using MRI. This abstract reports the use of MRI to assess the distribution of ischemia caused by coronary artery disease in patients with chest pain before infarction. Gadolinium enhancement and rapid image acquisition are required to demonstrate regional perfusion defects with this technique. The technique is promising, because the dynamic perfusion study can be done in combination with MRI anatomical and functional imaging to provide a total cardiac imaging evaluation with 1 modality. However, as an assessment of cardiac perfusion, further work needs to be done comparing this approach to CT, angiography, and radionuclide scintigraphy to define the optimum combination of studies in terms of accuracy, efficacy, cost, and convenience.—R.A. Clark, M.D.

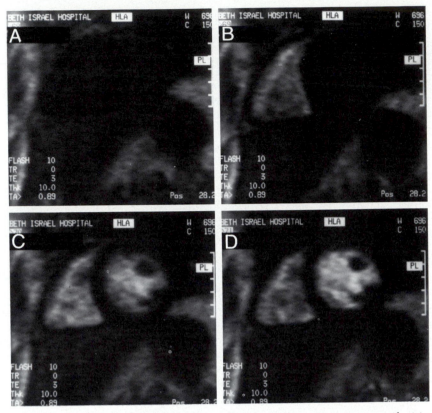

Fig 2–3.—A-G, series of 7 ECG-gated ultrafast gradient-refocused echo short-axis images after injection of Gd-DTPA. Note the sequential appearance of increased signal in the right ventricular cavity, left ventricular cavity, and left ventricular myocardium, with recirculation to the right ventricular cavity (**G**). TE, echo time; ThK, slice thickness; TR, repetition time. (Continued.) (Courtesy of Manning WJ, Atkinson DJ, Grossman W, et al: *J Am Coll Cardiol* 18:959–965, 1991.)

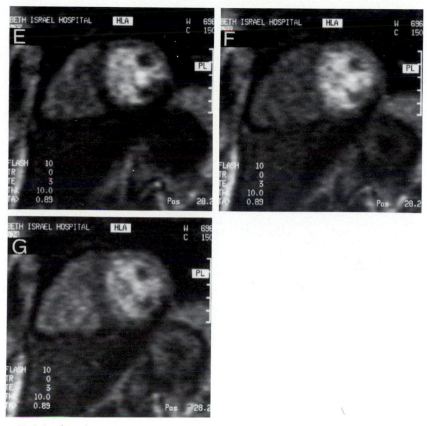

Fig 2–3.—*(cont.)*

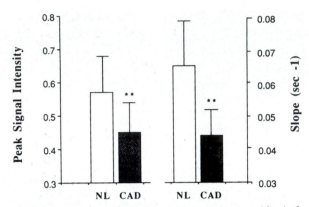

Fig 2–4.—Peak signal intensity (mean ± SD) and rate of signal increase (*slope*) of regional myocardium. *Abbreviations:* CAD, myocardial region supplied by a diseased vessel; NL, regional myocardium supplied by a nondiseased vessel. (Courtesy of Manning WJ, Atkinson DJ, Grossman W, et al: *J Am Coll Cardiol* 18:959–965, 1991.)

Estimating the Size of Myocardial Infarction by Magnetic Resonance Imaging

Turnbull LW, Ridgway JP, Nicoll JJ, Bell D, Best JJK, Muir AL (Royal Infirmary, Edinburgh, Scotland)
Br Heart J 66:359–363, 1991   2–3

Background.—The outcome for patients with acute myocardial infarction depends on the extent of myocardial damage and residual left ventricular function. A method was developed to examine infarct size with MRI and compare it with pyrophosphate PET.

Methods.—The patients were 14 men and 5 women who had had their first myocardial infarction. None had been treated with thrombolytic drugs. Five to 7 days after the onset of symptoms, the patients underwent both MRI and pyrophosphate scanning to measure the size of the infarct. The patients also had measurement of creatine kinase MB release and assessment of ventricular performance by radionuclide ventriculography.

Results.—Both techniques showed the infarct clearly and identically. Volume measurements of the infarct agreed well, with a mean difference of 2.7 cm³. Correlations with creatine kinase MB release were highest when total rather than peak release was used. There was also a close correlation between the imaging studies and the patients' subsequent ventricular performance.

Conclusion.—In patients with acute myocardial infarction, MRI is an accurate technique of measuring infarct size. It agrees well with pyrophosphate scanning, ventricular function assessments, and total creatine kinase MB release. Use of a 128 × 128 pixel matrix and reduced slice thickness should improve precision, though they will lengthen examination time.

▶ This article confirms that estimation of infarction size is comparable using either SPECT pyrophosphate imaging or MRI. However, MRI offers no immediate advantage unless it can be combined with other cardiac imaging evaluations (an added value) or can be offered more cheaply or conveniently (not yet widely possible). Nevertheless, MRI now has to be considered a real option in the evaluation of patients before or after (or both) myocardial infarction.—R.A. Clark, M.D.

Right and Left Ventricular Stroke Volume Measurements With Velocity-Encoded Cine MR Imaging: In Vitro and In Vivo Validation
Kondo C, Caputo GR, Semelka R, Foster E, Shimakawa A, Higgins CB (Univ of California Med Ctr, San Francisco; General Electric Med Systems, Milwaukee)
AJR 157:9–16, 1991   2–4

Background.—With velocity-encoded cine (VEC) MRI, pulsatile blood flow can be segmented into many time frames throughout the cardiac cycle and flow velocity at each frame determined. To confirm the accuracy of flow velocity measurements obtained with VEC MRI, data were compared with independent measurements in a flow phantom and in human studies.

Methods.—Both the in vitro and in vivo studies used an MR imager operating at 1.5 tesla. Velocity-encoded cine MRI was performed by using a flip angle of 30 degrees, an echo time (TE) of 13 msec, and a repetition time (TR) of 27 msec. The flow phantom was made of a tube 6 mm in internal diameter, with water as the circulating fluid. The human subjects, 12 volunteers between the ages of 21 and 56 years, had no history of cardiac disease. Six underwent Doppler echocardiography, as well as cine and VEC MRI studies.

Results.—Constant flow velocities generated in a phantom (range, 20–408 cm/sec) were correctly determined by VEC MRI. Peak systolic velocities in the main pulmonary artery determined by VEC MRI showed a good correlation with measurements obtained with continuous-wave Doppler echocardiography. There was also a good correlation between stroke volumes measured at the aorta by VEC MRI and continuous-wave Doppler imaging. In addition, VEC MRI measurements of aortic and pulmonary flow yielded left and right ventricular stroke volumes that correlated well with left ventricular stroke volumes determined by short-axis cine MR images. Interobserver and intraobserver variabilities were small for both left and right ventricular stroke volumes obtained with VEC MRI.

Conclusion.—Velocity-encoded cine MRI is an accurate means of measuring flow velocity of both in vitro constant and in vivo pulsatile flows. Under normal flow conditions, VEC MRI can be used to measure right and left ventricular stroke volumes. Further technical development may make the technique applicable in cases of extremely fast or disordered flow.

▶ Because it can provide anatomical, functional, and perfusion imaging in 1 setting, MRI has a potential advantage over other noninvasive modalities in cardiac imaging. Ultrasound and CT can accurately assess anatomy and function, but they cannot easily provide perfusion information; scintigraphy can assess all 3 parameters, but with different isotope injections and often at separate examinations. Last year's abstracts demonstrated the evaluation of cardiac anatomy and valvular function with MRI. Other abstracts in this year's section confirm the capability of MRI for evaluation of myocardial perfusion. This article confirms the capability of MRI to quantify myocardial function accurately by measuring flow velocity and clinically important ventricular stroke volumes. The comprehensive noninvasive cardiac evaluation appears to be an option with MRI; whether this efficacy is realized in practice depends on the local availability and expertise of competing modalities and the clinical necessity of a comprehensive evaluation in a given patient.—R.A. Clark, M.D.

Biomagnetic Localization of Ventricular Arrhythmias

Moshage W, Achenbach S, Göhl K, Weikl A, Bachmann K, Wegener P, Schneider S, Härer W (University of Erlangen-Nuremberg, Siemens, Erlangen, Germany)
Radiology 180:685–692, 1991   2–5

Introduction.—Multichannel, superconducting quantum interference device systems are capable of measuring the magnetic fields caused by electrical activity of the human heart. This technique could allow noninvasive localization of the underlying electrical activity.

Methods.—Magnetocardiography (MCG) was used to study 10 patients with spontaneous premature ventricular complexes, 3 with ventricular tachycardia, and 4 normal individuals with induced paced beats. Each patient underwent a 2- to 15-minute MCG recording. Localization results were anatomically assigned by use of MRI (Fig 2–5).

Results.—The origins of the arrythmias were localized from the magnetic field distribution at the beginning of the ectopic beats after correction for superimposed repolarization activity. In the patients with paced beats, there was an error of a few millimeters from the position of the catheter tip. In the patients with premature ventricular complexes and ventricular tachycardia, results were either confirmed with endocardial mapping or associated with ischemic lesions.

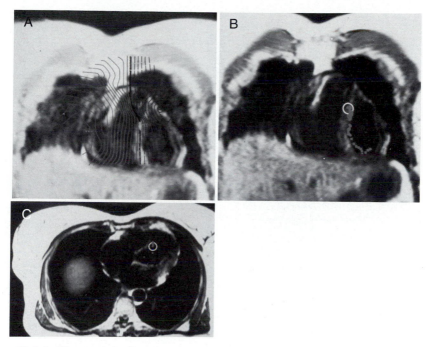

Fig 2–5.—Biomagnetic localization results in a patient with a parasystolic focus high in the interventricular septum, verified with an endocardial catheter mapping procedure. The magnetic field distribution recorded at the onset of the premature ventricular complex and the magnetocardiographic localization result (*arrow*) projected on the corresponding cross-section of an MRI **(A)** show that the ectopic focus (*circle*) lies high in the interventricular septum. The localization results during the first milliseconds of the ectopic beat form a path that indicates the spreading excitation moving distally along the interventricular septum in frontal view **(B)** and axial view **(C)**. (Courtesy of Moshage W, Achenbach S, Göhl K, et al: *Radiology* 180:685–692, 1991.)

Conclusion.—Multichannel MCG is a completely noninvasive technique of localizing ventricular arrythmias, which may ultimately improve treatment and prevention of life-threatening arrythmias.

▶ This technique will be beyond the capability of most MRI facilities. Nevertheless, I have included the article for review because it is innovative, and because it offers a view of the broad vistas that MRI may achieve as a comprehensive cardiac evaluation modality.—R.A. Clark, M.D.

Arterial Imaging

Lower-Extremity Vascular Grafts Placed for Peripheral Vascular Disease: Prospective Evaluation With Duplex Doppler Sonography
Gooding GAW, Perez S, Rapp JH, Krupski WC (San Francisco VA Med Ctr, San Francisco)
Radiology 180:379–386, 1991

2–6

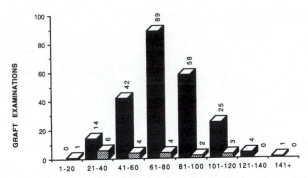

Fig 2–6.—Average PSV (in cm/sec; values shown at bottom) in grafts that were occluded by the time of the subsequent examination (*diagonal bars*) (20 examinations) compared with the average PSV in patent grafts (*black bars*) (233 examinations). In a total of 264 graft examinations, PSV was not calculated in 2 examinations; no PSV was calculated and a 2-degree occlusion was noted in 9 examinations; grafts were patent in 233 examinations; and in 20 examinations, occlusion was shown in the next study. (Courtesy of Gooding GAW, Perez S, Rapp JH, et al: *Radiology* 180:379–386, 1991.)

Background.—The use of ultrasound (US) technology in detecting abnormal flow patterns in vascular grafts can aid in predicting impending graft failure and allowing for intervention before occlusion develops. The utility of duplex US surveillance of inguinal grafts was prospectively examined in patients with peripheral vascular disease of the lower extremity.

Methods.—The study population was 85 men with 92 vascular grafts placed for peripheral vascular disease of the lower extremity. They underwent a total of 264 duplex Doppler examinations over 2.5 years.

Results.—Abnormal grafts had several different waveforms (Fig 2–6). Absence of diastolic flow and an average peak systolic velocity (PSV) of 32 cm/sec or less were signs of impending graft failure. The sensitivity of an average PSV of 40 cm/sec or less in predicting graft occlusion was 33% and the specificity was 94%. In 96% of the native femoral arteries, the PSV was higher than that in the graft. There was a normal PSV and increased diastolic flow associated with arteriovenous shunting.

Conclusion.—In this prospective study, vascular graft stenoses in patients with peripheral vascular disease were associated with high PSV locally in the graft or low PSV with absent diastolic flow. The sensitivity of duplex Doppler US in predicting graft failure will undoubtedly be increased with further refinements such as the addition of color.

▶ The ability to predict which vascular grafts are at risk for thrombosis before occlusion is attractive. Previous work has implied that low blood velocity (< 40 cm/sec) with absent forward diastolic flow is an indicator of graft failure. This study challenges that previous figure, because two thirds of the graft failures in this series were not predicted by that value. The authors offer another "magic number," 32 cm/sec, because this value or less was always associated with impending occlusion in their series. Although the concept is attractive and the technique is improving, more experience and refinement is necessary to improve accuracy (as evidenced by the next abstract).—R.A. Clark, M.D.

Does Postoperative Surveillance With Duplex Scanning Identify the Failing Distal Bypass?

Robison JG, Elliott BM (Med Univ of South Carolina, Charleston, NC)
Ann Vasc Surg 5:182–185, 1991   2–7

Background.—Disagreement remains as to the usefulness of routine postoperative noninvasive surveillance in patients who have had arterial reconstruction of the lower extremities. However, grafts at risk of thrombosis can be identified with increased sensitivity and specificity by duplex scanning. An experience with graft flow velocity surveillance was reviewed in an attempt to identify impending graft failure.

Methods.—During a 2-year period, 54 patients who had undergone lower extremity bypasses were evaluated by duplex scanning. The sample was made up of 43 men and 11 women, 45 of whom had infrapopliteal bypasses and 9 of whom had femoropopliteal bypasses. The indication for reconstruction was limb salvage in every case. Vascular laboratory parameters used were graft flow velocities, ankle/brachial indices, and toe pressure measurements.

Results.—Surveillance identified 3 patients with grafts at risk for stenosis: 1 had no evidence of arteriographic stenosis, 1 had symptoms of reduced flow velocity, and 1 had occlusion of the graft during follow-up. There were 8 cases of graft failure, 6 resulting from occlusion and 2 from an associated stenosis. All had graft flow velocities of more than 45 cm/sec. Unheralded graft occlusion developed in 6 patients less than 3 months after graft flow velocity was measured. Bypass to the dorsalis pedis artery was done in 4 of these patients.

Conclusion.—In patients undergoing lower extremity arterial reconstruction, graft flow velocity measurement may not predict impending graft failure. Sudden occlusion may result from several factors, especially in the pedal arteries. It would be helpful to use hemodynamic monitoring to predict graft failure, but it will require more sensitive or refined measurements.

▶ In this series of 54 patients, 6 with postoperative flow velocities greater than 45 cm/sec had graft failure, and 2 more had identified stenoses. This abstract would challenge somewhat the clinical usefulness of this procedure. Abstract 2–6 set a flow limit of 32 cm/sec, below which graft failure always occurred; nothing in this abstract refutes that figure. The problem occurs when higher flow grafts fail, which they obviously do. Therefore, at present, although very low flow is a sign of graft failure, further refinement of the technique is necessary to identify the higher flow grafts at risk. More experience, with evaluation of waveforms and color techniques, may improve this procedure.—R.A. Clark, M.D.

Does Color-Flow Imaging Improve the Accuracy of Duplex Carotid Evaluation?

Londrey GL, Spadone DP, Hodgson KJ, Ramsey DE, Barkmeier LD, Sumner DS (Southern Illinois Univ School of Medicine, Springfield, Ill)
J Vasc Surg 13:659–663, 1991   2–8

Objective.—Addition of color-flow technique to duplex scanning permits the visualization of blood flow within vessels. This study was designed to show whether adding color-flow imaging makes carotid sonography more accurate.

Study Design.—Results were compared for 2 laboratories, 1 using color flow and the other using standard duplex imaging. In other respects, the laboratories used identical techniques. A total of 307 internal carotid arteries were assessed by both color-flow imaging and standard angiography. Routine duplex scanning and angiography were carried out in 206 instances.

Findings.—Better agreement with angiography was found for color-flow than for conventional duplex scanning (86.6% vs. 79.6%). The color-flow study overclassified fewer vessels, but there was no difference in the number underclassified. The standard duplex study was less specific than color-flow imaging and had a lower positive predictive value. Sensitivity and negative predictive value were, however, generally comparable (Tables 1 and 2).

Conclusion.—Color-flow imaging may be preferable to standard duplex imaging because of more precise placement of the pulsed Doppler sample volume. Color-flow images clearly show the course of the vessel to be sampled and help differentiate external and internal carotid vessels. The absence of flow in occluded vessels is demonstrated more confidently using the color-flow technique.

TABLE 1.—Accuracy of Standard Duplex Examination

% Stenosis	Sensitivity	Specificity	Predictive value Positive	Negative	Accuracy
≤ 14 vs ≥ 15	98%	81%	89%	97%	92%
≤ 49 vs ≥ 50	100%	90%	87%	100%	94%
≤ 79 vs ≥ 80	87%	96%	82%	97%	94%
≤ 99 vs 100	100%	99%	82%	100%	99%

(Courtesy of Londrey GL, Spadone DP, Hodgson KJ, et al: *J Vasc Surg* 13:659–663, 1991.)

TABLE 2.—Accuracy of Color-Flow Examination

Predictive value

% Stenosis	Sensitivity	Specificity	Positive	Negative	Accuracy
≤14 vs ≥15	96%	93%	96%	93%	95%
≤49 vs ≥50	99%	94%	91%	99%	96%
≤79 vs ≥80	92%	97%	89%	98%	96%
≤99 vs 100	100%	99%	92%	100%	99%

(Courtesy of Londrey GL, Spadone DP, Hodgson KJ, et al: *J Vasc Surg* 13:659-663, 1991.)

▶ Color-flow imaging makes vascular ultrasound easier to perform and inter-pret. Despite some reports to the contrary, I have been convinced that color-flow imaging improved accuracy compared with duplex scanning. This study confirms previous reports indicating that, in experienced hands, there is probably little improvement in accuracy. However, for generalists like me, who do vascular ultrasound and can use all the help we can get, this report supports the concept that "easier" can translate to "better."—R.A. Clark, M.D.

Intravascular Sonography in the Detection of Arteriosclerosis and Evaluation of Vascular Interventional Procedures

Engeler CE, Yedlicka JW, Letourneau JG, Castañeda-Zúñiga WR, Hunter DW, Amplatz K (Univ of Minnesota, Minneapolis)
AJR 156:1087–1090, 1991   2–9

Background.—Miniaturized sonographic transducers with crystal thicknesses less than .1 mm have been produced. This technology was evaluated in the detection of arteriosclerosis by intravascular sonography (Fig 2–7). The effects of vascular interventional procedures on the arterial wall were also assessed.

Methods.—The subjects were 13 renal donors (mean age, 38 years); 12 patients with peripheral vascular disease symptoms; and 15 patients who had undergone 23 interventional vascular procedures (Fig 2–8). All patients had intravascular sonography of the aorta and ipsilateral iliac artery in real time under fluoroscopic guidance. A catheter-based miniature sonographic device with a 20-MHz transducer was used. The results of this study were compared with those of angiography.

Results.—Several arterial wall abnormalities in 8 of the 13 renal donors were shown by sonography but not angiography, including fatty streaks, diffuse or asymmetric intimal thickening, and focal calcified lesions. In the patients with peripheral vascular disease, more extensive arteriosclerotic changes were evident on sonography than on angiography, especially in analysis of the composition of the arteriosclerotic ab-

Arteriosclerosis

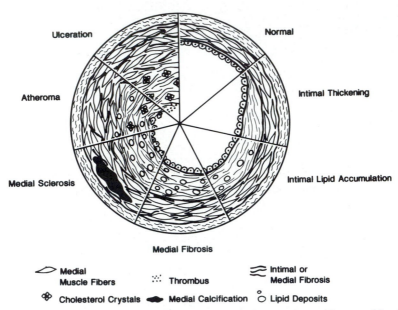

Fig 2–7.—Schematic representation of pathologic spectrum of arteriosclerosis. (Courtesy of Engeler CE, Yedlicka JW, Letourneau JG, et al: AJR 156:1087–1090, 1991.)

normality and determination of the degree of underlying diffuse arterio-sclerotic disease. In the patients who had had angioplasty or atherectomy, sonography demonstrated plaque fractures, intramural dissections, or atherectomy grooves.

Conclusion.—Intravascular sonography appears to have value in reducing the need for angiography to monitor progress or complications of vascular interventions. Intravascular sonography can differentiate the layers of the arterial wall, show vascular calcification, and characterize the diseased vessel and confirm the effect of angioplasty.

▶ This report describes the clinical usefulness of intravascular ultrasound to monitor the progress of vascular interventions. For this use, and for diagnostic purposes, intravascular sonography holds great promise. This article demonstrates high-quality images using a catheter-based sonographic device that can be introduced simply through a no. 7 French sheath and guided fluoroscopically to the area of interest. The equipment has been simplified over the last few years, and there are fewer technical barriers to the procedure. It is likely that the 1994 YEAR BOOK's abstracts will include more clinical trials of this technique.—R.A. Clark, M.D.

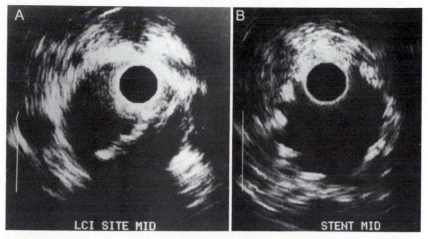

Fig 2–8.—Man, 46, with diabetes. **A,** sonogram shows a large, calcified flap with acoustical shadowing inferiorly in the common iliac artery after angioplasty. The pressure gradient is 20 mm Hg across the lesion. **B,** there was a good sonographic result after stent placement and there was no pressure gradient. (Courtesy of Engeler CE, Yedlicka JW, Letourneau JG, et al: *AJR* 156:1087–1090, 1991.)

Histopathologic Validation of Angioscopy and Intravascular Ultrasound

Siegel RJ, Ariani M, Fishbein MC, Chae J-S, Park JC, Maurer G, Forrester JS (Cedars-Sinai Med Ctr, Los Angeles)
Circulation 84:109–117, 1991   2–10

Introduction.—Angioscopy and ultrasonography can provide images of the arterial intima and media. However, no histopathologic validation of these images has been reported, nor has there been any comparison of the 2 techniques.

Methods.—An in vitro study of 70 postmorten human arterial segments was conducted to provide a histopathologic basis for interpretation of angioscopic and ultrasonographic images. The specimens were examined using no. 7 to 9 French fiberoptic angioscopes and 20- to 30-MHz intravascular ultrasound imaging catheters. After each specimen was classified by 3 observers according to both techniques, histologic classification was performed.

Results.—In normal vessels, both techniques (alone or together) had a sensitivity, specificity, and accuracy of at least 95%. Angioscopy had the better positive predictive value because of incorrect ultrasonographic interpretations of normal anatomy in vessels with thrombi. In stable atheromatous vessels, each technique had a sensitivity, specificity, and accuracy of more than 90%, but both tended to misclassify disrupted as stable atheroma. This resulted in a predictive value of 74% for angioscopy and 78% for ultrasonography. Sensitivities for disrupted atheroma were similarly moderate, but specificity, accuracy, and predictive value were high. Each technique had a high specificity, accuracy, and predictive value for thrombus, including a 100% sensitivity for angioscopy. The sensitivity of ultrasonography was only 57% because of false negative interpretation of laminar clots in normal vessels and the inability to differentiate disrupted or stable atheroma from intraluminal thrombus.

Conclusion.—Angioscopy and ultrasonography show good agreement with histologic analysis of arterial intimal and medial structure. When both techniques are concordant, agreement with histologic classification is 92%.

▶ This report nicely confirms the histologic basis for imaging findings and also classifies succinctly the angioscopic and intravascular sonographic findings for 4 categories of arterial pathologic conditions: normal, stable atheroma, disrupted atheroma, and thrombus. Angiographers know that these types of pathologic conditions are not always separable with standard imaging techniques. The combination of angioscopy and intravascular sonography was very accurate in identifying them. This article should be read by anyone using these techniques or contemplating the usefulness of these procedures.—R.A. Clark, M.D.

Evaluation of Traumatic Aortic Injury: Does Dynamic Contrast-Enhanced CT Play a Role?
Morgan PW, Goodman LR, Aprahamian C, Foley WD, Lipchik EO (Med College of Wisconsin, Milwaukee)
Radiology 182:661–666, 1992   2–11

Purpose.—In patients with blunt thoracic trauma, injuries to the aortic arch and great vessels are serious problems that require early diagnosis

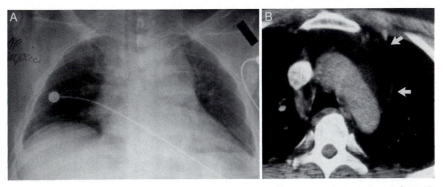

Fig 2–9.—Mediastinal widening secondary to excess mediastinal fat. **A,** supine chest radiograph demonstrates mediastinal widening with loss of definition of aorta and apparent left apical cap. This radiograph was considered likely to be positive for mediastinal hemorrhage. **B,** mediastinal CT scan helps exclude mediastinal hemorrhage and explain plain radiographic findings on the basis of mediastinal fat (*arrows*). (Courtesy of Morgan PW, Goodman LR, Aprahamian C, et al: *Radiology* 182:661–666, 1992.)

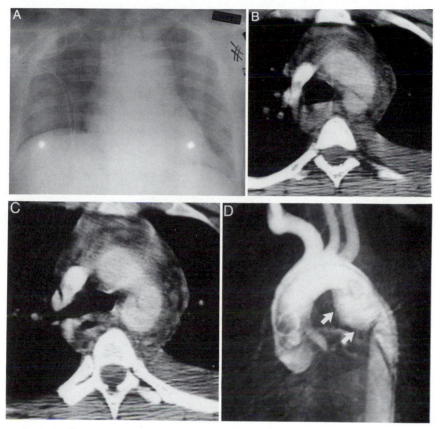

Fig 2–10.—Traumatic aortic rupture. **A,** equivocal chest radiograph demonstrates mediastinal widening in a supine patient. **B** and **C,** mediastinal CT scans demonstrate aortic irregularity, an intraluminal flap, and mediastinal hemorrhage. **D,** thoracic aortogram helps confirm presence of traumatic pseudoaneurysm (*arrows*).(Courtesy of Morgan PW, Goodman LR, Aprahamian C, et al: *Radiology* 182:661–666, 1992.)

and operation. Questions remain about the usefulness of CT in the classification of patients with blunt mediastinal injury. The value of 5-mm contrast-enhanced CT in patients with low-to-moderate probability of aortic laceration was examined.

Methods.—The study included 160 patients with substantial deceleration injury. Those with probable thoracic artery injury underwent immediate thoracotomy. Those who were clinically stable with at least 1 sign of mediastinal injury underwent thoracic aortography. Those with low-to-moderate probability of mediastinal injury had abdominal and mediastinal CT. If there was CT evidence of mediastinal hemorrhage, thoracic angiography was done.

Results.—Findings on admission chest radiographs were normal, with no evidence of mediastinal hemorrhage, in 132 patients. In 22 of 28 patients with abnormal findings on chest radiographs, CT helped exclude mediastinal hemorrhage (Fig 2–9); and 19 were treated without angiography. Mediastinal hematoma was found at CT in 6 cases, but there was only 1 aortic laceration at angiography (Fig 2–10).

Conclusion.—In patients with low-to-moderate risk of mediastinal hemorrhage, 5-mm contrast-enhanced CT can help exclude this diagnosis and reduce the need for angiography. Patients with normal chest radiographs are unlikely to have mediastinal hemorrhage. For patients at high risk of aortic laceration, angiography is recommended.

▶ Considerable interest has evolved recently in the evaluation of suspected traumatic aortic injury by CT before (or instead of) the traditional aortogram. Purists (and often surgeons) have long held that there was no substitute for aortography. This report describes a rational alternative; aortography only for those who have mediastinal hemorrhage identified by thin-section CT. In this series, CT helped exclude mediastinal hemorrhage in most patients with abnormal chest radiographs after trauma. This abstract and the confirming article referenced below (1) would suggest that CT can safely discriminate candidates for aortography and could preclude most patients from undergoing the invasive procedure.—R.A. Clark, M.D.

Reference

1. Raptopoulos V, et al: *Radiology* 182:667, 1992.

Aortic Dissection: Atypical Patterns Seen at MR Imaging
Wolff KA, Herold CJ, Tempany CM, Parravano JG, Zerhouni EA (Johns Hopkins Med Insts, Baltimore)
Radiology 181:489–495, 1991   2–12

Background.—In aortic dissection there is usually an intimal flap that separates the true and false lumina. However, some less well-recognized patterns of dissecton can occur. The MRI appearances of these atypical patterns were studied.

Methods.—Sixty-four cases of aortic dissection were reviewed; the mean age of the 36 male and 28 female patients was 48 years. Thirty-six had the Marfan syndrome or other connective tissue disorders, and 20 had a known history of hypertension. Each patient underwent T1-weighted and gradient-echo MRI of the entire aorta.

Findings.—In 9 cases, the only thoracic sign of dissection was thickening of the aortic wall. None of these patients had connective tissue disorders. Three patients showed an intimal flap in the abdominal aorta, but the absence of any flap led to false negative angiographic results in 3 of the remaining 6. This atypical appearance was present in 29% of acute vs. 7% of chronic dissections. An intimal flap was identified at follow-up in 2 patients who initially had the atypical appearance.

Conclusion.—In some cases of aortic dissection the sole manifestation may be thickening of the aortic wall. Magnetic resonance imaging of the entire aorta should be done for patients with suspected aortic dissection because it may show an identifiable flap only in the abdomen or atypical patterns may be recognized that may be missed by angiography.

▶ The more I read about and do MRI evaluation of suspected aortic dissection, the more anxious I become. All sorts of artifacts may mimic typical aortic dissection, and now we are shown that many dissections are atypical in their MRI appearance. On a positive note, if one learns the atypical appearances from this article, then evaluation becomes more sensitive; the atypical patterns will usually be missed at angiography.—R.A. Clark, M.D.

Imaging of the Renal Arteries: Value of MR Angiography
Debatin JF, Spritzer CE, Grist TM, Beam C, Svetkey LP, Newman GE, Sostman HD (Duke Univ, Durham, NC)
AJR 157:981–990, 1991   2–13

Introduction.—Renal artery stenosis can be assessed most accurately with conventional arteriography and intra-arterial digital subtraction angiography. To permit screening for potentially correctable renovascular disease, a sensitive, specific, noninvasive, easily available, and relatively inexpensive method is desirable. In the past, assessment of renovascular disease with MR angiography has been variably successful. In a prospective study, 4 MR angiographic image sets were evaluated and the results were compared with those of conventional arteriography in visualizing renal arteries.

Methods.—Within 48 hours of routine convention arteriography, 32 patients underwent MR angiography of the renal arteries. The studies were performed in 24 patients to evaluate possible renovascular hypertension and in 8 for possible donor nephrectomy. Axial 2-dimensional (2-D) phase contrast, coronal 2-D phase-contrast, coronal 2-D time-of-flight, and combined axial and coronal 2-D phase-contrast image sets were evaluated independently by 3 radiologists for image quality and visualization of dominant and accessory renal arteries and renovascular disease. The proximal 35 mm of the renal arteries were analyzed and compared with findings from conventional arteriograms adequate for diagnosis.

Results.—Axial and coronal phase-contrast images complemented one another (Fig 2–11) and when combined, resulted in visualization of 13 of 15 lesions diagnosed with conventional angiography, for a sensitivity of 87% and a specificity of 97%. Because signal loss from turbulent flow distal to a stenosis exaggerates the stenosis, 1 mild and 1 moderate le-

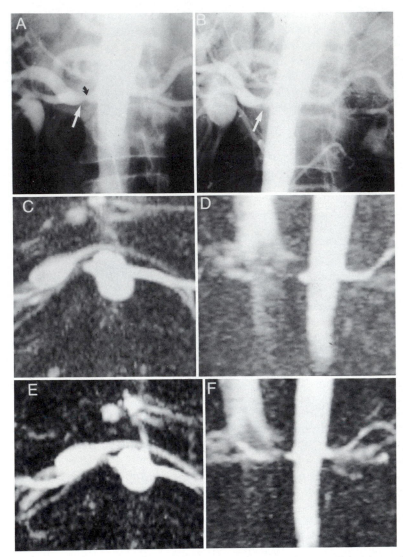

Fig 2–11.—A, a conventional arteriogram shows high-grade stenosis (75% to 99%) in the proximal right renal artery (*arrow*) of a man, 35. **B,** arteriogram shows reduction to a moderate lesion (*arrow*) after percutaneous transluminal angioplasty. **C** and **D,** axial (**C**) and coronal (**D**) preangioplasty maximum-pixel-intensity projection (*MIP*) phase-contrast images show extended area of signal void (greater than 5 mm) in the proximal right renal artery with reconstitution of signal distally. **E** and **F,** axial (**E**) and coronal (**F**) postangioplasty MIP phase-contrast images show a reduced area of signal void (less than 5 mm) corresponding to a moderate lesion (50% to 75%). Stenosis was correctly detected and graded on phase-contrast MR angiography both before and after angioplasty. (Courtesy of Debatin JF, Spritzer CE, Grist TM, et al: *AJR* 157:981–990, 1991.)

sion were overestimated; 1 moderate lesion was underestimated by most observers. All 3 observers agreed in the detection of severe lesions.

Conclusion.—Magnetic resonance angiography is promising as a noninvasive screening tool for the visualization of renal arterial disease. Increased experience should improve accuracy of estimations of lesions. Further studies on the usefulness of MR angiography in the evaluation of distal renal artery disease, especially fibromuscular dysplasia, are needed.

▶ This report suggests that MR angiography holds promise for evaluation of renovascular disease. The technique has limitations, however. The more commonly used time-of-flight technique was not very sensitive for detection of pathologic conditions. The best technique in this series was combined axial and coronal phase-contrast imaging. Although this approach makes sense (2-dimensional imaging allows better visualization of eccentric stenoses), the quality of MR angiography images is not yet so high that lesions identified in only 1 view can be confidently reported for clinical use. Moreover, MR angiography limits its evaluation to the proximal 3 cm of the artery; intrarenal vessels are not evaluated. Nevertheless, I agree with the authors that the technique holds great promise and deserves further refinement.—R.A. Clark, M.D.

Arterial Revascularization

Standards for Evaluating and Reporting the Results of Surgical and Percutaneous Therapy for Peripheral Arterial Disease
Rutherford RB, Becker GJ (Univ of Colorado, Denver; Baptist Hosp, Miami)
Radiology 181:277–281, 1991   2–14

Background.—It is often difficult to compare studies and evaluate treatments, because authors do not use standard reporting procedures and standard definitions for results such as patency and success rates. This study outlines some of the problems with current failure to use uniform standards and reporting procedures and details new standards recommended by the Society for Vascular Surgery (SVS) and the North American Chapter of the International Society for Vascular Surgery (ISCVS).

Recommendations.—The SVS/ISCVS recommended 14 standards for evaluating and reporting the results of treatment of peripheral vascular disease. These standards have been modified to reflect comment from authors and to accommodate new concepts. Very briefly, the standards are as follows: First, criteria for exclusion should be specific and not based on failure to complete treatment, failure to improve, or similar criteria. Second, using pretreatment status, acute ischemic limbs should be categorized as viable, threatened, or irreversible (Table 1). Third, chronic ischemic limbs should be categorized as asymptomatic, mild, moderate, or severe claudication; rest pain; major and minor tissue loss (Table 2). Fourth, changes in limb status should be graded from +3 to

TABLE 1.—Clinical Categories of Acute Limb Ischemia

Category	Description	Capillary Return	Muscle Weakness	Sensory Loss	Doppler Signals	
					Arterial	Venous
Viable	Not immediately threatened	Intact	None	None	Audible AP more than 30 mm Hg	Audible
Threatened	Salvageable if promptly treated	Intact, slow	Mild, partial	Mild, incomplete	Inaudible	Audible
Irreversible	Major tissue loss, amputation required regardless of treatment	Absent (marbling)	Profound, paralysis (rigor)	Profound, anesthetic	Inaudible	Inaudible

Abbreviation: AP, ankle pressure.
(Courtesy of Rutherford RB, Becker GJ: *Radiology* 181:277–281, 1991.)

TABLE 2.—Clinical Categories of Chronic Limb Ischemia

Grade	Category	Clinical Description	Objective Criteria
I	0	Asymptomatic, no hemodynamically significant occlusive disease	Normal results of treadmill†/stress test
	1	Mild claudication	Treadmill exercise completed, postexercise AP is greater than 50 mm Hg but more than 25 mm Hg less than normal
	2	Moderate claudication	Symptoms between those of categories 1 and 3
	3	Severe claudication	Treadmill exercise cannot be completed, postexercise AP is less than 50 mm Hg
II	4	Ischemic rest pain	Resting AP of 40 mm Hg or less, flat or barely pulsatile ankle or metatarsal plethysmographic tracing, toe pressure less than 30 mm Hg
III	5	Minor tissue loss, nonhealing ulcer, focal gangrene with diffuse pedal ischemia	Resting AP of 60 mm Hg or less, ankle or metatarsal plethysmographic tracing flat or barely pulsatile, toe pressure less than 40 mm Hg
	6	Major tissue loss, extending above transmetatarsal level, functional foot no longer salvageable	Same as for category 5

Abbreviation: AP, ankle pressure.
† Five minutes at 2 mph on a 12-degree incline.
(Courtesy of Rutherford RB, Becker GJ: *Radiology* 181:277–281, 1991.)

—3 on a scale ranging from marked improvement to marked worsening, including major amputation. Fifth, initial failures should be classified as (1) treatment aborted because of complication, (2) treatment completed but not technically successful, or (3) treatment technically successful without clinical improvement. Sixth, results reported as initial success and late patency must also report overall success rate. Seventh, patency should be determined by objective studies (e.g., CT and/or other specific indicies, observations, and postmortem examination). Eighth, primary patency is defined as uninterrupted patency with no procedures performed on or at the margins. Ninth, primary patency excludes procedures performed either before or after thrombosis. Secondary patency requires restored flow through most of the original graft. Tenth, assisted primary patency can be reported, but findings must also include true primary and secondary patency rates. Eleventh, the life-table method should be used for analyzing patency. Twelfth, procedural mortality should be reported using the 30-day limit with some exceptions. Thirteenth, pertinent nonvascular complications should be reported along with vascular complications. Finally, risk factors that affect outcome should be recorded, graded, and compared.

Conclusion.—The quality of published reports of revascularization procedures for lower extremity ischemia can be significantly improved by the adoption of uniform reporting standards. Such uniformity would allow meaningful comparisons of various treatment modalities.

▶ It is very difficult, if not impossible, to compare balloon angioplasty efficacy studies from different institutions or to compare surgical with nonsurgical revascularization studies because of case selection bias and clinical evaluation variances. Moreover, it is difficult to compare accepted treatments with new therapeutic modalities. This article recommends standards for reporting and evaluating results, based on precise definition of terms and objective criteria for outcome measurement. These recommendations are consistent with standards recommended by our surgical colleagues (1, 2). These standards are long overdue. All physicians involved in cardiovascular medicine should become familiar with and use these standards in their own practices and in the evaluation of the scientific literature for practice guidance.—R.A. Clark, M.D.

References

1. Rutherford RB, et al: *J Vasc Surg* 4:80, 1986.
2. Porter JM, et al: *J Vasc Surg* 8:172, 1988.

The Use of Angioplasty, Bypass Surgery, and Amputation in the Management of Peripheral Vascular Disease
Tunis SR, Bass EB, Steinberg EP (Johns Hopkins Univ, Baltimore)
N Engl J Med 325:556–562, 1991   2–15

Introduction.—Although percutaneous transluminal angioplasty has become a popular alternative to peripheral bypass surgery in patients with peripheral vascular disease of the lower extremities, some experts

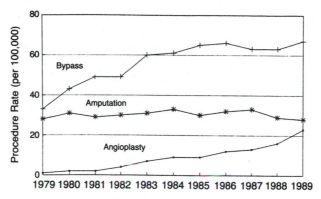

Fig 2–12.—Adjusted annual rates of angioplasty, bypass surgery, and amputation for peripheral vascular disease of the lower extremities in Maryland, 1979 through 1989. Rates have been adjusted for age and sex and are expressed as number of procedures per 100,000 Maryland residents. $P < .0001$ for the increase in the rate of angioplasty between 1979 and 1989. $P < .001$ for the increase in the rate of bypass between 1979 and 1989. (Courtesy of Tunis SR, Bass EB, Steinberg EP, et al: N *Engl J Med* 325:556–562, 1991.)

believe that the results of angioplasty are not as long lasting as those of surgery. Researchers sought to determine the extent to which angioplasty is used and the impact of this procedure on the surgical management of peripheral vascular disease.

Methods.—Study data were derived from the records of hospital discharges in Maryland between 1979 and 1989. Information was obtained on all angioplasty procedures, peripheral bypass operations, and lower extremity amputations performed for peripheral vascular disease during this period.

Findings.—Between 1979 and 1989, the estimated annual rate of angioplasty for peripheral vascular disease of the lower extremities rose from 1 to 24 per 100,000 Maryland residents (Fig 2–12). Yet the adjusted annual rate of peripheral bypass surgery increased as well, from 32 to 65

Total Hospital Charges and Number of
Hospital Days Associated with Angioplasty
and Peripheral Bypass Procedures
Performed for Peripheral Vascular Disease
of the Lower Extremities in Maryland

YEAR	CHARGES	DAYS
1979	$14.7 million	20,695
1984	$25.8 million	31,280
1989	$30.5 million	33,830

Note: Costs are in 1989 dollars. Changes and days have been adjusted for age.
(Courtesy of Tunis SR, Bass EB, Steinberg EP, et al: N *Engl J Med* 325:556–562, 1991.)

per 100,000. The adjusted annual rate of lower extremity amputation remained stable, at approximately 30 per 100,000. There was a substantial increase in the number of hospital days and in total charges associated with revascularization procedures (table). The charges increased from $14.7 million in 1979 (in 1989 dollars) to $30.5 million in 1989.

Conclusion.—The use of percutaneous transluminal angioplasty instead of peripheral bypass surgery in selected patients with peripheral vascular disease was expected to substantially reduce costs and the need for amputation. In Maryland, however, surgical procedures have increased, costs have risen, and the amputation rate remains unchanged. These findings may reflect increased diagnosis and an expansion of the indications for angioplasty and bypass surgery.

▶ For years, radiologists have argued that peripheral angioplasty was more cost-effective and equally efficacious when compared with surgical revascularization. This has been difficult to prove, however, because so few prospective randomized studies have been done comparing surgical and nonsurgical alternatives. Moreover, radiologists have often claimed that angioplasty may be useful in limb salvage, when definite revascularization was not possible. This provocative article challenges these views. In Maryland (from 1979 to 1989), the increased use of peripheral angioplasty was associated with an increased use of surgical bypass procedures and no decrease in amputations. These results would also imply that the increased use of both angioplasty and surgery did nothing for the limb salvage rate. A full discussion of the analyses and limitations of the study, as well as opposing viewpoints, can be had by reading the article and subsequent letters to the editor with replies by the authors (1). This article should stimulate the performance of controlled clinical trials in which outcomes are evaluated prospectively.—R.A. Clark, M.D.

Reference

1. Letters to the editor: *New Engl J Med* 326:413–415, 1992.

Clinical Outcome and Health Care Costs in Renal Revascularization—Percutaneous Transluminal Renal Angioplasty Versus Reconstructive Surgery
Weibull H, Bergqvist D, Jendteg S, Lindgren B, Persson U, Jonsson K, Bergentz SE (Lund University, Malmö, Sweden; Swedish Inst for Health Economics, Lund, Sweden)
Br J Surg 78:620–624, 1991   2–16

Background and Methods.—Studies have shown that percutaneous transluminal renal angioplasty (PTRA) may be more cost-effective than surgery in elderly atherosclerotic patients. However, if recurrence and complication rates are higher, clinical outcome is affected, and initial

Health Care Costs in SEK Per Patient in 1988

Period	PTRA group		Operated group	
	Median	Range	Median	Range
Diagnostic evaluation and preprocedure preparation	23 900	9 900– 44 500	23 400	3 500– 43 200
Procedure	4 600	4 600– 37 200	26 000	20 600– 80 700
Postprocedure	10 400	3 100– 30 200	17 200	6 200– 63 000
Follow-up	26 200	2 000–166 000	6 100	1 600– 64 000
Total	65 100	30 700–250 800	72 700	42 100–227 000

Abbreviation: SEK, Swedish Crowns (SEK 100 = U.S. $15).
(Courtesy of Weibull H, Bergqvist D, Jendteg S, et al: *Br J Surg* 78:620–624, 1991.)

cost savings may be lost. Here investigators compared clinical outcome and health care costs in 21 patients treated with PTRA and 16 patients treated with reconstructive surgery. Median follow-up for both groups was 48 months.

Results.—Of 21 PTRAs, 19 were wholly or partially successful, and 2 were impossible to perform. Six restenoses occurred at 4 to 24 months. Four patients received repeat PTRA, and 2 underwent surgery. In the group that had initial surgery, there were no recurrences. At the end of follow-up, patency in the PTRA group was 69% compared with 100% in the surgical group. Ninety percent of patients receiving PTRA had reduced primary or secondary hypertension, while 81% of surgical patients had improvement in hypertension.

Costs for diagnosis and pretreatment were the same in both groups, but procedural and postprocedural costs were lower in the PTRA group (table). Follow-up costs were greater in the PTRA group, however, because of recurrences and their treatment. The total median cost of reconstructive surgery was 12% higher than for PTRA. This difference was not significant.

Conclusion.—Reconstructive surgery and PTRA should be considered complementary not competitive procedures, both technically and economically. For initial treatment, PTRA should be tried. If PTRA fails, surgery should be undertaken. Using this strategy, about 50% of patients would require only a single PTRA procedure. The remainder would need repeat PTRA or surgery, but this approach would probably keep costs at the lowest possible level.

▶ Very few scientific articles have attempted to verify the claim that angioplasty is more cost-effective than surgical revascularization. Cost-effectiveness studies are complex because relevant costs include more than those of the initial procedures alone; incurred costs and costs of morbidity and mortality are to be included. This report calculates costs and outcomes for surgical and nonsurgical renal revascularization and finds that there is no significant difference. Although the procedure costs were lower in the angioplasty group, follow-up costs were higher because of recurrences and their treatment. The article suggests a rational alternative (i.e., initial angioplasty), with all recurrences treated with surgery. More studies of cost-effectiveness are needed in interventional radiology. Because we are often the ones who claim a cost-benefit advantage over surgery, we have the responsibility to do the studies to prove or disprove the claims.—R.A. Clark, M.D.

Percutaneous Iliac Artery Stent: Angiographic Long-Term Follow-Up
Long AL, Page PE, Raynaud AC, Beyssen-BM, Fiessinger JN, Ducimetière P, Relland JY, Gaux JC (Unité INSERM 258; Hôpital Broussais, Paris)
Radiology 180:771–778, 1991   2–17

Background and Methods.—Various procedures can be used in combination with percutaneous transluminal angioplasty (PTA) to improve results. Investigators have reported promising early and midterm results with the use of vascular endoprostheses for treatment of iliac arterial lesions, but long-term results remain unknown. Here investigators conducted a prospective study of 49 patients with 53 lesions in 52 iliac arteries. All patients were treated with PTA. Self-expanding, flexible endoprostheses were inserted in 47 lesions, and 5 prostheses were balloon expandable. Indications for insertion of endoprostheses were total occlusions in 28%, dissections in 42%, restenoses after PTA in 21%, and unsatisfactory PTA in 9%.

Results.—In all cases, stents were successfully inserted. Recanalization of total occlusion achieved smooth dilatation. Stents also sealed the 2

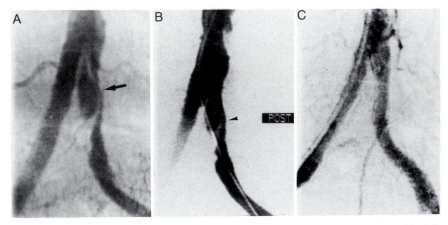

Fig 2–13.—Anteriograms demonstrate PTA-induced dissection of the proximal segment of the left common iliac artery. **A,** typical depiction of segmental occlusive dissection is shown (*arrow*). **B,** after ballon inflation, appearance is not satisfactory (*arrowhead*). **C,** three years later, good patency of the area with the Wallstent is seen, without hyperplasia. (Courtesy of Long AL, Page PE, Raynaud AC, et al: *Radiology* 180:771–778, 1991.)

dissected channels in these cases (Fig 2–13). However, the stent failed to expand in 16 cases, necessitating complementary intrastent angioplasty. Despite additional interventions, the stent still failed to expand in 7 cases, even after several balloon inflations. There was 1 aortic protrusion, 1 acute thrombosis of the stent that was resolved with urokinase, and 3 distal embolizations that were resolved with urokinase and aspiration. During 15-month follow-up, 2 patients died, 1 after occlusion. There were 3 other occlusions, 1 of which was resolved with local thrombolysis. There were 7 cases of hyperplasia, and 3 stenoses occurred at the end of the stent because of incomplete coverage of the lesion. Surgeons performed complementary procedures in 6 of these cases.

At 12 months, primary patency was 85.3%, whereas at 18 months, primary patency was 80.9%. Secondary patency was 96.1% at both 12 and 18 months. Excluding the patients who died, 54% of the limbs were asymptomatic at the end of the study, and 38% were improved. The clinical success rate was 92%, and there were no amputations.

Conclusion.—These findings confirm the long-term usefulness of treatment with intravascular stents as adjuncts to balloon angioplasty in the percutaneous treatment of iliac obstruction. Complete coverage of the lesion is necessary to avoid complications of early thrombosis or restenosis.

▶ This article and the next 3 abstracts present an overview of the current state of revascularization using stents. Three of the articles describe results with the more commonly used self-expanding Wallstent; 1 article studies the balloon-expanded Palmaz stent. This first series, using the Wallstent, has a heavy selection bias; patients were poor risk or had had previous angioplasties or complications. Nevertheless, the outcomes were respectable, and the study confirms the usefulness of the stent as an adjunct to balloon angioplasty.—R.A. Clark, M.D.

Arterial Stent Placement With Use of the Wallstent: Midterm Results of Clinical Experience

Zollikofer CL, Antonucci F, Pfyffer M, Redha F, Salomonowitz E, Stuckmann G, Largiadèr I, Marty A (Kantonsspital Winterthur, Winterthur, Switzerland; University Hospital, Zurich, Switzerland; Kantonsspital Frauenfeld, Frauenfeld, Switzerland)
Radiology 179:449–456, 1991   2–18

Background.—Restenosis and occlusion of dilated or recanalized arteries continue to be problems in patients undergoing percutaneous transluminal angioplasty (PTA). An expandable endovascular stent for preventing such recurrences was investigated.

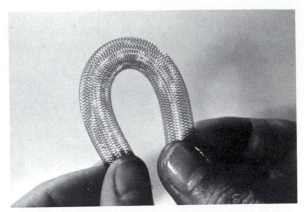

Fig 2–14.—Fully expanded stent. The tubular braided mesh with its longitudinal flexibility is well demonstrated. (Courtesy of Zollikofer CL, Antonucci F, Pfyffer M, et al: *Radiology* 179:449–456, 1991.)

Methods.—A self-expandable Wallstent made of surgical-grade stainless steel alloy filaments was used for 31 patients (Fig 2–14). Twenty-six patients had iliac and 15 had femoropopliteal artery stenoses or occlusions. All lesions were complex, including residual stenoses and dissections after previous PTA or iliac artery surgery and long-segment femoropopliteal occlusions with inadequate response to percutaneous recanalization.

Results.—In the iliac artery group, 96% of lesions remained patent after a mean follow-up of 16 months. However, in the femoropopliteal artery group, only 6 of 11 available stents were patent at a mean of 20 months (Fig 2–15). At least 1 secondary intervention was needed by 4 of these patients.

Conclusion.—In patients with complex iliac artery lesions that cannot be treated by simple balloon dilatation, self-expanding endoprostheses may be a valuable method of treatment. In long femoral artery lesions, however, this technique should be used with caution and with as short a stent as possible.

▶ This article also confirms that the stent is a useful adjunct to balloon angioplasty. It wisely advises that long lesions not be approached.—R.A. Clark, M.D.

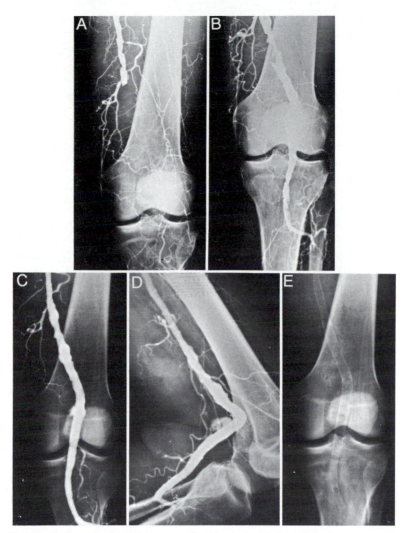

Fig 2–15.—Radiographs obtained in a man, 67, with a 1-month history of claudication stage IIB. **A,** femoral angiogram shows 25-cm occlusion of the femoropopliteal axis. **B,** after recanalization with local thrombolysis and PTA, there is a persistent stenosis at the femoropopliteal junction and in the distal popliteal artery, as well as an occlusion in the tibiobibular trunk and the anterior tibial artery. Also, a previously unknown recanalized popliteal artery aneurysm is shown. **C** and **D,** control angiograms in anteroposterior and lateral projections 5 days after placement of a 6-mm and an 8-mm Wallstent into the distal popliteal artery just proximal to the now recanalized trifurcation. Three 10-mm overlapping stents were also implanted into the distal femoral and the proximal-to-middle popliteal arteries. There is marked smoothening of the luminal surface compared with that in **B,** and the popliteal artery aneurysm is partly thrombosed. Note the flexibility and perfect adaptation of the stent while the knee is bent in the lateral projection. **E,** overlapping of fully expanded stents is shown 1 week after placement. (Courtesy of Zollikofer CL, Antonucci F, Pfyffer M, et al: *Radiology* 179:449–456, 1991.)

Palmaz Stent in Atherosclerotic Stenoses Involving the Ostia of the Renal Arteries: Preliminary Report of a Multicenter Study

Rees CR, Palmaz JC, Becker GJ, Ehrman DO, Richter GM, Noeldge G, Katzen BT, Dake MC, Schwarten DE (Univ of Texas Health Science Ctr, San Antonio, Tex; Indiana Univ, Indianapolis; University of Freiburg, Freiberg, Germany; Baptist Memorial Hosp, Miami; St Vincent's Hosp, Indianapolis)
Radiology 181:507–514, 1991   2–19

Background.—Angioplasty has a limited role in treating atheromatous renal artery lesions, and surgery often is risky in these patients. The Palmaz renal stent therefore was evaluated in 28 hypertensive patients who had atherosclerotic disease involving the ostia of the renal arteries (Fig 2–16).

Methods.—Twenty patients had stents placed to treat elastic recoil immediately after conventional angioplasty. Eight others had restenosis after percutaneous angioplasty.

Results.—In all patients but 1, there was less than 30% residual stenosis after stenting. Five patients had complications. Hypertension was absent in 3 patients at follow-up 1 to 25 months after treatment, and 15 others were improved. Renal function improved in 5 of 14 patients with an initial serum creatinine of 1.5 mg/dL or higher and stabilized in 5 others. Follow-up angiography demonstrated restenosis in 7 of 18 patients (Fig 2–17).

Conclusion.—Renal stenting will benefit many patients with renal ostial artheromatous disease who respond poorly to conventional angioplasty.

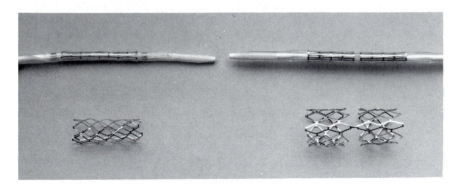

Fig 2–16.—Photograph of 2 stents. The stent on the left was used in the first 17 patients. Strut thickness is .0064 cm. Its unexpanded length on the 5-F balloon angioplasty catheter is 1.5 cm. The stent may be expanded to approximately 6 mm; in this photograph, the expanded stent is 1.35 cm long and 4.7 mm in diameter. The stent on the right was used in the last 11 patients. Strut thickness is .0102 cm, and unexpanded length on the 5-F balloon angioplasty catheter is 2 cm. The stent may be expanded to approximately 8 mm (manufacturer recommends no more than 7 mm). In this photograph, the expanded stent is 7 mm in diameter and 1.75–1.96 cm long (the expanded stent is shorter on the side with articulation). Articulation was added to enhance the flexibility of the longer stent. (Courtesy of Rees CR, Palmaz JC, Becker GJ, et al: *Radiology* 181:507–514, 1991.)

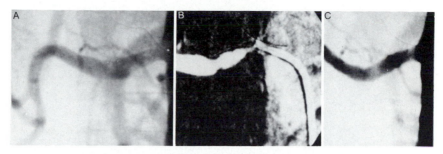

Fig 2–17.—Angiograms of a patient with restenosis. **A,** good initial result with stent placement. **B,** angiogram at 6 months shows restenosis within the stent. The stent extends from the ostium to the distal aspect of the stenosis. **C,** the stent can be seen on a misregistered image after partial clearance of contrast material. **D,** repeat PTA yielded a good technical result, but severe restenosis was seen again on an angiogram obtained 8.5 months later (not shown). (Courtesy of Rees CR, Palmaz JC, Becker GJ, et al: *Radiology* 181:507–514, 1991.)

▶ Abstracts 2–17 and 2–18 studied the results of vascular stents in the peripheral arterial circulation. In this multicenter trial, the balloon-expanded Palmaz stent was used to treat renal ostial lesions. I am not convinced that the stents offered much value in these patients. Renal ostial lesions are poor candidates for balloon angioplasty alone, and one would hope that angioplasty aided by stenting would improve results. However, the results shown here are not striking and, by design, they must be compared with historical controls. I am concerned that, if these results were compared with equivalent patients treated with balloon angioplasty alone, there would be no significant difference in outcomes. Nevertheless, the procedure holds some promise, and a controlled trial is warranted.—R.A. Clark, M.D.

Follow-Up Results After Stent Placement in Failing Arteriovenous Shunts: A Three-Year Experience

Vorwerk D, Günther RW, Bohndorf K, Kistler D, Gladziwa U, Sieberth HG (Technical University of Aachen, Aachen, Germany)
Cardiovasc Intervent Radiol 14:285–289, 1991   2–20

Background.—Arteriovenous access shunts for chronic hemodialysis have a high complication rate that may lead to shunt failure. Percutaneous transluminal angioplasty (PTA) is an effective treatment for shunt stenoses, but the addition of endovascular prostheses might improve both technical success and long-term patency of treated vessels.

Methods.—Surgeons treated 17 patients with 18 arteriovenous shunts. All patients had undergone unsuccessful balloon dilation before stent implantation was considered. All patients received self-expandable endoprostheses. Flexible introducing catheters allowed implantation even in curved vessels. Patients received heparin during the procedure. Subsequent hemodialysis was performed through the treated shunt. All patients with chronic renal failure received heparin during hemodialysis.

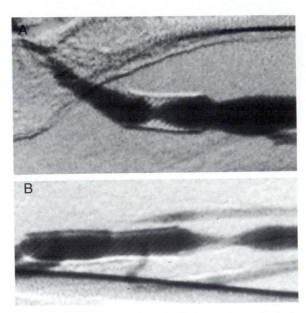

Fig 2–18.—A, concentric restenosis within the stent of a Brescia-Cimino fistula close to the elbow. **B,** new stenosis adjacent to the stent in a Brescia-Cimino forearm fistula. (Courtesy of Vorwerk D, Günther RW, Bohndorf K, et al: *Cardiovasc Intervent Radiol* 14:285–289, 1991.)

Results.—Stent placement was technically successful, with early patency in 17 of 18 shunts. Immediately after stenting, thrombosis occurred in 3 shunts, but 2 were successfully treated. At 1- to 31-month follow-up, 14 of 17 shunts remained open. Two patients died within 18 months, but their shunts remained functional until death. Three shunts were abandoned during follow-up. Eleven patients required either percutaneous or combined surgical and percutaneous intervention because of restenosis or reocclusion. Seven patients had restenoses within the stents (Fig 2–18). Six patients required multiple reinterventions. Although patency decreased to 27% at 18 months (table), when reinterventions were considered, patency increased to 77% at 18 months.

Conclusion.—Stent placement in arteriovenous shunts may be useful to overcome acute problems associated with balloon dilation. However, use of stents does not prevent restenosis.

▶ In the previous article, the problem did not lie with the stent or the interventionalists, but with the lesion itself, the renal ostial stenosis, which seems to preclude adequate nonsurgical treatment of any type. Similarly, stenoses of arteriovenous shunts are lesions that resist balloon angioplasty and commonly recur. As such, they are appropriate candidates for stent placement as an adjunct to angioplasty. This abstract shows how difficult it is to manage problems that do not respond to angioplasty with adjunct techniques. Stent placement was not useful in preventing restenoses, but it did help manage acute problems. Sometimes the fault does not lie in ourselves, but in the stars.—R:A. Clark, M.D.

Dialysis Shunt and Stent Patency Rates

Shunt patency rate without repeat interventions (n = 17)

Follow-up period	No. of shunts	No. failed	No. lost to follow-up	Cumulative patency (%)
1 month	17	3	—	82.4
3 months	14	4	0	58.9
6 months	10	3	1	40.3
12 months	6	0	2	40.3
18 months	4	1	2	26.9

Stent patency rate without repeat interventions (n = 17)

1 month	17	—	—	100.0
3 months	17	1	1	93.9
6 months	15	6	3	52.2
12 months	6	0	0	52.2
18 months	6	2	3	29.0

(Courtesy of Vorwerk D, Günther RW, Bohndorf K, et al: *Cardiovasc Intervent Radiol* 14:285–289, 1991.)

Total Peripheral Artery Occlusions: Conventional Versus Laser Thermal Recanalization With a Hybrid Probe in Percutaneous Angioplasty: Results of a Randomized Trial

Belli A-M, Cumberland DC, Procter AE, Welsh CL (Northern General Hospital, Sheffield, England)
Radiology 181:57–60, 1991   2–21

Background.—In part, laser-assisted angioplasty was developed to improve the success rate in crossing peripheral vascular occlusions. Newer techniques are more sophisticated and more costly, but there are few

Technical Success Rates in Femoropopliteal Occlusions

Occlusion Length (cm)	Laser Success				Conventional Treatment Success			
	No. of Patients	Laser Only	Laser and Wire	Total	No. of Patients	Wire Only	Wire and Probe	Total
1–5	18	16 (89)	1 (6)	17 (94)	12	9 (75)	2 (17)	11 (92)
6–10	12	8 (67)	2 (17)	10 (83)	18	14 (78)	2 (11)	16 (89)
>10	4	4 (100)	0	4 (100)	4	2 (50)	2 (50)	4 (100)
Total	34	28 (82)	3 (9)	31 (91)	34	25 (74)	6 (18)	31 (91)

Note: *Numbers in parentheses* are percentages.
(Courtesy of Belli A-M, Cumberland DC, Procter AE, et al: *Radiology* 181:57–60, 1991.)

reported clinical trials evaluating specific laser systems in comparison to cheaper conventional percutaneous angioplasty.

Methods.—Investigators randomized 81 patients with 84 occlusive lesions in the iliac and femoropopliteal segments to receive either laser recanalization or conventional recanalization. Only patients suitable for an ipsilateral femoral approach were chosen. Investigators used a 2.5-mm hybrid laser probe for all laser recanalizations. The laser source was either a continuous-wave argon generator or a continuous-wave neodymium yttrium–aluminum-garnet (Nd:YAG) generator. Successful laser recanalization was followed by balloon dilation using a standard technique. A 0.035 Medrad was used in patients treated with conventional recanalization. A variety of alternative guidewires were utilized if the Medrad wire failed. This procedure was also followed by balloon dilation. Procedures were considered technically successful if less than 50% residual stenosis was detected at angiography. Clinical success was defined as relief of symptoms and improved peripheral pulses as long as 2 weeks after the procedure.

Results.—The laser probe failed to traverse 6 of 34 femoropopliteal occlusions treated by this method (table), but 82% of recanalizations were successful. There was 1 acute reocclusion, for a clinical success rate of 79%. When both a probe and a guidewire were used, the technical success rate was increased to 91%, and the clinical success rate to 85%. With conventional recanalization, the guidewire failed to traverse 9 of 34 femoropopliteal occlusions, for a technical success rate of 74%. There was 1 acute reocclusion, for a clinical success rate of 71%. Again, combining the 2 procedures increased the primary technical rate to 91%. The number of patients with iliac occlusions was small, but the laser achieved an initial technical success rate of 0%, whereas the conventional procedure had technical and clinical success rates of 67%. Using both procedures increased the success rate to 14% in the laser category. The 1 iliac artery not recanalized by the conventional procedure could not be recanalized by combined procedures.

Conclusion.—Better guidewires and catheters improve primary success rates of conventional recanalization. There was no statistically significant difference between the laser and conventional recanalization for femoropopliteal occlusions. However, use of both techniques increased primary success rates somewhat.

▶ Too often, new techniques are adopted before the science has demonstrated efficacy, because the technology and the promise are available. Various types of lasers, drills, and probes have been used in recent years to improve primary recanalization for angioplasty; however, few randomized controlled trials have been done to evaluate efficacy. Quite often, the success or failure of a new technique is decided by the marketplace, at a substantial cost to all concerned. Unfortunately, randomized trials often follow the marketplace decision. This is 1 such example of a very good, well-designed trial that confirms what has been learned at great cost in the marketplace: in the aggregate, laser recanalization offers little over the standard guidewire. However, for some patients in whom the primary device fails (laser or guidewire), the second device succeeds. It is a hard lesson that we continue not to learn.—R.A. Clark, M.D.

Peripheral Arterial Obstructions: Analysis of Patency 1 Year After Laser-Assisted Transluminal Angioplasty

Nordstrom LA, Castaneda-Zuniga WR, Von Seggern KB (Park Nicollet Heart Ctr, St Louis; Univ of Minnesota, Minneapolis)
Radiology 181:515–520, 1991   2–22

Introduction.—Laser-assisted percutaneous transluminal angioplasty (PTA) involves direct, coaxial delivery of argon laser energy with a specially designed balloon catheter. Data were reviewed on the durability of results of the technique in various patient subgroups.

Methods.—The 68 procedures were performed in 63 nonconsecutive patients whose conditions ranged from life-style-limiting claudication to limb-threatening ischemia. Technical success required a reduction in the lesion to less than 50% stenosis together with a 0.15 or greater improvement in the ankle-brachial index (ABI) immediately after treatment. Alleviation of symptoms combined with the sustained improvement of ABIs constituted clinical success. The mean follow-up period was 12 months.

Results.—Most (87%) of procedures were technical successes, characterized by a significant increase in mean posttreatment ABI. The success rates ranged from 71% for occluded iliac segments to 100% for femoropopliteal stenoses. The 10 complications included 3 thermal perforations and 2 emboli. The overall patency at 1 year was 75%. Patients with claudication had a 1-year patency rate of 85%; the procedure had a less durable success at follow-up for patients with limb-threatening ischemia (23%).

Conclusion.—Laser-assisted angioplasty appears to be a viable treatment option for patients with claudication and long peripheral artery occlusions. Because the final result is achieved with balloon angioplasty, the prevalence of eventual restenosis may not be altered.

▶ This series reports respectable results with laser-assisted balloon angioplasty. The only comparison available is with historical controls; the results are very similar. This article does not claim that laser-assisted angioplasty is better than balloon angioplasty alone. It wisely tempers its conclusions and claims only that this technique is 1 of several that may be helpful in some subgroups of patients.—R.A. Clark, M.D.

Results and Follow-Up After Percutaneous Pulsed Laser-Assisted Balloon Angioplasty Guided by Spectroscopy

Geschwind HJ, Aptecar E, Boussignac G, Dubois-Randé J-L, Zelinsky R, Poirot G, Tomaru T (Hôpital Henry Mondor; INSERM U 2, Créteil, France)

Circulation 83:787–796, 1991 2–23

Introduction.—Because laser-assisted balloon angioplasty is a recently developed technique, few data are available on the long-term outcome of patients treated for occluded peripheral arteries. The early and late results of laser angioplasty in patients whose arteries could not be recanalized by conventional techniques were reviewed.

Methods.—The 66 patients had a mean age of 60 years; 60 were men. There was total occlusion of the iliac artery in 11 patients, of the superficial artery in 53, and of the tibial artery in 2. The mean length of the occlusion was 8.8 cm, and the mean duration of the procedure was 90 minutes. Previous attempts to cross the occlusion with guidewires had failed. The system consisted of a pulsed dye laser operated at 480 nm, 2 μsec/pulse, 5 Hz, 50 mJ/pulse coupled into a .021-in. laser catheter.

Results.—The occluded artery was successfully recanalized in 54 (82%) patients. The mean Doppler ankle-brachial index increased from .59 before to .97 after laser angioplasty. There was a higher primary success rate in iliac (91%) than in superficial femoral arteries (79%). Noncalcified lesions had a higher success rate (88%) than calcified lesions (71%). Early success did not differ significantly for long and short lesions. At a mean follow-up of 18 months, the peripheral arteries of 32 (64%) patients were considered patent. Complications included 7 early reocclusions that could be recanalized and 8 perforations that did not require surgical treatment.

Conclusion.—The cost of laser angioplasty is high, but the technique is effective for recanalization of totally occluded arteries that cannot be treated by conventional means. Given the severity of the lesions, the long-term patency rate was acceptable, especially for patients who did not experience early reocclusion.

▶ This is the third of 3 articles (Abstracts 2–21, 2–22, and 2–23) chosen to give the reader an overview of the state of laser-assisted angioplasty. The technique is occasionally useful, but it does not offer much benefit in aggregate compared with standard guidewire recanalization. This article is interesting in its use of laser spectroscopy to monitor the angioplasty procedure. I don't think this addition has proved useful or efficacious, but it is an intriging investigational approach.—R.A. Clark, M.D.

Combination Balloon-Ultrasound Imaging Catheter for Percutaneous Transluminal Angioplasty: Validation of Imaging, Analysis of Recoil,

and Identification of Plaque Fracture

Isner JM, Rosenfield K, Losordo DW, Rose L, Langevin RE Jr, Razvi S, Kosowsky BD (Tufts Univ, Boston)
Circulation 84:739–754, 1991   2–24

Background.—Intravenous ultrasound (IVUS) appears to have promise as an adjunct to percutaneous revascularization. A combination balloon-ultrasound imaging catheter (BUIC) that combines diagnostic and therapeutic functions in a single catheter was assessed in patients undergoing percutaneous transluminal angioplasty (PTA).

Methods.—The BUIC included a 20-MHz ultrasound transducer inside an angioplasty balloon, located halfway between its proximal and distal ends. This device was used to perform PTA in 10 patients with peripheral vascular disease. Before and after this investigative procedure, each site was also evaluated by standard IVUS.

Results.—There was no significant difference in cross-sectional area or luminal diameter as measured by BUIC and IVUS before PTA. After PTA, there was still no significant difference in cross-sectional area as measured by the 2 techniques, and luminal diameter measurements were identical. When measured immediately after deflation, cross-sectional area and luminal diameter were significantly smaller than the area of the balloon and diameter at full inflation; this suggested significant elastic recoil of the site. Percent recoil was 28.6% in the 9 evaluable patients, including 1 patient with a recoil of 61%. Six patients had plaque fractures identified on-line, all of which were initiated at inflation pressures of 2 atm or less.

Conclusion.—In vivo catheter-based IVUS imaging through an angioplasty balloon appears to be feasible and potentially useful in humans. This technique can allow quantitative and qualitative analyses of changes in the lumen, plaque, and vessel wall before, during, and after PTA. The ability to recognize plaque fracture on-line could allow modification of the procedure to prevent a flow-limiting dissection.

▶ Abstract 2–23 attempted to use laser spectroscopy to monitor balloon angioplasty results. This abstract has taken another novel approach to determine the endpoint of balloon dilatation and plaque fracture. It describes the use of a combination angioplasty balloon and an intravascular ultrasound device to permit sonographic imaging of the lumen immediately after balloon deflation. Plaque, plaque fracture, thrombus, and arterial recoil can be detected, and quantitative measurements of lumen can be made with the balloon catheter still in place. This approach is very interesting and holds promise for efficient sonographic monitoring of balloon angioplasty.—R.A. Clark, M.D.

Segmentally Enclosed Thrombolysis in Percutaneous Transluminal Angioplasty for Femoropopliteal Occlusions: A Report From a Pilot Study

Jørgensen B, Tønnesen KH, Nielsen JD, Holstein P, Bülow J, Jørgensen M, Andersen E (Bispebjerg Hospital, Univ of Copenhagen, Copenhagen, Denmark; Medi-Tech, Jyllinge, Denmark)
Cardiovasc Intervent Radiol 14:293–298, 1991   2–25

Background.—Femoropopliteal lesions present a particular challenge to the surgeon performing percutaneous transluminal angioplasty (PTA). Recurrences are common during the first year, and long-term patency rates vary from 26% to 58%. A double-balloon catheter should maintain

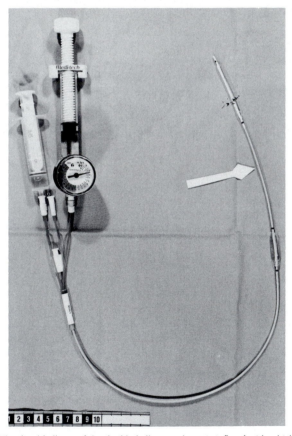

Fig 2–19.—The distal balloon of the double-balloon catheter is inflated with a high-pressure device for dilatation purposes. The proximal balloon inflated with a syringe is used during enclosure only. There is 1 connection for each of the balloons, 1 for the central lumen, and 1 for the sideport centered between the balloons (*arrow*). (Courtesy of Jørgensen B, Tønnesen KH, Nielsen JD, et al: *Cardiovasc Intervent Radiol* 14:293–298, 1991.)

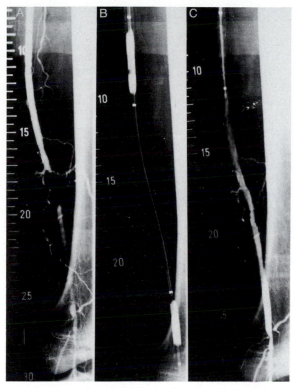

Fig 2–20.—The steps in segmentally enclosed thrombolysis. **A**, a 2-cm occlusion with possible adjacent thrombus before recanalization. **B**, after recanalization and dilatation, the double-balloon catheter is placed with a balloon at each end of the relevant segment. The balloons are inflated, and enclosed thrombolysis is continuing. **C**, completion arteriogram after segmentally enclosed thrombolysis. The tip of the double balloon is at the upper end of the arteriogram. (Courtesy of Jørgensen G, Tønnesen KH, Nielsen JD, et al: *Cardiovasc Intervent Radiol* 14:293–298, 1991.)

recombinant tissue plasminogen activator (rt-PA) and heparin within the vascular segment between the balloons for a short period of time. This principle of segmentally enclosed thrombolysis (SET) should prevent subsequent coagulopathy.

Methods.—Fifteen women and 19 men underwent PTA and SET for chronic femoropopliteal occlusions. The procedures were performed for intermittent claudication, rest pain, or gangrene. Twenty-three patients had critical limb ischemia. Patients received 500 mg of acetylsalicylic acid twice daily beginning 3 days before PTA and continuing indefinitely thereafter. Surgeons obtained segmental enclosure with a double-balloon catheter (Fig 2–19). For dilation purposes, the distal balloon was inflated with a high-pressure device. The proximal balloon was inflated with a syringe and used during enclosure only. The interballoon distance included possible thrombi adjacent to the occlusion (Fig 2–20). After the dilated segment was sealed off, 1 mg/mL of rt-PA and 200 IU/mL of heparin were injected between the balloons. After 30 minutes, the catheter was removed. Heparin treatment was maintained for 24 hours.

Results.—Alpha-2-Antiplasmin was initially reduced by 13%. Two hours after SET, it had normalized, suggesting that only small amounts of free plasmin were liberated during thrombolysis. There were no clinically relevant changes in plasma fibrinogen. There were 2 puncture site hemorrhages, but these did not coincide with the coagulopathy induced by SET. At 1 year, patency was 80%. Only 9% of patients experienced early rethrombosis. In contrast, 41% of patients who underwent standard PTA in a previous study experienced rethrombosis.

Conclusion.—The procedure under study combined recanalization, dilation, and thrombolysis. The procedure was quick, and it required no more staff or repeated arteriography than conventional PTA. Use of the double-balloon catheter and SET may allow treatment of chronic occlusions that might not be amenable to other procedures.

▶ There are as many ways to do direct thrombolysis as there are interventional radiologists. This report offers us *adjuvant* thrombolysis, to borrow a term from our oncology colleagues. The concept advanced here is that for arterial occlusions, prophylactic thrombolysis, given for 30 minutes at the angioplasty site, and contained at the site between 2 balloons, will reduce the incidence of early rethrombosis. The authors make a strong case for their thesis, because their rethrombosis rate with adjuvant thrombolysis was significantly less than their own historic rate without thrombolysis. The main limitation of their study is the lack of prospective randomization. However, their results are encouraging, and further study is warranted.—R.A. Clark, M.D.

Embolization/Infusion Therapy

Transcatheter Occlusion of Pulmonary Arterial Circulation and Collateral Supply: Failures, Incidents, and Complications

Remy-Jardin M, Wattinne L, Remy J (Hôpital Calmette, Lille, France)
Radiology 180:699–705, 1991   2–26

Background.—Definitive treatment of vascular lesions can be achieved by transcatheter occlusion of the pulmonary arterial circulation. There have been few reports of damage to the pulmonary parenchyma during surgery or angiography. Failures and complications of embolotherapy or occlusion of the pulmonary arterial circulation were reviewed.

Patients.—The experience included 45 patients. All had occlusion of the pulmonary arterial branches with steel coils; 19 had pulmonary arteriovenous malformations, 17 had hemoptysis orginating from the pulmonary artery (PA), and 1 had a massive parenchymal shunt. In 8 patients with hemoptysis and systemic-to-pulmonary arterial antegrade shunt resulting from chronic thromboembolism, the bronchial artery supply to the lungs was embolized with small particles.

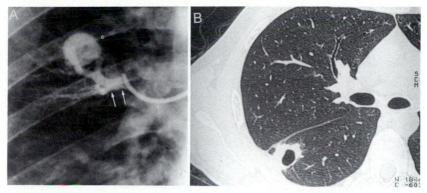

Fig 2–21.—Pulmonary infarction 1 month after vaso-occlusion of a peripheral pulmonary arteriovenous malformation in the apical segment of the right lower lobe. **A,** selective angiogram (anteroposterior view) shows the lateral subsegmental artery of the apical segment of the right lower lobe. Coils were deposited in the common trunk (*arrows*) for the 2 feeding arteries of the aneurysm and a few peripheral branches to the normal lung. **B,** a CT scan of the apical segment of the right lower lobe 4 months later shows pulmonary infarction demonstrated by a pleural-based and excavated nodule in the lateral subsegment associated with homolateral chest pain. (Courtesy of Remy-Jardin M, Wattinne L, Remy J: *Radiology* 180:699–705, 1991.)

Findings.—There were several examples of asymptomatic incidents, including catheterization failures, vascular damage, partial occlusion, partial thrombus recanalization, ectopic coil deposition, and delayed bacterial contamination of the thrombus. A few patients had transient clinical and radiologic signs of pulmonary infarction; this never occurred in patients undergoing complete occlusion of the main right or left PA, inferior right or left PA, or segmental branches, only after complete occlusion of the PA and bronchial artery embolization.

Discussion.—The severity of complications depends on the presence or absence of communications between the PAs and systemic arterial circulation. Parenchymal effects are more likely to be detected on CT than on chest radiography (Fig 2–21).

▶ Most of us do not see many patients who require occlusion of PAs. Therefore, when we see such a patient, we need the experience of those who have accumulated a large experience. This report nicely outlines the spectrum of findings one may encounter with this procedure.—R.A. Clark, M.D.

Intraperitoneal Hemorrhage From Hepatocellular Carcinoma: Emergency Chemoembolization or Embolization

Okazaki M, Higashihara H, Koganemaru F, Nakamura T, Kitsuki H, Hoashi T, Makuuchi M (Fukuoka University, Fukuoka, Japan; Shinsyu University Medicine, Nagano, Japan)

Radiology 180:647–651, 1991   2–27

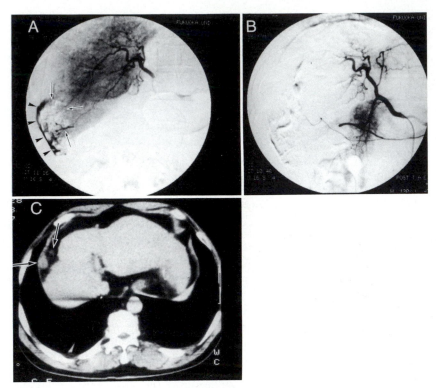

Fig 2–22.—In a patient without tumor thrombus in the portal vein (serum total bilirubin level, 1 mg/dL), extravasation of contrast material is shown. **A,** right hepatic arteriogram shows some tumor vessels, avascular areas (*arrows*), and linear extravasation of contrast material in the subcapsular area (*arrowheads*). **B,** hepatic arteriogram obtained after embolization with Lipiodol and gelatin sponge particles reveals occlusion of the right hepatic artery and retention of Lipiodol and contrast material in the subcapsular space. **C,** a CT scan obtained 2 months after embolization shows newly developed soft tissue masses around the liver (*arrows*). Exploratory laparotomy was performed after the patient's condition stabilized. Intraperitoneal dissemination was verified at histologic examination, and hepatectomy was not done. The patient died of peritonitis carcinomatosa 153 days after embolization. (Courtesy of Okazaki M, Higashihara H, Koganemaru F, et al: *Radiology* 180:647–651, 1991.)

Background.—Spontaneous hemorrhage of hepatocellular carcinoma (HCC) is a critical and life-threatening condition for which aggressive surgical management carries a high mortality. Emergency embolization was done in 38 patients with massive spontaneous bleeding from HCC.

Patients.—The patients all had emergency embolization with or without administration of anticancer drug and iodized oil over an 8-year period. Twenty-four patients, comprising group A, had a serum total bilirubin value of 3 mg/dL or less, and 14, comprising group B, had a serum bilirubin level greater than 3 mg/dL before embolization. After the clinical diagnosis was made, each patient had arterial portogaphy to evaluate the presence of a tumor thrombus, followed by hepatic arteriography and embolization (Fig 2–22).

Outcome.—Hemostasis was obtained in all patients. Group A patients survived a mean of 165 days compared with 13 days for group B; the correlation between bilirubin level and prognosis was significant. Presence of a tumor thrombus in the portal vein was associated with a poor prognosis, but prognosis was no different for patients with tumor thrombus vs. those without.

Conclusion.—In patients with intraperitoneal hemorrhage resulting from HCC, emergency embolization appears to be an effective treatment. Prognosis depends on the patient's serum bilirubin level before embolization.

▶ I admit that this is a rare occurrence and most radiologists will never encounter this entity; but it's a pet topic of mine because I have treated 2 such patients with embolization. Give me a break and let me have this one! I hope the article is as interesting to you as it was to me.—R.A. Clark, M.D.

Abdominal Venous Intervention and Imaging

Diagnosis of Portal Vein Thrombosis: Value of Color Doppler Imaging
Tessler FN, Gehring BJ, Gomes AS, Perrella RR, Ragavendra N, Busuttil RW, Grant EG (Univ of California, Los Angeles)
AJR 157:293–296, 1991   2–28

Background.—Real-time or duplex Doppler sonography can be used to make a noninvasive diagnosis of portal vein thrombosis (PVT). Color Doppler imaging (CDI) may be able to overcome some of the limitations of gray-scale and duplex Doppler. The accuracy of CDI in diagnosing PVT was assessed.

Methods.—During a 2-year period, 215 patients underwent CDI evaluation of the hepatic vasculature. If CDI could not demonstrate flow, duplex Doppler of the portal vein was done. The final study group comprised 75 patients who had angiographic or surgical confirmation of portal vein patency or thrombosis. On CDI, the sole criterion for diagnosing PVT was absence of color within the portal vein.

Results.—Sonographic and angiographic or surgical findings agreed in 69 patients, 8 of whom had PVT. In 1 case, a vein shown to be patent on sonography was thrombosed at surgery; in 5 cases, veins shown to be thrombosed on sonography were patent at angiography or surgery. Sensitivity was 89%, specificity 92%, and accuracy 92%. The false negative rate was .11, the negative predictive value was .98, and the positive predictive value was .62.

Conclusion.—Color Doppler imaging is useful in assessment of portal vein patency. No further study is needed if sonography shows a patent vein, but confirmatory studies are needed if thrombosis is indicated.

Most errors with DCI appear to occur in patients with patent vessels but sluggish flow.

▶ The best modality for the evaluation of abdominal venous thrombosis is dictated by local conditions (i.e., availability and expertise). This article offers a rational approach to the work-up: start with color Doppler sonography. If patency is shown, stop. If flow cannot be demonstrated, then the study is equivocal and further evaluation is necessary. The next study is dictated by local conditions. Magnetic resonance imaging is a good second-line technique (1), as are CT and angiography.—R.A. Clark, M.D.

Reference

1. Martinoli C, et al: *J Comput Assist Tomogr* 16:226, 1992.

Diagnosis of Abdominal Venous Thrombosis by Means of Spin-Echo and Gradient-Echo MR Imaging: Analysis With Receiver Operating Characteristic Curves

Arrivé L, Menu Y, Dessarts I, Dubray B, Vullierme M-P, Vilgrain V, Najmark D, Nahum H (Hôpital Beaujon, Clichy, France; Hôpital Saint-Louis, Paris, France)
Radiology 181:661–668, 1991   2–29

Objective.—The accuracy of spin-echo (SE) and gradient-echo (GRE) MRI for diagnosing abdominal venous thrombosis was studied in 72 patients clinically suspected of having thrombosis.

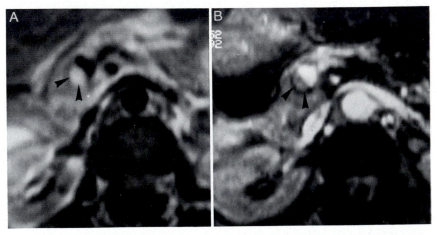

Fig 2–23.—Magnetic resonance images of nonobstructing thrombus of the superior mesenteric vein. **A,** SE (600/20) image shows blood clot thrombus (*arrowheads*) with high signal intensity. **B,** GRE (60/19) image shows clot (*arrowheads*) with intermediate signal intensity. (Courtesy of Arrivé L, Menu Y, Dessarts I, et al: *Radiology* 181:661–668, 1991.)

Methods.—Images of 292 abdominal veins were reviewed in a blinded manner by 3 radiologists using 7 levels of confidence. Corroborative studies demonstrated thrombosis in 95 instances. Both SE and GRE images were acquired in all patients.

Results.—Blood clot thrombus (Fig 2–23) was present in 86 vessels, and tumor thrombus was present in 9 others. Analysis of receiver operating characteristic curves showed that SE images alone were 76% sensitive at a specificity of 90% and 63% sensitive at a specificity of 95%. With GRE images alone, the sensitivities were 74% and 58%, respectively. Combining the 2 types of image yielded sensitivities of 88% at 90% specificity, and 82% at 95% specificity.

Conclusion.—Combining SE and GRE imaging can help determine whether confusing patterns of intravascular signal intensity represent a patent or thrombosed vessel. The MR approach remains limited in assessing small vascular structures because of suboptimal spatial resolution.

▶ The combination of SE and GRE MRI increases the accuracy of the diagnosis of abdominal venous thrombosis; however, remember that sonography and CT are also valid techniques. Should MRI be the primary imaging modality? I don't know, and there are no data available to answer the question. However, it seems reasonable to start with sonography or CT and to use MRI as a problem-solving modality.—R.A. Clark, M.D.

MR Angiography in Portal Hypertension: Detection of Varices and Imaging Techniques

Johnson CD, Ehman RL, Rakela J, Ilstrup DM (Mayo Clinic and Found, Rochester, Minn)
J Comput Assist Tomogr 15:578–584, 1991   2–30

Background.—The ability of MRI to show vascular structures has been used to image flowing blood, detect vascular disease, and depict flow direction. The use of MRI to detect upper abdominal varices noninvasively could aid in diagnosing and managing patients with chronic liver disease. The use of time-of-flight MR angiography in detecting varices was compared with conventional portography and endoscopy in patients with chronic liver disease. Magnetic resonance tomographic images were also compared with projection angiograms.

Methods.—Findings on conventional arterial portography, which is considered the gold standard, were compared with MR findings in 8 patients. The varices were graded by size and extent on a scale of 0–3.

Findings.—Splenic varices were detected by MRI in all patients, but the varices were scored larger on portography in 6 of 11 comparisons. All esophageal and left gastric varices were identified by MRI, and left gastric varices were rated within 1 grade of those seen at portography (Fig 2–24). In 26 patients examined with upper endoscopy, MR images

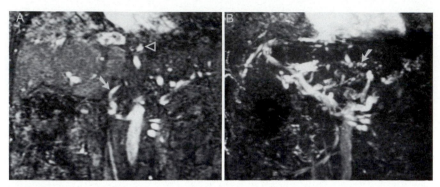

Fig 2–24.—A, esophageal varices: comparison of tomographic and projection images. Tomographic coronal image demonstrates left gastric (*arrow*) and esophageal varices (*arrowhead*). **B,** projection image demonstrates left gastric varices (*arrow*), but the presence of esophageal varices is equivocal. Differences in inspiratory effort between single-slice images may account for poorer visualization on projection angiogram. (Courtesy of Johnson CD, Ehman RL, Rakela J, et al: *J Comput Assist Tomogr* 15:578–584, 1991.)

rated varices significantly larger than endoscopy in 8 of 12 comparisons. In 2 patients, varices not seen endoscopically were detected by MRI. Portography visualized extraperitoneal varices in only 1 patient, whereas MRI identified the extraperitoneal varices in 6 of 8 patients. Axial and coronal MRI detected varices equally well. There were no significant differences when tomographic images were compared with projection images.

Conclusion.—Using limited-flip-angle, gradient-refocused acquisitions, MRI is a simple, accurate means of demonstrating varices in patients with portal hypertension. The tomographic single-slice images were generally as good as projection images except in the visualization of extraperitoneal varices. The extraperitoneal varices were better seen on projection axial images than on single-slice axial images, although the difference was not statistically significant.

▶ Abstracts 2–28 and 2–29 addressed the evaluation of portal vein thrombosis. This report evaluates MR angiography in portal hypertension. It appears that any MRI technique is adequate to detect varices: axial, coronal, tomographic, or projection images. I am a believer in MRI for this purpose. The global view that MRI provides makes this evaluation much easier than using any other modality.—R.A. Clark, M.D.

Percutaneous Transjugular Portosystemic Shunt
Zemel G, Katzen BT, Becker GJ, Benenati JF, Sallee S (Baptist Hosp of Miami, Miami)
JAMA 266:390–393, 1991   2–31

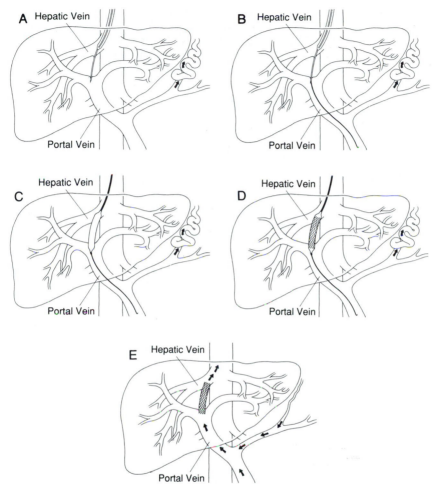

Fig 2–25.—**A,** modified Ross needle is advanced from an hepatic to a portal vein via a transjugular approach (*arrows* indicate hepatofugal flow in an enlarged coronary vein). **B,** guidewire is advanced through the needle into the superior mesenteric vein. **C,** an 8-mm angioplasty balloon is advanced over the guidewire and expanded across the hepatic parenchymal tract. **D,** Palmaz stent, mounted on an 8-mm angioplasty balloon, is expanded to bridge hepatic and portal veins. **E,** final appearance of stent resulting in an intrahepatic shunt from portal to hepatic vein. Coronary vein is smaller and demonstrates a return to hepatopetal flow. (Courtesy of Zemel G, Katzen BT, Becker GJ, et al: *JAMA* 266:390–393, 1991.)

Introduction.—Surgical portosystemic shunts effectively prevent rebleeding in variceal hemorrhage secondary to portal hypertension, but they are associated with a high rate of morbidity and mortality. Researchers evaluated a new technique—the Palmax balloon expandable stent—for creation of a transjugular intrahepatic portosystemic shunt (TIPS).

Patients.—During a 9-month period, 8 patients with cirrhosis received a TIPS (Fig 2–25) for control of hemorrhage. Bleeding occurred in 7 patients from esophageal varices and in the remaining patient from hemorrhoids. Shunt patency and recurrent variceal hemorrhage were assessed during a mean follow-up period of 5 months.

Results.—The procedures were performed without technical failure and achieved brisk flow in the shunt and complete decompression of the gastroesophageal varices. Immediately after placement, the average pressure gradient was reduced from a mean of 36 to 11 mm Hg. Liver functions showed no deterioration during the first 4 months. All shunts remained patent through the follow-up period, although the patient with hemorrhoidal bleeding required shunt enlargement by balloon angioplasty.

Conclusion.—This early experience with TIPS suggests that the procedure is an effective means of portal decompression for the treatment of variceal hemorrhage. In patients with end stage liver disease, use of a TIPS may allow time for a suitable donor to be found.

▶ The systemic decompression of portal hypertension has traditionally been done surgically with various operative shunt procedures. Surgical morbidity and mortality can be significant, depending on the procedure done and patient selection. A host of alternative procedures have been evaluated, including endoscopic sclerotherapy and angiographic embolization, but surgical decompression has the lowest frequencies of rebleeding. Charles Dotter described the approach to nonsurgical intrahepatic decompression as far back as 1969, but shunt patency could not be maintained. The current crop of vascular stents (e.g., Wallstent and Palmaz) has generated renewed interest in this technique, such as the Ring et al. (1) article describing the use of the Wallstent in the same procedure. This article describes encouraging results using the Palmaz stent. The results are preliminary, however, with mean follow-up less than 1 year. Nevertheless, the technique has great promise for management of this difficult disease.—R.A. Clark, M.D.

Reference

1. Ring EJ, et al: *Ann Intern Med* 116:304, 1992.

Gastrointestinal Intervention and Imaging

Liver Metastases: Results of Percutaneous Ethanol Injection in 14 Patients
Livraghi T, Vettori C, Lazzaroni S (Ospedale Civile, Milan, Italy; Ospedale Briolini, Gazzaniga, Italy)
Radiology 179:709–712, 1991   2–32

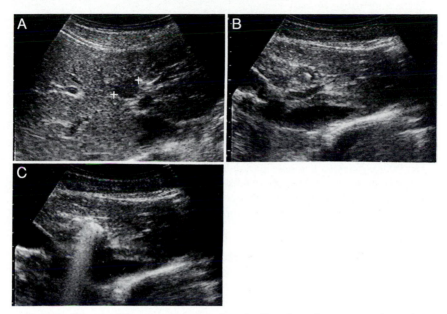

Fig 2–26.—Transverse US sections through the liver. **A,** solitary, hypoechoic metastasis (*cursors*), 1.8 cm in diameter, from bronchial carcinoid before the treatment. **B,** the tip of the needle is recognizable as it extends into the lesion before the ethanol injection. **C,** just after the injection, the lesion is completely perfused and appears as a highly hyperechoic area. (Courtesy of Livraghi T, Vettori C, Lazzaroni S: *Radiology* 179:709–712, 1991.)

Background.—High 3-year survival rates have been reported for the therapeutic use of percutaneous ethanol injection (PEI) under ultrasound (US) guidance in treating small hepatic cell carcinoma (HCC). Treatment with PEI may be an appropriate therapeutic option because it allows selective treatment of a localized tumor and does not spread outside the tumor (Fig 2–26). The therapeutic efficacy of PEI was assessed in liver metastases of different origins in a series of 14 patients.

Methods.—The 14 patients had 21 liver metastases 1.0 to 3.8 cm in diameter. The primary cancer was colorectal adenocarcinoma in 7 patients, adenocarcinoma of the stomach in 4 patients, abdominal leiomyosarcoma in 1 patient, gastrinoma of unknown origin in 1 patient, and bronchial carcinoid in 1 patient. Percutaneous ethanol injection under US guidance was performed in the outpatient department. Therapeutic efficacy was indicated by US, CT, fine-needle biopsy, and serologic markers.

Results.—There were no complications in a total of 175 treatment sessions. Complete response was obtained in 11 tumors, of which 9 were less than 2 cm in diameter, and in 4 lesions from endocrine metastases. The patients had a maximum, recurrence-free follow-up of 38 months and carcinoembryonic antigen values decreased in all patients but 1 for a 2–6 month period.

Conclusion.—The use of PEI was safe in the treatment of HCC, despite the higher risk of bleeding because of superimposed cirrhosis. All the endocrine metastases achieved complete remission, probably because of small size, slow growth, and likely, hypervascularity. The applicability of PEI, a localized treatment, is obviously limited in metastatic disease. The primary indications for PEI are single, metachronous, nonoperable metastasis of adenocarcinoma and endocrine metastases.

▶ This article is 1 of several describing the usefulness of this technique. However, I cannot find many suitable patients for the procedure. Patients with multiple lesions are not candidates; a single, metachronous, nonoperable metastasis is ideal. In many institutions, almost all single lesions are operable, and for those patients whose conditions are not operable, their medical conditions make ethanol treatment superfluous.—R.A. Clark, M.D.

Ultrasound-Guided Hepatic Cryosurgery in the Treatment of Metastatic Colon Carcinoma: Preliminary Results
Onik G, Rubinsky B, Zemel R, Weaver L, Diamond D, Cobb C, Porterfield B (Presbyterian-Univ Hosp, Pittsburgh; Univ of California, Berkeley; Allegheny Gen Hosp, Pittsburgh)
Cancer 67:901–907, 1991   2–33

Background.—Colorectal carcinoma has a preferential spread to the liver attributable to the portal venous anatomy. Surgical resection is the

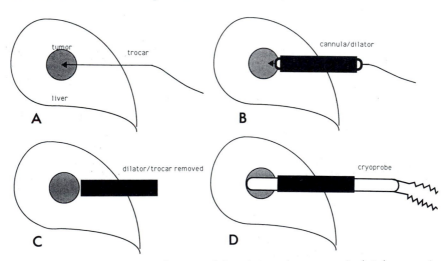

Fig 2–27.—**A,** diagram showing the steps and the technique of cryosurgery. A relatively atraumatic trocar is first placed into the tumor, guided by intraoperative ultrasound. The trocar is small enough that if a mistake occurs in the placement, it can be removed and replaced without causing major damage. **B,** a larger cannula and dilator is placed over the trocar. **C,** the dilator and trocar are removed, leaving the cannula down to the surface of the tumor. **D,** the cryoprobe is placed through the cannula into the tumor. (Courtesy of Onik G, Rubinsky B, Zemel R, et al: *Cancer* 67:901–907, 1991.)

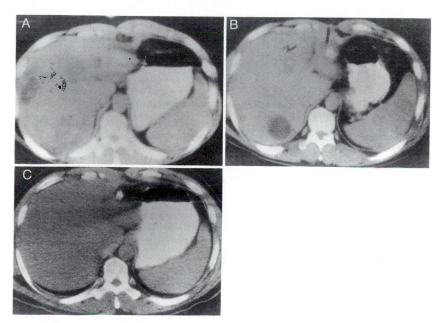

Fig 2–28.—A patient with 7 different metastatic lesions from colon carcinoma to the liver. **A,** immediately after cryosurgey, multiple lesions can be seen. High-density regions within each lesion represent intraparenchymal hemorrhage. **B,** 3 months after cryosurgery, lesions are smaller with low-density areas. **C,** 1 year after cryosurgery, no lesions are visible. (Courtesy of Onik G, Rubinsky B, Zemel R, et al: *Cancer* 67:901–907, 1991.)

only modality to offer long-term, disease-free survival in up to 30% of patients, but an estimated 25% or less of patients with hepatic metastasis are candidates for resection. Cryosurgery, the in situ freezing of cancer, may be advantageous in treating multiple hepatic lobes because it is a focal treatment that sacrifices less normal tissue than surgical resection. It could also be used to treat tumors in difficult locations because it does not affect large vessels.

Methods.—Eighteen patients with unresectable metastatic colon carcinoma confined to the liver were treated with cryosurgery coupled with intraoperative ultrasound to place the cryoprobes and monitor the freezing process (Fig 2–27). After cryosurgery, frozen tumors are left in situ to be reabsorbed.

Results.—The number of lesions frozen in each patient ranged from 1 to 12, with a mean of 6 lesions. Fourteen patients had bilobar disease, 3 had previous right lobectomies with recurrences in their remaining left lobes before cryosurgery, and 1 had unilobar disease. After cryosurgery, 4 patients were in complete remission at a mean follow-up of 28.8 months (Fig 2–28). Of the remaining 14 patients, 4 were not adequately treated at the time of cryosurgery, and 10 had recurrence of the disease. The mean survival of the 14 patients with recurrence was 21.4 months. Two of 14 patients are still alive.

Conclusion.—Ultrasound-guided hepatic cryosurgery was a safe and effective treatment for metastatic colon carcinoma to the liver, including bilobar and multiple lesions. Compared with present nonsurgical treatments for this disease, cryosurgery offered a possibility of complete remission, but its use should be reserved for patients with inoperable lesions.

▶ This approach to hepatic meatastases makes more sense to me than ethanol injection. It is done as an operative procedure, guided by sonography, in patients whose conditions would otherwise be inoperable. However, the concept of focal treatment for diffuse liver disease is problematic and certainly requires more investigation, including trials with nonoperative treatment controls.—R.A. Clark, M.D.

Shock Wave Lithotripsy of Gallstones: Results and 12-Month Follow-Up in 174 Patients
Torres WE, Baumgartner BR, Nelson RC, Morris SJ (Crawford Long Hosp, Atlanta)
Radiology 179:699–701, 1991   2–34

Background.—There have been several reports of biliary extracorporeal shock-wave lithotripsy (ESWL) with a variety of techniques. Previously, there was no reported difference in stone clearance in patients treated with the adjuvant oral chemolytic agent ursodeoxycholic acid (UDCA) placebo at 6 months. The 12-month results in 174 patients were reported.

Methods.—Patients were randomized to receive UDCA or placebo for 6 months after ESWL. Forty patients were retreated for fragments larger than 5 mm at 6 weeks after ESWL.

Results.—At 6 months, the stone-free rate for patients with initially noncalcified stones was 31% for UDCA patients and 21% for placebo patients. At 12 months, the rates were 36% and 23%, respectively. Neither of these differences was significant. Among patients who originally had a single noncalcified gallstone measuring a maximum of 20 mm, 12-month stone-free rates were 60% in the UDCA group and 33% in the placebo group. The rate of stone clearance was greater for UDCA patients than placebo patients with noncalified stones measuring 11–20 mm.

Conclusion.—For some patients with gallstones, ESWL is a safe and effective treatment. Stone-free rates are higher in patients treated with UDCA than in those treated with placebo. Those patients with a single noncalcified stone measuring no more than 20 mm seem to benefit most from lithotripsy.

▶ This report, from 1 of the centers involved in the Dornier National Biliary Lithotripsy Study, provides us with the most recent data from this American trial. The overall stone-free rate at 1 year for all patients with noncalcified stones was only 36% with the addition of oral UDCA (it was only 23% without this added medication). Better results were obtained in certain patient subgroups, but even in the best subgroup (single noncalcified stone < 20 mm in diameter), only 60% were stone free at 1 year. Although lithotripsy remains an alternative therapy for certain patients, it does not appear to be the answer for most patients to the problem of cholelithiasis.—R.A. Clark, M.D.

Extracorporeal Shock Wave Treatment of Common Bile Duct Stones: Experience With Two Different Lithotriptors at a Single Institution
den Toom R, Nijs HGT, van Blankenstein M, Laméris JS, Schröder FH, Terpstra OT (Erasmus University, Rotterdam, The Netherlands)
Br J Surg 78:809–813, 1991   2–35

Background.—Extracorporeal shock-wave lithotripsy (ESWL) was first reported for the treatment of kidney stones in 1980. It is now the treatment of choice for urolithiasis, and its use has been expanded to include fragmentation of gallbladder stones, common bile duct stones, and pancreatic duct stones. The results of the use of a first- or second-generation lithotriptor in patients with retained common bile duct stones are reported.

Methods.—Sixty-two patients (mean age, 75 years) were treated with 2 different lithotriptors. A lithotriptor operated on the electrohydraulic principle with waterbath (Dornier HM-3) was used on 13 patients who were treated with the use of general anesthesia. A second-generation electromagnetic lithotriptor (Siemens Lithostar) was used on 49 patients. One Lithostar patient was treated using general anesthesia, 43 received analgesia and sedation, and 5 had no analgesia at all.

Results.—The patients treated with Lithostar had more sessions and needed more shock waves compared with patients treated with HM-3. Fragmentation was achieved in 86% of the patients treated with Lithostar and 100% of patients treated with HM-3. Of the 42 patients treated with Lithostar, 10 patients underwent common bile duct exploration without complications. The side effects included 11 patients with transient hematuria after treatment with the HM-3 and 1 patient in each group with a subcapsular hematoma of the right kidney. None of the patients had biliary complaints at follow-up.

Conclusion.—Extracorporeal shock-wave lithotripsy is a nonsurgical alternative to surgery when endoscopic extraction of common bile duct stones fails. Treatment of 62 patients with 2 different lithotriptors resulted in stone clearance in 79% of the patients who otherwise would have been subjected to surgical exploration.

▶ Extracorporeal shock wave lithotripsy is a useful alternative treatment for common bile duct stones, an entity that can resist effective therapy by many modalities. This report confirms that either of the 2 most commonly available types of machines is safe and effective; this approach is indicated at least for the patient who is considered for repeat surgery or catheter intervention.—R.A. Clark, M.D.

Malignant Biliary Obstruction: Percutaneous Use of Self-Expandable Stents
Laméris JS, Stoker J, Nijs HGT, Zonderland HM, Terpstra OT, van Blankenstein M, Schütte HE (Erasmus University, Rotterdam, The Netherlands)
Radiology 179:703–707, 1991   2–36

Background.—Percutaneous transhepatic biliary drainage (PTBD) provides palliative treatment in patients with inoperable malignant biliary obstruction not amenable to endoscopic drainage. The problem is that currently available endoprostheses used for internal drainage often become blocked by tumor or sludge, a particularly unfortunate occurrence in these patients whose life expectancy is very brief. Self-expandable metallic stents might combine the advantages of large stent diameter with those of a small delivery catheter.

Methods.—Investigators implanted 83 self-expandable stents in 30 men and 39 women with inoperable malignant biliary obstruction. Forty-one patients had common bile duct (CBD) obstruction, and 28 had hilar lesions. The stent diameter was 1 cm, and length varied from 3.5 to 10.5 cm. Balloon dilation of the stenosis before insertion of the stent was performed in the first 5 patients only. The patients underwent plain abdominal radiography to confirm the position and degree of stent expansion.

Results.—Of the 41 patients with CBD obstruction, 27 died a median 3.2 months after stent insertion. Two patients had recurrent cholangitis and jaundice within 12 months, and 1 underwent reintervention. One to 8 months after stent placement, 14 patients were alive without jaundice. Thirteen of 28 patients with hilar lesions died a median 4.3 months after stent placement. Fifteen were alive a median 8.1 months after placement, but 8 developed recurrent jaundice and cholangitis within 6 months. Stents malfunctioned because of tumor overgrowth at the proximal end in 5 patients, tumor ingrowth in 1 patient, and tumor overgrowth at the distal end in 2 patients. Five patients in this group underwent reintervention. Four patients had stent-related complications.

Conclusion.—Placement of self-expandable stents in patients with CBD and hilar obstructions is a safe and effective procedure for percutaneous drainage. The rate of reinterventions is similar to that reported for conventional endoprostheses.

▶ This may be the year of the stent. We have read articles of stent use in almost every vascular and nonvascular lumen. The biliary tract is appropriate for stenting, and this report describes typical results of the use of stents in malignant biliary obstruction. Reintervention was required in 18% of the patients in this series, which seems to be a higher rate than that required with Silastic endoprostheses. My own experience is similar in this respect. It may be time to begin a randomized trial comparing stents and endoprotheses for management of malignant obstruction, because short-term palliative management should minimize the need for reinterventions.—R.A. Clark, M.D.

Treatment of Critically Ill Patients With Sepsis of Unknown Causes: Value of Percutaneous Cholecystostomy
Lee JM, Saini S, Brink JA, Hahn PF, Simeone JF, Morrison MC, Rattner D, Mueller PR (Massachusetts Gen Hosp, Boston)
AJR 156:1163–1166, 1991   2–37

Background.—Diagnosing acute cholecystitis clinically, radiographyically, or by percutaneous aspiration of the gallbladder is difficult in critically ill patients with severe intercurrent illness. A trial of percutaneous cholecystostomy was therefore done in intensive care unit patients with persistent, unexplained sepsis after a complete clinical, laboratory, and radiologic search showed no other source of infection.

Patients.—Twenty-four patients with persistent high fevers despite antibiotic therapy were enrolled in the study. Eighteen patients had elevated white blood cell (WBC) counts, 11 had vague abdominal tenderness, and 15 had septic shock requiring vasopressors. All patients had distended, spherical gallbladders on sonography. Six had gallstones, 8 had wall thickening, 3 had pericholecystic fluid, and 4 had Murphy's sign. A senior abdominal surgeon evaluated all patients and agreed to a trial of percutaneous cholecystostomy.

Outcomes.—Fourteen patients, or 58%, responded to percutaneous cholecystostomy, as indicated by a decrease in the WBC count, defervescence, and the ability to be weaned off vasopressors. Four patients had positive bile cultures. Of the 10 patients who did not respond to treatment, 5 eventually died of unrelated causes. Three of the 10 were eventually found to have a respiratory source of infection. Catheter insertion was not associated with any complications. Two patients suffered bile leaks when the percutaneous cholecystostomy catheter was removed, but there were no serious consequences.

Conclusion.—A trial of percutaneous cholecystostomy in critically ill patients with persistent unexplained fever and a distended tense gallbladder on sonography appears to be worthwhile. These patients often have nonspecific clinical and sonographic findings of acute cholecystitis.

▶ In most of my comments throughout this section, I have tried to emphasize the need for controlled trials to answer clinical questions and have pleaded for data rather than technology to guide practice. In reality, we all know that this ideal can rarely be realized. Instead, we all make educated, informed practice decisions before all the data are in. This article is interesting in that it concerns a topic, all too common in clinical interventional radiology, that does not lend itself well to controlled trials or defined measurements of outcomes. One of the authors, Peter Mueller, M.D., told me of this concept several years ago, and he convinced me it was worth investigating. I have subsequently used percutaneous cholecystostomy as a last resort in patients with unexplained sepsis, despite unclear indications for the procedure. I have become a believer in this approach, and I am glad to see it finally reach print. Critically ill patients commonly develop enlarged gallbladders with sludge; this may become a source for infection. If one sees more ominous sonographic signs, the indications for the procedure are clearer. However, bile aspiration should be performed in the right clinical setting, even if the sonographic signs are equivocal.—R.A. Clark, M.D.

Intraarterial Portography With Gadopentetate Dimeglumine: Improved Liver-to-Lesion Contrast in MR Imaging
Pavone P, Giuliani S, Cardone G, Occhiato R, Di Renzi P, Petroni GA, Buoni C, Passariello R (University of L'Aquila, L'Aquila, Italy)
Radiology 179:693–697, 1991   2–38

Background.—Special CT techniques have improved liver-to-lesion contrast and tumor detection in evaluation of liver disease. Authors have

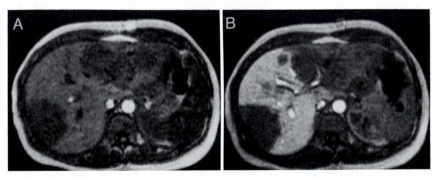

Fig 2–29.—Multiple metastases from colon carcinoma were seen in this female patient. **A**, precontrast GRE sequence shows the metastases with good intrinsic contrast. **B**, image acquired after intra-arterial injection of gadopentetate dimeglumine shows a significant increase in liver signal intensity, with no change in lesion signal intensity. Liver-to-lesion contrast is markedly improved. (Courtesy of Pavone P, Giuliani S, Cardone G, et al: *Radiology* 179:693–697, 1991.)

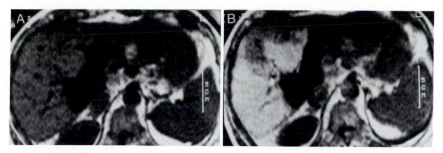

Fig 2–30.—Residual hydatid cyst at the hepatic hilum (RASE sequence). **A,** residual hypointense cyst is evident with excellent intrinsic contrast on the baseline image. There is no significant difference in signal intensity between the right and left lobes of the liver. **B,** postcontrast image displays very high signal intensity enhancement of the normal part of the liver. The contrast with the cystic lesion is increased. There is no increase in signal intensity of the left lobe, confirming the diagnosis of left portal-vein occlusion. Segmental branch involvement is also present, with hypointense areas in the anterior surface of the right side of the liver. L = left. (Courtesy of Pavone P, Giuliani S, Cardone G, et al: *Radiology* 179:693–697, 1991.)

reported that CT arterial portography (CTAP) is the most reliable procedure, with a sensitivity of up to 84%. In this study, investigators applied the CTAP technique to MRI to evaluate the liver-to-lesion contrast after intra-arterial injection of gadopentetate dimeglumine into the superior mesenteric artery.

Methods.—Nine women and 3 men with hepatic lesions received a low dose of injected gadopentetate dimeglumine during MRI with gradient-echo or rapid acquisition spin-echo images. In all cases, the images were acquired during the first passage of the contrast medium through the liver parenchyma.

Results.—In all but 1 case, there was a very strong increase in liver signal intensity on postcontrast images. However, the liver lesions did not show any significant improvement in signal intensity (Fig 2–29). Signal intensity was enhanced over the noise of the liver compared with that of focal lesions. Liver-to-lesion contrast evaluation, performed in 10 patients, showed a corresponding strong increase in contrast. Investigators found improved liver-lesion detection with visual evaluation. In 3 patients, previously undetectable lesions were well delineated. In 1 patient with an ambiguous angiographic evaluation, the postcontrast MR images showed no increase in signal intensity of the left lobe, confirming the diagnosis of left portal-vein occlusion (Fig 2–30). There were no allergic reactions to the medium.

Conclusion.—This report confirms the direct correlation between liver-to-lesion contrast and lesion detection. The findings justify further evaluation of a larger series of patients to determine the sensitivity of this procedure in detecting liver lesions and to compare the technique with CT.

▶ Computed tomography with intra-arterial portography enhancement has become a very useful and very sensitive method to detect small hapatic metastases. It should not be surprising, therefore, that MRI with intra-arterial portography enhancement would soon follow. The technical complexity of this approach remains daunting, and it is not likely to soon become an every-day procedure. However, it has some logic behind it and, given the results reported here, may deserve further study.—R.A. Clark, M.D.

Percutaneous Dilatation of Benign Biliary Strictures: Single-Session Therapy With General Anesthesia
Lee MJ, Mueller PR, Saini S, Hahn PF, Dawson SL (Massachusetts Gen Hosp, Boston)
AJR 157:1263–1266, 1991   2–39

Background.—Percutaneous biliary stricture dilatation (PBSD) is an important alternative to surgery for patients with benign biliary strictures, but it is an uncomfortable procedure that requires several sessions over up to 14 days. The use of general anesthesia to allow performance of PBSD in a single session was assessed.

Patients and Methods.—Fourteen patients were treated, 11 with anas-tomotic and 3 with iatrogenic strictures. Multiple strictures were present in 4 cases. Eleven patients underwent transhepatic cholangiography, and 3 had T-tube cholangiography to confirm the strictures. Eleven had transhepatic dilatation and three had T-tube dilatation. Balloons measur-ing 8 to 12 mm in diameter were manually inflated for 3 minutes for an average of 5 inflations per stricture. All patients had stenting catheters left across the stricture areas for a mean of 10 days.

Outcome.—The mean overall hospital stay was 5.7 days, 3.6 days for the 11 patients without complications vs. 13.7 days for the 3 patients with complications. Complications included cholangitis, liver hematoma, and hepatic artery pseudoaneurysm, the latter requiring embolization. Long-term patency was achieved in all patients but 1, for a mean of 3.2 years. The recurrent stricture was seen at 1.5 years.

Conclusion.—General anesthesia can be used to perform PBSD in a single session. The long-term patency rates are excellent, the hospital stay is shorter, and the procedure is pain free.

▶ Some years ago I might have quarreled with the conclusions of this study, that general anesthesia could be appropriate for biliary interventions. How-ever, after seeing many cases of biliary dilatation requiring repeated, often painful sessions, I think this may be an acceptable answer to a difficult prob-lem. Intrabiliary lidocaine is another technique that gives pain relief, but the effect is shorter acting. This report makes good sense.—R.A. Clark, M.D.

Invasive Treatment of Pancreatic Fluid Collections With Surgical and Nonsurgical Methods

Szentes MJ, Traverso LW, Kozarek RA, Freeny PC (Virginia Mason Med Ctr, Seattle)
Am J Surg 161:600–605, 1991

2–40

Introduction.—As many as 18% of patients with pancreatitis have pancreatic fluid collections, such as pseudocysts, peripancreatic accumulations, and intrapancreatic collections, develop. An experience with 75 patients having a total of 109 pancreatic fluid collections was reviewed. Those with phlegmon or necrosis at initial diagnosis were excluded. Sixty-five patients had 1 or more drainage procedures.

Outcome.—Fifty-nine patients were observed for a mean of 10 months after drainage. The majority of them were initially managed nonoperatively. Surgical drainage was performed in 34 patients. Morbidity rates were 20% to 25% for patients having invasive nonsurgical drainage, those having both invasive drainage and surgery, and those treated only by surgery. Rates of successful drainage exceeded 80% in all groups. The mortality rate was 8% in patients having invasive nonsurgical drainage and 5% in those having both forms of drainage. None of those having surgery alone died.

Conclusion.—Nonoperative invasive methods are an effective approach to treating pancreatic fluid collections, especially in patients whose fluid collections are unrelated to alcoholism or biliary tract disease and are symptomatic or persistent.

▶ Management of pancreatic fluid collections that require drainage can be a frustrating experience. Each case should be individualized, with guidelines as outlined in this article. No one approach will succeed in every patient; alternatives should be available based on patient need.—R.A. Clark, M.D.

Radiologic Placement of Peritoneal Dialysis Catheters: Preliminary Experience

Jacobs IG, Gray RR, Elliott DS, Grosman H (Oshawa General Hospital, Oshawa, Ont, Canada; Wellesley Hospital, Toronto, Ont, Canada)
Radiology 182:251–255, 1992

2–41

Background.—Surgical and percutaneous placement of catheters for peritoneal dialysis are the most popular placement methods, although neither has proved to be clearly superior. Initial experience with percutaneous placement under fluoroscopic guidance performed by radiologists was reviewed.

Patients and Procedure.—Forty-five catheters were placed in 32 patients with an average age 64 years during an 11-month period. Most were placed to provide permanent access for long-term peritoneal dialy-

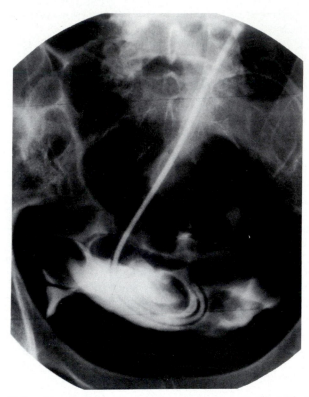

Fig 2–31.—Well-positioned catheter. (Courtesy of Jacobs IG, Gray RR, Elliott DS, et al: *Radiology* 182:251–255, 1992).

sis. The procedures were done under local anesthesia and with the use of a Hawkins needle. The first 15 catheters had a high rate of proximal cuff extrusion; thereafter, the deep cuff of each catheter was sutured to the rectus muscle or fascia. Beginning with the eighteenth insertion, a permanent bend, or "U" neck, was made between the 2 cuffs, which were then thickened.

Results.—Each catheter showed immediate, excellent function (Fig 2–31). There were 6 complications of placement, including bowel perforation associated with peritonitis in 1 patient. Delayed complications included a 20% incidence of cuff extrusion, a 20% incidence of obstruction, and a 7% incidence of peritonitis that required catheter removal (table).

Conclusion.—Percutaneous placement appears to be a safe alternative to surgical placement of peritoneal dialysis catheters. More experience is needed to determine the benefits of fluoroscopic guidance. Complications may be reduced by further refinements in the catheter itself.

Results of Catheter Placement

Complication or Result of Catheter Placement	No. of Episodes, Procedure, or Status	No. of Catheters Removed	Mean Time to Catheter Failure or Removal	Comments
Failure associated with catheter insertion	2	2	5 d	None
Proximal cuff extrusion	9	9	2 mo 5 d	None
Obstruction to flow	9*	6	28 d	3 catheters were manipulated back into the pelvis
Peritonitis	7[†]	3[‡]	2 mo 11 d[§]	None
Dialysate leak	3	0	12 d	All resolved with conservative therapy
Hernia	1	0	NA	Also has umbilical and bilateral inguinal hernias
Elective removal	9	9	2 mo 24 d	None
Functioning	16	0	3 mo 15 d[¶]	None

Abbreviation: NA, not applicable.

* One repositioned catheter eventually was removed because of recurrent malpositioning. Eight different catheters were repositioned or removed.

† Seven different catheters were associated with at least 1 episode of peritonitis, although some catheters were associated with up to 3 episodes.

‡ Catheters were removed because of infection unresponsive to conservative management.

§ Mean time to catheter removal.

¶ Mean time that catheters which were not removed have functioned.

(Courtesy of Jacobs IG, Gray RR, Elliott DS, et al: *Radiology* 182:251–255, 1992.)

▶ I have found the placement of peritoneal catheters in the absence of ascities to be very difficult and painful for the patient. Our own experience has been focused in the placement of catheters for peritoneal chemotherapy, yet the problems are similar. Although this article shows the feasibility of the procedure, more refined equipment and technique are necessary before this technique gains wide acceptance.—R.A. Clark, M.D.

Genitourinary Intervention and Imaging

Renal Carcinoma: Detection of Venous Extension With Gradient-Echo MR Imaging

Roubidoux MA, Dunnick NR, Sostman HD, Leder RA (Duke Univ, Durham, NC)
Radiology 182:269–272, 1992

2–42

Objective.—Intravascular growth of renal adenocarcinoma is a common finding. The only chance for cure is surgery, which relies on accurate delineation of the superior extent of the tumor. The use of limited flip-angle, gradient-recalled echo (GRE) MRI in the detection of venous extensions of renal adenocarcinoma was evaluated.

Methods.—The preoperative GRE MRI scans of 26 patients with renal adenocarcinoma were reviewed. All were specially referred for MR imag-

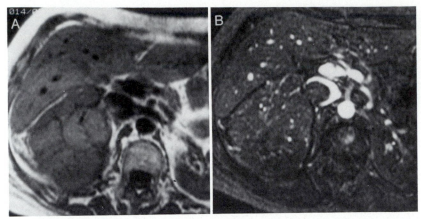

Fig 2–32.—Thrombus in inferior vena-cava is not as easily identified on (**A**) T₁-weighted image, as on (**B**) gradient-recalled acquisition in steady state image. (Courtesy of Roubidoux MA, Dunnick NR, Sostman HD, et al: *Radiology* 182:269–272, 1992.)

ing. Findings on MR imaging were compared to the patients' surgical and pathologic findings.

Results.—The GRE MRI technique correctly identified 13 of 13 cases of vena cava thrombus (Fig 2-32). Four of 5 patients who had intrahepatic caval extension into the right atrium were correctly identified using MRI. Renal vein thrombus was identified in 23 of 26 cases.

Conclusion.—With the use of GRE MRI sequences, vascular structures in patients with renal adenocarcinoma can be accurately assessed for surgical planning. The use of spin-echo and gradient-recalled acquisition in the steady state allows precise localization and more confident location of thrombi. A prospective study to determine whether GRE imaging alone is sufficient to detect thrombi may be useful.

▶ The accurate assessment of renal tumor extension to the renal vein and vena cava is important preoperative information. This study confirms our clinical experiences that MRI is an excellent method for venous imaging. However, MRI probably remains a second-line modality reserved for those cases with equivocal sonography or CT. See also the article by Kallamn et al. (1).—R.A. Clark, M.D.

Reference

1. Kallman DA, et al: *J Comput Assist Tomogr* 16:240, 1992.

Transurethral Balloon Dilatation of the Prostatic Urethra: Effectiveness in Highly Selected Patients With Prostatism
Wasserman NF, Reddy PK, Zhang G, Kapoor DA, Berg P (Dept of VA Med

Ctr, Minneapolis)
AJR 157:509–512, 1991

2–43

Background.—Some patients with moderately severe benign prostatic hyperplasia (BPH) are successfully treated with transurethral balloon catheter dilatation of the prostate (TUDP). Because it is an inexpensive and relatively low-risk treatment, some practitioners might apply TUDP nonselectively as first treatment for symptoms of bladder outlet obstruction; however, more careful selection of patients might lead to greater clinical improvement and better use of the technique for those who would most benefit.

Methods.—Investigators separated 91 patients with signs and symptoms of prostatism attributable to BPH into 2 groups. Group 1 included 42 patients with an initial mean symptom score of 16.8, residual urine of 249 mL, a maximal flow rate of 7.9 mL/sec, and nomogram of maximal flow rate of −1.5. The 49 patients in group 2 were less symptomatic, with an initial mean symptom score of 14.5, residual urine of 105 mL, maximal flow rate of 10.7 mL/sec, and nomogram of maximal flow rate of −.8. These differences were significant, but there was no significant difference in either mean age or mean prostate size between groups. Investigators performed TUDP under local anesthesia or intravenous sedation. Either a single- or double-balloon catheter was used. Follow-up was 6–48 months. The follow-up procedures included repeat symptom scoring, uroflometry, and measurement of residual urine.

Results.—At mean follow-up of 22 months, 80% of patients in group 2 had improved symptom scores, whereas only 43% of patients in group 1 had improved symptom scores (table). In both groups, improvement in symptom scores was significant.

Outcome of Transurethral Balloon Dilatation of the Prostate in 2 Groups of Patients With Benign Prostatic Hyperplasia

Outcome	No. (%)		
	Group 1	Group 2	Total
Improved	18 (43)	39 (80)	57 (63)
Unimproved			
Prostatectomy	15	5	20
Retention	5	1	6
Worse symptom score	1	4	5
Stable symptom score	2	0	2
Stent	1	0	1
Subtotal	24 (57)	10 (20)	34 (37)
Total	42	49	91

Patients in group 1 had more severe urethral obstruction than did those in group 2. The follow-ups ranged from 6 to 48 months (mean, 22 months).
(Courtesy of Wasserman NF, Reddy PK, Zhang G, et al: *AJR* 157:509–512, 1991.)

Conclusion.—The TUDP procedure appears to be more effective in patients with less severe symptoms and with less pronounced signs of obstruction than in patients with more marked prostatism. The best results are likely to occur in patients with symptom scores less than 20 who have prostates weighing less than 40 g, scant median-lobe hyperplasia, and residual urine less than 150 mL or nomogram of Q_{max} below -2.

▶ This study is very useful, because it identifies a subset of patients who are likely to respond to balloon dilatation of the urethra (i.e., those with more moderate symptoms and less marked signs of obstruction). This approach then makes efficacious sense, with less symptomatic patients treated with dilatation, and those who progress to or have more advanced disease treated with transurethral resection.—R.A..Clark, M.D.

Impassable Ureteral Strictures: Management With Percutaneous Ureteroneocystostomy
Cornud FE, Casanova J-MP, Bonnel DH, Helenon OR, Hanna SM, Chretien YR, Dufour BF, Moreau J-FM (Hôpital Necker, Paris, France)
Radiology 180:451–454, 1991   2–44

Background and Methods.—In the management of ureteral stenoses, stent placement by conventional methods is precluded if the ureter is totally obstructed or otherwise not negotiable by a guidewire. Investigators evaluated a technique for treatment of impassable ureteral stenoses that uses electrocautery to establish a neotract between the ureter and the bladder or ileal loop. This procedure was performed in 16 of 227 patients scheduled for percutaneous placement of a ureteral stent who had impassable stenoses. Eight stenoses were benign, and 8 were caused by malignant retroperitoneal neoplasms. Angioplasty was used for dilation of the tract for placement of the double-J stent.

Results.—Surgeons established neotracts and placed stents in all 16 patients (Fig 2–33). In 2 patients, the whole tract was established with cutting current. These patients experienced complications—digestive tract fistulas—because of interposition of bowel loops and left colon, respectively. Both patients had malignant stenoses that involved the iliac portion of the ureter.

Conclusion.—Percutaneous ureteroneocystostomy is a safe procedure if the electrode is placed near the bladder or ileal loop. The procedure may be useful as an alternative to surgery or permanent neophrostomy or as initial treatment of benign anastomotic stenoses.

▶ I am no longer amazed by successful procedures that were once unthinkable. The limits of interventional radiology are the limits of only our own imagination. The human body, and particularly the retroperitoneum, tolerates a great deal. Controlled trauma in any form can be beneficial, be it balloon an-

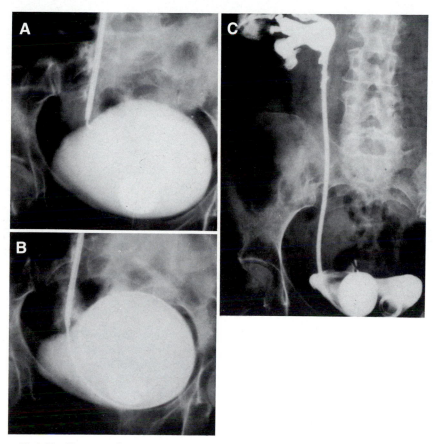

Fig 2–33.—Urograms of ureteroneocystostomy procedure used to bypass a complete stenosis, related to a gynecologic carcinoma, of the distal portion of the right pelvic ureter. **A,** the tip of the wire is close to the bladder wall. A coaxial 12-F Amplatz dilator passed over the 7-F catheter facilitates forward pressure when cutting current is applied. The bladder is fully distended with contrast medium injected through a Foley catheter kept in the bladder to control the degree of distention. **B,** the 7-F catheter is coiled into the bladder, after application of cutting current. **C,** 2 days later, antegrade urogram shows patency of the double-J stent, without leakage of contrast medium. (Courtesy of Cornud FE, Casanova J-MP, Bonnel DH, et al: *Radiology* 180:451–454, 1991.)

gioplasty, surgery, or ureteroneocystostomy using electrocautery. This is a creative, novel solution to a difficult clinical problem.—R.A. Clark, M.D.

Percutaneous Nephrostomy Tube Placement: An Outpatient Procedure?

Cochran ST, Barbaric ZL, Lee JJ, Kashfian P (Univ of California, Los Angeles)
Radiology 179:843–847, 1991   2–45

Background.—Percutaneous nephrostomy (PCN) has traditionally been done as an inpatient procedure. A variety of reasons, including economic considerations, prompted the performance of 56 PCNs (55 patients) on an outpatient basis.

Methods.—None of the 30 women and 25 men had signs of sepsis at the time of the procedure. The median age of the group was 52 years. Most procedures were done to relieve obstructions or to develop a tract for future percutaneous nephrolithotomy. Relationships between the development of sepsis and use of antibiotics, results of urinalysis, and type of kidney stone were evaluated.

Results.—Four patients needed parenteral medication for pain and 3 had bleeding, which resolved spontaneously. Shaking chills or fever, which were taken as a sign of sepsis, occurred in 12 cases. These patients were treated with antibiotics. Sepsis was more common than the reported rates of 1.4% to 4.5%. Likelihood of sepsis was reduced by antibiotics; in high-risk patients the use of antibiotics during and after PCN reduced signs of sepsis from 50% to 9%.

Conclusion.—It appears that PCN is more safely performed as an inpatient procedure. Guidelines are provided for avoiding sepsis, which is the major complication when PCN must be done on an outpatient basis.

▶ In an age when we are pushed to provide virtually any invasive procedure to outpatients, this study is a welcome sight. I agree with the conclusion of this study; for patient safety, urinary and biliary interventions should usually be inpatient procedures. The guidelines offered here for outpatient studies are reasonable and worth our consideration.—R.A. Clark, M.D.

Vascular Complications

Arteriographic Complications in the DSA Era
Waugh JR, Sacharias N (Alfred Hospital, Prahran, Vict, Australia)
Radiology 182:243–246, 1992   2–46

Introduction.—Although the incidence of arteriographic complications in patients who underwent investigation of cerebrovascular disease has recently been reviewed, most of the studies took place before the advent of digital subtraction angiography (DSA). The prevalence of complications of intra-arterial DSA was assessed prospectively in 2,475 consecutive patients who underwent intra-arterial DSA at a 650-bed Australian teaching hospital.

Methods and Findings.—Four hundred seven procedures were done on an outpatient basis. There were 939 cerebral procedures (Table 1). The overall incidence of systemic complications was 1.8% (Table 2). There was a .3% incidence of permanent neurologic deficit. In no case did a patient require hemodialysis for renal failure. There was a .4% incidence of minor allergic reactions and a .16% incidence of death within 24 hours. All of these patients died of complications of myocardial

TABLE 1.—Types of Arteriographic
Procedures (Intra-Arterial DSA)

Procedure Type	No. of Patients	% of Total
Cerebral ($n = 939$ [37.9%])		
Carotid bifurcation disease*	300	12.1
Selective intracranial lesion†	622	25.1
Selective interventional cerebral	17	0.7
Other diagnostic‡	1,252	50.6
Other interventional§	284	11.5
Total	2,475	100.0

* Arch only, 69%; selective, 31%.
† Aneurysm, arteriovenous malformation, tumor, and others.
‡ All peripheral extremity studies, renal studies, and others.
§ Angioplasty, embolization, and others.
(Courtesy of Waugh JR, Sacharias N: *Radiology* 182:243–246, 1992.)

TABLE 2.—Comparison of
Complications Associated With
Intra-Arterial DSA With Prevalence of
Complications Associated With
Conventional Angiography

Complication Type	Prevalence Associated with IA-DSA	Prevalence Associated with Conventional Angiography
Local	7.3	4.1*–23.2†
Systemic	1.8	2.2*–9.4‡
Neurologic deficit		
Transient	0.6	0.2†–5.6§
Permanent	0.3	0.2†–5.7§
All cases	0.9	0.4†–11.3§

Notes: All numbers are percentages. Data for intra-arterial DSA are from this study. Data for conventional angiography are from literature.
* From Swanson PD, et al: *JAMA* 237:2202, 1977.
† From Olivecrona H: *Neuroradiology* 14:175, 1977.
‡ From Reilly LM, et al: *Surgery* 96:909, 1984.
§ From McIvor J, et al: *Br J Radiol* 60:117, 1987.
(Courtesy of Waugh JR, Sacharias N: *Radiology* 182:243–246, 1992.)

TABLE 3.—Postarteriographic
Complications

Complication Type	No. of Patients	% of Total
Local (n = 181 [7.3%])		
Hematoma	153	6.18
Requiring transfusion*	5	0.20
Requiring surgery	0	0.00
Dissection (without sequelae)	11	0.44
Thrombosis (postangioplasty surgery)[†]	10	0.40
Embolus (fractured balloon catheter)[†]	1	0.04
Infected pseudoaneurysm	1	0.04
Systemic (n = 45 [1.8%])		
Nausea, vomiting, vasovagal attack	17	0.69
Allergic reaction (minor)	10	0.40
Angina	6	0.24
Acute renal dysfunction[‡]	5	0.20
Death within 24 h[§]	4	0.16
Other (eg, transient rigor)	3	0.12
Neurologic deficit		
Transient (<24 h)	3	0.3[¶]
Reversible (<10 d)	3	0.3[¶]
Permanent	3	0.3[¶]

* Four of these cases were related to interventional procedures.
† Related to interventional procedures.
‡ None of these patients required hemodialysis.
§ None of these patients died during procedure.
¶ Number of patients undergoing arch or cerebral arteriography, 939.
(Courtesy of Waugh JR, Sacharias N: *Radiology* 182:243–246, 1992.)

events; the contribution of DSA to these deaths could be assessed. Although there was a 7.3% rate of local complications (Table 3), they resulted in additional therapy in only .7% of cases.

Discussion.—Intra-arterial DSA is a safe imaging modality with low complication rates. The incidence of stroke in this study was .3%, compared with 1% and 2.4% in 2 recent studies with data drawn from the conventional film angiography era.

▶ It has been a while since a study documented arteriographic complications; the results, using modern equipment and catheters, are welcome. This study allows all of us to compare (or to benchmark, in the current jargon) our own quality assurance data with a large published series.—R.A. Clark, M.D.

Repair of Postcatheterization Femoral Pseudoaneurysms by Color Flow Ultrasound Guided Compression

Fellmeth BD, Baron SB, Brown PR, Ang JGP, Clayson KR, Morrison SL, Low RI (Sacramento Radiology Med Group, Carmichael Cardiology Consultants, Mercy San Juan Hosp, Sacramento, Calif)
Am Heart J 123:547–551, 1992   2–47

Background.—A well-recognized complication of cardiac catheterization is pseudoaneurysm. Rates of up to 6.25% have been reported, and it may become even more common with percutaneous use of large cannu-

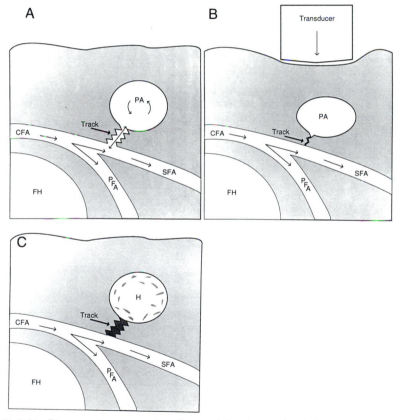

Fig 2–34.—Diagrammatic representation of events during ultrasound-guided compression repair of pseudoaneurysm. **A,** common femoral artery bifurcation region is shown in long orientation. Pseudoaneuryem (PA) cavity with swirling flow is seen just superficial to vessel at puncture site. *Abbreviation: FH* femoral head. **B,** color flow transducer is positioned over the artery defect, and downward manual force has opposed wall of track, arresting flow into and out of pseudoaneurysm cavity. Compression repair is in progress. **C,** compression has been released, and hemostatic plug of thrombosis has closed the artery defect. Pseudoaneurysm is now simple hematoma (H) that will resolve spontaneously. (Courtesy of Fellmeth BD, Baron SB, Brown PR, et al: *Am Heart J* 123:547–551, 1992.)

las. Nonsurgical treatment of this complication by using color flow ultrasound-guided compression has been reported.

Patients and Procedure.—Fourteen femoral pseudoaneurysms in 12 patients with a mean age of 74 years were treated over a 6-month period. Most had undergone cardiac catheterization for diagnostic purposes. When signs of pseudoaneurysm, such as expanding groin hematoma, were noticed, each patient underwent duplex sonography and color flow imaging. When contraindications were absent, the patients underwent compression repair under real-time color flow monitoring (Fig 2–34). Color flow imaging was repeated in 24–72 hours to recheck successfully treated lesions.

Results.—Only 1 lesion was found to be noncompressible; the other 13 were all treated successfully. One recurrence after 24 hours was retreated successfully. The median time of compression for successful procedures was 22 minutes. Titrated intravenous sedation was sufficient for pain control in most cases. Two procedures were done on an outpatient basis.

Conclusion.—The success rate with treating postcatheterization femoral artery pseudoaneurysms by using color flow–guided compression was 93% in this series. This procedure temporarily eliminates the extraluminal flow; the defect is then sealed by a hemostatic plug, converting the lesion to a hematoma, which resolves spontaneously. This is a useful alternative to surgical treatment.

▶ Ultrasound-guided compression is a surprisingly simple solution to a potentially serious vascular complication. Several recent articles have confirmed the usefulness of this approach (1, 2). If you haven't had the opportunity to use this technique, file it away for future reference. It works and it's easy.—R.A. Clark, M.D.

References

1. Fellmeth BD, et al: *Radiology* 182:570, 1992.
2. Fellmeth BD, et al: *Radiology* 178:671, 1991.

3 Neuroradiology

Introduction

The neuroradiology contributions over this past year have been varied, with the major focus being further observations on brain and spine MRI to include several new observations. There have been further clarifications of the use of MR in diagnosis and management of multiple sclerosis. I have broken down the neuroradiology abstracts into 8 subsets to bring more order to the presentation.

Vascular and angiographic manuscripts dealt with MR angiography in evolution. The focus was comparison of phase contrast technique with time of flight vascular imaging. There is a large series with short-term follow-up dealing with the management of arterial venous malformations with radiosurgery. One article emphasized the importance of timing for imaging the dura and vascular sinuses intracranially to minimize the risk of a false diagnosis of sagittal sinus thrombosis. Two articles dealt with a CT pattern of nonaneurysmal subarachnoid hemorrhage. The subgroup dealing with stroke had a presentation comparing the value of CT and MR in the diagnosis of acute stroke. There was an excellent histopathologic study of état criblé. Further discussion was presented on the dense middle cerebral artery as a sign in patients with cerebrovascular accident.

A varied group of papers dealt with changes of the intracranial CNS. Two articles discussed the varied appearance of CNS lymphoma. The MR changes of sarcoid and cryptococcosis were well presented in 2 separate articles. A single article deals with the spectrum of gray matter heterotopias. Three articles dealing with the radiologic management of epilepsy emphasize computer superimposition to compare anatomical studies with physiologic studies. A morphometric analysis of the hippocampus was used as a technique for selecting patients for temporal lobe surgery for partial complex features. The management of late-onset seizures and efficacy of MR were also presented. There was a group of 3 papers dealing with reversible and nonreversible basal ganglia signal change in various systemic diseases.

Presentations dealing with multiple sclerosis stress the selection of subgroups of multiple sclerosis for frequent monitoring of therapy with MRI after Gd. The histopathologic change of multiple sclerosis and other basal ganglia ischemic change have been well presented. Two manuscripts presented the corpus callosum change in multiple sclerosis, with a suggestion of this change as specific for multiple sclerosis.

Ultrasound manuscripts dealt with the transcranial applications in thrombolytic therapy for stroke and intracranial vascular spasm after subarachnoid hemorrhage. Two unrelated papers dealt with a bimodal waveform and aortic insufficiency and a second neck ultrasound presentation on specific ultrasound findings for carotid body tumors.

The manuscripts dealing with sella and suprasellar pathologic conditions dealt with changes in diabetes insipidus and pituitary gland change in normal pregnancy and postpartum. There was a presentation discussing the nonspecific cause for the bright signal in the posterior pituitary gland in normal subjects. There was a series describing hamartomas of the tuber cinereum assessed with MRI.

The ear-nose-throat and orbit presentations dealt with a biopsy technique of Meckel's cave, aggressive skull-based change with inflammatory disease of the paranasal sinuses. Two articles dealt with follow-up change in management of acoustic neuroma, both surgical and radiosurgical management.

To summarize, the neuroradiology publications presented new observations in disease states with MRI and further technical advances with MR techniques, primarily in vascular imaging.

Joseph F. Sackett, M.D.

Vascular Disease

Evaluation of the Carotid Artery Bifurcation: Comparison of Magnetic Resonance Angiography and Digital Subtraction Arch Aortography

Kido DK, Barsotti JB, Rice LZ, Rothenberg BM, Panzer RJ, Souza SP, Dumoulin CL (Univ of Rochester Med Ctr, Rochester; General Electric Corporate Research and Development Ctr, Schenectady, NY)
Neuroradiology 33:48–51, 1991   3–1

Background.—Magnetic resonance angiography (MRA) may be a useful alternative to invasive methods of screening the carotid arteries for significant atherosclerotic disease. A study was conducted to determine the accuracy of MRA and digital subtraction angiography (DSA) aortography in evaluating the carotid bifurcation for atherosclerotic disease compared with selective carotid angiography.

Methods.—The subjects were 18 patients who had DSA aortograms with right and left posterior oblique projections of carotid bifurcations. There were 13 men and 5 women, with a mean age of 67 years. The images were prepared as "road maps" before selective carotid arteriography. The MRAs consisted of a series of phase-sensitive projection images and a series of axial gradient echo recall acquisition in steady-state images. The MRAs and their corresponding selective invasive angiograms were interpreted by a panel of physicians with no knowledge of history or clinical findings.

Results.—A total of 34 sets of carotid images were obtained. The MRA stenosis ratings matched the angiographic ratings exactly in 12 carotids, were off by 1 step in 1, and off by 2 or more steps in 9. Compared with carotid angiography, MRA had a sensitivity of 73% and specificity of 91%. The DSA arch aortographic ratings matched exactly in 17 carotids, were off by 1 step in 11, and off by 2 or more steps in 6. Sensitivity of arch aortography was 27% and specificity 100%.

Conclusion.—Compared with selective angiography, MRA and DSA aortography are not highly accurate in diagnosing carotid bifurcation stenosis. Though MRA would not have to be as specific and sensitive as the invasive technique, lower accuracy could be accepted because of the lower risk. Magnetic resonance angiography does not appear to be sufficiently accurate, however, and arch DSA is even further from meeting criteria for accuracy.

▶ I am surprised that MRA performed better than DSA aortography, but I am not surprised at MRA having poor sensitivity when compared with selective carotid DSA. The MR techniques, of course, have improved, and the smaller voxel size and shorter echo times reduce the dephasing artifact with MRA. A new assessment is in order.—J.F. Sackett, M.D.

Natural History of the Cavernous Angioma
Robinson JR, Awad IA, Little JR (Cleveland Clinic Found, Cleveland)
J Neurosurg 75:709–714, 1991   3–2

Background.—It may be very difficult to diagnose and follow up cavernous angioma before surgical excision. Such lesions are not well imaged by cerebral angiography or CT. For this reason, little is known about their incidence and natural history. Magnetic resonance imaging was used to explore the clinical findings and natural history of this lesion.

Patients.—Over a 5-year period, 66 of 14,305 consecutive patients undergoing MRI had 76 lesions with an appearance typical of presumed cavernous angioma. Thirty-six patients were males and 30 were females, their mean age being 34.6. Eighty-six percent of the patients were followed up clinically for a mean of 26 months, resulting in 143 lesion-years of clinical survey.

Findings.—The most common sites were the frontal and temporal lobes, and the most common findings were seizure, focal neurologic deficit, and headache. There were MRI evidence of occult bleeding in most cases, but only 7 of 57 symptomatic patients had overt hemorrhage, and only 1 patient had overt hemorrhage during follow-up. The bleeding rate was thus .7% per year per lesion. The risk of overt hemorrhage was significantly greater in females. Fourteen patients underwent surgery, most for intractable seizures; the diagnosis was confirmed in every case. No deaths were directly attributable to cavernous angioma.

Conclusion.—Magnetic resonance imaging is valuable in the diagnosis and follow-up of cavernous angioma. It also allows study of the natural history of this lesion, assisting in treatment planning and prognosis.

▶ This is a nice 5-year follow-up study of 66 cavernous angiomas. This study emphasizes the benign nature of these lesions.—J.F. Sackett, M.D.

Assessment of Carotid Artery Patency on Routine Spin-Echo MR Imaging of the Brain
Lane JI, Flanders AE, Doan HT, Bell RD (Thomas Jefferson Univ, Philadelphia)
AJNR 12:819–826, 1991   3–3

Background.—The diagnostic value of intraluminal signal changes on spin-echo (SE) MRI of the brain has been debated. The utility of these signal changes in the diagnosis of compromised arterial flow was determined to critically assess their specificity and sensitivity in detecting occlusive and preocclusive disease.

Methods.—The routine SE MR studies of the brain in 12 patients with 13 angiographically demonstrated occlusions and in 14 patients with 16 high-grade stenoses of the carotid arteries were retrospectively studied.

Findings.—The partial flow void phenomenon was a reliable indicator of decreased flow within a partially collapsed lumen. The appearance of normal flow void on SE MR images of the brain did not exclude significant atherosclerotic stenosis of the extracranial vessels. The finding of isointense intraluminal signal from the skull base to the supraclinoid bifurcation on all pulse sequences is specific for complete occlusion. Six of 13 proved occlusions had significant degrees of hyperintense intraluminal signal indistinguishable from that observed consequent to slow flow distal to high-grade stenoses. Atherosclerotic occlusion may contain varying degrees of hyperintense intraluminal signal that may be caused by occlusion or the high signal produced by slow flow. Magnetic resonance imaging detected only 5 of 16 proved high-grade stenoses.

Conclusion.—On SE MR images, isointense intraluminal signal is specific for atherosclerotic occlusion, and conventional angiography is not necessary to confirm the diagnosis. However, occlusion cannot always be distinguished from high-grade stenosis when hyperintense intraluminal signal is encountered, and invasive angiography or MR angiography in combination with Doppler sonography may be needed to exclude marginal patency.

This manuscript sheds further light on the complexity of diagnosing a total vascular occlusion on SE MRI. The recommendations that the authors make are reliable in our practice as well.—J.F. Sackett, M.D.

Hemifacial Spasm: MR Imaging Features

Tash R, DeMerritt J, Sze G, Leslie D (Yale Univ, New Haven, Conn)
AJNR 12:839–842, 1991   3–4

Background.—Although controversial, much evidence supports the hypothesis that hemifacial spasm is caused by compression of the seventh cranial nerve at its anterior caudal root exit zone (REZ) by mechanisms including vascular loops, aneurysms, arteriovenous malformations, veins, and cerebellopontine angle masses. In patients who do not respond to conservative treatment, microvascular decompression is often performed, but this treatment also is controversial. Because both CT and angiography have limitations in evaluating the course of the seventh nerve from the REZ to the internal auditory canal and the relationship of the seventh nerve to the vertebrobasilar system, the utility of MRI of the REZ of the seventh cranial nerve and surrounding vascular structures was investigated.

Methods.—Thirteen patients with hemifacial spasm and 70 asymptomatic patients with vascular compression of the REZ of the seventh nerve were studied by MRI. The relationship of the REZ of the seventh nerve to surrounding vascular structures was determined.

Results.—Magnetic resonance imaging clearly demonstrated the course of the seventh nerve from the REZ to the internal auditory canal and its relationshp to the vertebrobasilar system. In all 13 symptomatic patients, a vascular structure at the REZ was detected. In the control group, 21% of the seventh nerves showed contact between the REZ and a vascular structure and 1% contact and deformity of the REZ.

Conclusion.—This study of a small group of patients provides preliminary evidence that MRI should be the initial screening procedure for all patients with hemifacial spasm. Neurovascular compression cannot be identified with certainty as the cause of the symptoms.

▶ This standard imaging technique could be complemented with MR angiography. It is likely that the root exit zone does need to be involved for persistent hemifacial spasm.—J.F. Sackett, M.D.

Persistent Nidus Blood Flow in Cerebral Arteriovenous Malformation After Stereotactic Radiosurgery: MR Imaging Assessment

Quisling RG, Peters KR, Friedman WA, Tart RP (Univ of Florida, Gainesville, Fla)
Radiology 180:785–791, 1991   3–5

Background.—Stereotactic radiosurgery and embolization therapy is the current multimodality therapy for arteriovenous malformations (AVMs) of the brain. Pretreatment and posttreatment uses of MRI in this approach include identification of the exact location of the AVM,

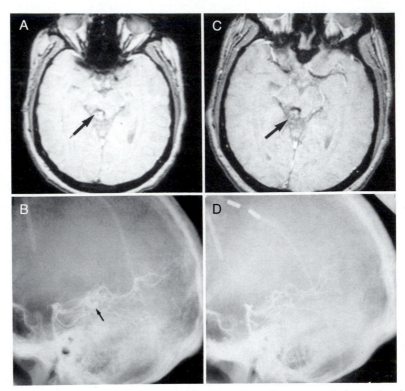

Fig 3–1.—Flow-compensated enhancement of residual nidus in the presence of subacute thrombus. **A,** axial gradient-recalled echo (GRE) image obtained with flow compensation. The image was obtained 18 months after treatment, but 2 months after the development of spontaneous partial thrombosis in efferent arteriovenous malformation circulation (e.g., clotted venous varix). Comparison of GRE images without (not illustrated) and with flow compensation revealed clear evidence of enhancement along the right lateral aspect of the matrix (*arrow*) and no intensity change along the left aspect (*arrowhead*). The former was considered residual flow, and the latter was considered residual thrombus. Flow-through residual nidus (*arrow*) was documented angiographically (see **B**). **B,** lateral vertebral angiogram obtained after the MR image shown in **A.** Residual transnidus blood flow (*arrow*) is evident in the dorsal mesencephalic region, confirming what was predicted with MRI (see **A**). **C,** axial GRE image obtained with flow compensation 22 months after treatment. This section was obtained in the same manner and at the same level as **A,** but 4 months later. It demonstrates persistent hyperintensity compared with the residual clot on the left (*arrowhead*), but no marginal enhancement on the right (*arrow*) lateral aspect. Magnetic resonance imaging findings were indicative of complete arteriovenous malformation thrombosis that was confirmed angiographically (see **D**). **D,** lateral vertebral angiogram obtained after the MR image shown in **C.** No residual transnidus blood flow can be detected, as was correctly predicted by images with and without flow-compensated GRE imaging protocol. (Courtesy of Quisling RG, Peters KR, Friedman WA, et al: *Radiology* 180:785–791, 1991.)

estimation of flow characteristics, and estimation of residual AVM nidus blood flow. A noninvasive method to assess residual transnidus blood flow is desirable because obliteration of flow through the malformation occurs in 75% to 85% of cases within 2 years. Whether AVM MRI can accurately depict the presence of residual flow across an AVM nidus, enable assessment of the progressive diminution of transnidus flow over

time, and enable determination of when complete thrombosis has occurred, was examined.

Methods.—A comparative analysis was conducted of 85 posttreatment
MR images and 27 follow-up cerebral arteriograms in 34 patients treated
with stereotactic radiosurgery. The comparison determined whether
measured nidus volumes determined at MRI matched those obtained
with cut-film angiography. Two-dimensional gradient-recalled echo
(GRE) acquisitions were performed in tandem first without flow compensation and then immediately after with flow compensation.

Findings.—Tandem, flow-compensated GRE images predicted transnidus flow or lack of flow in most complex matrix AVMs. The flow was
determined from apparent signal intensity differences between tandem 2
dimensional GRE images obtained first without and then with gradient
moment flow nulling, with empirically derived pulse parameters (Fig
3–1).

Conclusion.—The use of flow-compensated GRE techniques provided
a means to monitor the reduction in AVM matrix size and assess the extent of persistent arteriovenous shunting, or transnidus blood flow.

▶ This application of MR GRE imaging is an alternative to MR angiography
to detect persistent flow in the nidus of cerebral AVMs. Using a velocity encoding technique, one can determine reduction in flow serially after stereotactic radiotherapy.—J.F. Sackett, M.D.

**3DFT MR Angiography of the Carotid Bifurcation: Potential and Limi-
tations as a Screening Examination**
Masaryk AM, Ross JS, DiCello MC, Modic MT, Paranandi L, Masaryk TJ
(Univ Hosps of Cleveland, Cleveland Clinic Found, Cleveland)
Radiology 179:797–804, 1991   3–6

Background.—The ability of MR angiographic techniques to demonstrate stenoses has been questioned because of potential signal loss leading to underestimation of vascular dimensions, overestimation of stenoses, and potentially complete loss of definition of lumen.
Three-dimensional Fourier transform (3DFT) time-of-flight MR angiography was used and compared with intra-arterial digital subtraction angiography (DSA) in the diagnosis of arteriosclerotic disease of the carotid
bifurcation.

Methods.—Thirty-eight patients were initially studied with DSA for
suspected arteriosclerotic disease of the carotid bifurcation. In 65 of 75
carotid arteries visualized with DSA, 3DFT MR angiograms were obtained. Results of both techniques were reviewed by 2 independent observers on 2 occasions.

Results.—Changes in percentage area of stenosis were depicted by
both modalities without statistically significant difference. The 3DFT

time-of-flight MR angiography demonstrated the capability to approximate changes in arterial lumen similar to that of DSA. There was good intraobserver and interobserver consistency in interpretation.

Discussion.—Magnetic resonance angiography and MRI perfusion methods appear to have potential for providing important information on arteriosclerotic cerebrovascular disease.

▶ The authors point out the limitations of this technique and emphasize the need for reduction of echo time and voxel size to limit the spin dephasing.—J.F. Sackett, M.D.

Physiologic Mechanisms Underlying the Delayed Delta Sign
Ulmer JL, Elster AD (Bowman Gray School of Medicine, Winston-Salem, NC)
AJNR 12:647–650, 1991   3–7

Background.—Sagittal sinus thrombosis is usually diagnosed by the presence of the negative delta sign on contrast-enhanced CT scans. However, a similar appearance has been detected in patients who underwent cranial scanning more than 30 minutes after contrast injection. To determine the rate at which this might occur, cranial CT scanning with and without contrast infusion was performed prospectively in 100 patients without indications of sinovenous occlusive disease.

Results.—Hypodensity of the superior sagittal sinus was directly related to the elapsed time between contrast injection and CT scanning. In the 50 patients scanned within 30 minutes of contrast injection, hypodensity was observed in only 8%; whereas in the 50 patients scanned after 30 minutes, hypodensity was observed in 58%. In 5 of these patients, the sagittal sinus was sufficiently hypodense that it was possible that this would have been confused with a true negative delta sign if only postcontrast images were available. One volunteer was scanned successively from 5 to 55 minutes after contrast administration to determine the time course of the appearance of sinus hypodensity. Immediately after contrast administration, marked intravascular enhancement occurred. However, by 45 to 55 minutes, the dura again became denser than the sinus. This suggests that the distribution of the contrast material reaches an equilibrium before the delayed scans take place.

Conclusions.—Some delayed postcontrast CT brain images may have an appearance similar to that observed with sagittal sinus thrombosis. This hypodensity has been termed the delayed delta sign. Caution should be exercised to avoid confusion.

▶ This important relationship between the postcontrast attenuation coefficient between the lumen of the venous sinus and the dura must be understood by all those interpreting cranial CT scans. Understanding this phenomenon will eliminate the possibility of a false positive diagnosis of sagittal sinus thrombosis.—J.F. Sackett, M.D.

Intracranial Aneurysms and Vascular Malformations: Comparison of Time-of-Flight and Phase-Contrast MR Angiography
Huston J III, Rufenacht DA, Ehman RL, Wiebers DO (Mayo Clinic and Found, Rochester, Minn)
Radiology 181:721–730, 1991   3–8

Background.—Flowing blood has a distinct appearance when visualized with MRI. Time-of-flight (TF) and phase-contrast (PC) MR angiography have been used to provide projection angiographic images of flowing blood. This study compares and contrasts 3-dimensional PC and 3-dimensional TF MR angiographic techniques in patients with intracranial aneurysms and vascular malformation. Results were compared with conventional angiography.

Methods.—Twenty-seven patients with 14 aneurysms and 17 vascular malformations previously identified by conventional angiography were examined with both TF and PC MR angiography of the head.

Findings.—Three-dimensional PC and 3-dimensional TF angiography had unique advantages and disadvantages (Figs 3–2 through 3–4). A 3-dimensional TF data acquisition was performed in approximately half the time required for a 3-dimensional PC data acquisition and involved less reconstruction time. Three-dimensional PC imaging depicted the patent lumen of the aneurysms, whereas 3-dimensional TF imaging depicted the patent lumen and a subacute thrombus if present. The 3-dimensional PC techniques were superior in depicting aneurysms larger than 15 mm, allowed velocity resolution of vascular lesions, and yielded functional flow information by directly depicting collateral flow to vascular lesions. The 3-dimensional TF techniques were susceptible to saturation effects and artifacts from air-bone susceptibility gradients and hemosiderin, whereas the 3-dimensional PC technique had the disadvantage of aliasing artifacts.

Conclusion.—Advantages of the 3-dimensional PC imaging techniques compared with the 3-dimensional TF imaging techniques include variable velocity sensitivity, a superior ability to depict the patent lumina of vessels, low sensitivity to saturation effects, superior background suppression, and functional flow information.

▶ This is an excellent comparison of TF and PC vascular imaging. If one understands the limitations of each technique, they can be used in a complementary fashion in any single patient examination.—J.F. Sackett, M.D.

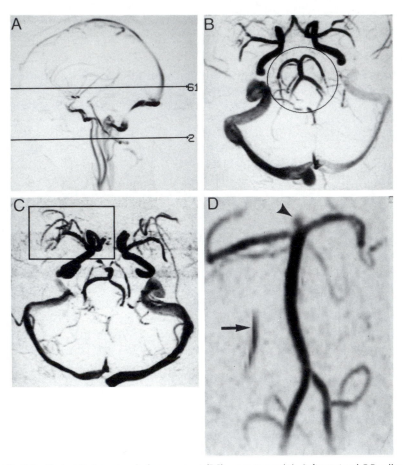

Fig 3–2.—Sagittal 2-dimensional phase-contrast (PC) scout image (**A**), 3-dimensional PC collapse image with posterior subvolume outlined (**B**), 3-dimensional collapse image with right carotid subvolume outlined (**C**), and 3-dimensional PC posterior subvolume (**D**), of a man, 70, with a 4-mm basilar tip aneurysm (*arrowhead* in **D**), obtained with the use of 60 sections 1 mm thick. Images include the posterior inferior cerebellar arteries. Note the segment of right internal carotid artery partially included in the posterior subvolume (*arrow* in **D**) and black-and-white-reversed photographic technique. (Courtesy of Huston J III, Rufenacht DA, Ehman RL, et al: *Radiology* 181:721–730, 1991.)

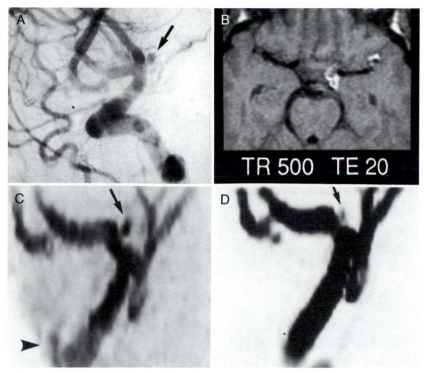

Fig 3–3.—Images of a man, 43, with a 3-mm left anterior cerebral artery aneurysm. **A,** conventional angiogram (lateral oblique view with the head turned to the right) shows aneurysm (*arrow*). **B,** T1-weighted image shows subarachnoid hemorrhage containing methemoglobin, but there is no evidence of an aneurysm. *TR* = repetition time, *TE* = echo time. The 3-dimensional time-of-flight (TF) (**C**) and 3-dimensional phase-contrast (**D**), projection images (both obtained with the use of 28 sections .7 mm thick) demonstrate the aneurysm (*arrow*) equally well (lateral oblique views with the head turned to the left). An air-bone susceptibility gradient is evident on the 3-dimensional TF angiogram (*arrowhead* in **C**). Some of the signal intensity adjacent to the aneurysm on the 3-dimensional TF angiogram is caused by the subarachnoid hemorrhage containing methemoglobin. (Courtesy of Huston J III, Rufenacht DA, Ehman RL, et al: *Radiology* 181:721–730, 1991.)

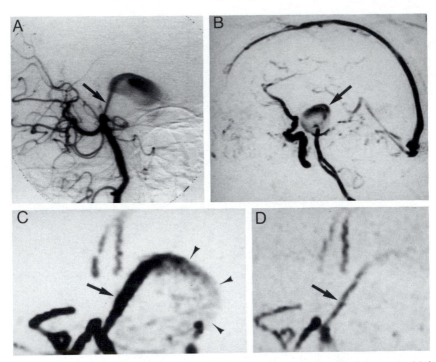

Fig 3–4.—Images of a woman, 30, with a giant fusiform aneurysm (30 mm) of the proximal left posterior cerebral artery. **A,** the flow jet (*arrow*) is demonstrated on an early arterial image obtained with digital subtraction angiography. **B,** sagittal 2-dimensional phase-contrast (PC) image obtained in the midline with 30-cm/second maximum velocity encoding demonstrates the giant aneurysm (*arrow*). **C,** a 3-dimensional PC projection image obtained with the use of 60 sections .7 mm thick demonstrates the flow jet (*arrow*) and aneurysmal lumen (*arrowheads*). **D,** a 3-dimensional time-of-flight (TF) projection image obtained with the use of 60 sections .7 mm thick demonstrates the flow jet (*arrow*) but does not depict the lumen. The 3-dimensional TF collapse image also failed to depict the lumen. Note the wider arterial lumina on the 3-dimensional PC image compared with those on the three-dimensional TF image. (Courtesy of Huston J III, Rufenacht DA, Ehman RL, et al: *Radiology* 181:721–730, 1991.)

Outcome in Patients With Subarachnoid Haemorrhage and Negative Angiography According to Pattern of Haemorrhage on Computed Tomography

Rinkel GJE, Wijdicks EFM, Hasan D, Kienstra GEM, Franke CL, Hageman LM, Vermeulen M, van Gijn J (University of Utrecht, Utrecht, The Netherlands; University of Rotterdam, Rotterdam, The Netherlands; University of Amsterdam, Amsterdam; St Elisabeth Hospital, Tilburg, The Netherlands; DeWever Hospital, Heerlen, The Netherlands)
Lancet 338:964–968, 1991   3–9

Background.—Cerebral angiography is normal in 15% of patients with spontaneous subarachnoid hemorrhage, and such patients do better than those with positive angiograms. However, patients with negative angio-

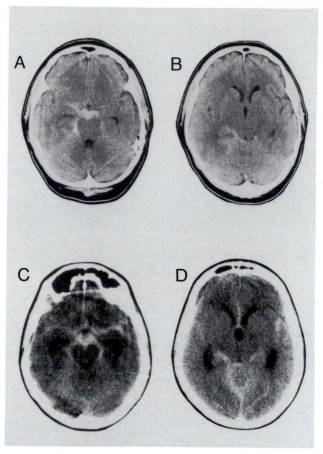

Fig 3–5.—Noncontrast-enhanced CT scans showing 2 patterns of hemorrhage on CT. **A** and **B**, perimesencephalic pattern of hemorrhage, with accumulation of subarachnoid blood in the cistern around the midbrain (interpeduncular, ambient, and suprasellar cisterns). **C** and **D**, aneurysmal pattern of hemorrhage, with subarachnoid blood in the cisterns around the midbrain and also in the anterior interhemispheric fissure and both sylvian fissures. (Courtesy of Rinkel GJE, Wijdicks EFM, Hasan D, et al: *Lancet* 338:964–968, 1991.)

grams can still have rebleeding and cerebral ischemia. Patients with the "perimesencephalic nonaneurysmal hemorrhage" variant, who have a normal angiogram and accumulation of blood in the cisterns around the midbrain, have an excellent outcome. Outcome in a large series of patients with and without the perimesencephalic pattern on CT was compared.

Patients.—The subjects were 113 patients, mean age 51 years, with angiogram-negative subarachnoid hemorrhage admitted during a 7½-year period. All patients were investigated by CT using a third-generation scanner within 72 hours of the event. All patients were followed up for at least 6 months, and mean follow-up was 45 months. Computed tomography showed the perimesencephalic pattern in 77 patients and a pattern indistinguishable from that of proven aneurysmal bleeding in 36 (Fig 3–5).

Outcome.—There were no deaths or disabilities resulting from hemorrhage in the patients with the perimesencephalic pattern. Of patients with the aneurysmal pattern, 4 had rebleeding and 9 died or were disabled as a result of the hemorrhage. Overall, 97% of the perimesencephalic group had a good outcome (i.e., all but 2 who died of carcinoma) compared with 75% of those in the aneurysmal group.

Conclusion.—Two distinct subgroups of patients with angiogram-negative subarachnoid hemorrhage were identified—those with a perimesencephalic pattern on CT, in whom prognosis is excellent, and those with an aneurysmal pattern, who are prone to rebleeding, cerebral ischemia, and residual disability. Only patients with the latter pattern should have repeated angiographic studies in search of an occult aneurysm.

▶ Identifying this perimesencephalic subarachnoid hemorrhage may, indeed, be a technique for selecting patients who do not require follow-up angiography in the face of subarachnoid hemorrhage.—J.F. Sackett, M.D.

Non-traumatic Subarachnoid Hemorrhage With Normal Angiogram: Long-Term Follow-Up and CT Predictors of Complications
Ferbert A, Hubo I, Biniek R (Rheinisch-Westfälisch Technische Hochschule, Aachen, Germany)
J Neurol Sci 107:14–18, 1992   3–10

Background.—Before the use of CT, more than 20% of patients with nontraumatic subarachnoid hemorrhage (SAH) showed no specific cause such as aneurysm or an arteriovenous malformation (AVM). The use of CT has reduced this figure to 15% to 18% of patients with SAH. The outcome in these patients is sometimes much better than in those with an aneurysm. Patients who had suffered from SAH and in whom angiography did not reveal an aneurysm were investigated.

Method.—A total of 91 patients underwent a neurological examination, a CT scan, and an angiogram in the acute phase. Thirty-one of these patients did not show subarachnoid blood. The patients were treated with antifibrinolytic therapy including 12×2 g ϵ-aminocaproid acid (EACA), nimodipine, or unspecific therapy. Forty-nine patients were reexamined 6 months to 11.8 years after SAH, and the remainder of the 85 patients available for follow-up were sent a questionnaire on outcome. Six of the 91 patients had been treated for SAH within the previous 2 weeks.

Findings.—Clinical outcome showed 79 of 91 patients were free from neurologic signs. Most were completely symptom free, but some complained of headache or occasional forgetfulness. Three patients had mild neurologic deficits and 1 had severe neurologic deficits on follow-up. Five patients had died of SAH. The patients who died or had complications showed the greatest amount of blood in the frontal interhemispheric fissure in the initial CT. None of the 3 different therapeutic regimens was superior.

Conclusion.—The prognosis is generally good for patients with nontraumatic subarachnoid hemorrhage (SAH) in whom no aneurysm is found, but an unidentified aneurysm must be considered, and repeat angiogram is warranted if blood is found in the anterior part of the basal cisterns. Repeat angiogram is not necessary when the hemorrhage is in the prepontine cistern. None of the 3 therapies was considered superior, so EACA therapy is not recommended for further use.

▶ This is another example of the interpeduncular cistern hemorrhage. This manuscript, again, emphasizes the benign nature of this manifestation of subarachnoid hemorrhage.—J.F. Sackett, M.D.

Transarterial Platinum Coil Embolization of Carotid-Cavernous Fistulas
Halbach VV, Higashida RT, Barnwell SL, Dowd CF, Hieshima GB (Univ of California San Francisco Hospitals, San Francisco)
AJNR 12:429–433, 1991   3–11

Background.—Direct carotid-cavernous fistulas (CCFs) are most often solitary connections between the cavernous carotid artery and the cavernous sinus, most often occurring as the result of closed head injury accompanied by basal skull fracture. Transarterial balloon embolization has become the treatment of choice. When it is unsuccessful, transvenous embolization or direct surgical exposure and embolization with copper wire or balloons have been described. A new technique of transarterial embolization uses platinum coils.

Method.—In 227 embolization procedures for symptomatic CCFs, 5 were accomplished by placement of platinum coils in the cavernous sinus from a transarterial route. In 4 of the 5 patients, prior transarterial balloon procedures had failed, and in the fifth patient, a woman with Ehlers-Danlos syndrome, a previous transvenous embolization attempt was unsuccessful.

Results.—In 3 patients, there was complete closure of the CCF, and the parent artery was preserved. In 1 patient, internal carotid occlusion was performed after a portion of the platinum coil projected through the fistula and into the parent artery. In the patient with Ehlers-Danlos syndrome, closure of the anterior drainage was achieved, but the platinum coils migrated distally with transient aggravation of ocular symptoms. It was not possible to occlude the remaining cortical drainage with platinum coils, but a balloon successfully closed the small remaining fistula.

Conclusion.—Problems with displacement or migration of the platinum coils in treatment of CCFs may be alleviated with the development of shorter, more thrombogenic, retrievable or detachable coils such as the prototype electrothrombosis coils.

▶ The platinum coil technique for treating CCF appears to be a successful alternative when transarterial balloon placement is not successful.—J.F. Sackett, M.D.

The Case for Conservative Management of Venous Angiomas
Kondziolka D, Dempsey PK, Lunsford LD (Univ of Pittsburgh, Pittsburgh)
Can J Neurol Sci 18:295–299, 1991   3–12

Background.—Venous angiomas are malformations of normal venous drainage that may develop in the absence of normal venous pathways to drain brain tissue. They are associated with intracranial hemorrhage, seizures, or progressive neurologic deficits or detected as incidental findings in patients with headaches or unrelated neurologic disorders. Venous angiomas drain normal cerebral tissue within a functionally normal arterial territory and obliteration or resection can lead to venous infarction or intracranial hemorrhage.

Methods.—Fourteen male and 13 female patients with venous angiomas were managed conservatively with clinical observation and no neurosurgery or radiosurgery. Diagnosis was confirmed by cerebral angiography in 24 patients and by MRI in 3 patients. Their characteristic angiographic appearance is a radiating collection of medullary veins deep within the brain parenchyma. Clinical observation ranged from 3 months to 26 years (mean, 3.7 years).

Findings.—The venous angioma was associated with the onset of neurologic symptoms in 7 patients with hemorrhage, 3 with hemorrhage and seizures, 2 with seizures, 1 with an extrapyramidal movement disorder, and 1 with motor deficit. In 13 patients, the lesions were incidental findings in evaluation for headache or unrelated neurologic symptoms. Ten venous angiomas were in the posterior fossa and 7 were in the cerebellum, but location did not correlate with symptomatic manifestation. None of the patients with hemorrhage required surgical evacuation, and no patient died or had significant morbidity.

Conclusion.—Conservative nonmicrosurgical, nonradiosurgical management of venous angiomas is recommended as a management strategy. Surgical resection should be considered only in patients with recurrent symptomatic hemorrhage associated with progressive neurologic deterioration.

▶ Most venous angiomas are incidental findings in patients who have CT or MRI for other reasons. I agree with the authors' recommendation that only recurrent hemorrhage is an indication for therapy for these reasonably common lesions.—J.F. Sackett, M.D.

Contrast-Enhanced MR of Cerebral Arteritis: Intravascular Enhancement Related to Flow Stasis Within Areas of Focal Arterial Ectasia
Lazar EB, Russell EJ, Cohen BA, Brody B, Levy RM (Chatham TWP, NJ; Northwestern Univ, Chicago)
AJNR 13:271–276, 1992   3–13

Introduction.—In MRI, the "intravascular enhancement sign" usually results from slow flow in partly occluded or collateral vessels near an infarction. This sign may also be seen in arteritis with ectatic change.

Case Report.—Man, 31, had AIDS diagnosed at the time of orchiectomy 2 years previously. He had had hepatitis B infection, testicular carcinoma, and *Pneumocystis carinii* pneumonia, and in the past year had been injecting methamphetamine intravenously and using oral amphetamines. He came to attention with acute headache, dizziness, and anomia. Magnetic resonance imaging showed a tiny focal area of prolonged T2 in the left posterior temporal lobe. After discontinuation of azidothymidine (AZT) therapy, his headaches improved, and a follow-up MRI scan 4 months later showed reduction in size and intensity of the high-signal focus. When AZT was resumed, the patient had transient right facial weakness, aphasia, and confusion; CT showed multiple punctate foci at the periphery of the cerebral hemispheres, and MRI showed multiple, scattered foci of enhancement in a superficial pattern (Fig 3–6). When cerebral angiography

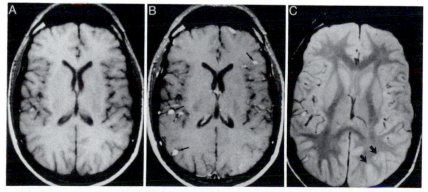

Fig 3–6.—Enhancement of slow flow in areas of arterial ectasia on MRI. **A** and **B**, pre- and post-Gd-DTPA infusion images (spin echo, 600/20/2) demonstrate focal nodular enhancement in many sulcal sites (*arrows*) corresponding to areas of arterial ectasia later revealed by angiography. **C**, axial section at level identical to that shown as **A** and **B** above (spin echo, 2,200/20/1). There is a hyperintense cortical infarct in the left parietooccipital cortex (*arrows*), and there are several sulcal/cortical lesions. (Courtesy of Lazar EB, Russell EJ, Cohen BA, et al: *AJNR* 13:271–276, 1992.)

was done 2 months later, extensive alternating regions of medium and small vessel aneurysmal dilatation and stenosis were noted, corresponding to the nodular areas of enhancement noted on CT. The patient died of *P. carinii* pneumonia after suffering further cerebral infarctions and a new seizure disorder. Autopsy showed multifocal distentions randomly distributed within the leptomeningeal branches of the cerebral arteries. Small, recent infarcts in the cerebral hemispheres partly correlated to the arterial ectasia. The histologic changes suggested drug-induced arteritis.

Discussion.—A patient with AIDS had probable amphetamine-induced cerebral arteritis, which was documented by cerebral angiography. Areas of focal arterial ectasia may show MRI enhancement, probably because of slow flow. The diagnosis of cerebral arteritis must include angiography.

▶ This is an unusual MR finding of high signal on spin-echo sequence, secondary to slow flow in aneurysmally dilated arteries with amphetamine-induced arthritis.—J.F. Sackett, M.D.

Stereotactic Radiosurgery for Arteriovenous Malformations of the Brain
Lunsford LD, Kondziolka D, Flickinger JC, Bissonette DJ, Jungreis CA, Maitz AH, Horton JA, Coffey RJ (Univ of Pittsburgh, Pittsburgh)
J Neurosurg 75:512–524, 1991   3–14

Background.—The best option for eliminating the risk of hemorrhage in arteriovenous malformations (AVMs) is microsurgical resection, but this carries a high risk of a new neurologic deficit. For some carefully selected patients, stereotactic radiosurgery is successful in the complete obliteration of AVMs. A 3-year experience with stereotactic radiosurgery using a 201-source cobalt 60 gamma unit was analyzed.

Patients.—Two hundred twenty-seven patients, almost equally divided between men and women, underwent this treatment for angiographically visible AVMs. Sixty-three percent had prior hemorrhage, 46% had headache, 31% had seizures, and 45% had neurologic deficits. Sixteen percent of the patients had had a previous surgical resection. Embolization was done first in an attempt to reduce the size of the AVM in 21%. According to the Spetzler and Martin grading system, 28% of the lesions were grade VI (inoperable), 10% were grade IV, 40% were grade III, 19% were grade II, and 4% were grade I. Computer imaging–integrated isodose plans were used for single-treatment irradiation. One hundred sixty-one patients were followed up with MRI every 6 months.

Outcome.—The AVM nidus was totally covered in 95% of patients, the most important factors for dosing being location and volume of the AVM. Of 17 patients who had MRI evidence of complete obliteration, angiography at 3 months confirmed obliteration in 14. At 2 years, complete angiographic obliteration was confirmed in 37 of 46 patients, mean confirmation being after 17 months. At 2 years, all lesions with a volume less than 1 cm³ were obliterated compared with 85% of those measuring 1 to 4 cm³ and 58% of those greater than 4 cm³. At mean of 10.2 months postoperatively, MRI showed postirradiation changes in 24% of patients with only 26% of these having symptoms. There were 2 patients with new, permanent, treatment-related neurologic deficits and 2 deaths from repeat hemorrhage during the latency period before obliteration.

Conclusion.—For some patients with AVM, especially those previously considered inoperable, stereotactic radiosurgery appears to be a useful method of obliteration. The location and volume of the AVM have much to do with the success and risk of complications of the procedure. The procedure was recommended for AVMs in critical brain locations, particularly those less than 10 mm³ in volume.

▶ This is an extensive controlled study of a large number of patients treated with radiotherapy for AVMs. Our experience is similar in a smaller patient group, but long-term follow-up is necessary to determine success in controlling the hemorrhagic sequelae of brain AVMs.—J.F. Sackett M.D.

Long-Term Results of Radiosurgery for Arteriovenous Malformation: Neurodiagnostic Imaging and Histological Studies of Angiographically Confirmed Nidus Obliteration

Yamamoto M, Jimbo M, Kobayashi M, Toyoda C, Ide M, Tenaka N, Lindquist C, Steiner L (Tokyo Women's Medical College, Tokyo, Japan; Karolinska Hospital, Stockholm, Sweden; Univ of Virginia, Charlottesville, Va)
Surg Neurol 37:219–230, 1992   3–15

Introduction.—Stereotactic radiosurgery with a gamma unit is being used in the treatment of cerebral arteriovenous malformations (AVMs), but little long-term follow-up has been reported. Twenty-five cases of cerebral AVM treated with stereotactic radiosurgery with a gamma unit were followed up for 26 to 154 months. Findings at CT scans and MRI, as well as angiographic studies, were available.

Results.—Complete nidus obliteration was confirmed by angiography in 73% of the cases receiving full-dose irradiation. There was no mortality related to the radiation treatment. Both CT and MRI revealed that increased enhancement of the nidus after administration of contrast or Gd could persist after angiographically confirmed obliteration of the nidus.

Conclusion.—Because of the risk and burden to the patient of angiography, it is recommended that MRI be the first step in the follow-up of radiosurgically treated AVM. Angiography should be used only as the final confirmation.

▶ At Wisconsin, we have had similar good results. We have found that quantitative MR angiography will select the patients who have fistula formation, and these patients are excluded from radiosurgery.—J.F. Sackett, M.D.

Hyperperfusion Syndrome After Carotid Endarterectomy: CT Changes

Harrison PB, Wong MJ, Belzberg A, Holden J (St Paul's Hospital, Vancouver, BC, Canada)
Neuroradiology 33:106–110, 1991   3–16

Background.—Neurologic problems during and after carotid endarterectomy (CEA) may occur in as many as 10% of patients. Two patients who had headache and seizures suggesting hyperperfusion syndrome after CEA were examined with CT.

Case.—Woman, 79, reported a 1-year history of light-headedness, falling to the left side, and a probable transient ischemic attack affecting her left arm. On arteriography severe bilateral internal carotid stenoses with a left subclavian occlusion were demonstrated. A right CEA was done without complication. After surgery, the patient complained of a mild headache. However, analgesics re-

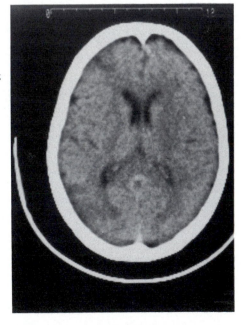

Fig 3–7.—Unenhanced CT demonstrates right frontal and parietal minor cortical and subcortical low density changes on day 5. (Courtesy of Harrison PB, Wong MJ, Belzberg A, et al: *Neuroradiology* 33:106–110, 1991.)

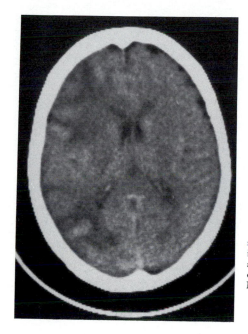

Fig 3–8.—A repeat CT scan on day 14 showed low density changes more extensively involving the right cerebral white matter, associated with greater mass effect. (Courtesy of Harrison PB, Wong MJ, Belzberg A, et al: *Neuroradiology* 33:106–110, 1991.)

lieved the headache, and she was discharged on day 2. Three days later, she was found unconscious in her home. She had several seizures involving her left arm, which later generalized. Repeat angiography showed carotid patency. Unenhanced CT indicated low-density changes in the right frontal and parietal cortical and subcortical areas (Fig 3–7). She was discharged using corticosteroid medication 13 days after admission. The next day, however, she was readmitted with left-sided focal seizures, and a dense, left hemiparesis developed. A repeat CT scan demonstrated low-density changes more extensively involving the right cerebral white matter associated with greater mass effect (Fig 3–8). Three days later she reported having an intense headache and then became comatose. A scan showed punctate regions of hemorrhage and a 3-cm right frontal pole hematoma. The substantial hemisphere mass effect and subcortical hypodensity worsened, with the overlying cortex apparently less involved (Fig 3–9). The patient died 20 days after surgery. At autopsy, fibrinoid necrosis of the small arteries and arterioles within the viable cortex adjacent to the bleeding, as well as a right frontal hematoma, was seen. Also noted were intraluminal fibrin deposition, marked endothelial swelling, and red blood cell extravasation. The changes resembled those seen in malignant hypertension.

Conclusion.—The CT scans of the 2 patients showed ipsilateral mass effect and white matter hypodensity. Although infarction is said to be the most common neurologic event after CEA, autopsy or cerebral

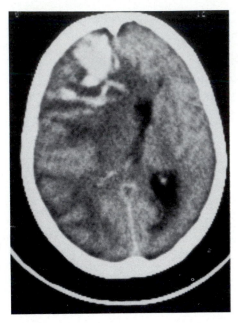

Fig 3–9.—By day 17, punctuate areas of hemorrhage and a 3-cm hematoma had occurred in the right frontal lobe. Hemispheric mass effect and hypodensity had worsened. (Courtesy of Harrison PB, Wong MJ, Belzberg A, et al: *Neuroradiology* 33:106–110, 1991.)

blood flow studies in these patients suggested that the changes resulted from hyperperfusion rather than infarction.

▶ This entity appears difficult to separate from ischemic infarction. Cerebral blood flow studies are probably the only accurate way of making this diagnosis. The CT findings are really nonspecific.—J.F. Sackett, M.D.

Stroke

Angiography in Patients With Occlusive Cerebrovascular Disease: Views of a Stroke Neurologist and Neuroradiologist
Caplan LR, Wolpert SM (New England Med Ctr Hosp, Boston)
AJNR 12:593–601, 1991   3–17

Background.—There is continued disagreement about the use of cerebral angiography. Although the need for this procedure is reduced, it remains critical in evaluation of several conditions.

Myths.—It is not true that angiography is indicated only for patients who will undergo surgery. Treatment should be based on the nature of the vascular lesion, and the physician should determine the patient's problem before selecting or excluding treatments. Further, all large extracranial arteries need not be visualized in patients with ischemia; it is not true that disease at any site can lead to ischemia at another. This perception is related to subclavian steal syndrome, which results from decreased antegrade flow, rather than reversed flow. Similarly, the aortic arch need not be opacified to demonstrate all arteries and thus ensure that proximal occlusive lesions near the arch are not missed. Angiography is safe for use in patients with vertebrobasilar disease, and patients may be studied in the acute phase of ischemic stroke with no increase in risk.

Rules.—It is true that angiography should be used only when it can answer questions that cannot be answered by less invasive means. It should be done only after neuroimaging and noninvasive sonographic tests have been performed. The angiographer should always study the vessel supplying the ischemic zone first, rather than in a nonsymptomatic vessel, in case complications require stopping the procedure. Ideally the responsible clinician should make decisions on vessel imaging or opacification in sequential fashion. In all cases, the amount of contrast material and the length of the procedure should be minimized. The best and most useful studies can be obtained only by close cooperation between clinicians and angiographers. Finally, problems or complications should be identified as early as possible through frequent examinations between injections.

Conclusion.—It must be emphasized that these recommendations represent the authors' own biases and will change as techniques, data, and experience dictate.

▶ The authors present an excellent discussion of this controversial topic. Their division of myths and rules is amusing; some of the rules may be myths and vice versa. I agree with most of their biases, however.—J.F. Sackett, M.D.

Diagnosis of Acute Cerebral Infarction: Comparison of CT and MR Imaging
Bryan RN, Levy LM, Whitlow WD, Killian JM, Preziosi TJ, Rosario JA (The Johns Hopkins Hosp, Baltimore; Baylor College of Medicine, Houston)
AJNR 12:611–620, 1991   3–18

Introduction.—There is yet no imaging technique that allows precise diagnosis and delineation of acute cerebral infarction. The appearance's of early stroke on MRI and CT scans were compared in a prospective study of 31 patients who met the standard clinical criteria for acute stroke.

Methods.—The patients were studied within 24 hours of the ictus. Follow-up examinations were performed 7 to 10 days later in 20 patients, and the findings were correlated with the initial studies.

Results.—For the diagnosis of acute stroke, MRI was significantly more sensitive than CT (82% vs. 58%). On the initial MRI scans, increased signal intensity caused by acute infarcts were visible on proton density- or T_2-weighted images, but changes on proton density–weighted images were more conspicuous, especially for portions of strokes involving peripheral gray matter. In addition, proton density–weighted images showed better anatomical delineation when the internal and external capsules, thalamus, and basal ganglia were involved. On follow-up examination, MRI identified 95% and CT identified 82% of the stroke regions. Of these, 54% were larger or better defined than on initial studies.

For the assessment of acute hemorrhage, both studies were in agreement in delineating acute hemorrhage. Two basal ganglia hematomas were detected, as reflected by decreased signal intensity on T_2-weighted images and gradient-echo images and increased density on CT. In another acute hemorrhage in the basal ganglia, increased signal intensity on T_1-weighted images was evident. This latter hemorrhagic pattern differed from that of the usual hematoma and reflected ischemic lesions with damaged capillary endothelium through which there was leakage into the surrounding parenchyma (ischemia petechial infarction). On follow-up studies, MRI detected more evidence of hemorrhage than CT.

Conclusion.—Magnetic resonance imaging appears to be more sensitive than CT in the diagnosis of acute cerebral infarction. In addition, MRI allows differentiation of any associated hemorrhage.

▶ This is an excellent prospective study comparing MRI and CT in patients with acute stroke. There are no real surprises, but the overall accuracy of MRI is surprisingly good. A cost-effectiveness study is probably the next step to determine whether the added cost of the MR examination is a cost-effective approach.—J.F. Sackett, M.D.

The Morphologic Correlate of Incidental Punctate White Matter Hyperintensities on MR Images
Fazekas F, Kleinert R, Offenbacher H, Payer F, Schmidt R, Kleinert G, Radner H, Lechner H (Karl-Franzens University, Graz, Austria)
AJNR 12:915–921, 1991   3–19

Background.—Incidental punctate white matter hyperintensities (WMHs) are sometimes seen on MRI studies of elderly patients. Postmortem examinations were performed on the brains of 6 such patients in an attempt to define the morphologic correlate of WMH.

Methods.—The patients, aged 52 to 63, had WMHs as their only abnormal finding (2 individuals) or WMHs unrelated to brain tumor (4 patients). Brains were removed after death and fixed for at least 3 weeks. Four brains were rescanned by MRI. The investigators optimized identification of the lesions by cutting the specimens parallel to the MRI plane and examining whole-hemisphere microscopic sections.

Results.—Most of the WMHs could be seen on postmortem scans, but few would have been identified without knowledge of the in vivo findings. Histologic examination revealed areas of reduced myelination, atrophy of the neuropil around fibrohyalinotic arteries, and different stages of perivenous damage. The most extensive form of perivenous damage included large areas with marked rarefaction of myelinated fibers. In 1 patient, edematous glial swelling in foci of ganglion cell heterotopia caused subcortical WMHs.

Conclusion.—The morphologic substrate of WMH is probably minor perivascular damage without infarction. Analysis of such small lesions will require histologic correlations with MRI scans taken in living patients or with studies of unfixed material.

▶ This is another histologic analysis of white matter intensities in the elderly. This is an example of état criblé. The histologic changes are fibrohyalinosis in a fluid-filled space. There is surrounding demyelination, which is probably what is seen on T_2-weighted images.—J.F. Sackett, M.D.

Thrombus Localization With Emergency Cerebral CT
Tomsick T, Brott T, Barsan W, Broderick J, Haley EC, Spilker J (Univ of Cincinnati, Cincinnati; Univ of Virginia, Charlottesville, Va)
AJNR 13:257–263, 1992   3–20

Background.—In CT the hyperdense middle cerebral artery sign (HMCAS) is a known marker of thrombus in the middle cerebral artery. The sign may be common enough to serve as a predictor of infarct volume. The prevalence of the HMCAS was determined in 55 patients with an acute stroke, and the HMCAS was correlated with arteriographic findings and infarct volume.

Methods.—All of the 55 patients who suffered acute ischemic stroke had CT to exclude cerebral hemorrhage and were then treated with intravenous tissue plasminogen activator (t-PA). Mean dose was 57.96 mg; t-PA was always given within 90 minutes of the onset of stroke. With no knowledge of clinical or arteriographic findings, initial and subsequent scans were examined for the presence of the HMCAS. In patients who survived, infarct volumes were measured by pen-trace technique up to 3 months after the stroke.

Results.—Nineteen patients had the HMCAS, for a rate of 34.5%. One of the signs was false positive. Fourteen of the patients underwent arteriography, which confirmed the predicted middle cerebral artery segment in 12. Mean infarct size in patients with the HMCAS was 132 mL vs. 52 mL in those without the sign.

Conclusion.—In patients with stroke examined by CT, the HMCAS predicts middle cerebral artery occlusion and subsequent large infarct size. This is so despite prompt treatment with t-PA. Combined with immediate arteriography, the HMCAS could suggest the need for more aggressive therapy such as intra-arterial thrombolysis.

▶ The new scanners have an improved low-contrast resolution that makes it more likely to make a false positive diagnosis of HMCAS. One really should use Hounsfield numbers to ensure that the dense middle cerebral artery is, indeed, from thrombosis.—J.F. Sackett, M.D.

Early Computed Tomographic Findings for Thrombolytic Therapy in Patients With Acute Brain Embolism
Okada Y, Sadoshima S, Nakane H, Utsunomiya H, Fujishima M (St Mary's Hospital, Kurume, Japan; Kyushu University, Fukuoka, Japan)
Stroke 23:20–23, 1992   3–21

Background.—Some clinical trials of thrombolytic treatment for acute brain infarction have resulted in unfavorable outcomes. In such cases, conversion to hemorrhagic infarction or frank hemorrhage caused clinical worsening or death. Recombinant tissue plasminogen activator (rt-PA) has been shown to be effective in patients with acute myocardial infarction. After CT and angiography, rt-PA was given to patients with acute brain embolism to assess the clinical indications for this therapy.

Methods.—Ten patients received rt-PA, 20 to 30 MU for 1 hour, intravenously. Neurologic outcomes and findings on CT and angiography were assessed.

Results.—In 4 patients, symptoms ameliorated within 24 hours after onset. In 2 patients, occluded arteries reopened just after rt-PA infusion. Initial CT scans in 4 cases showed early indications of brain ischemia—an obscure margin of the lentiform nuclei, reduced tissue attenuation, or effacement of cortical sulci. In those 4 patients, occluded arteries did not reopen; 1 had a massive brain hemorrhage with clinical deterioration. Of the remaining 6 patients, 2 improved clinically with recanalization soon after treatment, suffering slight hemorrhagic complications. One-month outcomes were favorable in 5 patients and poor in 3. Two patients died.

Conclusion.—Thrombolytic treatment with rt-PA may be safe and effective in patients with no early CT findings within 3 hours of embolic stroke onset. However, the number of patients in this series was too small to draw definitive conclusions. Further hemodynamic and follow-up studies are needed.

▶ These are promising early results for thrombolytic therapy in stroke.—J.F. Sackett, M.D.

Brain

CT Appearance of Primary CNS Lymphoma in Patients With Acquired Immunodeficiency Syndrome

Goldstein JD, Zeifer B, Chao C, Moser FG, Dickson DW, Hirschfield AD, Davis L (Albert Einstein College of Medicine, Bronx, NY)
J Comput Assist Tomogr 15:39–44, 1991   3–22

Introduction.—Patients with AIDS often have neurologic problems. Cranial CT scans often show intracerebral mass lesions, which can result from different causes, but can have similar clinical and radiographic appearances.

Methods.—To determine whether AIDS-related primary lymphoma has a characteristic pattern on CT scans, cranial CT scans from 32 patients with AIDS were reviewed. In 1985–1990, all patients were found by biopsy to have primary CNS lymphoma. Computed tomography was performed using a GE 9800 or GE 8800 device; 21 patients had examinations both with and without intravenously administered contrast medium, 6 had a contrast-only scan and 5 had only a noncontrast scan.

Results.—A total of 58 mass lesions were recorded, ranging from 1.5 to 7 cm in diameter. They were usually found in the cerebral lobes and central gray matter. The lesions varied greatly in size, location, and number. Most were isodense or hyperdense to gray matter on noncontrast scans, with varying degrees of edema and mass effect seen in almost all patients. All were enhanced but with different patterns. Ring enhancement was most frequently observed. In 11 patients, CT was performed after radiotherapy. Treatment resulted in a decrease in size of all tumors, and reduction or resolution of edema and mass effect occurred in 10 of 11 patients. Areas of contrast enhancement decreased or disappeared, and all but 2 lesions became hyperdense. At the sites of the lesions, tissue retraction occurred after radiotherapy, with focal dilatation of adjacent CSF spaces. Interval increases in the size of the ventricular systems and the cortical sulci revealed generalized volume loss in most patients after treatment.

Conclusion.—Because of the diversity of CT appearances of primary CNS lymphoma in these patients, the CT findings are not diagnostic. Biopsy is necessary. After radiation therapy to these lesions, their CT appearance is consistent with regression.

▶ Paleation for primary CNS lymphoma in AIDS patients is excellent with radiotherapy. This article shows the varied appearance of CNS lymphoma and underlines the need for biopsy for proper patient selection for radiotherapy.—J.F. Sackett, M.D.

Studies of Primary Central Nervous System Lymphoma With Fluorine-18-Fluorodeoxyglucose Positron Emission Tomography

Rosenfeld SS, Hoffman JM, Coleman RE, Glantz MJ, Hanson MW, Schold SC
(Duke Univ, Durham, NC)

J Nucl Med 33:532–536, 1992   3–23

Background.—Primary CNS lymphoma (PCNS-L) is an uncommon, aggressive malignancy with a strong association with immunosuppression. It consists of a dense, predominantly lymphoid infiltrate that manifests as uniformly enhancing lesions that are frequently periventricular and can involve the corpus callosum on contrast-enhanced CT or MRI. However, similar radiologic findings may be present, and the use of ^{18}F-2-fluoro-2-deoxy-D-glucose (FDG) and PET allows the evaluation of lesions on their metabolic activity. The results of FDG-PET imaging of biopsy-proved gliomas were compared with those of patients with PCNS-L. The effects of corticosteroids on the CT and FDG-PET imaging of PCNS-L were also examined.

Method.—Ten patients with biopsy-proved primary CNS lymphoma were studied with FDG-PET. The FDG uptake ratios of PCNS-L were compared with ratios from a series of biopsy-diagnosed gliomas organized by histologic grade. One patient with PCNS-L had scans before and approximately 3 weeks after treatment with dexamethasone. Corticosteroid therapy substantially reduced the uptake of FDG.

Findings.—Primary CNS lymphomas demonstrated high FDG uptake on PET, supporting the finding that highly aggressive nonglial tumors can show marked FDG accumulation. When that finding is combined with findings on meningioma and malignant gliomas, the implication is that high FDG uptake by a CNS tumor correlates with clinically aggressive behavior, regardless of histologic type. The CT and FDG-PET scans of PCNS-L showed uniformly enhancing or active lesions, respectively, with close anatomical correlation between the 2 imaging modalities. The accumulation of FDG in primary CNS lymphoma is similar to that seen in anaplastic gliomas and is significantly more prominent than in low-grade astrocytomas. Primary CNS lymphoma, like gliomas, suppresses the metabolism of both contiguous and distant but functionally linked areas of the brain. Corticosteroids overall have no significant effect on FDG uptake of PCNS-L.

Conclusion.—Because PCNS-L resembles malignant glial tumors in its FDG-PET appearance, radiologic findings are not pathognomonic for PCNS-L. However, FDG-PET may be helpful in narrowing the differential diagnosis in cases in which PCNS-L is a consideration.

▶ This study involving PET confirms the active metabolic nature of these aggressive neoplasms; FDG-PET would likely be a method of monitoring therapy in primary CNS lymphoma.—J.F. Sackett, M.D.

CNS Sarcoidosis: Evaluation With Contrast-Enhanced MR Imaging
Seltzer S, Mark AS, Atlas SW (George Washington Univ, Washington Hosp
Ctr, Washington, DC; Univ of Pennsylvania, Philadelphia)
AJNR 12:1227–1233, 1991   3–24

Background.—Symptomatic involvement of the CNS has been found
in 5% of patients with sarcoidosis, and CNS involvement is 1 of the
more common causes of sarcoid-related mortality. Studies with unenhanced MRI and contrast-enhanced CT suggest that MRI without contrast enhancement may miss meningeal involvement in neurosarcoidosis.
The appearance of CNS sarcoidosis on the contrast-enhanced MR images in 14 patients is studied.

Methods.—Fourteen patients with CNS sarcoidosis were studied with
T_1- and T_2-weighted precontrast and postcontrast sequence and T_1-
weighted postcontrast sequences.

Findings.—In 5 of 14 patients, CNS findings were the initial clinical
manifestation of neurosarcoidosis; and in 9 of 14 patients, the diagnosis
of neurosarcoidosis was suggested only after administration of a contrast
agent (Fig 3–10). Eight of 12 patients with intracranial sarcoidosis and 1
of 2 patients with spinal sarcoidosis had meningeal involvement that was
not apparent on the unenhanced scans. Eight patients had enhancing
lesions that were not apparent or were poorly seen on unenhanced

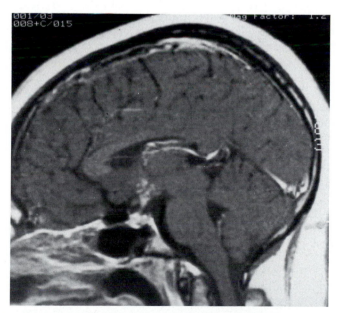

Fig 3–10.—A woman, 18, with amenorrhea. A sagittal postcontrast T1-weighted image shows punctate enhancement of hypothalamus. (Courtesy of Seltzer S, Mark AS, Atlas SW: *AJNR* 12:1227–1233,
1991.)

scans. In 3 patients, enhancing extra-axial masses mimicking meningiomas on postcontrast T_1-weighted images were of very low intensity on unenhanced T_2-weighted images. In this series, enhancement of intra-axial lesions was uncommon.

Conclusion.—The addition of gadopentetate dimeglumine greatly enhanced the sensitivity of MRI in the detection of CNS sarcoid lesions. After the addition of the contrast agent, meningeal, parenchymal, optic nerve, and ependymal sarcoid lesions not seen on unenhanced MRI scans were detected. The routine use of contrast agent is recommended when CNS sarcoidosis is suspected, especially if unenhanced studies are normal or nonspecific.

▶ Figure 3–10 shows the typical appearance on CNS sarcoidosis after intravenous Gd MR examination. Gadolinium MR scanning is the best technique to demonstrate CNS sarcoidosis.—J.F. Sackett, M.D.

Intracranial Cryptococcosis in Immunocompromised Patients: CT and MR Findings in 29 Cases
Tien RD, Chu PK, Hesselink JR, Duberg A, Wiley C (Univ of California San Diego Med Ctr)
AJNR 12:283–289, 1991   3–25

Purpose.—*Cryptococcus neoformans*, the only *Cryptococcus* species known to be pathogenic in human beings, is a common cause of CNS infections in immunocompromised patients. Computed tomographic and MR imaging studies were obtained in 29 immunocompromised men with documented intracranial cryptococcal infection.

Patients.—The study patients ranged in age from 19 to 57 years. Twenty-eight patients had AIDS or AIDS-related complex, and 1 had diabetes mellitus. All 29 patients had cranial CT studies, and 26 of them received iodinated contrast medium. Ten patients also had MR studies, and 4 of them received gadopentetate dimeglumine contrast medium. Three patients died between 4 and 7 days after the imaging studies, and the postmortem autopsy findings were correlated with the MR and CT studies.

Results.—Nine patients had normal CT studies, 13 had various degrees of central or cortical atrophy, 3 had nonenhancing small lesions in the brain, 2 had enhancing lesions in the right front lobe, and 2 had small foci of calcification in the leptomeningeal spaces. All 10 patients who underwent MRI had abnormal findings, and 4 different patterns were observed. Three patients had parenchymal cryptococcoma. Four patients had numerous clustered tiny foci that were hyperintense on T_2-weighted images and were nonenhancing on postcontrast T_1-weighted images; they were located relatively symmetrically in the basal ganglia bilaterally and in the midbrain, representing dilated Virchow-Robin spaces.

One patient had multiple miliary enhancing parenchymal and lepto-meningeal nodules. Two patients had a mixed pattern of dilated Virchow-Robin spaces with mixed lesions, such as cryptococcoma and miliary nodules. The dilated Virchow-Robin space lesions in the 2 patients who were given contrast medium did not enhance, whereas the lesions in the other 2 patients who received contrast medium were enhanced. The postmortem results in all 3 patients who died revealed dilated Virchow-Robin spaces filled with fungi in basal ganglia and small numbers of surrounding perivascular chronic inflammatory cells, primarily macrophages. The pathologic findings correlated well with the dilated space lesions seen on MRI.

Conclusion.—Magnetic resonance imaging provides valuable information about CNS abnormalities in immunocompromised patients with intracranial cryptococcal infections.

▶ This manuscript shows the varied manifestation for cryptococcosis in immune-compromised patients. In general, the organism involves the leptomeninges and, rarely, parenchymal infection.—J.F. Sackett, M.D.

Enhancement of Pineal Cysts on MR Images
Mamourian AC, Yarnell T (Milton S Hershey Med Ctr, Hershey, Pa; Geisinger Wyoming Valley Med Ctr, Wilkes Barre, Pa)
AJNR 12:773–774, 1991   3–26

Background.—Benign pineal cysts can resemble solid tumors on MRI after administration of gadopentetate dimeglumine. Six such cases are reported.

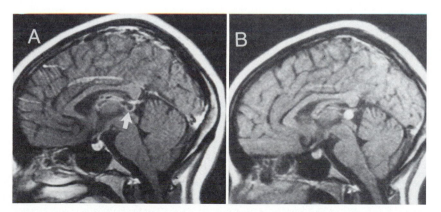

Fig 3–11.—A, magnetic resonance image obtained immediately after injection of contrast material shows the typical rim enhancement of a pineal cyst (*arrow*). **B**, MR image obtained 1 hour after injection of contrast material. The cyst appears uniformly hyperintense. (Courtesy of Mamourian AC, Yarnell T: *AJNR* 12:773–774, 1991.)

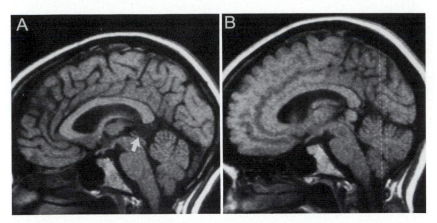

Fig 3–12.—A, unenhanced MR image shows a sharply marginated pineal cyst (*arrow*) with low signal intensity. **B,** on delayed image obtained after administration of contrast material, cyst enhances but appears isointense with corpus callosum. (Courtesy of Mamourian AC, Yarnell T: *AJNR* 12:773–774, 1991.)

Methods.—Imaging used either a 1- or 1.5-T MRI unit with contrast medium. All 6 patients were studied for signs and symptoms not referable to the pineal region. In no case was pathologic confirmation available; CT correlation was available in 1 case.

Results.—The pineal cysts were sharply marginated in all cases, having low intensity on T_1-weighted images, and hyperintensity of T_2-weighted images. Administration of contrast resulted in a rim of rapid enhancement at the margin (Fig 3–11) and, in 2 cases, small areas of rapid focal enhancement within the cyst. In all cases, enhancement of the entire cyst occurred 60 to 90 minutes after injection of contrast. In 4 cases, the cysts appeared uniformly hyperintense at that time. In 2 cases that did not show rapid focal enhancement, cysts eventually enhanced uniformly but were isointense with corpus callosum (Fig 3–12). In the case in which CT correlation was available, a densely calcified partial rim around the cyst was seen on the CT scan.

Conclusions.—Recognition of benign pineal cysts is not always easy, especially with unenhanced MRI. After administration of contrast material, the degree of enhancement depends in part on the time elapsed between injection and imaging. Images obtained with unintentional delays may be interpreted as showing a solid enhancing lesion. If sagittal images are obtained first, they will show the typical rim enhancement.

▶ The authors stress the importance of timing of the post-Gd injection imaging of pineal cysts. The pineal, of course, is not protected by the blood-brain barrier. Early rim enhancement occurs with these cysts, and late more homogeneous enhancement occurs on delayed scans.—J.F. Sackett, M.D.

Clinical Manifestations of Hydrocephalus Caused by Impingement of the Corpus Callosum on the Falx: An MR Study in 40 Patients

Jinkins JR (Univ of Texas Health Science Ctr, San Antonio, Tex)
AJNR 12:331–340, 1991   3–27

Background.—Hydrocephalus results in impairments in motor and cognitive functions, but the clinical signs and symptoms vary in degree and character. This review was undertaken to see whether any specific MRI correlates of the signs and symptoms of hydrocephalus could be found.

Methods.—Forty adults with hydrocephalus according to MRI evidence were the subjects of studies using spin-echo MRI techniques. T_1- and T_2-weighted double-echo acquisitions in 2 or 3 orthogonal planes were made. All standard MRI criteria for hydrocephalus, including the presence of dilated lateral ventricles, an upwardly elevated corpus callosum, and outwardly expanded cerebral hemispheres, were required for inclusion in this study.

Results.—Twenty-four of the 40 patients had dorsal flattening or thinning of the posterior body of the corpus callosum (or both) (Figs 3–13 through 3–15). This finding has not previously been described in hydrocephalus. Twenty-one of these 24 patients (87.5%) showed imbalance, gait disturbance, memory deficits or dementia, incontinence, or psychopathologic behavior. In contrast, 16 subjects with ventricular dilatation did not show this callosal abnormality. Although most of these 16 pa-

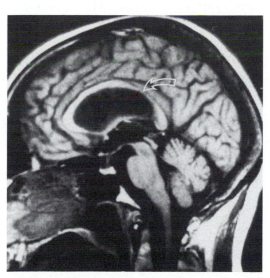

Fig 3–13.—Moderate callosal impingement in hydrocephalus. Sagittal T_1-weighted section shows mild curvilinear flattening of the dorsal surface of the posterior body of the corpus callosum (*arrow*). (Courtesy of Jinkins JR: *AJNR* 12:331–340, 1991.)

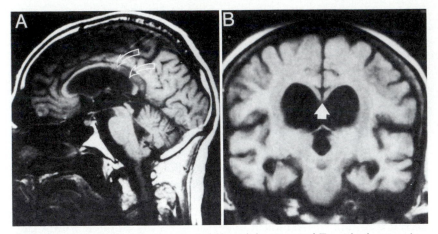

Fig 3–14.—Marked callosal impingement in hydrocephalus. **A,** sagittal T₁-weighted section shows marked flattening and thinning of the posterior body of corpus callosum (*arrows*). **B,** a coronal T₁-weighted image shows stretching of the fibers of the corpus callosum over the posterior falx with associated extreme thinning and a focal loss of callosal signal (*arrow*). (Courtesy of Jinkins JR: *AJNR* 12:331–340, 1991.)

tients were seen with nonspecific symptoms such as headache and visual impairment not likely related to hydrocephalus per se, only 1 had symptoms of hydrocephalus (dementia). Imaging showed that all 16 patients had smooth and uninterrupted, curvilinear upward expansion of the entire corpus callosum.

Conclusion.—Many of the symptoms of hydrocephalus seem linked to dorsal flattening and thinning of the posterior corpus callosum. This im-

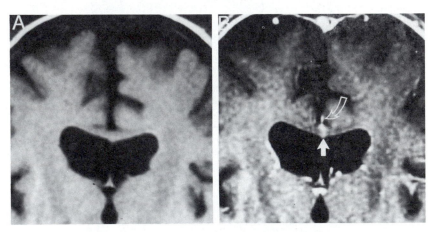

Fig 3–15.—Blood-brain barrier breakdown in callosal impingement. **A,** unenhanced T₁-weighted coronal image immediately anterior to the point of maximal callosal thinning. **B,** an enhanced T₁-weighted image shows vertical transcallosal enhancement (*straight arrow*), indicating a focal disruption of the blood-brain barrier within the corpus callosum. Punctate enhancement within the inferior sagittal sinus (*curved arrow*). (Courtesy of Jinkins JR: *AJNR* 12:331–340, 1991.)

plies that this process is pathogenetic. When the rigid-free surface of the falx cerebri impinges on the caudal extent of the upwardly expanding corpus callosum and supracallosal hippocampal formation, it may result in neuroelectrically active axonal dysfunction. This radiating callosal/hippocampal commissuropathy and fornicopathy may, in turn, result in the clinical symptoms of hydrocephalus because of a dynamic associational, commissural, and projectional cerebral disconnection.

▶ This study shows the value of the various planes that MRI uses to define brain structure. The neuropsychologic sequela of the corpus callosum lesion are likely masked by the changes secondary to hydrocephalus.—J.F. Sackett, M.D.

Deep Gray Matter Hypointensity Patterns With Aging in Healthy Adults: MR Imaging at 1.5 T
Milton WJ, Atlas SW, Lexa FJ, Mozley PD, Gur RE (Univ of Pennsylvania, Philadelphia)
Radiology 181:715–719, 1991   3–28

Introduction.—Magnetic resonance imaging is extremely sensitive to the presence of iron in the brain. A study of young patients imaged at 1.5 T showed that hypointensity in certain areas increased with increasing age. This finding parallels the documented accumulation of iron in deep gray matter structures during childhood and early adulthood. The physicians of this study sought to derive standards for normal patterns of brain hypointensity on long repetition time/echo time MRI in healthy adults.

Methods.—Thirty volunteers were selected to represent each age decade from the 20s through the 70s. All images were obtained with a 1.5-T system. Results were expressed as the volume of hypointensity for the dentate nucleus, substantia nigra, red nucleus, globus pallidus, and putamen.

Results.—Areas of hypointensity in the red nucleus, substantia nigra, and dentate nucleus were similar for the 6 decades. The globus pallidus showed an increased volume of hypointensity in the middle-aged and elderly subjects compared with the young adults. Hypointensity in the putamen was only seen in the elderly subjects; no subject, regardless of age, show hypointensity in the thalamus or caudate nucleus.

Conclusion.—The volumes of hypointensity reflect, at least approximately, the presence of ferric iron in deep gray matter structures. Cerebral disease should be considered in patients whose patterns of hypointensity in these areas differ from normal patterns.

▶ This study allows the understanding of iron deposition in normal subjects. These standards have not been well understood previously. The authors do state that if this normal pattern is seen to develop in an accelerated fashion or the distribution in a different location, that degenerative CNS disease should be considered.—J.F. Sackett, M.D.

Gray Matter Heterotopias: MR Characteristics and Correlation With Developmental and Neurologic Manifestations
Barkovich AJ, Kjos BO (Univ of California, San Francisco; Swedish Hosp, Seattle)
Radiology 182:493–499, 1992   3–29

Background.—Most reports of gray matter heterotopias have been concerned with their appearance and association with other abnormalities. The MR studies of 20 patients were reviewed to correlate patterns of heterotopias with clinical findings.

Observations.—The patients were 14 females and 6 males, median age 13 years. Seizures and developmental delay were the most common clinical manifestations. Eight had subependymal heterotopias (Fig 3–16), 6 had focal gray matter heterotopias, and 6 had diffuse subcortical heterotopias on MRI. Normal development was significantly more likely in those with subependymal heterotopias. Developmental delay was more likely in those with thick heterotopias and overlying cortical gyral anomalies. Motor dysfunction was significantly more likely in patients with thick focal gray matter heterotopias. Three patients had gray matter

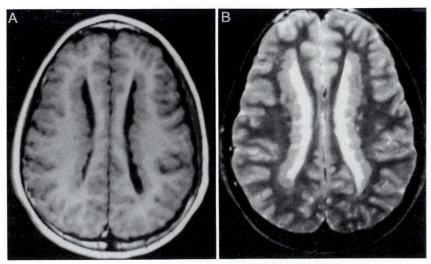

Fig 3–16.—Subependymal heterotopias. **A**, axial MR image (SE, 600/20) shows multiple ovoid nodules isointense to cortical gray matter, lining the lateral ventricles. The overlying cortex is normal. **B**, axial T2-weighted MR image (SE, 2,800/80) shows that the nodules remain isointense to gray matter. The patient's development was normal except for a seizure disorder that began at age 14 years. (Courtesy of Barkovich AJ, Kjos BO: *Radiology* 182:493–499, 1992.)

heterotopias in association with infoldings of dysplastic cortex, which contained blood vessels or CSF.

Conclusion.—Clinical findings can be associated with various MRI patterns in gray matter heterotopia. The infoldings of dysplastic cortex described could be mistaken for neoplasms if not carefully analyzed.

▶ This is an excellent review of the varied manifestations of gray matter heterotopias. These anomalies must be recognized and not confused with a neoplastic process.—J.F. Sackett, M.D.

MR Imaging of Tuberous Sclerosis: Pathogenesis of This Phakomatosis, Use of Gadopentetate Dimeglumine, and Literature Review
Braffman BH, Bilaniuk LT, Naidich TP, Altman NR, Post MJD, Quencer RM, Zimmerman RA, Brody BA (Memorial Hosp, Hollywood, Fla; Children's Hosp of Philadelphia, Philadelphia; Univ of Miami; Baptist and Children's Hosps, Miami, Miami)
Radiology 183:227–238, 1992   3–30

Introduction.—Tuberous sclerosis (TS) is a phakomatosis characterized by both dysplastic and neoplastic processes in organs derived from embryonic ectoderm, mesoderm, and endoderm. The findings on cranial MRI were reviewed in 42 patients with histopathologically confirmed TS. The 24 male and 18 female patients had a median age of 8 years.

Methods.—Both 1.5- and 0.5-T MR units were used. Spin-echo sequences were recorded with short and long repetition times. Seventeen patients were examined with intravenous gadopentetate dimeglumine.

Findings.—Cortical tubers were detected in all but 2 of the 42 patients. In most cases they were solely cerebral and bilateral. Most of those lesions were identified solely by their abnormal signal intensity. All but 3 patients had white matter lesions, which in general were more numerous in patients having numerous cortical tubers. Bands of abnormal signal intensity were more frequent than wedge-shaped lesions. Forty patients had subependymal nodules. Nine subependymal giant cell astrocytomas were found in 7 patients. Relatively few cortical tubers and white matter lesions enhanced after contrast injection. Subependymal nodules enhanced more frequently.

Implication.—The predominance of cortical tubers and white matter lesions supports the view that the cerebral manifestations of TS reflect the disordered migration of dysgenetic cells.

▶ In early CT days, it was believed that enhancement of subependymal tubers indicated malignancy. This is not the case with MRI after Gd. So 1 important finding from this article is that enhancement does not indicate neoplastic transformation into subependymal giant cell astrocytoma.—J.F. Sackett, M.D.

Proton Relaxation Enhancement Associated With Iodinated Contrast Agents in MR Imaging of the CNS

Jinkins JR, Robinson JW, Sisk L, Fullerton GD, Williams RF (Univ of Texas Health Science Ctr, San Antonio, Tex)
AJNR 13:19–27, 1992   3–31

Background.—Conventional radiologic and computed imaging methods may be used together in patient evaluation. Possible proton relaxation in MR images by iodinated x-ray contrast agents commonly used in clinical imaging of the CNS was evaluated.

Methods.—Two patients were examined after the intrathecal administration of Isovue, an iodinated nonionic contrast agent. Five other subjects with cranial tumors were evaluated after the intravenous administration of Renografin, an iodinated ionic contrast medium. Magnetic resonance images were obtained before administration and after excretion of the iodinated contrast agent. The basic relationship of T_1 and T_2 relaxation in regard to signal intensity was studied.

Findings.—The 2 patients who received subarachnoid iodinated contrast media demonstrated a relative reduction in T_1 or T_2 times (or both) using a spin-echo sequence. Four of the 5 patients with intracranial tumors had a visible MR effect after intravenous enhancement (Fig 3–17). During in vitro measurement of T_1 and T_2 while varying the concentration of the contrast media in saline solution, all iodinated contrast media showed progressively reduced relaxation times as the concentration of the agent was increased. That effect is probably attributable to the binding and exchange of surrounding water with the contrast molecules.

Conclusion.—Visible effects in MRI are observed with ionic or nonionic iodinated contrast agents administered within 2 hours of the MR study. The observed shortening effects of T_1 and T_2 may have important

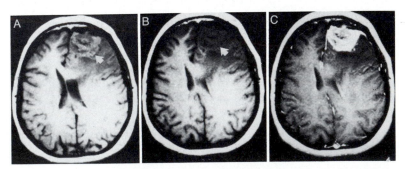

Fig 3–17.—**A,** postintravenous iodinated contrast-enhanced T_1-weighted image (500/15/2) demonstrating the greater relative T_1 shortening (hyperintense) within the matrix of a calcified frontal meningioma, compared with **B** (*arrow*). **B,** follow-up noncontrast axial T1-weighted image (500/15/2) 24 hours later reveals low intensity in the region of the poorly defined tumor (*arrow*) after clearing of the iodinated contrast media (calcifications proved on prior CT). **C,** immediate post-Gd-enhanced T_1-weighted image (500/15/2) illustrating the typical intense enhancement of tumor. (Courtesy of Jinkins JR, Robinson JW, Sisk L, et al: *AJNR* 13:19–27, 1992.)

implications in MRI. Administration of iondinated contrast media in the period immediately before MR scanning may be contraindicated in some cases because of the demonstrated alteration of MR signal intensity, which may lead to diagnostic inaccuracies.

▶ The T_1 and T_2 effects of iodinated contrast medium are important to understand because many patients will receive an MR examination the same day that they might have an iodinated contrast CT study. Intracranial lesions could be masked because of the reduced relaxation effect of the iodinated agent.—J.F. Sackett, M.D.

Computer-Assisted Superimposition of Magnetic Resonance and High-Resolution Technetium-99m-HMPAO and Thallium-201 SPECT Images of the Brain
Holman BL, Zimmerman RE, Johnson KA, Carvalho PA, Schwartz RB, Loeffler JS, Alexander E, Pelizzari CA, Chen GTY (Harvard Med School, Boston; Univ of Chicago, Chicago)
J Nucl Med 32:1478–1484, 1991   3–32

Background.—Though special purpose SPECT imaging systems now give excellent definition of small structures in the brain, it may be difficult to localize these structures precisely from the functional image. Previous reports have described a system for registering 3-dimensional CT, MRI, and PET data sets. This method was adapted to SPECT and MRI.

Methods.—The system employed axial T_2-weighted MRI scans, as well as transaxial technetium 99m–HMPAO and thallium 201 images acquired with an annular single-crystal brain stem. The images were merged by an objective registration program in which the images were translated, rotated, and rescaled. Fourteen individuals were studied: 5 normal volunteers; 4 patients with Alzheimer's disease; 2 with recurrent glioblastoma; and 1 each with stroke, arachnoid cyst, and head trauma.

Results.—Gray matter structures were seen as focal areas of high uptake in the normal subjects and in the patients with Alzheimer's disease and focal lesions. Areas observed as focal lesions on MRI appeared as perfusion defects on SPECT. On ^{201}T1 images, increased uptake corresponding to recurrent tumor could be seen in patients who had had surgical resection of glioblastoma, followed by interstitial brachytherapy. Average residuals were 6.0 mm^2. In 12 patients with normal thalamic anatomy, lateral thalamic displacement was 2.0 mm. The surface match was thus very good, although mean square excursions away from the surface may have been large when noise was large.

Conclusion.—A useful method was found for superimposing MRI and high-resolution SPECT scans of the brain. Regional function can be correlated with brain anatomy, and the technique may be useful for guiding biopsy. Implementation of this system would require department-wide networking and rapid processing.

▶ Superimposition techniques have more and more importance as we are trying to integrate changes with PET and SPECT imaging. These authors have found 1 useful technique.—J.F. Sackett, M.D.

Three-Dimensional Fast Low-Angle Shot Imaging and Computerized Volume Measurement of the Hippocampus in Patients With Chronic Epilepsy of the Temporal Lobe

Ashtari M, Barr WB, Schaul N, Bogerts B (Long Island Jewish Med Ctr; Long Island Campus for the Albert Einstein College of Medicine, New Hyde Park, NY)
AJNR 12:941–947, 1991   3–33

Introduction.—Patients with intractable temporal lobe seizures can be treated surgically. Decisions to perform a temporal lobectomy are based on the results of brain imaging procedures, EEG monitoring, and neuropsychologic testing.

Methods.—The value of 3-dimensional fast low-angle shot (FLASH) imaging and computer-assisted morphometry to determine hippocampal changes associated with unilateral temporal lobe seizures was assessed in 28 patients undergoing inpatient evaluation for intractable epilepsy. Ictal and interictal electroencephalographic (EEG) evidence showed that the seizures originated from the left temporal lobe in 17 patients and in the right temporal lobe in 11. The control group included 28 age- and sex-matched normal volunteers. Contiguous 3.1-mm coronal FLASH images were obtained in both groups and hippocampal volumes calculated with a computerized mensuration system (Fig 3–18).

Results.—Patients with left temporal lobe seizures showed significant reductions (32%) in hippocampal volume; similarly, significant reductions in right hippocampal volume (35%) were apparent in patients with right temporal lobe seizures (Fig 3–19). Results of discriminant analysis were statistically significant and correctly classified 86% of patients into their respective groups.

Conclusion.—Unilateral temporal lobe seizures are accompanied by significant reductions in hippocampal volume ipsilateral to the seizure focus (Fig 3–20). Imaging with FLASH and computer assisted morphometry of the hippocampus provides the structural information required to confirm the laterality of the EEG seizure focus.

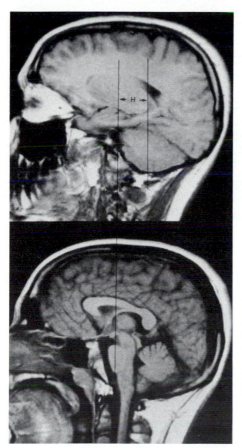

Fig 3–18.—Longitudinal (anteroposterior) landmarks of hippocampal (*H*) measures shown in sagittal orientation. The anterior landmark (*left line*) consists of slice posterior to mamillary body. Posterior landmark (*right line*) consists of slice where pulvinar (posterior portion of thalamus) can be seen. These landmarks include approximately 80% of hippocampal formation when measured on coronal sections. (Courtesy of Ashtari M, Barr WB, Schaul N, et al: *AJNR* 12:941–947, 1991.)

▶ Patients with intractable temporal lobe seizures have been studied with multiple modalities to select those with potentially surgically correctable lesions. This morphometric technique shows surprising accuracy.—J.F. Sackett, M.D.

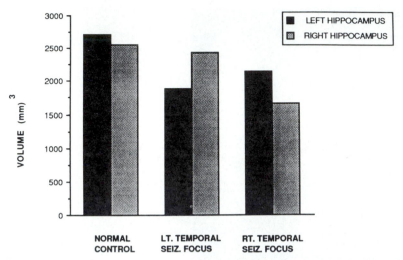

Fig 3–19.—Mean left and right hippocampal MR volumes for normal controls ($n = 28$), patients with left (*LT.*) temporal lobe seizures (*SEIZ.*) ($n = 17$), and patients with right (*RT.*) temporal lobe seizures ($n = 11$). (Courtesy of Ashtari M, Barr WB, Schaul N, et al: *AJNR* 12:941–947, 1991.)

Fig 3–20.—**A** and **B,** coronal FLASH images of right (*RH*) and left (*LH*) hippocampi in normal controls **(A)** and in a patient with left temporal lobe seizures **(B).** (Courtesy of Ashtari M, Barr WB, Schaul N, et al: *AJNR* 12:941–947, 1991.)

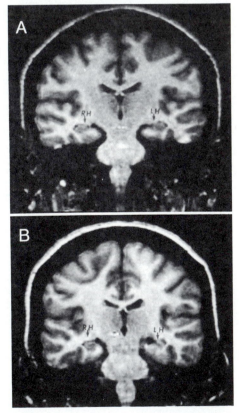

Magnetic Resonance Imaging and Late-Onset Epilepsy

Kilpatrick CJ, Tress BM, O'Donnell C, Rossiter SC, Hopper JL (Royal Melbourne Hospital, Parkville, Vict, Australia)
Epilepsia 32:358–364, 1991

3–34

Background.—It is generally thought that a structural cause is more likely to be identified in a patient investigated for late-onset epilepsy than in younger patients with seizure disorder. There have been no systematic studies of the usefulness of MRI in investigation of patients with late-onset epilepsy. A prospective study of the diagnostic value of MRI in cases were CT was nondiagnostic was performed.

Methods.—The subjects were 50 patients who had seizures beginning after age 25 years. All had CT scans, MRI, and electroencephalography. There were 32 women and 28 men, with a mean age of 52 years. Computed tomography was normal in 32, provided no definitive diagnosis in 12, or revealed irrelevant lesions in 6. The imaging studies were evaluated by a single neuroradiologist blinded to all clinical and laboratory data. An age- and sex-matched group of subjects without seizures was also investigated.

Results.—Of the 32 patients who had normal CT findings, MRI was also normal in 20 cases. Irrelevant ischemic lesions were demonstrated in 8 cases, and the cause of the seizures was found in 4. Of the 12 patients in whom CT was nondiagnostic, MRI clarified the diagnosis in 5 cases and was normal in 2 cases. All 6 patients who had irrelevant lesions on CT also had irrelevant lesions on MRI, though an additional, relevant lesion was found in 1 of these cases. Ischemic lesions were detected with MRI no more frequently in cases than in controls. Of 31 patients with either partial or focal electroencephalographic features, MRI was diagnostic in 10 cases; MRI was not diagnostic in 19 patients without focal features.

Conclusion.—Magnetic resonance imaging appears to be valuable in the study of patients with late-onset epilepsy in whom CT is normal or does not allow a definitive diagnosis. Imaging is particularly useful in patients with late-onset epilepsy and focal features.

▶ This is, of course, a different patient group than those with partial complex intractable seizures. Once again, it is no surprise that overall accuracy is better with MRI. This is another patient subgroup that a cost-effectiveness study would determine whether the cause of seizures found in 4 out of 50 subjects was treatable and worth the increased cost of the MR examination across the 50 subjects.—J.F. Sackett, M.D.

MR Imaging of Reversible Cyclosporin A-Induced Neurotoxicity

Truwit CL, Denaro CP, Lake JR, DeMarco T (Univ of California, San Francisco; US Army Academy of Health Sciences, Fort Sam Houston, Tex)
AJR 157:651–659, 1991   3–35

Introduction.—Some patients undergoing cyclosporine A therapy after organ transplantation experience neurotoxicity, usually manifested by seizures and altered mental status. The corresponding changes seen on imaging studies are areas of cerebral matter with hypoattenuation on CT and T_2 prolongation on MRI. Cyclosporine A toxicity occurred in 3 patients with reversible changes in the cerebral white matter.

Case Report 1.—Woman, 50, who underwent orthotopic liver transplantation received cyclosporin A, 750 mg orally twice daily for the first 2 postoperative days, and 1 g orally twice daily thereafter. On day 7 after transplantation, the patient had 2 focal seizures. Her serum cyclosporine A level increased precipitously over 2 days from 78 to 401 μg/L. At this time, a CT scan showed bilateral, nonenhancing areas of hypoattenuation in the occipital white matter; the next day, MRI showed bilateral nonenhancing areas of T2 prolongation in the occipi-

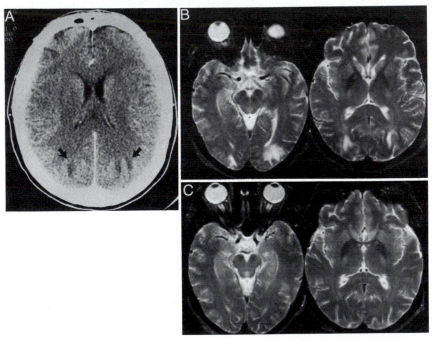

Fig 3–21.—Patient 1. **A,** an axial 5-mm enhanced CT scan on the day of seizures reveals hypoattenuation of occipital white matter (*arrows*). The overlying cortex is uninvolved. **B,** axial spin-echo T2-weighted MRIs, 2,800/80/1 (TR/TE/excitations), 1 day after seizures reveal high signal intensity in occipital white matter corresponding to CT findings. **C,** axial images 16 days after seizures reveal normal white matter. (Courtesy of Truwit CL, Denaro CP, Lake JR, et al: *AJR* 157:651–659, 1991.)

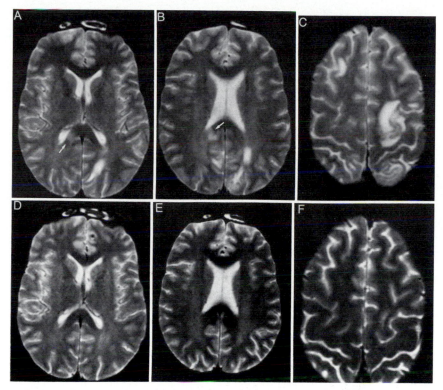

Fig 3–22.—Patient 3. **A–C,** axial spin-echo T2-weighted MR images, 2,500/80/1 (TR/TE/excitations), 4 days after an initial episode of cyclosporine A neurotoxicity, reveal multiple foci of hyperintensity in subcortical white matter, as well as in right splenium (*arrows*). **D–F,** follow-up T2-weighted images (2,308/80/1) 12 days later reveal complete resolution of white matter abnormalities. (Courtesy of Truwit CL, Denaro CP, Lake JR, et al: *AJR* 157:651-659, 1991.)

tal white matter (Fig 3–21). Cyclosporine A was withheld for 2 days and restarted on postoperative day 9 at a dose of 200 to 300 mg orally twice daily. Preoperative serum cholesterol levels ranged from 40 to 58 mg/dL; postoperative serum creatinine values were normal. The white matter appeared to be normal on MRI 16 days after the seizures.

Case Report 2.—Man, 36, underwent cardiac transplantation with unremarkable perioperative and postoperative periods until an episode of severe systemic hypertension (210/110 mm Hg) suddenly developed 4 weeks after transplantation. At this time he also experienced confusion and seizures, suggesting cyclosporine A neurotoxicity. His serum cyclosporine A level on admission was 348 μg/L. His serum cholesterol, magnesium, and creatinine levels were normal. The MRIs taken the day after admission showed nonenhancing areas of T_2 prolongation in the occipital white matter. Cyclosporine A was withheld for 3 days, and his serum level decreased to 169 μg/L. At this time, MRI showed nearly complete resolution of the abnormalities.

Case Report 3.—Woman, 33, who underwent heart and lung transplantation for cystic fibrosis, was receiving cyclosporine A, 100 mg, 3 times daily, with no unusual complications until postoperative day 29, when she experienced seizures and severe headache. Her serum cyclosporine A level was 636 µg/L. Phenytoin therapy was instituted, and cyclosporine A was temporarily withheld. Examinations with CT and MRI showed multiple areas of hypoattenuation in the cerebral white matter that appeared to be resolved 12 days later (Fig 3–22). On postoperative day 84, she experienced a generalized tonic-clonic seizure; MRI showed subcortical white matter lesions of the cerebral hemispheres and new lesions of the corpus callosal genu and splenium and the midbrain and pons. Her cyclosporine A serum level at this time was 116 µg/L. Follow-up MRI on postoperative day 99 showed complete resolution of abnormalities in the white matter.

Conclusion.—Reversible cyclosporine A–induced neurotoxicity seems to coincide with reversible changes in cerebral white matter seen on CT and MRI. Based on these 3 patients, cyclosporin A toxicity does not seem related to reduced serum cholesterol levels.

▶ This remarkable white matter change does, indeed, seem to be reversible and related to cyclosporine A serum levels. This reversible phenomenon must be separated from other nonreversible CNS lesions in the immune-suppressed patients to include lymphoma and infection. There does not appear to be a specific pattern in these 3 patients to allow such a definite separation from the irreversible CNS changes from the latter diseases.—J.F. Sackett, M.D.

Chronic Acquired Hepatic Failure: MR Imaging of the Brain at 1.5 T
Brunberg JA, Kanal E, Hirsch W, Van Thiel DH (Univ of Michigan, Ann Arbor, Mich; Univ of Pittsburgh, Pittsburgh)
AJNR 12:909–914, 1991   3–36

Introduction.—Although histologic changes in the CNS of patients with chronic hepatic failure are well defined, neuroradiologic alterations are less well known.

Methods.—The results of MRI of the brain in 42 patients with chronic, severe non-Wilsonian hepatic failure who were candidates for possible orthotopic liver transplantation were reviewed. In addition to MRI, CT studies of the abdomen and laboratory results were available. Patients were also examined for the presence or absence of encephalopathy at the time of MRI.

Results.—In 30 patients, T_1-weighted images showed symmetrically increased signal intensity throughout the globus pallidus. The increase was mild in 24 patients and of marked severity in 6. Signal intensity in the putamen was bilaterally symmetric and increased mildly in 17 patients and markedly in 4. Patients with increased signal intensity in the

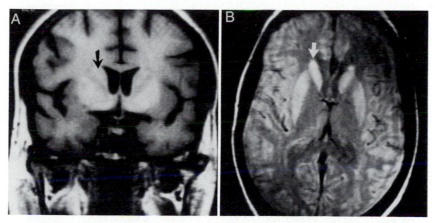

Fig 3–23.—Man, 53, with postoperative biliary obstruction. **A,** T1-weighted MRI (600/20) shows increased signal intensity in caudate (*arrow*), globus pallidus, and putamen. **B,** at 3,000/25 there is increased signal intensity in the heads of the caudate nuclei (*arrow*) and in the putamen. The T2-weighted images were normal. (Courtesy of Brunberg JA, Kanal E, Hirsch W, et al: *AJNR* 12:909–914, 1991.)

globus pallidus or putamen on T_1-weighted images did not demonstrate altered intensity in a similar distribution on T_2-weighted sequences. Increased signal intensity surrounding the red nuclei was present in 17 patients. In 1 patient who had mildly increased intensity in the caudate nuclei (Fig 3–23), there was markedly increased signal intensity in the globus pallidus, putamen, and mesencephalon surrounding the nuclei.

Conclusion.—Characteristic findings of chronic hepatocellular dysfunction include increased signal intensity in the basal ganglia, pituitary gland, and mesencephalon surrounding the red nuclei. The cerebral cortex or cerebellum did not show alterations in signal intensity. The MRI findings did not correlate with neurologic status, histologic liver diagnosis, or laboratory indices of hepatic or thyroid function. The cause of the increased intensity on T_1-weighted images remains uncertain.

▶ This unusual increased T_1 signal in globus pallidus is not well understood. Follow-up MR scans after liver transplant would be of interest to see whether these findings are modified.—J.F. Sackett, M.D.

Reversible MRI and CT Findings in Uremic Encephalopathy
Okada J, Yoshikawa K, Matsuo H, Kanno K, Oouchi M (Chiba University, Chiba, Japan; Honda Mem Hospital, Kooriyama, Japan)
Neuroradiology 33:524–526, 1991   3–37

Introduction.—In patients with renal failure uremic encaphalopathy may occur. The pathogenesis of this condition is not well understood.

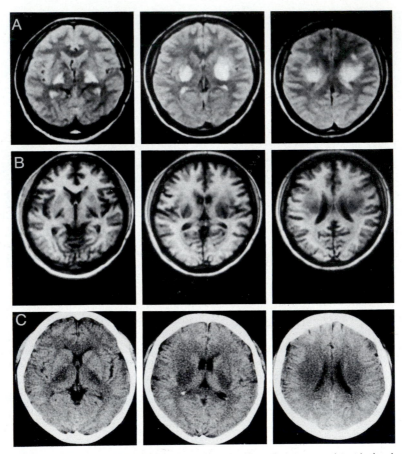

Fig 3–24.—A, T2-weighted SE MRI scan showed increased signal intensity involving the basal ganglia, internal capsules, and the periventricular white matter. **B**, T1-weighted IR MRI showed hypointensities in those areas. **C**, CT showed reduced alteration in same zone. (Courtesy of Okada J, Yoshikawa K, Matsuo H, et al: *Neuroradiology* 33:524–526, 1991.)

One patient had uremic encephalopathy with reversible abnormalities that were observable on CT.

Case Report.—Woman, 35, with chronic glomerulonephritis had uremic encephalopathy. On CT examination the basal ganglia, internal capsules, and periventricular white matter were hypodense, with a low signal intensity on T_1-weighted MRI and a high signal intensity on T_2-weighted MRI (Fig 3–24). After dialyses her condition improved, and the CT and MRI findings returned to normal.

Conclusion.—Reversible abnormalities were detected by CT and MRI in a patient with uremic encephalopathy. These reversible abnormalities may have been caused by ischemic changes, but cerebral metabolism disorders and uremic toxins may also have contributed.

▶ This is another example of the nonspecific change after systemic illness of basal ganglia on MRI. In this particular entity, the MR findings proved to be reversible with correction of the renal failure.—J.F. Sackett, M.D.

Hyperintense Basal Ganglia on T1-Weighted MR Images in Patients Receiving Parenteral Nutrition

Mirowitz SA, Westrich TJ, Hirsch JD (Washington Univ, St Louis)
Radiology 181:117–120, 1991   3–38

Background.—Patients with gastrointestinal disorders may receive total parenteral nutrition (TPN) for extended periods. One such patient was found to have atypical patterns of signal intensity on T_1-weighted MR images of the brain. A prospective study was done to determine whether such changes are found in other patients receiving TPN.

Methods.—Two men and 7 women (mean age, 58.9 years) who had received TPN for a mean of 5.3 years underwent MRI. The findings were compared with those in 25 control patients who underwent MRI for various medical indications.

Results.—All patients showed hyperintensity on T_1-weighted MR images of the basal ganglia. Specifically, the globus pallidus was hyperintense compared with the adjacent internal capsule in all 9 patients but in none of the control subjects. The abnormal signal intensity seen in patients receiving TPN was bilateral and symmetric. Administration of gadopentetate dimeglumine did not lead to enhancement. The T_2-weighted spin-echo and gradient-echo images and CT scans were normal. The relative signal intensity of the globus pallidus varied considerably among the patients but did not appear to be a function of duration of TPN treatment.

Conclusions.—Patients undergoing long-term TPN had T_1-weighted MR images showing symmetric hyperintensity in the basal ganglia. These abnormalities may be the result of abnormal deposition of manganese or other trace elements.

▶ The authors have identified another abnormality of basal ganglia related to systemic disease. Again, the cause in this clinical setting is uncertain.—J.F. Sackett, M.D.

Multiple Sclerosis

Magnetic Resonance Imaging in Monitoring the Treatment of Multiple Sclerosis: Concerted Action Guidelines

Miller DH, Barkhof F, Berry I, Kappos L, Scotti G, Thompson AJ (Institute of Neurology, London, England; Free University Hospital, Amsterdam, The Netherlands; Rangueil Hospital, Toulouse, France; Kantonsspital Basel, Basel, Switzerland; Istituto Scientifico HS Raffaele, Milan, Italy)
J Neurol Neurosurg Psychiatry 54:683–688, 1991   3–39

Background.—Although therapeutic outcome in multiple sclerosis (MS) has historically been assessed by clinical disability, serial Gd-enhanced MRI can disclose significant disease that is clinically silent in the early relapsing-remitting and secondary progressive phases of MS. This imaging technique can thus be an important tool in monitoring the effects of treatment. Guidelines for the use of MRI to monitor treatment trials in MS were reviewed.

MRI System.—Systems used should have a field strength of 0.5 T or more, and serial scans should be done on the same equipment with accurate repositioning. The axial slice orientation is the most widely accepted. Standard T_2-weighted spin-echo imaging produces the best signal/noise ratio. Gadolinium enhancement is recommended for use in patients with relapsing-remitting or secondary progressive disease.

Patient Selection.—In patient selection, it is important to consider the 4 main clinical subgroups, namely, early relapsing-remitting, an illness of less than 10 years with relapses and remissions but no progressive deterioration; benign, with minimal or no disability after at least 10 years; secondary progressive, with progressive deterioration after a relapsing-remitting course; and primary progressive, with progression from the outset and no relapses or remissions. The latter type is present in only 5% to 10% of patients, and in studies they must be separated out from patients with relapsing-remitting and secondary progressive MS.

Design and Analysis of Results.—In trials, the ultimate determination of efficacy must be done on clinical grounds in parallel with MRI. Monitoring of the spinal cord and optic nerves is not recommended. Open, uncontrolled studies are of little value. A useful effect may be noted on enhanced scans at 6 months, compared to 2 years for clinical monitoring. Analysis of results must address control of image quality, quantitative analysis, and relaxation time measurement.

Discussion.—More study is needed to determine the best monitoring technique and the long-term value of monitoring. Also, more sensitive and quicker methods of demonstrating spinal cord lesions are needed.

▶ This article emphasizes the complexity of monitoring progression of patients with MS. Their breakdown into 4 subgroups may assist in patient selection for MRI, with the identification of primary progressive MS being a category that may require frequent scanning early in the disease after intravenous contrast enhancement.—J.F. Sackett, M.D.

Multiple Sclerosis: Histopathologic and MR and/or CT Correlation in 37 Cases at Biopsy and Three Cases at Autopsy

Nesbit GM, Forbes GS, Scheithauer BW, Okazaki H, Rodriguez M (Mayo Clinics and Mayo Found, Rochester, Minn)
Radiology 180:467–474, 1991

3–40

Introduction.—Many authors have tried to correlate clinical signs and symptoms of multiple sclerosis (MS) with findings on imaging studies. However, few studies have attempted to correlate histologic confirmation of MS with imaging studies because biopsy is not often performed in MS patients. The records of 40 patients with biopsy- or autopsy-proved MS were retrospectively reviewed and the histopathologic findings were correlated with imaging studies.

Methods.—The patients ranged in age from 6 to 74 years. All had histologically confirmed inflammatory demyelination consistent with MS. Of the 40 patients, 8 underwent only CT, 10 only MRI, 22 both, and 5 contrast-enhanced CT and MRI. Pathologic specimens were always obtained within 14 days after the imaging studies. Complete data sets were available for 24 patients (60%).

Findings.—Seventeen patients (43%) had solitary demyelinating lesions and 23 (57%) had multiple lesions. In cases with multiple lesions, a biopsy of the predominant lesion was performed. The mean number of lesions was 3.2. More lesions were detected with MRI than with CT. Three predominant radiologic appearances of the demyelinating lesions were noted. Twenty-one patients (53%) had relatively small homogeneous lesions with no or minimal diffuse enhancement (Fig 3–25). Seventeen patients (42%) had lesions that appeared on CT as hypoattenuating structures and on short repetition time images as hypointense structures with contrast-enhanced rings (Fig 3–26). Four of these had lesions with hyperintensity and an additional rim of increased signal intensity on short repetition time, short echo time images compared with the signal intensity of normal white matter peripheral to a relative isointense ring (Fig 3–27). Two patients (5%) had ill-defined infiltrative lesions with mixed attenuation and signal intensity and scattered enhancement.

The radiologic appearance of lesions and their enhancement patterns correlated well with their histologic activity. Lesions with a more aggressive radiologic appearance all showed moderate to marked macrophage infiltration, whereas less aggressive-appearing lesions typically had less macrophage infiltration. All histologically inactive lesions appeared homogeneously hypoattenuating at CT, hypointense on short repetition time images, and hyperintense on long repetition time images.

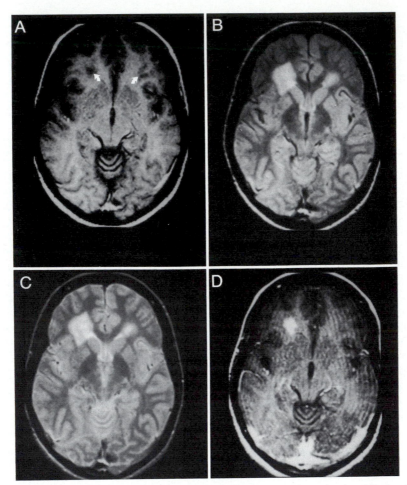

Fig 3–25.—In a patient with MS, images depict homogeneous brain lesion. **A,** short-TR, short-TE 600/30 MR image with 1 signal averaged shows ill-defined regions of low signal intensity in the white matter of both frontal lobes (*arrows*). **B,C,** long TR 2,000/35–70 MR images with 1 signal averaged show minimally inhomogeneous areas of increased signal intensity in corresponding areas. **D,** Gadolinium-enhanced 660/30 MR image with 1 signal averaged shows homogeneous central diffuse enhancement in the right frontal lesion. The left frontal lesion had similar enhancement on a contiguous section. (Courtesy of Nesbit GM, Forbes GS, Scheithauer BW, et al: *Radiology* 180:467–474, 1991.)

Conclusion.—There is excellent correlation between the patterns of contrast enhancement of MS lesions on MRI and their histologic activity. The level of contrast enhancement is related primarily to the degree of macrophage infiltration.

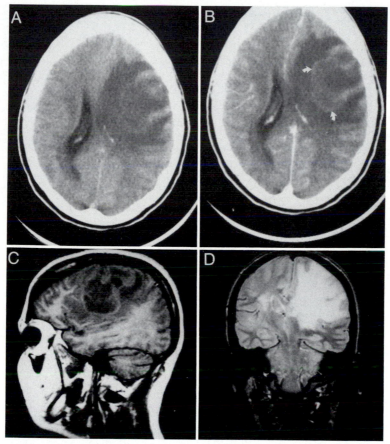

Fig 3–26.—Images of a patient with MS depict ring lesion. **A,** unenhanced CT image shows large low-attenuating lesion in the left frontal lobe, with an isoattenuating lobulated ring and extensive mass effect. Significant mass effect was seen only in this patient; minimal mass effect was noted in 3 others. **B,** after administration of iodinated contrast material, the isoattenuating ring is moderately enhanced (*arrows*). **C,** sagittal short-TR, short-TE 500/20 MR image with 2 signals averaged shows similar hypointense lesion with isointense ring. **D,** coronal long-TR 2,500/40–80 MR image with 1 signal averaged shows extensive increased signal intensity and mass effect in the same region. (Courtesy of Nesbit GM, Forbes GS, Scheithauer BW, et al: *Radiology* 180:467–474, 1991.)

▶ This is 1 of the few studies of MS with histopathologic correlation. In most subjects, the lesions were considered active, had varied radiologic appearances, but did show contrast enhancement. The authors describe 3

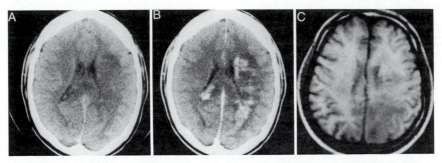

Fig 3–27.—Images of a patient with MS show infiltrative brain lesion. **A,** unenhanced CT scan shows ill-defined, large, low-attenuating region in the left frontal and parietal white matter, extending into the splenium of the corpus callosum. **B,** after administration of contrasting material, scattered central enhancement in the left cerebral white matter and right splenium are seen. **C,** axial short-TR, short-TE 600/20 MR image with 1 signal averaged shows infiltrative hypointensity in the left cerebral white matter and splenium. (Courtesy of Nesbit GM, Forbes GS, Scheithauer BW, et al: *Radiology* 180:467–474, 1991.)

distinct patterns for CT and MR presentation for clinically active MS.—J.F. Sackett, M.D.

Destructive Lesions in Demyelinating Disease
Youl BD, Kermode AG, Thompson AJ, Révész T, Scaravilli F, Barnard RO, Kirkham FJ, Kentall BE, Kingsley D, Moseley IF, Stevens JM, Earl CJ, McDonald WI (The Multiple Sclerosis NMR Research Group, Institute of Neurology and the National Hospitals for Nervous Diseases, London, England)
J Neurol Neurosurg Psychiatry 54:288–292, 1991   3–41

Background.—In patients suspected of having demyelinating disease, evidence that clinically, radiologically, or histologically suggests tissue destruction often presents diagnostic problems. This is because physicians may believe that the apparent development of tissue destruction is incompatible with the diagnosis of demyelinating disease. Three cases are presented in which the clinical and radiologic features suggested glioma, but biopsy proved a demyelinating process.

Case Report.—Boy, 16, had left-sided numbness, weakness, unsteadiness of gait, headache, and visual disturbance. An enhanced CT head scan was normal, but T₂-weighted MRI showed numerous discrete and periventricular hyperintensity lesions in the white matter. Abnormalities were also seen in both cerebellar hemispheres, the left side of the pons, and a small region adjacent to the right frontal horn. The patient had oligoclonal IgG bands present. Treated with methylprednisolone, he improved. After further symptoms developed, he was admitted to hospital where he transiently improved with methylprednisolone therapy. A CT scan showed a large ring-enhancing lesion in the right frontal lobe with mass effect and edema (Fig 3–28). A right frontal craniotomy was done to remove the wall of a cyst and surrounding tissue, based on the presumption of gli-

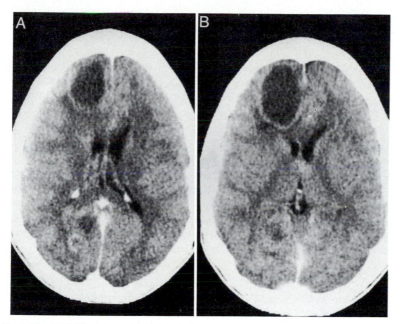

Fig 3–28.—Axial CT sections plain (**A**) and after intravenous contrast medium (**B**). There is a large low-density lesion that shows mass effect with a higher density rim that enhances. There is a small amount of surrounding edema. (Courtesy of Youl BD, Kermode AG, Thompson AJ, et al: *J Neurol Neurosurg Psychiatry* 54:288–292, 1991.)

oma. Histology results showed a subacute demyelinating lesion compatible with a plaque of multiple sclerosis (MS).

Additional Patients.—Two additional patients had probable acute disseminated encephalomyelitis. In 1, CT showed a high left frontoparietal lesion that enhanced in a ring pattern with contrast but without mass effect. A glioma was suspected, but aspiration biopsy samples were compatible with an acute demyelinating process. In the last case, T_2-weighted MRI showed small areas of high signal in the white matter of the cerebral hemispheres, discrete from the ventricles. Spinal cord biopsy material suggested a subacute or chronic demyelinating process. Multiple sclerosis could not be excluded.

Conclusion.—In all cases, surgical intervention was used. This was based on marked swelling or ring enhancement at CT, leading to the presumptive diagnosis of glioma. Histologic investigations ruled out neoplasia but instead identified an association of extensive tissue destruction with MS and acute disseminated encephalomyelitis. Because tissue destruction can occur in demyelinating disease, patients with known or possible MS and evidence of cysts or swelling of the brain or spinal cord and rapidly progressing neurologic dysfunction should be treated with corticosteroids. If this treatment fails, biopsy should be considered.

▶ This manuscript underlines the varied manifestation that MS may have in the brain. Ring enhancement with or without mass effect or diffuse enhancement with mass effect can both be manifestations of MS involving the brain. In our experience, a biopsy is required to make this proper diagnosis when the clinical manifestation and radiologic manifestation are confusing.—J.F. Sackett, M.D.

Abnormal Corpus Callosum: A Sensitive and Specific Indicator of Multiple Sclerosis
Gean AD, Vezina LG, Marton KI, Stimac GK, Peyster RG, Taveras JM, Davis KR (Massachusetts Gen Hosp; New England Deaconess Hosp, Boston; First Hill Diagnostic Imaging, Seattle; Hahnemann Med Ctr, Philadelphia)
Radiology 180:215–221, 1991   3–42

Introduction.—Different periventricular white matter diseases may have similar appearances on MRI. Magnetic resonance imaging has a high sensitivity for identifying multiple sclerosis (MS) lesions, but its diagnostic specificity is poor. The corpus callosum (CC) in patients with MS often has an abnormal appearance on MRI scans. A prospective study was undertaken to determine whether the detection of CC involvement on MRI might be specific for MS.

Patients.—Magnetic resonance imaging was performed in 42 patients with MS, aged 22 to 68 years, and in 127 patients with periventricular white matter disease of varying causes, aged 23 to 87 years. Image analysis was performed by neuroradiologists who had no knowledge of the patient's clinical history. Image analysis was limited to the region of the callosal-septal interface.

Results.—Thirty-nine MS patients (93%) had an abnormal callosal-septal interface that appeared as an irregular rim of hyperintensity along the inferior aspect of the CC at its junction with the pellucid septum (Fig 3–29). An abnormal callosal-septal interface was optimally demonstrated on long repetition time/short echo time midsagittal images, but it was also seen on axial and coronal images. In patients with more advanced MS, the focal CC lesions became confluent. A confluent appearance was always associated with some degree of CC atrophy. All CC lesions were seen in association with other white matter lesions. The remaining 3 MS patients (7%) had no focal abnormalities within the CC and were considered as having false negative callosal-septal interface examinations. The 3 patients with other periventricular white matter diseases (2.4%) who had CC lesions were considered as having false positive callosal-septal interface examinations. The appearance of the callosal-septal interface in these 3 patients differed from that in MS patients.

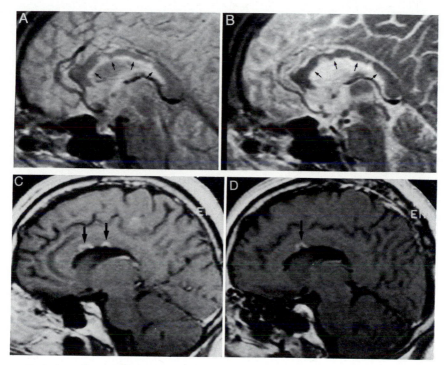

Fig 3–29.—A, long TR/short TE and (**B**) long TR/TE midsagittal images of a patient, 36, with multiple sclerosis. Note the irregular rim of hyperintensity in the region of the callosal-septal interface (*arrows*). The focal signal abnormalities abut the ventricular surface and extend into the overlying callosum. No significant atrophy of the corpus callosum is seen. **C** and **D,** short TR/TE sagittal images of same patient after intravenous administration of contrast agent with gadolinium core, demonstrating peripheral enhancement of the callosal-septal interface lesions (*arrows*). (Courtesy of Gean AD, Vezina LG, Marton KI, et al: *Radiology* 180:215–221, 1991.)

Conclusion.—The distinctive appearance of the callosal-septal interface as a nonuniform rim of hyperintensity along the inferior aspect of the CC on the midsagittal long repetition time/short echo time spin-echo image appears to be specific for MS.

▶ A corpus callosum change associated with the nonspecific white matter changes of MS appears to be a specific sign for MS. As with many specific signs, this must stand the test of time.—J.F. Sackett, M.D.

Spine

Effects of Magnetic Susceptibility Artifacts and Motion in Evaluating the Cervical Neural Foramina on 3DFT Gradient-Echo MR Imaging
Tsuruda JS, Remley K (Univ of California, San Francisco)
AJR 156:1069–1073, 1991

3–43

Background.—Anecdotal information has suggested that 3-dimensional Fourier transformation (3DFT) gradient-recalled echo (GRE) imaging usually provides excellent detail of the neural foramina, equal to that of CT, when used in the evaluation of cervical radiculopathy. In some patients, however, this technique has resulted in overestimations of the degree of neural foraminal stenosis. To try to find the reason for these errors, the effects of magnetic susceptibility and motion on the estimation of neural foraminal diameter using 3DFT GRE MRI were evaluated.

Methods.—This in vitro study was based on the use of a phantom cervical model, constructed from desiccated cadaveric vertebrae from the C5 through the T1 levels. After immobilization of the spinous processes in clay, the "vertebral column" formed was embedded in a water-based proteinaceous gel designed to give T_1 and T_2 relaxation properties similar to that of soft tissue. Thin-section CT was performed using a GE 9800 unit with axial 1.5-mm thick sections. Scanning at 1.5 T using a posterior planar surface coil was also performed, and multiple 3DFT GRE acquisitions were obtained with the echo time varied from 11 to 22 msec and the repetition time constant at 35 msec. The MR studies were repeated with gentle rocking of the phantom back and fourth 2 to 3 mm for 5-second periods separated by 30 seconds of stillness. Neural foraminal measurements were made from each type of study.

Results.—By underestimating the diameters of the neural foramina, MR studies consistently overestimated neural foraminal stenosis compared with CT findings. As the echo time values increased, the overestimations increased, from 8% at an echo time of 11 msec to 27% at an echo time of 22 msec. Overestimations were also increased by motion artifacts, which resembled osseous hypertrophy. Again, with motion, artifact increased with increased echo time.

Conclusion.—Imaging with short echo time 3DFT GRE MR can result in acceptable magnetic susceptibility artifacts, but imaging with longer echo times significantly increases the artifacts. Motion also degrades images qualitatively and quantitatively, especially with longer echo times. To reduce artifacts, 3DFT GRE MRI should involve the shortest possible echo time. This technique should not be used when patient motion is anticipated.

▶ This in vitro phantom study studies the variables to improve gradient-recalled steady-state MR compared with thin-section CT imaging. As might be predicted, CT remains that reference standard in determining bony foraminal stenosis.—J.F. Sackett, M.D.

Spinal Epidural Abscess: Evaluation With Contrast-Enhanced MR Imaging

Sandhu FS, Dillon WP (Univ of California, San Francisco)

AJNR 12:1087–1093, 1991

3–44

Background.—Diagnosis and treatment of spinal epidural abscess before the onset of neurologic deficits is crucial to prevent permanent deficits. Magnetic resonance imaging has replaced myelography with CT as the primary diagnostic method. Contrast-enhanced MRI increases the sensitivity and specificity of MR for spinal cord lesions. The pattern of enhancement after administration of gadopentetate dimeglumine was assessed and contrast-enhanced images were compared with routine T_1- and T_2-weighted images.

Methods.—The MR scans of 7 patients with spinal epidural abscess were reviewed retrospectively. The T_1-weighted precontrast and postcontrast images were analyzed and the T_1-weighted contrast-enhanced images were also compared with available T_2-weighted images.

Findings.—On MRI, the epidural infection was isointense to hypointense compared with the spinal cord on unenhanced T_1-weighted images, and increased in intensity on proton density–weighted and T_2-weighted images. After contrast administration, the infection enhanced homogeneously in 3 patients. In 1 patient, peripheral enhancement surrounded a central focus of low signal intensity (Fig 3–30). One abscess, which had infiltrated the posterior thoracic epidural fat, produced a decreased signal within the high-signal fat on T_1-weighted images. In 3 cases, the T_1- and T_2-weighted images were comparable, whereas in 2 cases, the T_1-weighted images were superior to the T_2-weighted images.

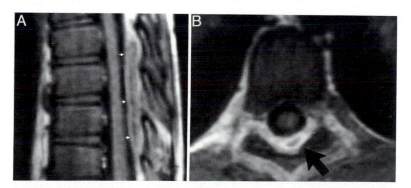

Fig 3–30.—Peripheral enhancement in the epidural abscess after contrast administration in a previously healthy 7-year-old boy who had increasing back pain and fever 1 week after being struck in the back while playing soccer. **A,** T1-weighted (600/20) sagittal image of the lower thoracic spine shows a focal oval low-signal-intensity area within the posterior epidural fat (*arrows*); **B,** a T1-weighted (600/20) contrast-enhanced axial image at the level of the abscess shows peripheral enhancement of epidural abscess (*arrow*) with a signal greater than adjacent epidural fat. (Courtesy of Sandhu FS, Dillon WP: *AJNR* 12:1087–1093, 1991.)

The enhanced images helped determine whether the abscess composition was liquid or solid.

Conclusion.—Contrast-enhanced MR images are useful in characterizing spinal epidural abscesses. Abscesses detected on routine T_1- and T_2-weighted images may have a nonspecific appearance. After administration of gadopentetate dimeglumine, there may be peripheral or homogeneous enhancement of the infection. The contrast-enhanced images aid in differentiating the composition of the abscess and separating the infectious component from surrounding CSF.

▶ The sensitivity of spinal MRI in detecting osteomyelitis has been described earlier. It is clear that MRI is also the technique of choice to detect spinal epidural abscess. The use of Gd increases the specificity.—J.F. Sackett, M.D.

Complications of Epidural Anesthesia: MR Appearance of Abnormalities
Sklar EML, Quencer RM, Green BA, Montalvo BM, Donovan MJD (Univ of Miami, Miami)
Radiology 181:549–554, 1991   3–45

Background.—Epidural anesthesia has supplanted spinal anesthesia because it is injected extradurally, lessening the risk of neurologic complications. However, some of the drug may enter the subarachnoid space or be unintentionally placed into the intradural space. Eight patients with acquired intradural arachnoid abnormalities caused by epidural anesthesia were evaluated, and the pathophysiologic mechanism for creating these abnormalities was examined.

Methods.—Eight women with arachnoiditis secondary to the administration of epidural anesthesia were evaluated with MRI, and 4 patients were evaluated with intraoperative ultrasound imaging. Seven of the 8 patients were referred from Latin America and 1 came from Italy.

Findings.—In 6 patients, subarachnoid cysts were found in the lower cervical and thoracic spine, and 7 patients had irregularity of the surface of the cord (Figs 3–31 and 3–32). Two patients had associated intramedullary cysts and myelomalacia. Magnetic resonance findings suggested arachnoiditis in 4 patients where it was unsuspected clinically. Magnetic resonance findings charactertistic of arachnoiditis are loculated collections of cerebrospinal fluid (subarachnoid cysts), irregularities of the surface of the cord, mass effect on the cord, and atrophied spinal cord. In 7 of the 8 patients, the suspected underlying mechanism for the intradural and cord abnormalities was a chemically induced arachnoiditis possibly caused by the preservative agents in the vials of anesthetic. In the eighth patient, an infection introduced at the time of the epidural injection was the cause of the abnormalities.

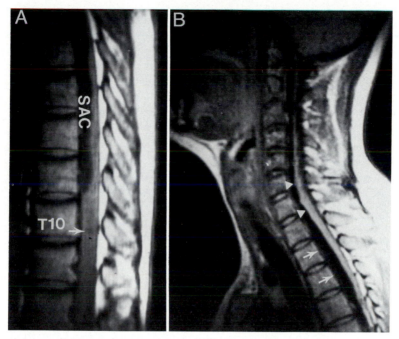

Fig 3–31.—Radiologic images of the cervical and thoracic spine obtained to rule out multiple sclerosis. **A,** ventral subarachnoid cyst extending from C-7 to T-10 displaces the cord posteriorly on this T1-weighted (1,000/20) image. *Arrow* points to small hypointense area that was found to represent a small intramedullary cyst with intraoperative spinal sonography. **B,** note the irregularity of the surface of the ventral cord in the cervical region (*arrowheads*) in this spin-echo (800/26) image. The subarachnoid cyst extended from T-10 superiorly to the C-7 level (*arrows*). The upper cervical spinal cord, although not seen in this section, was normal. (Courtesy of Sklar EML, Quencer RM, Green BA, et al: *Radiology* 181:549–554, 1991.)

Conclusion.—Magnetic resonance imaging enabled accurate characterization of subarachnoid cysts and arachnoiditis induced by epidural anesthesia. In 4 of 8 patients, MR was the first diagnostic examination to suggest the cause of symptoms. In 7 of 8 patients, the preservative agents in the epidural anesthetic appear to have caused arachnoiditis.

▶ We have had little prior understanding of the incidence and pattern of complications of epidural anesthesia. It is likely that the incidence of these complications is greater than previously thought. Magnetic resonance is, of course, the technique to detect postanesthesia arachnoiditis. Further studies are indicated to ensure that proper preservative agents are used with epidural anesthesia.—J.F. Sackett, M.D.

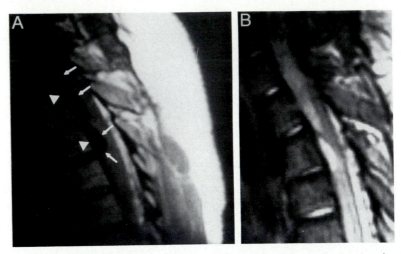

Fig 3–32.—Magnetic resonance images of a patient who had progressive numbness and weakness of the lower extremities after receiving epidural anesthesia for childbirth. On the (**A**) T1-weighted (800/20) and (**B**) T2-weighted (1,991/80) images, note the irregular ventral cord surface (*arrows* in **A**) and ventral CSF fluid collections (*arrowheads* in **A**). (Courtesy of Sklar EML, Quencer RM, Green BA, et al: *Radiology* 181:549–554, 1991.)

Symptomatic Chiari Malformation in Adults: A New Classification Based on Magnetic Resonance Imaging With Clinical and Prognostic Significance
Pillay PK, Awad IA, Little JR, Hahn JF (Cleveland Clinic Found, Cleveland)
Neurosurgery 28:639–645, 1991   3–46

Background.—Varying surgical anatomy at the craniovertebral junction has been noted in adults with Chiari malformation, with overlapping features of both types of hindbrain pathologic change and a lack of association with myelodysplasia or hydrocephalus. A new classification is based on MR imaging of symptomatic Chiari malformation in adults.

Patients and Methods.—Thirty-five consecutively seen adults aged 18 to 57 years with progressive symptoms were treated at 1 center over 3 years. Magnetic resonance imaging was done before and after surgery in all cases.

Findings.—Craniovertebral junction images confirmed herniation in all patients. Two anatomically distinct categories of the Chiari malformation in this age group were defined. Twenty patients, with concomitant syringomyelia, were classified as type A. The remaining 15 patients, with frank herniation of the brain stem below the foramen magnum but without evidence of syringomyelia, were classified as type B. Type A patients had a predominant central cord symptomatology. Patients with type B showed signs and symptoms of brain stem or cerebellar compression. The main treatment consisted of decompression of the foramen magnum, opening of the fourth ventricular outlet, and plugging of the obex. Significant improvement occurred after treatment in 45% of patients with type A and in 87% with type B. Postoperative reduction in syrinx volume was noted in 11 patients with type A, including all 9 with excellent results.

Conclusion.—Magnetic resonance imaging has enabled a classification of the adult Chiari malformation that is based on objective anatomical criteria. This classification has clinical and prognostic relevance. Patients with syringomyelia appear to respond less favorably to surgical intervention.

▶ These 35 subjects, who were symptomatic, had surgical management. Only half the patients with syringomyelia improved after surgery. This probably is related to the chronic nature of the syringomyelia and fixed myelopathy.—J.F. Sackett, M.D.

MR Imaging of Spinal Cord and Vertebral Body Infarction
Yuh WTC, Marsh EE III, Wang AK, Russell JW, Chiang F, Koci TM, Ryals TJ (Univ of Iowa, Iowa City, Iowa; Rancho Los Amigos Med Ctr, Downey, Calif; Harbor-Univ of California, Los Angeles Med Ctr, Torrance, Calif)
AJNR 13:145–154, 1992   3–47

Background.—Spinal cord infarctions are rare and difficult to diagnose. The MR findings associated with spinal cord and vertebral body infarctions were reviewed.

Patients and Methods.—Magnetic resonance examinations of 12 patients were performed 8 hours to 4 months after abrupt onset of symptoms of spinal cord ischemia. The 10 male and 2 female patients were aged 17 to 85 years.

Results.—The MR findings included abnormal cord signal, best seen on T_2-weighted images (Fig 3–33), and morphologic changes, best seen on T_1-weighted images.

Conclusions.—Magnetic resonance imaging is useful in the detection of spinal cord infarction and associated vascular and bony changes. The bone marrow abnormalities reflect the pathophysiology of the blood supply to the bone and cord and enhance diagnosis.

▶ Once again, MR has been shown to be sensitive for picking up a difficult to diagnose entity. Vertebral body changes from ischemia appear to occur concomitantly with spinal cord ischemic change.—J.F. Sackett, M.D.

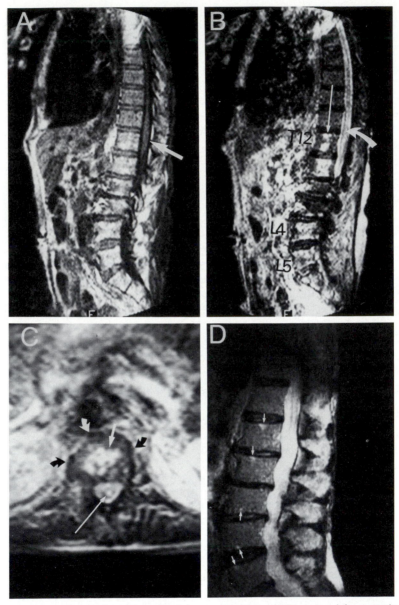

Fig 3–33.—Man, 76, had weakness of both lower extremities and T-7 sensory deficit immediately after bilateral aortoiliac bypass for abdominal aortic aneurysm. **A,** parasagittal T1-weighted image (350/20) shows enlargement (*arrow*) of the spinal cord. **B,** a parasaggittal T2-weighted image (2,000/100) shows abnormal signal (*curved arrow*) within the spinal cord from T-11–L-1 levels to conus. Abnormal bone marrow signal is also noted involving multiple vertebrae, especially T-12–L-1 levels, predominantly in areas near the end-plate and deep medullary portion of the vertebral body. Characteristic triangular ischemic areas (*straight arrow*) correspond to regions that are most vulnerable *(continued)*

Spinal Epidural Abscess: Evaluation With Contrast-Enhanced MR Imaging

Sandhu FS, Dillon WP (Univ of California, San Francisco)
AJR 158:405–411, 1992   3–48

Background.—A spinal epidural abscess, usually caused by *Staphylococcus aureus*, is relatively uncommon but can produce severe neurologic deficits and death if left untreated. Early symptoms may include fever and localized tenderness over the spine, but nonspecific symptoms may delay diagnosis. Magnetic resonance imaging has replaced myelography with CT as the primary diagnostic method. The pattern of enhancement of spinal epidural abscesses after administration of gadopentetate dimeglumine was identified and contrast-enhanced images and routine T_1- and T_2-weighted sequences were compared.

Method.—Seven patients with spinal epidural abscess were evaluated with T_1-weighted images before and after the administration of gadopentetate dimeglumine. The contrast-enhanced images were compared with available T_2-weighted images and unenhanced T_1-weighted images.

Findings.—On MRI, epidural abscesses characteristically appear as a mass isointense with the spinal cord on T_1-weighted images and high in signal intensity on T_2-weighted images. The MR images of the epidural infection were characteristic in 6 of the 7 cases. Patterns of contrast enhancement were a homogeneous increase in signal in the area of infection, peripheral enhancement surrounding a central focus of low signal intensity, or a combination of peripheral and homogeneous enhancement. In 3 cases, enhanced T_1-weighted images were equivalent to unenhanced T_2-weighted images in detecting the extent of epidural involvement. In 2 cases, the enhanced T_1-weighted images were superior to T_2-weighted images in differentiating the infectious component from surrounding CSF. In 1 case, contrast administration produced no discernible enhancement (Fig 3–34).

Conclusion.—Spinal epidural abscess can usually be detected on routine T_1- and T_2-weighted images with a characteristic image of a mass of low signal intensity on T_1-weighted images and homogeneous increased signal on T_2-weighted images. After administration of the contrast agent gadopentetate dimeglumine, there may be homogeneous or peripheral enhancement of the epidural infection. Enhanced images may demon-

Fig 3–33 (cont).
to ischemia. Other possibly involved vertebrae include L-4, L-5, and S-1. Flow-void phenomena of the abdominal aorta are not seen on parasagittal images because of complete aortic occlusion. Bone marrow abnormalities are not obvious on T1-weighted image (**A**). **C**, axial T2-weighted image obtained at pedicle level shows abnormal signal in central gray matter of spinal cord (*long straight arrow*). Abnormal bone marrow signal shows location of ischemia in the deep medullary portion (*short straight arrow*) of the vertebral body (*curved arrows*). **D**, a parasaggital T2-weighted image (2,000/100) obtained with surface coil 1 year later shows similar findings. However, these lesions (*arrows*) are much smaller, and the triangular area in most vulnerable regions now may represent true infarcted rather than ischemic areas. (Courtesy of Yuh WTC, Marsh EE III, Wang AK, et al: *AJNR* 13:145–154, 1992.)

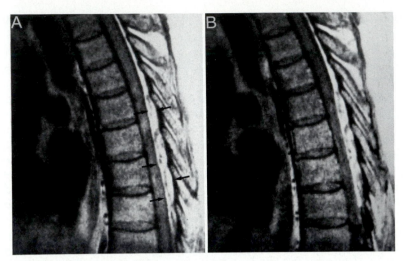

Fig 3–34.—Epidural abscess presenting as infiltration of the posterior epidural fat in a man, 57. **A** and **B,** T1-weighted (500/24/4) sagittal images of midthoracic spine were obtained before (**A**) and after (**B**) administration of gadopentetate dimeglumine. On both the unenhanced and enhanced images, multiple low-signal-intensity areas infiltrate and enlarge the posterior epidural fat over 3 vertebral segments (*arrows*). Mild mass effect on the thecal sac is evident by attenuation of CSF posterior to the cord. No significant enhancement is identified on contrast-enhanced images. Enhancement is not appreciated because of the high signal from the fat. Incidentally noted is high signal in the spinal cord, which represents motion artifact from adjacent great vessels. (Courtesy of Sandhu FS, Dillon WP: *AJR* 158:405–411, 1992.)

strate a drainable abscess and help differentiate the infectious component from surrounding CSF in some cases.

▶ Magnetic resonance scanning without intravenous contrast is usually diagnostic of epidural infection. The use of Gd may allow the selection of patients for abscess drainage, because this may be a technique for separating cellulitis from drainable abscess.—J.F. Sackett, M.D.

Ultrasound

Carotid Duplex Sonography: Bisferious Pulse Contour in Patients With Aortic Valvular Disease

Kallman CE, Gosink BB, Gardner DJ (VA Med Ctr, Univ of California, San Diego)
AJR 157:403–407, 1991   3–49

Introduction.—The bisferious waveform (defined as 2 systolic peaks) and retrograde diastolic flow are characteristic carotid Doppler patterns associated with aortic regurgitation. However, the presence of a bisferious pulse contour or retrograde diastolic flow has never been documented in the carotid duplex waveforms of patients with aortic valve disease. The presence of these carotid duplex waveform abnormalities was

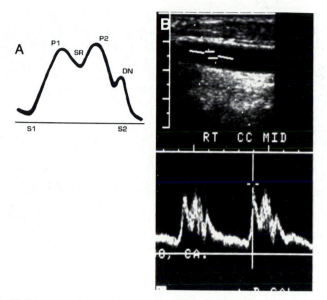

Fig 3–35.—Bisferious waveform with 2 systolic peaks. **A,** diagram shows 2 systolic peaks (*P1, P2*) separated by midsystolic retraction (*SR*). *Abbreviations: DN*, dicrotic notch; *S1*, first heart sound, resulting from artrioventricular valves closing and pulmonic and aortic valves opening; *S2*, second heart sound, caused by aortic and pulmonic valves closing. **B,** duplex tracing of external carotid artery in a man, 50, with moderate aortic regurgitation. (Courtesy of Kallman CE, Gosink BB, Gardner DJ: *AJR* 157:403–407, 1991.)

investigated in patients with known aortic valve disease and to correlate the findings with the severity of valve regurgitation.

Patients.—The study population consisted of 25 men and 1 woman, aged 33 to 90 years, who had preoperative duplex carotid sonography and echocardiography before undergoing coronary artery bypass grafting or valve replacement. All patients had aortic regurgitation or combined aortic regurgitation and stenosis. The carotid duplex sonograms of 20 age-matched patients with a variety of cardiovascular diseases but no evidence of aortic valvular disease were also studied. The carotid duplex sonograms were examined by 2 radiologists for the presence of the bisferious waveform and diastolic flow reversal.

Results.—Thirteen patients (50%) with aortic regurgitation had bisferious waveforms on their carotid duplex sonograms (Fig 3–35) and 5 patients (19%) had significant retrograde diastolic flow. Three patients with retrograde diastolic flow also had bisferious waveforms. The other 2 patients had diastolic flow reversal without bisferious waveforms. In all, 15 patients (57%) had abnormal waveforms. Four patients with abnormal waveforms who subsequently underwent aortic valve replacement had normal waveforms after the operation (Fig 3–36). None of the 20 control patients had characteristic systolic or diastolic abnormalities.

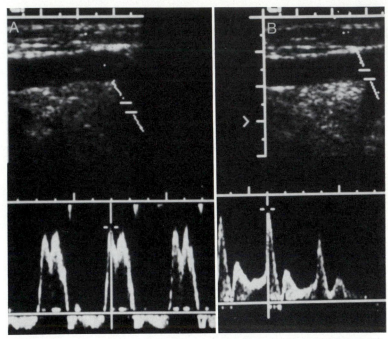

Fig 3–36.—Changes in carotid waveform after aortic valvular replacement in a man, 59, with severe aortic stenosis and moderate aortic regurgitation. **A,** initial duplex sonogram shows both a bisferious pattern and retrograde flow throughout diastole. **B,** a duplex sonogram obtained 8 days after aortic valvular replacement shows normal carotid waveforms with a single systolic peak and antegrade diastolic flow. (Courtesy of Kallman CE, Gosink BB, Gardner DJ: AJR 157:403-407, 1991.)

Conclusion.—Because up to one third of patients with aortic regurgitation may not have a detectable murmur, carotid duplex sonography may be useful in identifying previously unsuspected aortic valvular disease.

▶ This peculiar waveform in Doppler carotid sonography has characteristics that are reproducible and probably diagnostic of aortic insufficiency. Cardiac echo would, of course, be the next study.—J.F. Sackett, M.D.

Cerebral Vasospasm Evaluated by Transcranial Doppler Ultrasonography at Different Intracranial Pressures
Klingelhöfer J, Sander D, Holzgraefe M, Bischoff C, Conrad B (University of Göttingen, Göttingen, Germany; Technical University of Munich, Munich, Germany)
J Neurosurg 75:752–758, 1991   3–50

Background.—Transcranial Doppler (TCD) ultrasonography is a noninvasive method of diagnosis for cerebrovascular spasm in patients with subarachnoid hemorrhage and allows observation of its time course. The interdependence of the patient's clinical grade, vasospasm, intracranial pressure (ICP), and TCD ultrasonographic parameters was evaluated.

Methods.—Seventy-six patients with spontaneous subarachnoid hemorrhage underwent angiography. The mean flow velocity of blood in the middle cerebral artery and the index of cerebral circulatory resistance as a measure of the peripheral vascular flow resistance were determined. The ICP was measured with an epidural transducer in 41 patients.

Findings.—High ICP and a high mean flow velocity were never observed simultaneously. When the resistance index was less than .5, changes in the mean flow velocity sufficiently reflected the actual severity and time course of vasospasm. An increase in the resistance index above values of .6 with a simultaneously decreased mean flow velocity during the time course of vasospasm indicated increased ICP rather than a reduction in vasospasm. When the ICP is increased, evaluation of the severity and time course of vasospasm by TCD ultrasonography based solely on the mean flow velocity can lead to false negative results.

Conclusion.—The interdependence of clinical stage, cerebral vasospasm, ICP, and TCD ultrasonographic parameters were studied in patients with spontaneous subarachnoid hemorrhage.

▶ Transcranial Doppler will likely be the noninvasive technique of choice to evaluate cerebral vasospasm following subarachnoid hemorrhage. Portable dedicated equipment is required for this technique.—J.F. Sackett, M.D.

Carotid Body Tumors: US Evaluation
Derchi LE, Serafini G, Rabbia C, De Albertis P, Solbiati L, Candiani F, Musante F, Bertoglio C, Rizzatto G (Università di Genova, Genoa, Italy; Ospedale di Savona, Savona, Italy; Ospedale Molinette, Turin, Italy; Varese Ospedale, Busto Arsizio, Italy; Università di Padova, Padua, Italy; et al)
Radiology 182:457–459, 1992   3–51

Background.—Carotid body tumors are relatively rare lesions arising from the chemoreceptor tissue at the bifurcation of the common carotid arteries. The role of ultrasound (US) in the diagnosis of these tumors has not been thoroughly studied.

Methods and Findings.—Twenty patients with 23 carotid body tumors underwent US. Twenty-two of the tumors were visualized on US. The remaining lesion could not be distinguished from surrounding enlarged lymph nodes caused by thyroid cancer. The tumors were solid and slightly heterogeneous, ranging from 1.2 to 5 cm. They were found within the carotid bifurcation. In 8 patients with 9 carotid body lesions, pulsed Doppler analysis of blood flow within the tumor mass was possible. Low-resistance waveforms were obtained from many sites within the

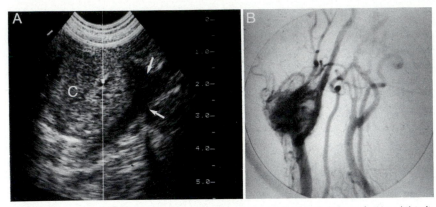

Fig 3–37.—**A,** sagittal ultrasound scan (7.5-MHz transducer) of right-sided chemodectoma (**C**) indicates a close relationship with the internal carotid artery. The tumor is solid, with many fine vascular channels. *Arrows* indicate the carotid bifurcation. **B,** digital subtraction angiogram of the same tumor demonstrates a hypervascular mass within the carotid bifurcation. (Courtesy of Derchi LE, Serafini G, Rabbia C, et al: *Radiology* 182:457–459, 1992.)

mass in all patients. Overall, a US diagnosis was possible in 18 of the 20 patients in this series (Fig 3–37).

Conclusion.—The diagnosis of a carotid body tumor must be considered when a solid mass is seen within the carotid bifurcation. Doppler analysis of the mass to assess intratumor blood flow is useful in differentiating carotid body tumors from other solid, nonhypervascular lesions.

▶ Ultrasound is an excellent technique for assessing neck masses. The US, in this case, demonstrates the relationship of the mass to the carotid bifurcation and the hyperechoic nature secondary to its vascularity.—J.F. Sackett, M.D.

Transcranial Doppler Sonography Monitoring of Local Intra-arterial Thrombolysis in Acute Occlusion of the Middle Cerebral Artery
Karnik R, Stelzer P, Slany J (Krankenanstalt Rudolfstiftung, Vienna, Austria)
Stroke 23:284–287, 1992   3–52

Background.—Thrombolytic therapy is being examined as a potential therapy for acute stroke, and knowledge of the timing of vessel reperfusion will be useful in adjusting the lytic regimen. Transcranial Doppler (TCD) ultrasonography was used as a noninvasive diagnostic monitoring tool during local intra-arterial lysis in a patient with acute embolic occlusion of the middle cerebral artery (MCA).

Results.—Local thrombolysis was performed with human tissue plasminogen activator at a dosage of 0.05 mg/kg/hr. The thrombolytic process was monitored by TCD ultrasonography. After the first 120 minutes a hemodynamically relevant residual stenosis was observed, and complete patency was obtained 180 minutes later.

Conclusion.—Transcranial Doppler ultrasonography may be useful for monitoring the thrombolytic treatment of occlusion of the MCA and determining patency.

▶ This is an innovative application of TCD sonography. This, again, emphasizes the importance of portable equipment that can be taken to the angiography suite.—J.F. Sackett, M.D.

Sella

High-Intensity Signals Within the Posterior Pituitary Fossa: A Study With Fat-Suppression MR Techniques

Mark LP, Haughton VM, Hendrix LE, Daniels DL, Williams AL, Czervionke LF, Asleson RJ (Med College of Wisconsin, Milwaukee)
AJNR 12:529–532, 1991   3–53

Background.—Many explanations are offered for the high-intensity signals seen near the posterior pituitary fossa on T_1-weighted MR images. They include a paramagnetic effect on phospholipids, fat in the sella outside the gland, a short-T_1 substance in neurosecretory granules, lipid in posterior-lobe pituicytes, and lipid in the dorsum sellae and posterior clinoid bone marrow.

Study.—The high-intensity signals were analyzed using fat-suppression MR imaging to define the contribution of fat. The sellae of 19 normal subjects and 2 cadavers were imaged using an experimental fat-water-suppression technique.

Observations.—Technically adequate fat- and water-suppression images were achieved in 19 subjects. Seventeen studies demonstrated suppression with water-suppression technique; 2 showed suppression with fat suppression; and 2 were indeterminate.

Discussion.—There may be more than 1 source of high-intensity signals in the posterior sella. Sources not suppressing with fat-suppression MRI appear to account for most cases. In a few cases, an artifact, fat pad, pituicyte lipid, or bone marrow may be responsible.

▶ This is 1 of 3 studies presented at the American Society of Neuroradiology meeting in March of 1989 dealing with the posterior pituitary signal. There is consensus that there is more than 1 source for this high-intensity signal.—J.F. Sackett, M.D.

MR Imaging of the Brain in Patients With Diabetes Insipidus

Tien R, Kucharczyk J, Kucharczyk W (Univ of California, San Francisco)
AJNR 12:533–542, 1991   3–54

Introduction.—Studies have reported that as many as 50% of cases of diabetes insipidus (DI) may result from head injury. If not promptly identified and treated, DI can lead to life-threatening hypernatremia and the need for continuous medical care. The MR studies of 26 patients with clinically proved DI were reviewed.

Methods.—The patients were 12 females and 14 males, with a mean age of 28 years. Both enhanced and unenhanced MR scans were analyzed by 2 neuroradiologists.

Results.—The MR scan results demonstrated a uniformly thickened pituitary stalk in the coronal and sagittal planes in 6 female patients. Four patients had a large, abnormal upper pituitary stalk on acute onset and persistence of DI. One of these individuals also had an isolated hypothalamic growth on MR enhancement. Two patients demonstrated a craniopharyngioma at the acute onset of DI, with enhanced MR verifying sellar and suprasellar masses accompanied by a large multicystic lesion in the posterior third ventricle. One patient, 12 years old, had a visual field defect along with the acute onset of DI, which was associated with a hypothalamic lesion. A patient with tuberculosis and acute onset of DI and seizures was found to have a uniformly thickened stalk and, after enhancement of the MR, some diffuse material in the basal cisterns and a spinal epidural abscess. Two patients with transient DI and visual problems had inhomogeneous sellar and suprasellar masses, later diagnosed as primary carcinomas. Three patients undergoing hypophysectomy for pituitary cancer all had transient DI, and 2 individuals injured in car accidents had this same disorder. A patient with an 8-year history of DI was diagnosed with Erdheim-Chester disease. Review of these patients found 10 individuals with uniformly thickened pituitary infundibulum. Twenty-two of the 26 patients showed no signs of the hyperintense posterior pituitary usually found in DI patients.

Conclusion.—In this series of patients, MRI suggested a specific diagnosis in most DI cases, particularly when coupled with clinical observations.

▶ Once again, MRI is the technique of choice to assess patients with DI. This is valuable for detecting infiltration of the pituitary stalk or transection of the pituitary stalk after trauma.—J.F. Sackett, M.D.

Size and Shape of the Pituitary Gland During Pregnancy and Post Partum: Measurement With MR Imaging

Elster AD, Sanders TG, Vines FS, Chen MYM (Wake Forest Univ, Winston-Sa-

lem, NC)
Radiology 181:531–535, 1991

Introduction.—Magnetic resonance imaging often aids in the diagnosis of pituitary disorders. Standard MR measurements for the size and shape of the pituitary glands have been published recently. The alterations in the pituitary gland's size and shape that occur during pregnancy and postpartum were investigated.

Methods.—Sixty-eight healthy women with no apparent pituitary disorders underwent MR evaluation over 2 years. Group 1 consisted of 17 pregnant women (median age, 24 years), group 2 consisted of 12 women up to 6 days after the birth, and group 3 included 15 women and volunteers imaged 1 week to 6 months after delivering an infant. Group 4 consisted of 30 control female subjects. The MRI was conducted at high-field strength in all cases.

Results.—The findings for the 17 percent subjects demonstrated a specific, significant increase in the height and convexity of the pituitary gland as the pregnancy continued. The gland became the largest and roundest during the days immediately after delivery. Figure 3–38 shows a significant expansion of the pituitary gland between 30-weeks' gestation and 4 days after the birth, whereas Figure 3–39 represents the largest gland found in this series of women (the MR image was taken 4 days after delivery). Promptly after the postpartum period, the size and shape of the pituitary gland decreased. The high signal intensity occurred in 11 of the 17 pregnant subjects, in 16 of 27 postpartum women, and in 20 of 30 controls.

Conclusion.—These findings establish specific figures and MRI guidelines for the size and shape of the pituitary gland during pregnancy and immediately after delivery. It is advised that 10 mm be used as the upper

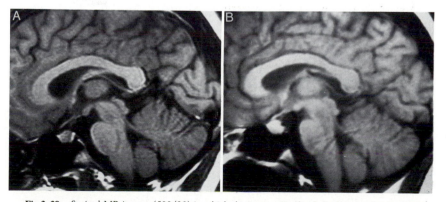

Fig 3–38.—Sagittal MR images (500/20) in which the increase in gland size between late pregnancy and postpartum is evident. **A,** at 30 weeks' gestation, the gland is 8.3 mm high and has a grade 4 shape. **B,** at 4 days post partum, the gland is noticeably larger (height, 10 mm; shape, grade 5). (Courtesy of Elster AD, Sanders TG, Vines FS, et al: *Radiology* 181:531–535, 1991.)

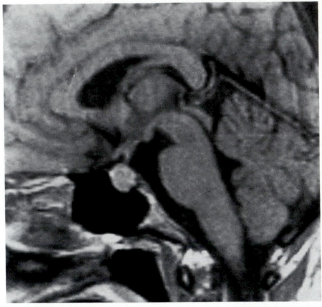

Fig 3–39.—Sagittal MR image (500/20) of the largest gland in this series of patients. The image was obtained at 4 days postpartum (height, 11.8 mm; shape, grade 5). (Courtesy of Elster AD, Sanders TG, Vines FS, et al: *Radiology* 181:531–535, 1991.)

limit for normal gland height during the last 2 trimesters of the pregnancy, whereas 12 mm would best serve as the upper limit for normal pituitary gland height during the last few weeks of pregnancy and the first week after delivery.

▶ This is the first quantitative measurement of physiologic change of the pituitary gland related to pregnancy. A gland height of 12 mm may be found in a postpartum phase of pituitary change.—J.F. Sackett, M.D.

Radiologic Characteristics and Results of Surgical Management of Rathke's Cysts in 43 Patients
Ross DA, Norman D, Wilson CB (Univ of Californfia, San Francisco; Univ of Michigan, Ann Arbor, Mich)
Neurosurgery 30:173–179, 1992   3–56

Objective.—Rathke's cysts are sellar and suprasellar structures found in up to one third of autopsies; they rarely are symptomatic. Experience was reviewed on the management of Rathke's cysts in 43 patients operated on in a 13-year period.

Patients and Management.—Forty patients underwent transsphenoidal surgery with drainage of the cyst contents and biopsy of the cyst wall.

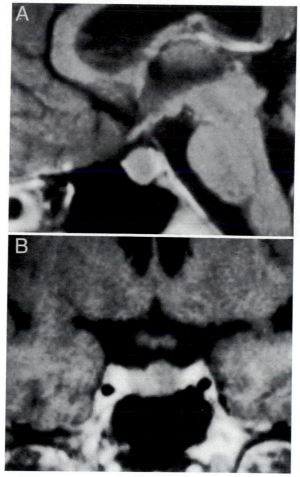

Fig 3–40.—T1-weighted MR images of well-circumscribed intrasellar Rathke's cyst measuring 9 mm in diameter and showing low intensity, located centrally and left of midline. There is displacement of pituitary stalk and normal gland to right. The lesion is indistinguishable from a pituitary microadenoma. (Courtesy of Ross DA, Norman D, Wilson CB: *Neurosurgery* 30:173–179, 1992.)

Biopsy specimens confirmed at Rathke's cyst in 26 of these patients. Patients with a Rathke's cyst recognized at surgery were followed up for a mean of about 5½ years.

Appearances.—Nineteen of the 30 cysts visualized on CT study and MRI were 3 to 10 mm in diameter. Two thirds of them were at an intrasellar site, and one third were suprasellar lesions. Most of the larger lesions had both intrasellar and suprasellar components. Most contrast CT studies demonstrated a low-density cyst. Two thirds of the MRI studies showed a high signal intensity cyst on short repetition time/echo time images, and one third showed a low signal intensity cyst (Fig 3–40). The

MRI studies done with contrast enhancement demonstrated both the intrasellar and suprasellar components. Imaging using long repetition time/echo time parameters yielded variable signal intensity values.

Recommendations.—Simple drainage by the transsphenoidal route and biopsy of the cyst wall are suggested for symptomatic Rathke's cysts. A single follow-up MRI study is appropriate unless symptoms or signs develop.

▶ Because of a varied cyst content, the MR image may show a varied MR signal from the cyst contents. Most Rathke's cysts are intrasellar in location.—J.F. Sackett, M.D.

Hamartomas of the Tuber Cinereum: CT, MR, and Pathologic Findings
Boyko OB, Curnes JT, Oakes WJ, Burger PC (Duke Univ Med Ctr, Durham, NC; Greensboro Radiology Associates, Greensboro, NC)
AJNR 12:309–314, 1991   3–57

Introduction.—Hamartoma of the tuber cinereum is a rare malformation that is usually found during investigation of precocious puberty or seizures. Both CT and MRI were used to evaluate 5 children having biopsy-proved hypothalamic hamartomas.

Findings.—The 3 patients with pedunculated hamartomas all had precocious puberty, whereas both of those with sessile lesions had seizures. Preoperative MRI demonstrated lesions that were isointense with gray matter on T_1-weighted images and hyperintense relative to gray matter on the second echo of T_2-weighted images. Intermediate (first-echo) T_2-weighted images demonstrated either isointensity or hyperintensity relative to gray matter. No contrast enhancement occurred on CT scanning. None of the lesions contained calcium.

Discussion.—Hamartomas of the tuber cinereum most closely resemble gray matter on T_1-weighted MR studies. The finding of a third ventricular mass having MR signal characteristics suggestive of gray matter in a child with precocious puberty or seizures should suggest the possibility of hamartoma of the tuber cinereum.

▶ This is a good description of the MR and CT findings of this entity. Once upon a time when skull films were used, a suprasellar calcification could be considered a hamartoma of the tuber cinereum. No calcifications were seen in this small group of patients.—J.F. Sackett, M.D.

ENT/Orbit

MR Imaging of Sjögren Syndrome: Correlation With Sialography and Pathology
Takashima S, Takeuchi N, Morimoto S, Tomiyama N, Ikezoe J, Shogen K,

Kozuka T, Okumura T (Osaka University, Osaka, Japan)
J Comput Assist Tomogr 15:393–400, 1991   3–58

Background.—Sjögren syndrome is characterized by dry eyes, dry mouth, and signs of a systemic autoimmune disease. Magnetic resonance imaging of the parotid glands in patients with this syndrome was performed to determine if there are any typical MRI features.

Methods.—Thirteen patients were studied. Their MRI results were compared with results of sialography and pathologic assessment. Signal intensity ratios of parotid to skeletal muscle were measured in the patients and in 10 healthy control subjects.

Results.—Both T_1- and T_2-weighted images demonstrated multiple hypointense mixed with hyperintense foci throughout the glands in the 6 patients with disease of intermediate severity. Inhomogeneous glands were observed in the 5 patients with early or advanced disease, and homogeneous glands were noted in the remaining 2 patients with the earliest stage of disease. Mean intensity ratios in T_2-weighted pulse sequences in the patients with salt-and-pepper appearances and inhomogeneous glands were significantly smaller than those of healthy subjects. Pathologic assessment suggested that focal lymphocytic aggregates associated with increased interlobular fibrosis were probably responsible for the hypointense foci and the reduction in intensity ratios (Fig 3–41).

Conclusion.—The salt-and-pepper appearance seen in this series may suggest Sjögren syndrome. The reduced intensity ratios combined with a typical clinical picture may enable a highly probable diagnosis of the disorder.

▶ It appears that parotid gland imaging can be correlated with early, intermediate, and late stages of Sjögren's syndrome. The clinical application of these findings remains to be defined.—J.F. Sackett, M.D.

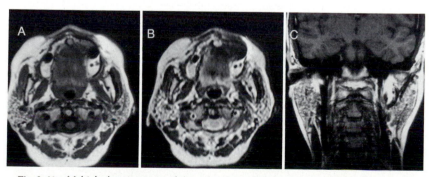

Fig 3–41.—Multiple hypointense and hyperintense spots 1–2 mm in diameter are distributed throughout the parotid glands on axial SE 600/15 (**A**) and SE 2,000/70 (**B**) and coronal SE 600/15 (**C**) images. Note the salt-and-pepper appearance of glands. (Courtesy of Takashima S, Takeuchi N, Morimoto S, et al: *J Comput Assist Tomogr* 15:393–400, 1991.)

Meckel Cave Lesions: Percutaneous Fine-Needle-Aspiration Biopsy Cytology

Dresel SHJ, Mackey JK, Lufkin RB, Jabour BA, Desalles AAF, Layfield LJ, Duckwiler GR, Becker DP, Bentson JR, Hanafee WN (Univ of California, Los Angeles)
Radiology 179:579–581, 1991   3–59

Background.—The percutaneous approach to Meckel's cave via the foramen ovale is an old technique, as is the use of fine-needle aspiration biopsy cytology for the diagnosis of head and neck lesions. Here, the 2 techniques are combined in a new procedure permitting diagnosis of deep lesions involving Meckel's cave in the middle cranial fossa. Without this method, lesions of this region might otherwise require craniotomy to permit tissue sampling sufficient for a histologic diagnosis.

Methods.—Two patients underwent percutaneous aspiration biopsy cytology of Meckel's cave lesions via the foramen ovale. The technique was performed on an outpatient basis after preliminary submentovertex, anteroposterior or Water, and lateral plain radiographs were obtained. With the patient supine, the head was rotated until optimal visualization of the foramen ovale occurred, using cephalic, angulated fluoroscopy. Lidocaine was injected at the site of needle entry and further injections were administered as a spinal needle was advanced toward the foramen ovale under intermittent fluoroscopic observation. Care was taken to avoid puncture of the internal carotid artery. Plain radiographs in different projections verified correct location of the needle tip within Meckel's cave. Multiple aspiration samples were then obtained, and cytopathologic reviews of samples were performed.

Results.—The first patient had been shown to have adenoid cystic carcinoma of the parotid gland and cervical lymphadenopathy. Computed tomography showed a mass in the anterior aspect of the cistern of the left cerebellopontine angle, with the ipsilateral foramen ovale enlarged. Magnetic resonance imaging showed an isointense mass within Meckel's cave. A Gd-enhanced MRI showed enhancement of the lesion, extending to the foramen ovale. Biopsy of the isointense area seen on T_2-weighted images was necessary to rule out a concurrent tumor of another origin. The needle was placed under fluoroscopic guidance, with its position confirmed by plain radiograph. A sample was easily aspirated, showing solid-pattern adenoid cystic carcinoma. In the second patient, CT and MRI showed a lesion in the right cavernous sinus and Meckel's cave. The needle was inserted into Meckel's cave, aspirate obtained, and lymphoma diagnosed after microscopic review. Both patients were discharged after 2 hours of observation, and neither suffered complications. Accurate needle penetration of the foramen ovale was easily achieved after the foramen ovale was identified with fluoroscopy.

Conclusion.—This combination of aspiration cytology with a percutaneous approach to Meckel's cave lesions permits tissue sampling with less patient morbidity and at less cost than otherwise possible. Use of this technique requires fluoroscopic guidance and verification of the position of the coaxial needle by plain radiographs in 3 views.

▶ This new application to foramen ovale placement of a needle is an excellent interventional technique for biopsy. This, indeed, would have far less patient morbidity than the standard surgical approach.—J.F. Sackett, M.D.

Simulated Aggressive Skull Base Erosion in Response to Benign Sinonasal Disease
Som PM, Lawson W, Lidov MW (City Univ of New York, New York)
Radiology 180:755–759, 1991   3–60

Introduction.—Inverted papilloma is a rare, benign neoplasm arising in the nasal cavity and paranasal sinuses. Its malignant potential is low, ranging from 3% to 13%. Nasal polyps and inverted papillomas tend to remodel the nasal vault and facial bones. However, when these benign masses press against the floor of the anterior cranial fossa and the walls of the sphenoid sinuses, the imaging appearance will simulate aggressive bone destruction, rather than bone remodeling. The imaging studies of 14 patients were reviewed to illustrate this diagnostic dilemma.

Methods.—The CT scans of 40 patients with inverted papillomas and 100 with nasal polyposis and mucoceles were reviewed. The scans of 2 patients with inverted papillomas and 12 with nasal polyposis and mucoceles showed evidence of aggressive bone destruction of the skull base (Fig 3–42). However, surgical exploration revealed that the growths pressing against the eroded bone were benign and had not invaded the destroyed bone. The CT scans of these 14 patients were compared with

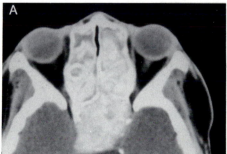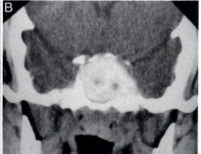

Fig 3–42.—Axial (**A**) and coronal (**B**) noncontrast CT scans of a patient with extensive polyposis. The ethmoid and sphenoid sinuses are completely filled. The ethmoid complex is widened; however, the laminae papyracea remain intact but are remodeled outward into the orbits. The walls of the sphenoid sinus are eroded. (Courtesy of Som PM, Lawson W, Lidov MW, et al: *Radiology* 180:755–759, 1991.)

those of a patient with inverted papilloma and carcinoma, a patient with esthesioneuroblastoma, and a patient with a nasoethmoid carcinoma.

Results.—The scans of all patients showed some remodeling of the walls of the nasal vault. The lesion extended into the maxillary sinus in 2 patients with inverted papillomas and in 10 patients with polyposis. The ethmoid sinuses were involved in all patients, and there was some lateral bowing without erosion of the lamina papyracea in all but 1. The frontal sinuses were involved in 1 patient with inverted papilloma and in 12 patients with polyposis, 3 of whom showed posterior sinus wall displacement and some degree of bone remodeling. In the other patients, the posterior sinus wall was either thinned or destroyed and not visualized on sectional imaging studies. Similarly, the floor of the anterior cranial fossa was primarily eroded, with little if any bone remodeling. The bone erosion in the patient with inverted papilloma and carcinoma could not be distinguished from that in the patient with solely inverted papilloma.

Conclusion.—Patients with nasal polyposis and mucoceles or patients with inverted papillomas that simulate an incurable carcinoma on imaging studies should be operated on for cure because benign disease will be found in most cases.

▶ The importance of recognizing that benign disease can mimic malignant destruction is most important. The signs of remodeling are often difficult to detect when there is associated bony destruction in benign sinonasal disease.—J.F. Sackett, M.D.

MR Imaging in Rhinocerebral and Intracranial Mucormycosis With CT and Pathologic Correlation

Terk MR, Underwood DJ, Zee C-S, Colletti PM (Univ of Southern California; LAC+USC Imaging Science Ctr, Los Angeles)
Magn Reson Imaging 10:81–87, 1992 3–61

Background.—Mucormycosis is a rare, often fatal opportunistic fungal infection that is most commonly seen in persons with diabetes but can occur in drug abusers, immunocompromised individuals, and those with a number of other conditions. Because of its quick progression, it is vital to detect the infection at an early stage. In 3 patients with mucormycosis, MRI and CT were useful in diagnosis.

Case Report.—Man, 22, with insulin-dependent diabetes had a 3-week history of headache, nasal stuffiness, and loss of vision in the left eye. On CT, a large, midline mass was seen involving the nasal septum and sinuses bilaterally (Fig 3–43). On MRI, signal void in the sinuses was noted, along with elevation of the planum sphenoidale extending to the sella turcica, erosion of the clivus, and displacement of the basilar artery. Surgical findings confirmed *Mucor* in the naso-ethmoid mucosa. The patient's vision returned to near normal.

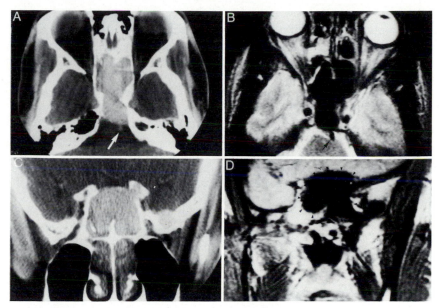

Fig 3–43.—**A,** contrast-enhanced CT depicting a soft tissue density mass in the region of the ethmoid and sphenoid sinuses with destruction of the clivus posteriorly and posterior displacement of the basilar artery (*arrow*). **B,** corresponding T_2-weighted axial MR image (TR/TE, 2,220/80) demonstrating low signal intensity within the ethmoid and sphenoid sinuses, corresponding to the enhancing soft tissue mass seen on CT. Note posterior displacement of the basilar artery (*arrow*). **C,** coronal CT revealing a soft tissue mass in the sphenoid sinus with bony destruction of the planum sphenoidale and the tuberculum sella. Note destructive lesion in left sphenoid wing with assoicated soft tissue mass. **D,** corresponding T_2-weighted coronal MR image (TR/TE, 1,800/80) demonstrating a low-signal-intensity mass (*arrows*) in the sphenoid sinus with destruction of the planum sphenoidale and tuberculum sella. (Courtesy of Terk MR, Underwood DJ, Zee C-S, et al: *Magn Reson Imaging* 10:81–87, 1992.)

Discussion.—Rhinocerebral infection is the most common manifestation of mucormycosis in persons with diabetes; focal intracerebral infection is generally seen in intravenous drug abusers. The low signal intensity of the mass in the patient described differs from previous descriptions of mucormycosis in the literature and could represent an interpretive pitfall.

▶ The MR manifestation of T_2 images is a destructive lesion invading the base of the skull from the sinuses with a hypointense signal on T_2.—J.F. Sackett, M.D.

Osteomyelitis of the Skull Base
Malone DG, O'Boynick PL, Ziegler DK, Batnitzky S, Hubble JP, Holladay FP
(Univ of Kansas, Kansas City, Kansas)
Neurosurgery 30:426–431, 1992   3–62

Introduction.—Osteomyelitis of the skull base is rare. Three cases of this condition illustrate the typical and atypical forms it can take.

Findings.—Typical cases are initiated by ear infections, with *Pseudomonas aeruginosa* as the usual pathogen. Headaches and earaches are typical symptoms and patients are frequently diabetic or immunocompromised. Atypical cases are more rare. Headaches are typically the only initial symptom. Diagnosis is difficult.

Management.—Gadolinium-enhanced MRI studies can be useful in diagnosis. Bone scans are useful as an initial screening tool. Gallium scanning is a sensitive method for detecting infection and can be used to evaluate therapeutic response. Indium-labeled white blood cell scans are useful for diagnosis and therapeutic evaluation. A bone biopsy and culture of the bony lesion itself may be necessary to determine the infectious organism. Antibiotics should be administered until 1 week after findings on the Ga scan are normal. A Ga scan should then be performed at 1 week and at 2 to 3 months after cessation of antibiotics to look for recurrence.

▶ This is an unusual diagnosis. This manuscript reviews the various imaging techniques to diagnose skull-based osteomyelitis. Magnetic resonance imaging is rather specific and will quantitate the intracranial extension.—J.F. Sackett, M.D.

Neuroimaging of Acoustic Nerve Sheath Tumors After Stereotaxic Radiosurgery
Linskey ME, Lunsford LD, Flickinger JC (Univ of Pittsburgh; Pittsburgh)
AJNR 12:1165–1175, 1991   3–63

Background.—Stereotaxic radiosurgery for acoustic tumors has given promising results in hearing preservation, frequency of cranial neuropathy, and tumor control. Previous reports have not described changes in tumor size objectively or documented the measurement criteria used. A method of measuring changes in tumor size was developed and used to evaluate tumor responses to radiosurgery.

Methods.—Eighty-eight patients with a total of 89 acoustic tumors were treated during a 3-year period. The median age was 60 years, and most of the younger patients had neurofibromatosis. All underwent stereotaxic radiosurgery with a 201-source cobalt 60 gamma unit. Patients were assessed with contrast-enhanced CT or MRI. Five different measurements were taken of each tumor to assess diameter and volume.

Results.—There was no change in tumor size for 73% of patients and an increase in tumor size for 4%. At 3 to 33 months postoperatively, an average decrease of 4.9 mm was observed in 22% of patients, and at least 1 year after treatment 36% of 50 patients had a decrease in tumor size. Seventy-nine percent of patients had a loss of tumor contrast enhancement 1 to 18 months postoperatively, and a delayed communicating hydrocephalus developed in 4 patients. At 5 to 15 months, 8 patients had an increased signal on T_2-weighted MRI, 5 in the adjacent cerebellar peduncle and 3 in the peduncle and dorsolateral pons. No such changes were detected with T_1-weighted MRI or with CT. At a mean of 14.6 months, the complication rate was low and the tumor control rate was 96%.

Conclusion.—In patients undergoing stereotaxic radiosurgery for acoustic tumors, MRI is the most sensitive means to assess tumor response, adjacent parenchymal signal changes, and ventricular size. The treatment is relatively safe, economical, nondisruptive, and effective. Long-term follow-up is needed to assess tumor control and complication rate.

▶ This is the first significant series with follow-up examination for patients who have had stereotaxic radiosurgery for acoustic nerve sheath tumors. The authors state that MRI is the technique to assess tumor size but realize that long-term follow-up will be required to assess long-term results and complication rate.—J.F. Sackett, M.D.

Gadolinium-Enhanced MR of the Postoperative Internal Auditory Canal Following Acoustic Neuroma Resection via the Middle Fossa Approach

Mueller DP, Gantz BJ, Dolan KD (Univ of Iowa, Iowa City, Iowa)
AJNR 13:197–200, 1992   3–64

Introduction.—Small acoustic neuromas can be surgically removed using the middle cranial fossa approach, which preserves both hearing and facial nerve function. A Gd-enhanced MR technique was used to identify recurrent tumors in patients undergoing the removal of small acoustic tumors.

Methods.—Of the 44 patients undergoing the excision of an acoustic neuroma through the middle cranial fossa approach, 13 had a postsurgical Gd-enhanced MR study. Nine of the MR examinations were performed routinely, and 2 were done because of existing abnormalities.

Results.—The MR studies showed that the surgical procedure shortened the distance between the internal auditory canal and the adjacent temporal lobe, but the cerebellopontine angle cisterns remained normal. Twelve of the 13 patients had enhancement at the operative site, which could be seen as early as 7 months and as late as 68 months after the procedure. Eight of the 13 patients had enhancement at about the superior margin of the internal auditory canal. Two patients underwent serial MR examinations, but no alterations in the enhancement outcome were observed over the study intervals.

Conclusion.—A single examination appears to provide little information in these patients. An MR follow-up should be scheduled with the initial baseline MR examination at about 2 months after the surgery and another examination about 2 years later. If the patient experiences a change in clinical status, an additional MR examination should be conducted, obtaining images in the axial and the coronal planes in particular.

▶ This manuscript underscores the difficulty of postoperative enhancement as a differential from recurrent neoplasm. The authors found postoperative enhancement as late as 68 months after surgery.—J.F. Sackett, M.D.

Selective MR Imaging Approach for Evaluation of Patients With Horner's Syndrome
Digre KB, Smoker WRK, Johnston P, Tryhus MR, Thompson HS, Cox TA, Yuh WTC (Univ of Utah School of Medicine, Salt Lake City; Univ of Iowa, Iowa City, Iowa)
AJNR 13:223–227, 1992   3-65

Objective.—The value of MRI in assessing patients with Horner's syndrome was examined in a prospective series of 33 patients, 13 with preganglionic and 20 with postganglionic Horner's syndrome. The diagnosis was confirmed by photography or video recording showing a distinct dilation lag or by cocaine drop testing.

Findings.—Six of the 13 patients with preganglionic Horner's syndrome had clinical evidence of central involvement, and 4 of them had abnormal MR studies showing lateral medullary infarction or a dolichoectatic basilar artery. Four of the patients without other central signs also had MR abnormalities. Three of the 20 patients with postganglionic Horner's syndrome had MR findings of carotid artery dissection. None of 7 patients with cluster headaches had abnormal MR findings. No patient whose Horner's syndrome had been present for longer than 2 months had an identifiable lesion.

Conclusions.—Patients with Horner's syndrome and central symptoms or signs should have MRI of the brain stem and upper cervical spinal cord. Patients with postganglionic Horner's syndrome for less than 2 months are the likeliest to exhibit abnormalities. Magnetic resonance imaging has not proved helpful in patients with chronic postganglionic Horner's syndrome, especially when cluster headaches are present.

▶ I believe this is a useful classification of Horner's syndrome, and separating the preganglionic subset will result in a more cost-effective imaging work-up for this group of patients.—J.F. Sackett, M.D.

Delayed Visual Loss due to Trauma of the Internal Carotid Artery
Weinstein JM, Rufenacht DA, Partington CR, Graves VB, Strother CM, Appen RE, Jacobson DM, Cox TA, Moster ML (Univ of Wisconsin, Madison, Wis; Marshfield Clinic, Marshfield, Wis; Univ of British Columbia, Vancouver, BC, Canada; Temple Univ, Philadelphia)
Arch Neurol 48:490–497, 1991   3–66

Introduction.—Visual loss resulting from optic nerve damage usually occurs immediately after closed head trauma. However, in some patients, visual deterioration will not be noted until 12 to 72 hours after the injury. Data were reviewed on 6 patients in whom visual loss occurred weeks to years after an episode of head trauma.

Case Report 1.—Man, 21, sustained basilar skull fractures in an automobile accident. He awoke 3 to 4 hours after the injury with complete loss of vision in the left eye and 20/20 vision in the right eye. Intractable keratopathy necessitated a complete left tarsorrhaphy, but the patient had no immediate visual complaints. He noticed progressive visual loss in the right eye 2 months later. An MRI scan obtained 6 months after injury revealed a large right carotid–cavernous fistula with massive expansion of the cavernous sinus. The patient underwent carotid occlusion with endovascular balloons, which resulted in collapse of the previously dilated cavernous sinus. The patient's visual acuity in the right eye improved to 20/20 6 weeks later.

Case Report 2.—Woman, 26, had sustained a basilar skull fracture and traumatic left optic neuropathy in an automobile accident 12 years before presentation. Her vision was normal after the injury, but 12 years later she reported the gradual onset of blurred vision. She was found to have a giant, partially thrombosed aneurysm of the left internal carotid artery. A permanent balloon occlusion of the artery was successfully performed. The patient's field defect in the right eye gradually and completely resolved during the next year.

Conclusions.—Of the 6 patients in this series, 5 had significant visual recovery after diagnosis and treatment of aneurysm or fistula. Patients with severe fractures of the sphenoid and ethmoid sinuses should be examined carefully for carotid artery injury. A traumatic aneurysm should be suspected in patients with delayed posttraumatic visual loss.

▶ This is an important cause of delayed onset visual deterioration. Although it is not always an urgent treatment situation, 5 of the 6 patients did have visual improvement with endovascular balloon therapy. Fat suppression orbital imaging with gadopentetate dimeglumine has become the pulse sequence of choice for orbital CT scanning.—J.F. Sackett, M.D.

Intra- and Paraorbital Lesions: Value of Fat-Suppression MR Imaging With Paramagnetic Contrast Enhancement

Tien RD, Chu PK, Hesselink JR, Szumowski J (Univ of California, San Diego; Oregon Health Sciences Univ, Portland, Ore)

AJNR 12:245–253, 1991   3–67

Introduction.—Conventional MR images do not optimally depict anatomical detail in areas of high fat content such as the orbit. Lesions in fatty regions can be depicted using gadopentetate dimeglumine, a paramagnetic contrast agent, in conjunction with a modified chopper fat-suppression technique.

Methods.—Magnetic resonance imaging of the orbit was carried out in 2 normal persons and 16 patients, all but 1 of whom received gadopentetate dimeglumine. In 8 patients, T_1-weighted fat-suppression images were acquired before and after contrast enhancement. A hybrid

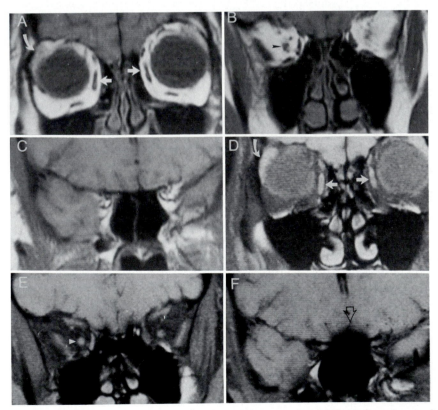

Fig 3–44.—Normal volunteer. Coronal T_1-weighted images (600/20/2) **(A–C)** and coronal T1-weighted images with fat suppression insert (D–F). (*Continued.*)

technique of fat suppression was used in the spin-echo mode of data acquisition.

Results.—Precontrast T_1-weighted hybrid images in normal persons demonstrated the optic nerve, muscle contour, and lacrimal gland (Fig 3–44). Irregular enhancement of the posterior chorioretina was clearly seen on axial postcontrast hybrid T_1-weighted images in acutely blind patients with global lesions. Intraconal lesions also were demonstrated on postcontrast images. Postcontrast hybrid T_1-weighted images were helpful in demonstrating enhancing tumors and their margins in patients with intraorbital masses.

Conclusion.—Fat-suppression T_1-weighted MRI is a useful means of assessing orbital and paraorbital lesions, particularly if contrast enhancement is used.

▶ Thin-section multiple projections and surface coil imaging also improve diagnostic accuracy of the orbit with MRI.—J.F. Sackett, M.D.

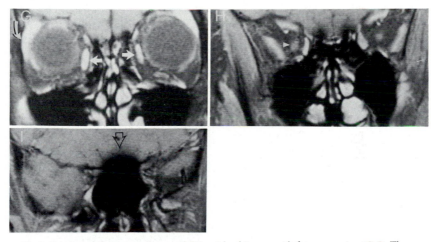

Fig 3–44.—(cont.) Postcontrast coronal T1-weighted images with fat suppression **(G–I).** The margins and outlines of extraocular muscles (*straight white arrows*), optic nerves (*arrowheads*), and lacrimal glands (*curved arrows*) are much better defined on fat-suppression images. Extraocular muscles enhance intensely, and they appear slightly larger than on conventional T_1-weighted images. Also, there is increased magnetic susceptibility artifact at ethmoid air cells and subfrontal regions on the fat-suppression images (*open black arrows*); however, the orbits are not affected significantly. (Courtesy of Tien RD, Chu PK, Hesselink JR, et al: *AJNR* 12:245–253, 1991.)

Magnetic Resonance Imaging of Choroidal Melanoma With and Without Gadolinium Contrast Enhancement

Bond JB, Haik BG, Mihara F, Gupta KL (Tulane Univ, New Orleans)
Ophthalmology 98:459–466, 1991   3–68

Background.—Treatment of the common and potentially life-threatening choroidal melanoma requires accurate determination of the extent of the tumor. Previous reports have shown that MRI is effective in delineating these tumors, but is less effective for imaging amelanotic tumors. These reports, however, were made before Gd contrast was widely available. Whether Gd enhancement results in superior imaging of choroidal melanoma by MRI was investigated.

Methods.—Thirty-four patients with choroidal melanoma were the subjects of this study. All underwent T_1-, T_2-, and proton density–weighted MRI, and 19 also underwent MRI with Gd contrast. The MRI studies used a 1.5-T superconducting MRI unit with an orbital surface coil, 3-mm slices, and axial, coronal, and oblique sagittal views.

Results.—In 6 of the 34 patients, T_1-weighted images did not show the presence of a tumor. T_2-weighted images failed to visualize tumors in 10 patients, and proton density–weighted images did not visualize tumors in 9 patients. T_1-weighted images resulted in higher contrast/noise ratios than T_2- and proton density–weighted images, thus providing better tu-

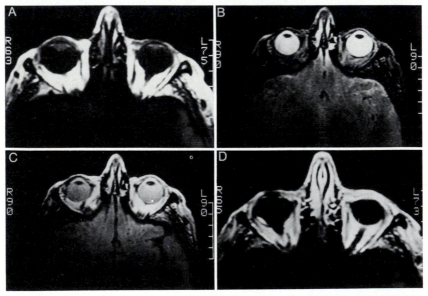

Fig 3–45.—A–C, axial T_1-weighted (TR 600 msec; TE 20 msec), T_2-weighted (TR 2,000 msec; TE 70 msec), and proton-density-weighted (TR 2,000 msec; TE 20 msec) images fail to detect tumor. **D,** axial Gd-enhanced (TR 600 msec; TE 20 msec) image detects a small tumor in the right eye. (Courtesy of Bond JB, Haik BG, Mihara F, et al: *Ophthalmology* 98:459–466, 1991.)

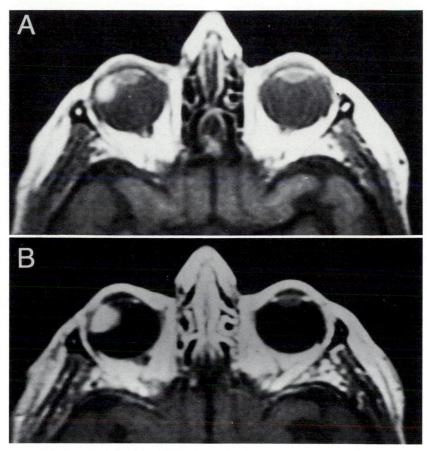

Fig 3–46.—**A,** an axial T$_1$-weighted (TR 600 msec; TE 20 msec) image shows ciliary body tumor. **B,** axial Gd-enhanced (TR 600 msec; TE 20 msec) image shows tumor more completely, with much higher signal intensity. (Courtesy of Bond JB, Haik BG, Mihara F, et al: *Ophthalmology* 98:459–466, 1991.)

mor delineation and detection. Gadolinium contrast further increased the contrast/noise ratio of T$_1$-weighted images. Tumors in 4 of 19 patients receiving contrast were visible only after enhancement (Fig 3–45), and tumors in 14 were seen completely and had higher signal intensity (Fig 3–46). Only 1 study with Gd failed to detect a tumor (2 × 5 mm) in the ciliary body. Gadolinium contrast permitted the detection of a retinal detachment not visualized without enhancement and helped delineate tumor from subretinal fluid in 2 patients. In 1 patient, however, enhancement made differentiation of tumor from chronic hemorrhagic detachment more difficult.

Conclusion.—The use of Gd contrast increases the sensitivity of MRI for detecting both melanotic and amelanotic melanoma. Optimal evaluation of choroidal melanoma is obtained with Gd-enhanced T_1-weighted MRI.

▶ This study shows the value of Gd enhancement in tumor delineation of choroidal melanoma. Because these lesions are intraocular, fat-suppression technique is not required. The separation of hemorrhagic retinal detachment and enhancing tumor can be a diagnostic dilemma.—J.F. Sackett, M.D.

The Acute Orbit: Differentiation of Orbital Cellulitis From Subperiosteal Abscess by Computerized Tomography
Handler LC, Davey IC, Hill JC, Lauryssen C (Groote Schuur Hospital, University of Cape Town, Cape Town, South Africa)
Neuroradiology 33:15–18, 1991   3–69

Introduction.—An acute orbital infection can threaten a person's visual acuity. Physicians may have to surgically intervene even when the patient has received antibiotic therapy. The clinical, radiologic, and tomographic data available on 65 patients with orbital inflammatory disease were reviewed to ascertain whether checking for cellulitis or subperiosteal abscess would alter treatment.

Methods.—The medical records of 65 patients, mostly children and adolescents, with acute postseptal orbital infection underwent reassessment. The patients had a mean age of 21 years. Based on the clinical information, 17 patients had orbital cellulitis and 48 had abscesses.

Results.—An orbital mass occurred in 48 of the 65 individuals. It was often attached to the medial wall of the orbit and contiguous with the displaced medial rectus muscle. The masses varied in size, 5 of them ex-

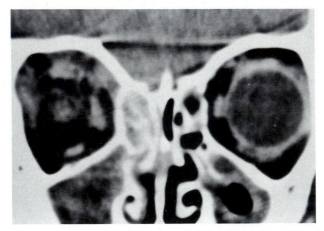

Fig 3–47.—Presumed subperiosteal abscess of 4 days' duration has extended under the orbital roof. Note the causative maxillary and ethmoid sinusitis. (Courtesy of Handler LC, Davey IC, Hill JC, et al: *Neuroradiology* 33:15–18, 1991.)

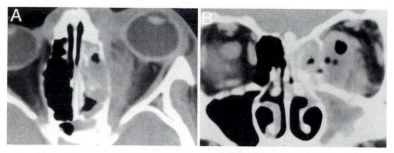

Fig 3–48.—Inflammatory mass. Axial (**A**) and coronal (**B**) views of phlegmon of 5 days' duration. No pus from the subperiosteal space was found at external ethmoidectomy, but *S. milleri* was isolated. There is maxillary frontal and ethmoid sinusitis. (Courtesy of Handler LC, Davey IC, Hill JC, et al: *Neuroradiology* 33:15-18, 1991.)

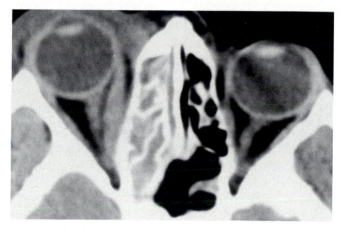

Fig 3–49.—Proven subperiosteal abscess of 2 days' duration. Nonhemolytic *Streptococcus* species was cultured from the pus. The orbital fat has the same μ as the other side. Note ethmoiditis and preseptal edema. (Courtesy of Handler LC, Davey IC, Hill JC, et al: *Neuroradiology* 33:15-18, 1991.)

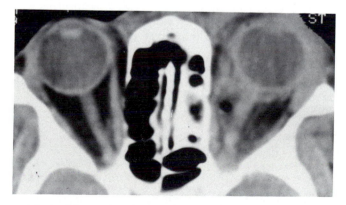

Fig 3–50.—Orbital cellulitis resulting from a stab wound to the orbit 2 days earlier. The lamina papyracea was disrupted on superior cuts. The increased density of the orbital fat was caused by contusion. (Courtesy of Handler LC, Davey IC, Hill JC, et al: *Neuroradiology* 33:15-18, 1991.)

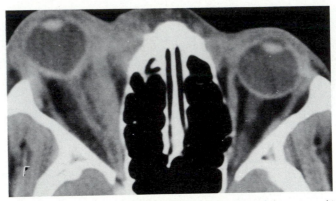

Fig 3–51.—Primary abscess of 5 days' duration. Sinuses were clear and there was no history of any potential cause. Pus from orbitotomy revealed mixed growth of P. *mirabilis* and a hemolytic *Streptococcus* species. Partial volume averaging accounted for nonvisualization of the left lamina papyracea. (Courtesy of Handler LC, Davey IC, Hill JC, et al: *Neuroradiology* 33:15–18, 1991.)

tending under the roof of the orbit (Fig 3–47) and 2 onto the floor (Fig 3–48). Most masses lay near the orbit's bony wall (Fig 3–49) and appeared to be homogeneous. If trauma appeared to be the cause of the cellulitis, a significant rise in the attenuation of orbital fat was present (Fig 3–50). The rectus muscles were frequently swollen, and a gas bubble occurred within the orbit in 17 patients with an orbital mass and in 4 with cellulitis. The CT diagnosis of orbital cellulitis correlated with the clinical diagnosis of the infection. Of the 48 patients with an orbital mass, follow-up surgery verified an abscess in 33 (Fig 3–51), and 9 had presumed abscesses. The latter patients responded more slowly to intravenous antibiotics. Sinusitis appeared to be the cause of infection in most patients, although infection was linked with orbital trauma in 10 and with dental extraction in 4.

Conclusion.—The pus from the infection was not drained in 15 patients. These 15 individuals eventually responded to intravenous antibiotics and maintained their visual acuity, but their hospital stays were longer than those of patients who had drainage of the infection site.

▶ This large number of patients with orbital inflammatory change supports a conservative approach to the therapy unless there is progression of proptosis or deterioration of ocular movement or vision.—J.F. Sackett, M.D.

4 Musculoskeletal System

Introduction

This year's selection of musculoskeletal articles is grouped under the topics of neoplasia, arthropathy, infection, trauma, and miscellaneous. The miscellaneous group includes those most interesting articles that don't fit our groupings but are still fascinating and informative. The technical areas of plain film radiography, CT, MRI, and nuclear medicine continue to lead our clinical investigations. As you would expect, MRI is still discovering aspects of the marrow space, soft tissues of the joint and musculoskeletal system, that prove very exciting; MRI continues to open new areas of investigation and understanding. Even with our concerns about medical economics, government regulations, and recognized problems with our health care system, it is still an exciting time for radiology, especially in the musculoskeletal system.

John E. Madewell, M.D.

Neoplasia

Chondromyxoid Fibroma: Radiographic Appearance in 38 Cases and in a Review of the Literature

Wilson AJ, Kyriakos M, Ackerman LV (Washington Univ, St Louis; State Univ of New York, Stony Brook, NY)
Radiology 179:513–518, 1991
4–1

Introduction.—The entity of the relatively rare, benign bone tumor chondromyxoid fibroma (CMF) is well known, but few reports of CMF in an appreciable number of patients have appeared in the literature. The radiographic evidence was reviewed in 38 cases of CMF to determine the frequency (Table 1) and range of diverse characteristics in these tumors.

Methods.—All cases of CMF were seen at Barnes Hospital, St Louis, or State University of New York Hospital, Stony Brook. The radiographic features in each case were recorded. The histologic material was examined independently.

Results.—The 19 female and 19 male patients had a mean age of 23 years. The tumors were found in 13 different bones (Table 2). Thirty

TABLE 1.—Sites of 38
Chondromyxoid Fibromas

SITE	NUMBER	PERCENT
Tibia	9	23.7
Femur	9	23.7
Fibula	4	10.5
Phalanx-Foot	3	7.9
Metatarsal	3	7.9
Ilium	2	5.3
Tarsal	2	5.3
Phalanx-Hand	1	2.6
Humerus	1	2.6
Ischium	1	2.6
Rib	1	2.6
Scapula	1	2.6
Skull	1	2.6
TOTAL	38	100.0

Note: *Numbers in parentheses* are percentages.
(Courtesy of Wilson AJ, Kyriakos M, Ackerman LV:
Radiology 179:513–518, 1991.)

were located in the long bones and short tubular bones; 16 were centered in the metaphysis, 13 in the diaphysis, and 1 in the epiphysis. Radiographs showed that all 38 CMFs had geographic bone destruction, with either partial or complete erosion of the cortex. One third of the lesions had complete cortical erosion accompanied by penetration into the soft tissue. In 26 cases there was a lobulated tumor margin, and in 25 there was a septated tumor (Fig 4–1). Nearly all tumors had well-delineated margins. Thirty-four produced cortical expansion, usually greater than 1 cm. Half the tumors were classified as elongated and the other half were classified as round.

Conclusion.—The diagnosis of CMF remains difficult because of the diverse nature of the sites affected. A diagnosis of CMF should be considered in patients with a solitary bone lesion with geographic destruction that has lobulated margins, cortical expansion, septations, or a sclerotic rim. A patient in the second or third decade who has 1 or more of these symptoms may be at increased risk for CMF.

TABLE 2.—Frequency of Radiographic Features of Chondromyxoid Fibroma

	Current Series (N=38)	Beggs & Stoker (N=31)	Combined (N=69)
Geographic bone destruction	38 (100%)	31 (100%)	69 (100%)
Well-defined margin	37 (97%)	22 (71%)	59 (86%)
Expanded shell	34 (89%)	13 (42%)	47 (68%)
Partial cortical erosion	26 (68%)	21 (68%)	47 (68%)
Lobulated margin	26 (68%)	14 (45%)	40 (58%)
Septation	25 (66%)	14 (45%)	39 (57%)
Eccentric medullary location	22 (58%)	19 (61%)	41 (59%)
Matrix calcification	1 (3%)	4 (13%)	5 (7%)
Sclerotic rim	31 (82%)	not stated	---
Round shape	19 (50%)	"	---
Elongated shape	19 (50%)	"	---
Metaphyseal centering	16 (53%)*	"	---
Central medullary location	14 (37%)	"	---
Diaphyseal centering	13 (43%)*	"	---
Complete cortical erosion	12 (32%)	"	---
Cortical centering	2 (5%)	"	---
Epiphyseal centering	1 (3%)*	"	---

* **Percentage of tubular bones**

Abbreviation: NS, not stated.
Note: Numbers in parentheses are percentages.
* Percentage of tubular bones.
(Courtesy of Wilson AJ, Kyriakos M, Ackerman LV: *Radiology* 179:513–518, 1991.)

▶ This rare benign bone tumor is most common around the knee but can be found anywhere in the skeleton. In may experience it is 1 of those benign tumors that can mislead you on the plain films by appearing very aggressive with ill-defined border and breakout but yet still be benign.—J.E. Madewell, M.D.

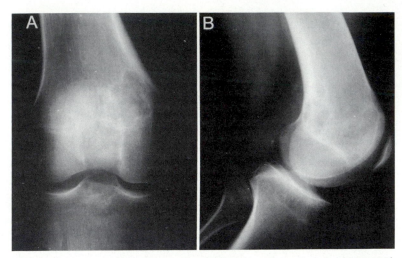

Fig 4–1.—Histologically proved eccentric CMF of distal femoral metaphysis in man, 23. **A,** frontal and **B,** lateral views. The tumor has typical location and the appearance of nonossifying fibroma. (Courtesy of Wilson AJ, Kyriakos M, Ackerman LV: *Radiology* 179:513–518, 1991.)

Benign Osteochondromas and Exostotic Chondrosarcomas: Evaluation of Cartilage Cap Thickness by Ultrasound

Malghem J, Vande Berg B, Noël H, Maldague B (St Luc University, Brussels, Belgium)
Skeletal Radiol 21:33–37, 1992   4–2

Background.—Differentiation of benign exostoses from exostotic chondrosarcomas can be achieved by detection and measurement of the cartilage cap. This can be done with CT or MRI. Ultrasound (US) is also useful; the cap appears as a hypoechoic layer covering the hyperechoic surface of the calcified part. The US findings in osteochondroma or exostotic chondrosarcoma were studied and compared with the CT, MRI, and pathologic findings.

Methods.—Thirty patients who had osteochondroma or exostotic chondrosarcoma underwent US with a 5-MHz linear-array transducer. These examinations were successful unless the lesion was located deeply. Twenty-two specimens were resected; these were cut perpendicularly to the surface to allow true measurement of the cap's thickness. Fourteen patients underwent CT and 10 had MRI. Linear regression analysis was done to correlate imaging measurements with the pathologic findings.

Results.—There were 22 proved benign exostoses and 2 proved exostotic chondrosarcomas. Histologic cap thickness was less than 5 mm in 15 of the benign cases and 15 and 70 mm in the chondrosarcomas. Ultrasound clearly showed a hypoechoic cap layer in all cases but 2 (Fig 4-2). The detection rate and measurement accuracy of US were higher

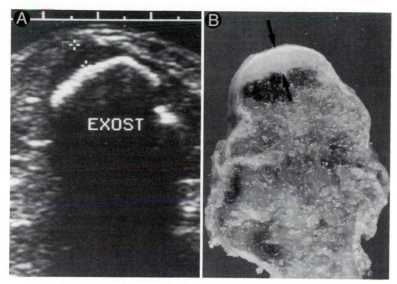

Fig 4–2.—Comparison between ultrasound and anatomical measurements: the 4-mm hypoechoic cap measured on ultrasound (**A**) corresponds to the 4-mm cartilage cap measured on the anatomical specimen (*arrows* on **B**). (Courtesy of Malghem J, Vande Berg B, Noël H, et al: *Skeletal Radiol* 21:33–37, 1992.)

than those of CT and comparable with those of MRI (table). Correlation coefficients were 0.978 for US, 0.985 for CT, and 0.982 for MRI.

Conclusion.—In patients with benign osteochondroma or exostotic chondrosarcoma, US is a useful technique for evaluating the cartilage cap. Caps thinner than 1 cm are usually benign, and those thicker than 2 cm are usually malignant. The cap may not be seen on US when it is oriented inward or located deep in the soft tissues, but these situations are relatively uncommon.

▶ Osteochondromas usually have characteristic features (stalk, cartilage cap, chondroid matrix) enabling one to diagnose them as benign lesions. However, occasionally osteochondrosarcoma can appear very similar or may even arise from a preexisting osteochondroma. It can be difficult to detect the potential of malignancy, but the amount and degree of soft tissue extension is very valuable. This article shows another way (US) to detect these extensions. It is more routine to determine soft tissue about cartilage tumors by the CT or MRI findings.—J.E. Madewell, M.D.

Comparison Between Cap Measurements on Pathologic Specimens,
Ultrasound Examinations, CT Scans, and MRI

Case no.	Location	Histological diagnosis	Cartilage cap thickness measured (in mm) on			
			Specimen	US	CT	MR
1.	Scapula	Benign	0	1		
2.	Femur (distal)	Benign	1	1		
3.	Tibia (proximal)	Benign	1	5	5	
4.	Tibia (proximal)	Benign	1	1	2	
5.	Metatarsus	Benign	1	1		
6.	Humerus (proximal)	Benign	2	3		
7.	Tibia (proximal)	Benign	3	3	3	
8.	Rib	Benign	3	4	3	
9.	Humerus (proximal)	Benign	3	3	*	
10.	Femur (distal)	Benign	3	3	*	3
11.	Femur (distal)	Benign	4	6	5	
12.	Scapula	Benign	4	3		2
13.	Femur (distal)	Benign	4	4		
14.	Femur (distal)	Benign	4	8		4
15.	Femur (proximal)	Benign	4	4		
16.	Femur (proximal)	Benign	5	7	*	
17.	Pubis	Benign	6	4	*	5
18.	Femur (distal)	Benign	6	6		5
19.	Femur (proximal)	Benign	8	22	20	22
20.	Ilium	Benign	13	11	11	12
21.	Scapula	Benign	13	15	18	16
22.	Humerus (proximal)	Benign	13	15		
23.	Metatarsus	Malignant	15	11	13	12
24.	Femur (distal)	Malignant	70	80	90	90

* Caps not clearly distinguishable from surrounding soft tissues.
(Courtesy of Malghem J, Vande Berg B, Noël H, et al: *Skeletal Radiol* 21:33–37, 1992.)

Hemorrhage Simulating Tumor Growth in Malignant Fibrous Histiocytoma at MR Imaging

Panicek DM, Casper ES, Brennan MF, Hajdu SI, Heelan RT (Memorial Sloan-Kettering Cancer Ctr, New York)
Radiology 181:398–400, 1991   4–3

Introduction.—Chemotherapy sometimes preceeds limb salvage surgery in patients with primary malignant neoplasms in the musculoskeletal area to reduce the possibility of recurrence and metastasis. Soft tissue tumors, however, can undergo intratumor hemorrhage and cell death on their own or as a result of some types of therapy. Three patients with malignant fibrous histiocytoma (MFH) had an enlarged mass found on

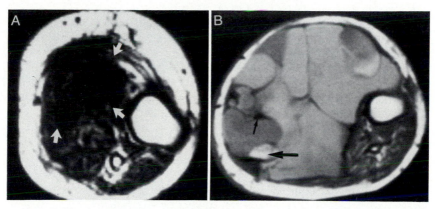

Fig 4–3.—Magnetic resonance images of high-grade MFH in the posterior proximal left calf. **A,** T_1-weighted axial MR image (600/17) obtained at 1 tesla before therapy demonstrates a poorly defined mass (*arrows*). **B,** a T_1-weighted axial MR image (617/20) obtained at 1.5 tesla 4 months later, after preoperative chemotherapy, shows that the overall mass enlarged considerably in the interval (12 × 7 × 6 cm before therapy, 28.5 × 16.5 × 14 cm after therapy). However, the original mass has largely been replaced by multiple locules that contain fluid with various signal intensities, ranging from hypointense (*small arrow*) to hyperintense (*large arrow*), consistent with hemorrhage. Pathologic examination of the gross specimen confirmed that it was largely necrotic, cystic tumor filled with blood clot. (Courtesy of Panicek DM, Casper ES, Brennan MF, et al: *Radiology* 181:398-400, 1991.)

physical examination. Magnetic resonance imaging served to define and characterize these masses.

Case Report.—Man, 64, had an MFH of the thigh. He underwent 2 cycles of chemotherapy preoperatively. During the presurgery preparations, the mass appeared enlarged and fluctuant. The MRI found the tumor measured 10 cm at the widest point before chemotherapy and 17 cm at this same point after the drug administration. T_1- and T_2-weighted MR images found the enlargement of the mass occurred because of extensive hemorrhage within the necrotic tumor tissue.

Results.—A clinical increase in the soft tissue of the MFR was found in the lower extremity in all 3 patients treated first with chemotherapy before surgery (Fig 4–3). The enlargement of the mass as seen on MRI resulted from excessive hemorrhaging and not from the growth of the tumor.

Conclusion.—These results suggest that tumor growth can be differentiated from intratumor hemorrhage by employing some imaging methodology, such as MR, in addition to the clinical examination of the patient. It is suggested that other imaging techniques (e.g., sonography) be used to assess an increase in the MFH mass. Thorough assessment of the growth can ascertain if the enlargement is the result of disease progression or treatment failure.

▶ Soft tissue sarcomas such as MFHs may enlarge very fast with extension and increased bulk of the tumor tissue. This can be associated with a worsening of the prognosis and breakthrough while the patient is on chemotherapy.

However, as pointed out in this article, we must be careful because this enlargement may also be caused by necrosis and hemorrhage within the tumor. The MRI can be very effective in differentiating these situations.—J.E. Madewell, M.D.

Metastatic Fractures of Long Bones
Korkala OL, Karaharju EO (University Central Hospital, Helsinki, Finland)
Int Orthop 15:105–109, 1991   4–4

Objective.—Primary stability is the goal of surgery for actual or imminent metastatic fractures; this is often achieved in the leg by endoprosthetic replacement, combined with tumor removal and cement fixation. These patients should have only the operation needed for the particular site being treated. The outcomes of the surgical treatment of 52 metastatic fractures of the long bones were reviewed, focusing on surgical complications and pitfalls and the patients' postoperative quality and length of life.

Patients and Outcomes.—The 52 fractures of the long bones were treated in 42 patients during a 4-year period (Table 1). The most common primary tumor sites were the breast, kidney, and other urogenital sites. Most complications occurred in shaft fractures treated by plating (Table 2). Results were more reliable using osteosynthesis with added methylmethacrylate cement or endoprosthetic replacement. Diaphyseal fractures were best treated by intramedullary nailing, preferably with cement. Of 37 patients with femoral fractures, only 27 could walk unaided or with crutches.

Discussion.—Life expectancy is improving for patients with metastatic disease; thus careful consideration is needed in selecting the best operation for metastatic fractures. Indications for osteosynthesis with a plate are limited. To gain immediate stability, cement should be used along with osteosynthesis or replacement of pathologic fractures.

▶ As life expectancy improves for patients with malignancies, we will most likely continue to see more metastases. Because the bone is a frequent site, the number of pathologic lesions will also increase. These lesions can result in pathologic fracture and early detection, and management is worthwhile in these patients.—J.E. Madewell, M.D.

TABLE 1.—The 52 Pathologic Fractures of 42 Patients According to Anatomical Location and Mode of Treatment

	EP	AP	LP	MN	PL	MNC	PLC	P/O	GR
Fem.neck	8	1							2
Fem.troch.	7	3							
Fem.subtr.		1		1	1		1		
Fem.shaft				3	1	3		1	
Fem.cond			2				1		
Hum.neck	1								
Hum.shaft				5	4		1		
Tibia							1	3	
Total	16	5	2	10	6	3	4	4	2
Compl.	3	–	–	1	4	–	–	1	2

Note: The total number of cases according to each individual therapy is counted, as are the cases with complicated healing, which are specified in Table 2. Abbreviations: EP, endoprosthesis; AP, angle-plate; LP, L-plate; MN, medullary nail; PL, plate (ASIF); MNC, medullary nail with cement; PLC, plate (ASIF) with cement; P/O, plaster cast or orthosis; GR, Girdlestone resection.
(Courtesy of Korkala OL, Karaharju EO: Int Orthop 15:105–109, 1991.)

TABLE 2.—Patients With Local Complications or Complicated Healing of the Fracture Site

Primary tumor	Fracture site	Operation	Complications and outcome
Breast	Fem.neck	Thompson HA	Cortex perforation by the prosthetic shaft. Not able to walk. Death at six weeks.
Breast	Fem.neck	Thompson HA	Walking with crutches. Prosthetic site fracture at 30 months. Death at 47 months.
Breast	Fem.neck	Girdlestone resection	Deep infection. Able to sit. Death at 50 months.
Breast	Fem.neck	Girdlestone resection	Loose hip. Not able to walk. Death at six months.
Prostate	Fem.trochanteric	Minneapolis HA	Not able to walk. Haematoma, prosthetic dislocation (not reduced). Death at 4 months.
Kidney	Fem.subtrochanteric	Intramed. nailing	Walking. Nonunion. Local tumour growth. Hip disarticulation at 39 months. Death at 45 months.
Urinary bladder	Fem.shaft	Plating	Continuous local growth. Walking with crutches. Proximal refracture. Death at two months.
Breast	Tibial shaft	Plaster cast	3rd pathological fracture. Walking with crutches. Nonunion. Death at 8 months.
Breast	Humeral shaft	Plating + resection	Walking. Plate loosening and nonunion at 12 months. Death at 22 months.
Thyroid	Humeral shaft	Plating + bone transplant	Walking. Plate loosening at 3 weeks, new plating. Death at six months.
Kidney	Humeral shaft	Plating	Walking. Plate loosening at 3 months. Orthosis. Death at 13 months.

Abbreviation: HA, hemiarthroplasty.
(Courtesy of Korkala OL, Karaharju EO: *Int Orthop* 15: 105–109, 1991.)

Cortical Bone Metastases

Hendrix RW, Rogers LF, Davis TM Jr (Northwestern Mem Hosp, Chicago)
Radiology 181:409–413, 1991   4–5

Introduction.—Peripheral appendicular skeletal metastases result from systemic arterial dissemination of tumor; thus, cortical metastases could occur with any tumor capable of dissemination in this way, not just bronchogenic carcinoma. Radiographs and bone scans of 27 patients with solitary or multiple cortical bone metastases were evaluated.

Methods.—Identified from a total of 1,237 bone scans, all patients had proved extraosseous malignancy, malignancy of undetermined origin with proved metastases, or serial radiographs showing progression. The cortical location of the lesion was established from its CT or radiographic appearance. Patients with multiple myeloma and 2 or more primary malignancies were excluded.

Findings.—The patients were 15 women and 12 men, aged 45 to 80 years, with cortical metastases from at least 6 tumor types (table). Three patients had a pathologic fracture at the metastatic site. The cortical lesion was the only metastasis detected in 8 patients, and in 1 patient it was the first sign of any abnormality. Seven patients had more than 1 cortical metastasis. Three of the 36 lesions were identified on radiography, with normal radioisotope uptake on bone scan (Fig 4–4).

Conclusion.—Cortical metastases to the long bones may result from a variety of tumors at a variety of sites and may be more common than previously thought. These lesions are important because they can quickly jeopardize the integrity of the weight-bearing bone and because they may indicate the only sign of metastatic disease.

▶ Cortical metastasis is not common, but it is certainly a recognized feature of metastatic disease and may be more common than we think. This article illustrates these features well and points out that cortical metastasis may

	Tumor Type		
Primary Tumor	No. of Patients ($n = 27$)	No. of Patients with Pathologically Proved Cortical Metastasis ($n = 14$)	No. of Cortical Metastases ($n = 36$)
Bronchogenic	8	3	16
Breast	9	3	10
Renal cell	5	3	5
Pancreatic	1	1	1
Laryngeal	1	1	1
Uterine leiomyosarcoma	1	1	1
Adenocarcinoma of unknown origin	2	2	2

(Courtesy of Hendrix RW, Rogers LF, Davis TM Jr: *Radiology* 181:409–413, 1991.)

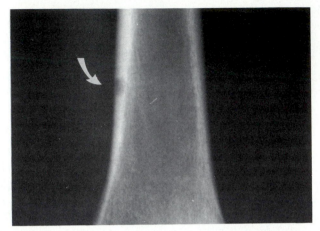

Fig 4–4.—Anteroposterior radiograph shows a 6-mm osteolytic, intracortical lesion in the distal femoral metadiaphysis (*arrow*) in a man, 45, with bronchogenic carcinoma. The lesion was not detected on a bone scan. This was the only bone lesion in the patient. A biopsy was performed because of clinical uncertainty of malignancy. (Courtesy of Hendrix RW, Rogers LF, Davis TM Jr: *Radiology* 181:409–413, 1991.)

compromise the bone's weight-bearing capacity quicker than marrow metastasis.—J.E. Madewell, M.D.

Upper Humeral Cortical Thickness as an Indicator of Osteopenia: Diagnostic Significance in Solitary Myeloma of Bone

Jackson A, Scarffe JH (University of Manchester; Christie Hospital and Holt Radium Institute, Manchester, England)
Skeletal Radiol 20:363–367, 1991   4–6

Background.—The localized plasma cell tumor solitary myeloma of bone presents solitarily and is histologically indistinguishable from multiple myeloma. Radiotherapy may yield long-term survival in many patients, but some will eventually have multiple myeloma. Features that might predict prognosis in solitary myeloma were investigated.

TABLE 1.—Criteria for Diagnosis of Solitary Myeloma of Bone

1. Histologically proven plasmacytoma of bone
2. No excess of plasma cells in bone marrow aspirate
3. X-ray evidence of only one or two solitary lesions at diagnosis
4. No anemia
5. No hypercalcemia
6. No impairment of renal function

(Courtesy of Jackson A, Scarffe JH: *Skeletal Radiol* 20:363–367, 1991.)

TABLE 2.—Distribution of Solitary Myeloma of Bone

Site	Number of cases
Axial tumors	
Skull	1
Cervical spine	1
Thoracic spine	16 *
Lumbar spine	4
Sacrum	2
Nonaxial tumors	
Clavicle	2
Femur	3
Humerus	1
Sternum	1
Pelvis	1

* One patient with a dorsal spine tumor also had a solitary lesion of the eighth rib.
(Courtesy of Jackson A, Scarffe JH: *Skeletal Radiol* 20:363–367, 1991.)

Methods.—The subjects were 32 patients seen over 10 years who met the diagnostic criteria for solitary myeloma of bone (Table 1). There were 19 men and 13 women, median age 62 years. The most common tumor site was the thoracic spine (Table 2). All underwent biochemical and hematologic assessment at baseline and at regular intervals during follow-up. Radiologic assessment was done at initial visitation and repeated annually. Local radiotherapy was given in each case. Osteopenia was assessed by comparing measured upper humeral shaft combined cortical thickness with normal values derived from a group of 413 controls.

Findings.—Six patients had the subjective diagnosis of osteopenia at diagnosis. Osteopenia and immunoparesis were the only independent, significant predictors of decreased survival. If either risk factor was present, median survival was only 27 months; excluding those patients, chance of 10-year survival was 80% to 90%.

Conclusion.—Osteopenia and immunoparesis appear to be significant predictors of decreased survival in solitary myeloma of bone. Patients with generalized osteopenia when first seen probably have widespread abnormal plasma cells even if their bone marrow studies are normal. This might explain their poor response to local chemotherapy and justify the use of systemic therapy.

▶ Osteopenia, as well as immunoparesis, seen in the solitary myeloma patient seem to be significant prognosticators of decreased survival.—J.E. Madewell, M.D.

Arthropathy

Sacroiliitis: MR Imaging Findings

Murphey MD, Wetzel LH, Bramble JM, Levine E, Simpson KM, Lindsley HB
(Univ of Kansas, Kansas City, Kan)
Radiology 180:239–244, 1991   4–7

Introduction.—Sacroiliitis occurs as a symptom of many diverse illnesses from spondyloarthropathies to rheumatoid arthritis to pyogenic arthritis. Overlying tissue may block the detection of physical signs. The MR image of normal sacroiliac joints was compared with that of joints with sacroiliitis, and findings on MRI were compared with those on CT scans.

Methods.—Seven volunteers (14 sacroiliac joints) and 17 patients (34 joints) with diagnosed or suspected sacroiliitis were evaluated with MRI. All patients had anteroposterior pelvis radiography and 16 underwent CT scans. The 3 female and 4 male volunteers had a mean age of 30 years, and the 8 female and 9 male study subjects had a mean age of 37 years.

Results.—In all 7 volunteers, MRI clearly delineated the synovial and the ligamentous sections of the sacroiliac joint. The joints demonstrated prominent sacral irregularities and marrow defects. Among the study subjects, 16 joints in 10 patients were diagnosed as having sacroiliitis by using the CT scan. Twenty joints in 12 articulations had abnormalities that led to the diagnosis of sacroiliitis (Fig 4–5). In 19 of the 20 joints the T_1-weighted image of the synovial area showed a reduction of the normal, thin zone in the intermediate signal intensity range. In 16 patients (20 joints) focal or linear sections in the synovial area had abnormally increased signal intensity on the T_2-weighted scans (Fig 4–6).

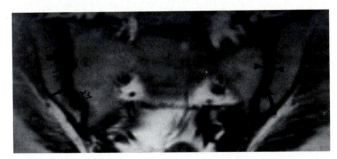

Fig 4–5.—Coronal MR image (600/25) of unilateral sacroiliitis associated with psoriatic arthritis in a woman, 47. There is a loss of cartilage in the right sacroiliac joint with replacement by inhomogeneous mixed signal- intensity tissue (*large straight arrow*) and widening of the right sacroiliac joint. Cortex has areas of increased signal intensity (*small straight arrows*), and the marrow margin adjacent to the right sacroiliac joint is irregular, representing erosions (*short arrows*). The contralateral joint shows normal cartilage (*curved arrow*), cortex, and marrow margin (*arrowheads*). (Courtesy of Murphey MD, Wetzel LH, Bramble JM, et al: *Radiology* 180:239–244, 1991.)

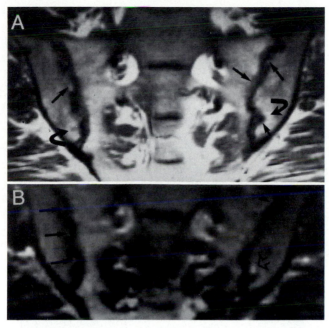

Fig 4–6.—Magnetic resonance images of psoriatic sacroiliitis in a woman, 31. **A,** a coronal MR image (600/25) shows cartilage replacement bilaterally. Adjacent irregularity of marrow margin and increased intensity in cortex representing erosions (*large straight arrows*) result in sacroiliac joint space widening. Deeper erosion (*small arrow*) is noted on the left, as is hyperintense reactive bone marrow (*curved arrows*). **B,** coronal MR image (2,100/90) shows both focal (*arrows*) and linear (*arrowhead*) increased signal intensity in the sacroiliac joints and in most inferior erosion on the left (*short arrow*). (Courtesy of Murphey MD, Wetzel LH, Bramble JM, et al: *Radiology* 180:239–244, 1991.)

Twenty-one of the 34 sacroiliac joints with possible sacroiliitis had pulse sequences that showed reduced marrow signal.

Computed tomography best demonstrated changes in bone production, whereas MRI best presented alterations in cartilage. Erosions were equally shown on CT scans and MR images in 10% of articulations. The conspicuity of erosions was improved at MRI in 81% of affected joints.

Conclusion.—Magnetic resonance imaging is the preferred method overall for assessing the sacroiliac joint, with increased signal intensity of the image being interpreted as joint erosions. Magnetic resonance imaging can lead to a diagnosis of sacroiliitis while assessing the lower back for causes of pain in this location.

▶ Magnetic resonance imaging is another follow-up method for further study of suspected abnormal sacroiliitis joints. It provides a look at the cartilage, which is only indirectly studied by other methods. The exact role of MRI evaluation in sacroiliitis joint disease needs further study, but it offers some interesting possibilities.—J.E. Madewell, M.D.

Spiking of the Tubercles of the Intercondylar Eminence of the Tibial Plateau in Osteoarthritis

Reiff DB, Heron CW, Stoker DJ (St George's Hosp, Royal National Orthopaedic Hospital, London, England)
Br J Radiol 64:915–917, 1991   4–8

Introduction.—Patients with osteoarthritis (OA) often have a narrowing of the joint space, osteophytes, sclerosis of the subchondral bone, as well as formation of a subchondral cyst. The literature also lists the spiking of the tubercles of the tibia's intercondylar eminence as an early sign of OA. The phenomenon of peaking of the tibial tubercles is studied to assess whether this occurrence influences OA in the knee.

Methods.—The radiographs of 55 patients with OA located in the knee were reviewed for joint space narrowing, for formation of the osteophyte, or for sclerosis of the bone. These results were compared to those gathered from 36 control subjects of similar age who underwent knee radiography. Two sets of assessments were collected for each tu-

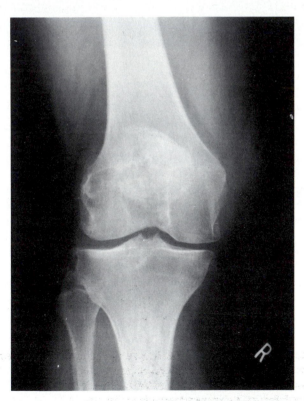

Fig 4–7.—Spiking of the tubercles of the intercondylar eminence of the tibial plateau in a patient with osteoarthritis of the knee joint. Osteophyte formation, diminution of joint space, and subarticular sclerosis are noted. (Courtesy of Reiff DB, Heron CW, Stoker DJ: *Br J Radiol* 64:915–917, 1991.)

bercle. The OA patients, 37 females and 18 males, had a mean age of 63.5 years, while the controls, 27 females and 9 males, had a mean age of 62.4 years.

Results.—The results demonstrated a significant difference between the mean of the angles evaluated for both the medial and lateral tubercles of each set of subjects. A significant difference also occurred between the height/width ratios of both tubercles. The usual radiograph in the OA patients showed a spiking of the tubercles (Fig 4–7).

Conclusion.—These findings indicate that the medial and lateral intercondylar tubercles represent important pivotal points of rotation of the femur on the tibia. The peaking of the tibial tubercles usually occur on radiographic assessment of OA of the knee, but the cause for this occurrence remains unknown. It is concluded that the lengthening of the medial and lateral tubercles of the intercondylar eminence, and the increase of their angles, that is, spiking or peaking, are characteristic of OA of the knee.

▶ An excellent and closer look at a very common problem (OA of the knee) using a universally available inexpensive technique (plain film radiography). In this day of MRI and CT, it is refreshing to see interesting applications of routine technique to common problems.—J.E. Madewell, M.D.

Radiographic Detection of Metal-Induced Synovitis as a Complication of Arthroplasty of the Knee
Weissman BN, Scott RD, Brick GW, Corson JM (Brigham and Women's Hosp; Harvard Med School, Boston)
J Bone Joint Surg [Am] 73-A:1002–1007, 1991   4–9

Introduction.—Metal-induced synovitis is a reported complication of total knee arthroplasty in which a hinged knee prosthesis is implanted. Metal-to-metal contact after total knee replacement may be caused by wear of a metal-backed tibial or patellar component or of a metal-to-metal bearing. The radiographs of 18 patients who had metal-induced synovitis after total knee arthroplasty were reviewed.

Patients.—Multiple sets of radiographs were available for 11 patients, and 1 set of radiographs was available for the other 7. All radiographs were examined for the presence of a dense line outlining a portion of the capsule or articular surface of the knee joint, called a metal-line sign (Fig 4–8). Histologic sections of resected synovial tissue were available for 15 patients. Bone and articular cartilage specimens were available for 8 patients.

Findings.—A metal-line sign associated with wear was found in the radiographs of 11 patients. Specimens for histologic examination were available for 9 of these. All 9 specimens showed dense dispositions of metal particles in the synovial tissue. In contrast, 5 of the 6 specimens

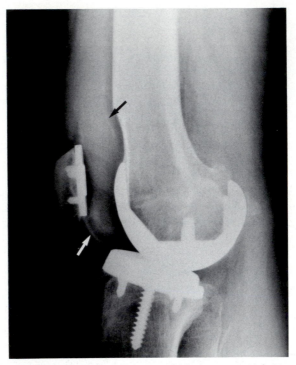

Fig 4–8.—Radiograph showing the metal-line sign. The linear increase in density corresponding to the joint capsule (*arrows*) indicates metal-induced synovitis. There is a moderate effusion. (Courtesy of Weissman BN, Scott RD, Brick GW, et al: *J Bone Joint Surg* 73-A:1002–1007, 1991.)

from patients who did not have a metal-line sign on their radiographs contained only slight amounts of metal in the synovial tissue, the sixth specimen contained a moderate amount of metal. The presence of the metal-line sign on radiographs was associated with metal-induced synovitis in 11 of 18 patients.

Conclusions.—The appearance of a radiographic metal-line sign after total knee arthroplasty is essentially diagnostic, particularly when it is seen on radiographs obtained 1 year or more after operation.

▶ Joint prosthesis is a frequent observation in our radiologic practices. This article gives us an interesting look into a very complex process. Its concepts should make us more critical when we read the prosthetic joint films in our daily practice.—J.E. Madewell, M.D.

Arthrography of Painful Hips Following Arthroplasty: Digital Versus Plain Film Subtraction

Walker CW, FitzRandolph RL, Collins DN, Dalrymple GV (Univ of Arkansas,

Little Rock, Ark)
Skeletal Radiol 20:403–407, 1991   4–10

Background.—Arthrography is more accurate than conventional radiography in detecting component loosening in patients with painful hip prostheses. Plain film manual subtraction images are commonly used to improve visualization of small collections of contrast medium, but digital subtraction can be a useful adjunct. These 2 subtraction techniques were compared for their ability to detect contrast collections suggestive of component loosening.

Methods.—Seventy-eight hip arthrograms from 69 patients, mean age 64 years, were reviewed. Digital and plain film manual subtraction images were available in each case and surgical correlation in 53 cases. Arthrographic technique emphasized achievement of high intra-articular pressure during injection to minimize false-negative results. If contrast medium extended along at least half the length of the femoral stem at the bone-cement or the cement-prosthesis interface, the femoral component was considered loose. All images were reviewed without knowledge of the surgical results.

Findings.—The 2 subtraction methods were in agreement in 88% of femoral components (Fig 4–9); when there was disagreement, loosening

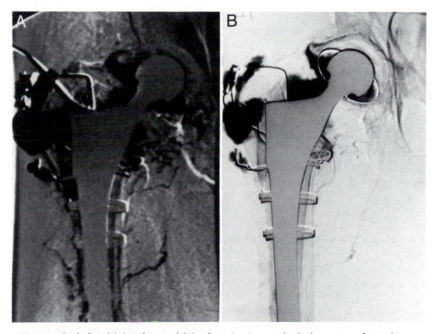

Fig 4–9.—Both digital (**A**) and manual (**B**) subtraction images clearly demonstrate femoral component loosening. There is a much more dramatic depiction of the contrast material on the digital image. (Courtesy of Walker CW, FitzRandolph RL, Collins DN, et al: *Skeletal Radiol* 20:403–407, 1991.)

264 / Diagnostic Radiology

Comparison of Digital and Manual Subtraction Methods in the
Detection of Component Loosening

	Femoral component		Acetabular component	
	Digital	Manual	Digital	Manual
True-positive	46	38	20	18
False-negative	2	10	4	6
False-positive	0	0	4	4
True-negative	5	5	16	16
Sensitivity	96%	79%	83%	75%
Specificity	100%	100%	80%	80%

Note: True positive cases were positive for loosening on both arthrography and at surgery. False negative cases were loose at surgery without arthrographic evidence of loosening. False positive cases were unstable arthrographically but intact at surgery. True negative cases were surgically and arthrographically intact.
(Courtesy of Walker CW, FitzRandolph RL, Collins DN, et al: *Skeletal Radiol* 20:403–407, 1991.)

was found on the digital subtraction image only. There was agreement in 80% of acetabular components. Digital subtraction was significantly better than manual subtraction in detecting femoral component loosening (table).

Conclusion.—Digital subtraction technique appears to improve detection of femoral component loosening in patients undergoing arthrography for a painful hip prosthesis. The technique does not increase examination time or radiation dose to the patient, and it can help to reduce misregistration artifact caused by patient motion. Loosening is still the most common complication of hip replacement.

▶ Detecting the loosened area about a prosthesis is important. Plain film radiograph and subtraction is a standard technique and reliable in the majority of cases; however, this article points out that there are some cases where digital subtraction detects more abnormalities.—J.E. Madewell, M.D.

Infection

Osteomyelitis: Characteristics and Pitfalls of Diagnosis With MR Imaging

Erdman WA, Tamburro F, Jayson HT, Weatherall PT, Ferry KB, Peshock RM (Univ of Texas, Dallas)
Radiology 180:533–539, 1991   4–11

Introduction.—Recent reports on the use of MRI to noninvasively diagnose osteomyelitis appear encouraging. The prospective and retrospective interpretations of MR images taken at .35 T were compared

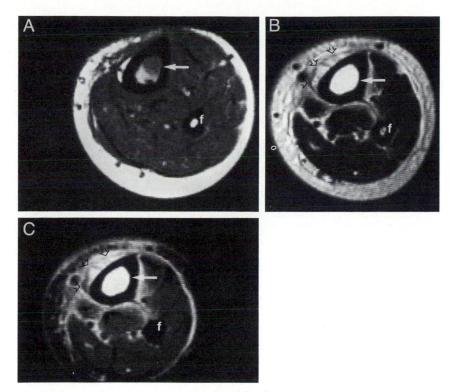

Fig 4–10.—Acute hematogeneous osteomyelitis of the tibia in a woman, 20. **A,** T1-weighted axial image (SE 500/30) shows infected tibial marrow as area of low signal intensity (*arrow*) compared with normal fibular marrow (*f*). **B,** T2-weighted image (SE 2,000/80) acquired 1 cm below the level of the image in **A** shows infected marrow (*arrow*) with higher signal intensity than normal (compare with marrow of fibula). Dark line of periosteum (*short arrows*) is elevated by pus (surgically proved), although the cortex of the bone is intact and shows no abnormal signal intensity. **C,** STIR axial image (IR, 1,500/30/100) demonstrates high contrast in infected tibial marrow (*arrow*) and in the inflamed surrounding muscle and subcutaneous tissue (high signal intensity). Normal fibular marrow (*f*) and subcutaneous fat are dark with use of this sequence. Short arrows indicate periosteum. (Courtesy of Erdman WA, Tamburro F, Jayson HT, et al: *Radiology* 180:533–539, 1991.)

with the final diagnosis in 110 patients originally suspected of having osteomyelitis.

Methods.—The records of all patients who had MRI for suspected osteomyelitis were assessed prospectively by 3 trained radiologists who were not aware of the final diagnosis. Two radiologists retrospectively analyzed the MR images. All patients underwent MRI in a 0.35-T superconducting instrument.

Results.—A total of 138 MR images were obtained on 130 patients, 20 of whom were later excluded. Eighty-one of the remaining 110 patients received a final diagnosis of osteomyelitis based on histopathologic or microbiologic tissue testing. Comparison of these results with the outcome of MRI showed 53 true positive interpretations, 14 false positive

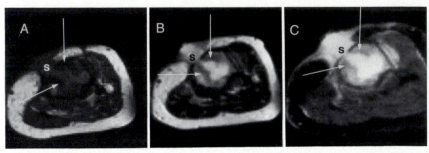

Fig 4–11.—Rim sign of chronic osteomyelitis in the tibia of a woman, 38, with 28-year history of draining sinus. **A,** T1-weighted (SE, 500-30); **B,** T2-weighted (SE, 2,000/80); and (**C**) STIR axial (IR, 1,500/30/100) images show a dark rim around the area of histopathologically proved chronic active infection (*arrows*). The rim presumably is fibrous tissue and is dark with use of all sequences. Disruption of the cortical bone at the sinus tract (S), cortical remodeling, and paucity of soft tissue inflammatory changes are further characteristics of chronic traumatic osteomyelitis. (Courtesy of Erdman WA, Tamburro F, Jayson HT, et al: *Radiology* 180:533–539, 1991.)

interpretations, 42 true negative interpretations, and 1 false negative interpretation, for an overall sensitivity of 98% and a specificity of 75%. All 12 patients with acute osteomyelitis had focal dark signal intensity in the marrow on T_1-weighted images and abnormal brighter-than-fat signal intensity on T_2-weighted and short-tan inversion recovery (STIR) imaging (Fig 4–10). Forty-two of 54 patients with osteomyelitis received a diagnosis of chronic disease. In 14 of 15 patients whose chronic osteomyelitis resulted from trauma a well-outlined rim of low signal intensity surrounded the area of focal active disease (Fig 4–11). Eighteen of 27 diabetic patients with foot problems had osteomyelitis, and 14 of the 110 patients had an infection of a joint space. Sixteen of the 110 eventually received a diagnosis of noninfectious pathologic condition, 8 of the 16 were interpreted as being false positive at MRI.

Conclusion.—Magnetic resonance imaging of patients with suspected osteomyelitis should include dark marrow signal intensity of a T_1-weighted image. The location and duration of infection influence the morphologic appearance of the disease on the MR image.

▶ There are many ways to study patients with osteomyelitis, including plain films, CT, and nuclear medicine. This article shows the authors' experience with MRI in patients suspected of having osteomyelitis.—J.E. Madewell, M.D.

Diagnosis of Osteomyelitis of the Foot in Diabetic Patients: Value of ^{111}In-Leukocyte Scintigraphy
Larcos G, Brown ML, Sutton RT (Mayo Clinic and Found, Rochester, Minn)
AJR 157:527–531, 1991   4–12

Introduction.—Some patients with diabetes may eventually have osteomyelitis. Several radiographic techniques using a variety of radioactive agents now contribute to the diagnosis and understanding of this condition in diabetics. The value of using indium 111–white blood cell (WBC) scintigraphy was examined in a large series of diabetic patients with possible osteomyelitis in the foot.

Patients and Methods.—Fifty-one patients were suspected of having osteomyelitis of the foot and had ^{111}In-WBC scintigraphy. The 20 women and 31 men had a mean age of 62 years. The protocol for the ^{111}In-WBC scan included cell preparation and labeling and then reinjection of the labeled cells into the patient. The scans were then taken within 24 hours of reinjection of the radiolabeled cells.

Results.—Fourteen of the 51 patients had osteomyelitis of the foot; 11 of the 14 were identified by the ^{111}In-WBC scanning procedure. Among the 37 scans from patients without osteomyelitis, 29 were rated true negative and 8 were rated false positive. The radiographs also demonstrated that 11 patients had neuropathic joint disease. Thirteen patients had ^{111}In-WBC and technetium 99m–methylene diphosphonate (MDP) absorbance. In 8 of 9 patients with confirmed osteomyelitis the uptake of ^{111}In-WBC was greater than that for ^{99m}Tc-MDP. The ^{111}In-WBC scinitigraphy technique also demonstrated a sensitivity for soft-tissue ulcers and antibiotic use, but poor spacial resolution of the images led to false positive and false negative results for some patients.

Conclusion.—The ^{111}In-WBC scintigraphic method provides acceptable sensitivity and specificity for the diagnosis of osteomyelitis of the foot in diabetics. This method also can aid in the detection of soft tissue ulcers, neuroarthropathy, and ingestion of antibiotics. However, ^{111}In-WBC scintigraphy should probably be correlated with other diagnostic methods such as radiographs or ^{99m}Tc-MDP scans.

▶ The difficulty of diagnosing osteomyelitis of the foot in diabetic patients is significant. This article demonstrates the authors' experience and value of ^{111}In-labeled leukocyte scintigraphy.—J.E. Madewell, M.D.

Trauma

Ipsilateral Femoral Neck and Shaft Fractures: An Overlooked Association
Daffner RH, Riemer BL, Butterfield SL (Allegheny Gen Hosp, Pittsburgh)
Skeletal Radiol 20:251–254, 1991   4–13

Background.—Most radiologists seem unaware of the combined fracture of the femoral shaft and ipsilateral femoral neck. Particularly from the standpoint of liability, it is important to be aware of this association; up to one third of femoral neck fractures may be initially missed.

Patients.—During a 6-year period, 304 patients with injuries of the femoral shaft and hip were seen at a trauma center. Fracture of the fem-

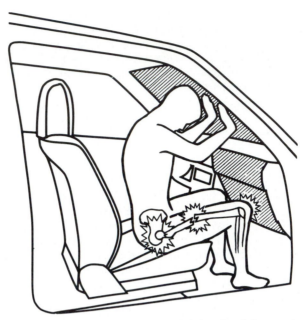

Fig 4–12.—Mechanism of injury in combined femoral shaft and neck fractures. Longitudinal compression of the femur occurs as the knee of an unrestrained front-seat occupant strikes the dashboard. If the force is not dissipated by the femoral shaft fracture, an injury to the hip occurs. (Courtesy of Daffner RH, Riemer BL, Butterfield SL: *Skeletal Radiol* 20:251–254, 1991.)

oral shaft and dislocated hip or fracture of the acetabulum were found in 253. Fifty-one had fractures of the femoral shaft and neck or trochanteric region; 31 of those had combined femoral shaft and trochanteric fractures and 20 had combined femoral shaft and neck fractures. Most of the injuries occurred in motor vehicle collisions, and all of those who were unrestrained drivers or front-seat passengers had knee injuries from hitting the dashboard (Fig 4–12).

Observations.—In all 31 cases of ipsilateral femoral shaft and trochanteric fracture, the latter injury was detected on initial radiographs. The diagnosis of hip fracture was delayed in 11 of 20 patients with ipsilateral femoral shaft and neck fractures. Two patients in each group had CT of the hip as well; the diagnosis still could not be made, even in retrospect. Treatment of the combined femoral shaft and neck fractures consisted of plating of the shaft and AO cancellous screws of the neck. There were no cases of avascular necrosis of the femoral head.

Conclusion.—Combined fractures of the femoral neck and shaft may be difficult to diagnose. Delays may result from lack of fracture separation in the initial evaluation period and from external rotation of the proximal femoral fragment because of the femoral shaft fracture. Despite the need for an additional operation, there appears to be no additional morbidity associated with missing the femoral neck fracture.

▶ We are always learning more about trauma. The authors have reviewed their large experience and demonstrate the association of ipsilateral femoral neck and shaft fractures.—J.E. Madewell, M.D.

Pisiform Fractures
Fleege MA, Jebson PJ, Renfrew DL, Steyers CM Jr, El-Khoury GY (Univ of Iowa, Iowa City, Iowa)
Skeletal Radiol 20:169–172, 1991   4–14

Background.—Pisiform fractures are frequently missed because of improper radiographic assessment and a tendency to focus on other, more obvious injuries. Disabling sequelae can result from delayed diagnosis. Ten patients with pisiform fracture were assessed.

Patients.—The patients were 2 women and 8 men, aged 22 to 59 years. The mechanism of injury was a direct blow in 5 patients and hyperextension in 5. Four patients had no associated injuries. The other 6 patients had olecranon fracture, radius fracture, clavicle fracture, multiple fractures, multiple lacerations, or bilateral fractures.

Radiography.—In 5 patients, the pisiform fracture could be seen on the posteroanterior radiographic view but not on the oblique or lateral views. In 1 patient, the fracture was seen only on the carpal tunnel view. The injury was seen on lateral and oblique views in another patient and on the lateral view alone in another patient. Radiographic data were not available for the remaining 2 patients.

Conclusion.—A high index of clinical suspicion and appropriate radiographic assessment help to correctly establish the diagnosis of pisiform fracture. A pitfall in radiographic interpretation is confusion with multiple ossification centers of the pisiform, a normal variant.

▶ The pisiform is a small bone that can easily be overlooked and fractures missed with resultant long-term disability. Even though uncommon, the pisiform fracture is 1 that we should not miss. The authors discuss and demonstrate their experience.—J.E. Madewell, M.D.

Calcaneal Insufficiency Avulsion Fractures in Patients With Diabetes Mellitus
Kathol MH, El-Khoury GY, Moore TE, Marsh JL (Univ of Iowa, Iowa City, Iowa)
Radiology 180:725–729, 1991   4–15

Introduction.—Calcaneal insufficiency avulsion (CIA) breakages, which usually occur near the posterior calcaneus, affect areas prone to fatigue fractures. Most calcaneal fractures in nondiabetic patients are found in the intraarticular area, but require very great force. Calcaneal

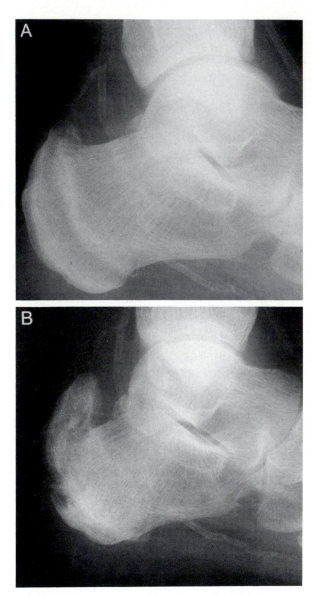

Fig 4–13.—Fracture associated with altered gait. Woman, 33, who had insulin-dependent diabetes for 18 years, had a great toe ulceration and walked without touching her forefoot to the ground. **A,** the next month, she noted pain and tenderness of 1 week duration, and an insufficiency fracture was visible on the radiograph. **B,** a radiograph obtained 6 weeks later shows that fragmentation has occurred. (Courtesy of Kathol MH, El-Koury GY, Moore TE, et al: *Radiology* 180:725–729, 1991.)

fractures in patients with diabetes mellitus and associated conditions from this fracture were studied.

Methods.—The radiographic and medical records of 21 individuals with diabetes underwent retrospective review for evidence of calcaneal fractures. The 21 patients, 11 women and 10 men, ranged in age 21 to 69 years. Displacement of the bones was measured on the radiographs. The results of this analysis were compared with the medical and radiograph information from 40 nondiabetic patients.

Results.—Fourteen of the 21 patients had evidence of CIA fracture while none in the control group demonstrated such a bone breakage. In the CIA fracture group, the mean age of fracture was 34.8 years and the mean age of onset of diabetes was 14.6 years. Eleven of the 14 had a 10-mm or more fragment displacement. Each patient in the CIA fracture group showed the clinical signs of neuropathy with 6 patients having Charcot arthropathy in the lower extremities. Eight of these patients had received a renal transplant. All patients with CIA fractures had normal serum calcium levels. Nine of these individuals had skin ulceration, however (Fig 4–13). The 7 patients with diabetes demonstrated many fracture patterns.

Conclusion.—The CIA fracture distinctly occurs in patients with diabetes, but the incidence of such fractures in this population cannot be calculated based on this select and small sample. Most of these diabetic patients experienced juvenile onset disease, followed by a long period of insulin dependence. The CIA fracture in diabetics often is complicated by many other medical conditions such as neuropathy, ulceration, walking problems, renal difficulties, and bone abnormalities.

▶ Insufficiency fractures of the calcaneus in diabetic patients are well known and differ from calcaneal fractures in the nondiabetic patient, as pointed out in this article.—J.E. Madewell, M.D.

Insufficiency Fractures of the Distal Tibia Misdiagnosed as Cellulitis in Three Patients With Rheumatoid Arthritis

Straaton KV, López-Méndez A, Alarcón GS (Univ of Alabama, Birmingham, Ala)
Arthritis Rheum 34:912–915, 1991   4–16

Introduction.—Aged patients with osteoporosis often have insufficiency fractures, sometimes without overt trauma. Patients with rheumatoid arthritis (RA) also can have insufficiency fractures, particularly near a proximal tibia joint. Three patients with RA had insufficiency or nondisplaced fractures of the distal tibia and symptoms that mimicked cellulitis.

Case Report 1.—Woman, 47, with RA and systemic lupus erythematosus took up to 60 mg of prednisone daily. She had pain, swelling, and erythema of the distal end of the lower left leg 2 weeks before reporting the symptoms. A radiograph showed an insufficiency fracture of the distal tibia.

Case Report 2.—Woman, 73, with advanced RA had increasing pain in the left ankle and distal portions of the lower left leg. A radiograph showed an insufficiency fracture of the distal tibia and a healed impacted fracture of the lateral malleolus. The break healed after 4 weeks in a cast.

Case Report 3.—Woman, 46, with advanced seropositive RA had pain and swelling of the right lower leg, accompanied by chills and mild fever for 2 weeks. A radiograph showed a nondisplaced break of the distal tibia. The fracture healed after 4 weeks in a cast.

Conclusion.—Patients with RA may have accelerated osteoporosis. Asians, whites, and postmenopausal women and those taking corticosteroids may have a higher risk for the early onset of this disease. Insufficiency fractures should be considered in the differential diagnosis of persistent pain in the distal portion of the lower extremity in patients with RA. Bone scans may be required to achieve a definitive diagnosis. A repeat radiograph usually documents healing.

▶ Insufficiency fractures in the compromised skeleton from osteopenia of any cause is well known. Pain is usually the presenting sign. This article reports 3 patients with RA who have insufficiency fractures of the tibia manifesting as cellulitis, which certainly is an unusual complex of symptoms for insufficiency fractures.—J.E. Madewell, M.D.

Diagnosis of Pelvic Fractures in Patients With Acute Pelvic Trauma: Efficacy of Plain Radiographs
Resnik CS, Stackhouse DJ, Shanmuganathan K, Young JWR (Univ of Maryland, Baltimore)
AJR 158:109–112, 1992   4–17

Background.—Computed tomography has been a valuable addition to the evaluation of acute pelvic trauma. However, in serious injuries, surgeons may rely heavily on plain x-ray films in deciding whether immediate external fixation is necessary. The efficacy of plain radiographs was investigated in detecting pelvic fractures and dislocations using CT as the gold standard.

Methods.—Studies of 50 patients with acute pelvic injuries were examined independently in blinded fashion. An anteroposterior radiograph and CT scan were obtained for all patients within 24 hours of admission. Most patients had other radiographic studies as well.

Findings.—Of 162 fractures and dislocations, only 9% were misdiagnosed on plain x-ray films. The patient's management was not altered by the misdiagnosis in any of these subtle injuries. Eighty percent of intraarticular fractures were not seen on plain x-ray films.

Conclusion.—Almost all clinically important pelvic fractures and dislocations can be adequately detected by plain radiography. After the patient's condition is stabilized, CT can be used to detect fractures within the joint. These findings disagree with the high rates of misdiagnosis found in previous studies.

▶ This article shows the importance and critical role plain films play in acute pelvic trauma. I think that CT is still useful in the detection of soft tissue abnormalities and intraarticular bone fragments and determination of fracture plains and fragment position.—J.E. Madewell, M.D.

Traumatic Trabecular Lesions Observed on MR Imaging of the Knee
Tervonen O, Snoep G, Stuart MJ, Ehman RL (Mayo Clinic and Found, Rochester, Minn)
Acta Radiologica 32:389–392, 1991   4–18

Introduction.—Magentic resonance imaging has proved useful in evaluating ligament and meniscus tears of the knee, particularly in patients with fractures and trauma to the bone. Trabecular lesion alterations usually appear as a signal loss on T_1-weighted images and as a signal increase on T_2-weighted images. Often radiographs and arthroscopic tests show negative results for these lesions. The clinical results of MRI changes in the trabecular lesion were presented.

Methods.—A total of 302 patients with a mean age of 29.1 years underwent MRI for ligament or meniscus tears. The patients also had general radiographs taken of the affected area before MRI. The functional status of the joint was also recorded.

Results.—Of the 302 patients, 31 had evidence of bone changes in the subcortical region that met the criteria for classification as a trabecular lesion. After exclusions for clinical reasons, 27 patients remained (19 women and 8 men with a mean age of 24.1 years) with symptoms of trabecular lesions. The mean time between the MRI and the trauma was 10 days. Trabecular injuries included 21 femoral lesions, 5 tibial lesions, and 1 fibular lesion. The trabecular lesion occurred by direct trauma in 3, a valgus injury in 12, a rotation problem in 3, and combined valgus injury and rotation problem in 5. At a mean follow-up of 56 days, 26 of the 27 patients demonstrated no symptoms of the trabecular lesion or trauma and 1 had moderate residual signs of the injury.

Conclusion.—The controversial term "trabecular lesion" usually means a bandlike area of heightened intensity on the contralateral site of the injury as seen on T_2-weighted MR images. It was concluded that such a trabecular lesion can occur from a tear in a ligament. Thus, a trabecular lesion appears to be a benign alteration in the bone caused by knee trauma that eventually heals without intervention.

▶ Magnetic resonance imaging certainly is giving us more information about the bone marrow space than we ever expected. This article continues to show the ability of MRI to detect subtle abnormalities, which the authors conclude as traumatic trabecular lesions associated with knee trauma, which heal without sequelae.—J.E. Madewell, M.D.

Follow-Up of Grade 2 Meniscal Abnormalities in the Stable Knee
Dillon EH, Pope CF, Jokl P, Lynch JK (Yale Univ, New Haven, Conn; Maine Med Ctr, Portland, Me)
Radiology 181:849–852, 1991   4–19

Background.—The MRI appearance of a grade 2 meniscal abnormality differs from that of a complete tear only in extent. Grade 2 lesions may progress to complete tears. A prospective follow-up study of grade 2 meniscal lesions was evaluated.

Methods.—Twenty-two patients with a total of 27 grade 2 lesions were restudied by MRI. All menisci had been proven not to be torn by arthroscopy. A 1.5-T imager with a 17-cm transmit-receive extremity coil was used to obtain images.

Results.—Mean time between images was 27.3 months. Six lesions seemed to have decreased in size, and 2 had disappeared altogether. No change was seen in 18, and 3 had become larger. Patients whose lesions disappeared were among the youngest, and those whose lesions increased in size were older and more active than the group average.

Conclusion.—A prospective MRI study suggests that grade 2 meniscal lesions remain stable up to 3 years after injury in most patients with intact anterior cruciate ligaments. Some may even decrease or disappear. Age and activity may be causative factors in the few lesions that do progress.

▶ We all see many grade 2 meniscal abnormalities in our MRI practices. This prospective study of 22 patients with grade 2 meniscal lesions and no tear at arthroscopy confirm that, at follow-up, most are unchanged, several increased in size, and a few disappeared.—J.E. Madewell, M.D.

Full-Thickness Tears of the Rotator Cuff of the Shoulder: Diagnosis With MR Imaging
Farley TE, Neumann CH, Steinbach LS, Jahnke AJ, Petersen SS (San Francisco Magnetic Resonance Ctr; Univ of California, San Francisco; Letterman Army Med Ctr, Presidio of San Francisco, Calif)
AJR 158:347–351, 1992   4–20

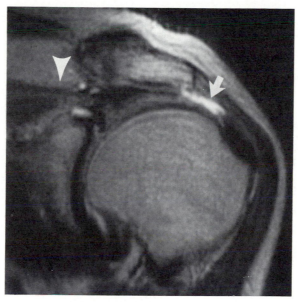

Fig 4–14.—A T$_2$-weighted MR image (1,800/70) shows a tendinous fluid-filled gap (*arrow*) in a man, 70, with a large tear of the supraspinatus tendon. This figure illustrates the MR findings in patients with tears larger than 2 cm. Note atrophy of the supraspinatus muscle and retraction of the musculotendinous junction (*arrowhead*). (Courtesy of Farley TE, Neumann CH, Steinbach LS, et al: *AJR* 158:347–351, 1992.)

Objective.—Magnetic resonance imaging is a useful technique for evaluation of the rotator cuff. Full-thickness tears of the cuff often require open surgery, whereas other injuries may be treated arthroscopically; thus, it is important to make the correct diagnosis. The MRI findings in complete-thickness tears of the rotator cuff were evaluated.

Methods.—Thirty-one of 102 shoulders examined by MRI were found to have full-thickness rotator cuff tears at arthroscopy and open surgery or arthroscopy/bursoscopy. In each case, images were obtained in the oblique coronal and axial planes. Each scan was examined by 2 experienced radiologists for the presence of fluid in the bursae, abnormal signal of the tendons, interruption of continuity or thinning of the tendons, and proximal retraction of the muscle-tendon junction (Fig 4–14).

Findings.—Twenty-nine shoulders had fluid in the subacromial bursae, and 22 had interruption of tendinous continuity. Twenty-seven had focally increased tendon signal equivalent to that of joint fluid, and 24 had musculotendinous retraction. Eighteen had muscular atrophy. The most specific indicator of a tear was supraspinatus muscle atrophy, and the most sensitive indicator was fluid in the subacromial bursa (table).

Discussion.—Specific MRI findings in full-thickness tears of the rotator cuff were evaluated. These studies must be done carefully, because

Efficacy of MR Findings in Predicting Full-Thickness Tears of the Supraspinatus Tendon

MR Findings	Sensitivity (%)	Specificity (%)	PPV	NPV	Accuracy (%)	95% Confidence Interval (%)
Grade 3, T2-weighted images	70	96	0.86	0.89	89	82–96
Grades 2 and 3, T2-weighted images	89	77	0.60	0.95	81	73–89
Thinning	85	89	0.74	0.94	88	81–95
Retraction	78	92	0.78	0.92	88	81–95
Atrophy	60	97	0.89	0.86	87	80–94
Bursal fluid	93	75	0.58	0.96	80	72–88

Note: n = 98. The 4 patients with a full-thickness tear involving only the subscapularis tendon were excluded from this analysis of the supraspinatus tendon. Grade 3 = increased signal intensity equal to that of water extending through the full width of the tendon and at least 1 cm in length; grade 2 = focally increased signal intensity equal to that of water but comprising less than the full width of the tendon.. All values are highly statistically significant to the $P < .0001$ level as determined by χ^2 analysis for independence. A confidence interval of 95% is calculated for accuracy. *Abbreviations: PPV*, positive predictive value; *NPV*, negative predictive value. (Courtesy of Farley TE, Neumann CH, Steinbach LS, et al: AJR 158:347–351, 1992.)

many diseases can alter the signal intensity of the cuff. T_2-weighted images were found most useful.

▶ The MRI finding of full-thickness tears of the rotator cuff are demonstrated, with the interruption of tendon continuity being the most specific.—J.E. Madewell, M.D.

Knees of Trained Long-Distance Runners: MR Imaging Before and After Competition

Shellock FG, Mink JH (Univ of California; Cedars-Sinai Med Ctr, Los Angeles)
Radiology 179:635–637, 1991   4–21

Background.—In a previous study, normal individuals who had jogged on a treadmill for 30 minutes showed subtle increases in intrameniscal signal intensity and visible joint effusions on a postexercise MR study. To determine whether such findings would be magnified in trained distance runners, the knees of 5 marathon runners were examined before and after competition.

Methods.—Four of the runners were asymptomatic before racing 17 to 50 miles. Twenty-four hours before and within 24 hours after the race, T_1-weighted coronal, proton-density T_2-weighted sagittal, and short T_1 inversion recovery sagittal images were obtained in the 5 runners.

Results.—The marathon runners showed no evidence of degenerative joint disease. All ligaments were normal before and after the race, and there was no increase in joint fluid after running. The MR images revealed no alterations in meniscal signal intensity. Three of the racers reported quadriceps or gastrocnemius pain (or both) after running.

Conclusion.—Trained long-distance runners, in contrast to recreational runners, appear to have adapted to the stresses of their activity. The absence of an increase of meniscal signal intensity in these trained athletes warrants further study in a larger group.

▶ Stress and the musculoskeletal system's adaptation related to time and conditioning are very dynamic processes. We know of MRI changes in recreational runners. This article demonstrates no MRI changes in trained long-distance runners and raises many interesting questions about adaptive mechanisms in the musculoskeletal system.—J.E. Madewell, M.D.

Indications for Radiography in Patients With Acute Ankle Injuries: Role of the Physical Examination

Auletta AG, Conway WF, Hayes CW, Guisto DF, Gervin AS (Med College of Virginia, Richmond, Va)
AJR 157:789–791, 1991   4–22

Background.—Ankle trauma accounts for approximately 10% of all emergency room visits, but ankle fractures are detected in only 13% of these injuries. There is growing concern about overuse of radiologic examinations in the evaluation of acute ankle trauma. A prospective study was conducted to determine whether a thorough but brief physical examination could reduce the need for radiologic investigations in patients with acute ankle trauma.

Study Design.—Two hundred one patients, aged 11 to 72 years, seen at the emergency department for acute ankle trauma within 24 hours were referred to the department of radiology for ankle radiographs. Radiology residents performed a brief but thorough physical examination on all patients before radiographs were taken. Based on the presence of gross deformity, instability, crepitation, focal bony tenderness, severe soft tissue tenderness, moderate or severe soft tissue swelling, and ecchymosis, the radiologist determined whether or not radiographs were indicated. Regardless of the results of the physical examination, all patients underwent ankle radiography.

Results.—Based on the results of physical examination, 100 patients had adequate indications for ankle radiography, including 29 fractures and 1 chronic tear of the deltoid ligament that required orthopedic intervention. The remaining 101 patients had inadequate indications for radiographs of the ankle, and only 1 of these had an ankle fracture — a small avulsion fracture of the dorsal aspect of the talus that was treated conservatively. There was no significant difference between the percentages of indicated studies ordered by an emergency department physician and by nonphysician triage personnel or between the percentages of clinically significant injuries detected on radiographs ordered by these 2 groups.

Conclusion.—A brief but thorough physical examination can eliminate the need for a large percentage of radiographs requested for the evaluation of acute ankle trauma without affecting the quality of patient care.

▶ An interesting article showing that thorough physical examinations may eliminate the need for radiograph study in some patients with acute ankle trauma.—J.E. Madewell, M.D.

Unidirectional Joint Communications in Wrist Arthrography: An Evaluation of 250 Cases
Wilson AJ, Gilula LA, Mann FA (Washington Univ, St Louis)
AJR 157:105–109, 1991   4–23

Introduction.—Wrist arthrography serves to establish the health of the intrasynovial intercarpal ligaments and the triangular fibrocartilage complex. The monitoring procedure also measures the state of the intracapsular extrasynovial ligaments, but indirectly. It has been claimed that if all

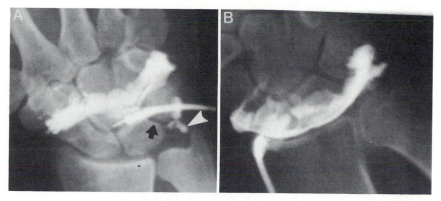

Fig 4–15.—A woman, 47, with undirectional tear of lunotriquetral ligament. **A,** midcarpal joint arthrogram shows contrast medium flowing from the midcarpal joint to the radiocarpal joint (*arrowhead*), between the lunate bone and triquetral bone the (*arrow*). **B,** arthogram after radiocarpal joint injection does not show communication. (Courtesy of Wilson AJ, Gilula LA, Mann FA: *AJR* 157:105–109, 1991.)

3 joint areas are not injected with contrast medium, serious injuries may be missed on diagnosis. A triple-joint wrist arthrography procedure was used that specifies injecting the medium into the midcarpal joint (MCJ) first.

Methods.—Two hundred fifty triple-joint wrist arthrographies were conducted between July 1987 and November 1989 in patients referred because of wrist instability or pain. Of the 250, 119 patients were female and 131 male, with a mean age of 26 years.

Technique.—The triple-joint wrist arthrography procedure prescribes the following contrast medium injection sequence; the MCJ, the distal radioulnar joint (DRUJ), and the radiocarpal joint (RCJ). After medium injection, the wrist underwent fluoroscopy through a range of motions.

Number (%) of Patients Studied for Radiocarpal to Distal Radioulnar Joint Communications

Age (years)	Patients with Communications			Total Patients
	Two Way	One Way	Total	
0–20	4 (21)	1 (5)	5 (26)	19
21–30	13 (13)	3 (3)	16 (16)	100
31–40	17 (23)	3 (4)	20 (27)	74
41–50	5 (13)	1 (3)	6 (16)	38
51–60	0 (0)	1 (8)	1 (8)	12
61–70	1 (20)	0 (0)	1 (20)	5
>70	0 (0)	0 (0)	0 (0)	2
Total	40 (16)	9 (4)	49 (20)	250

(Courtesy of Wilson AJ, Gilula LA, Mann FA: *AJR* 157:105–109, 1991.)

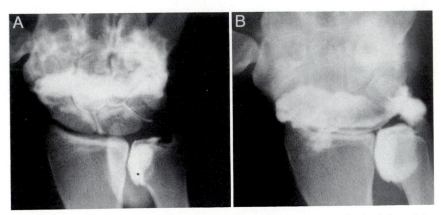

Fig 4–16.—A man, 23, with unidirectional triangular fibrocartilage tear. **A,** distal radiolunar joint arthogram does not show any communication between the distal radioulnar joint and the radiocarpal joint. **B,** arthrogram after radiocarpal joint injection reveals a communication between 2 joints confirming a tear in triangular fibrocartilage. (Courtesy of Wilson AJ, Gilula LA, Mann FA: *AJR* 157:105–109, 1991.)

Results.—Seventy-six patients had 123 communications between the RCJ and the MCJ, whereas 174 patients showed no signs of such a communication. Thirty-five of 38 patients had communications in 1 direction only, usually with the medium flowing from the MCJ to the RCJ (Fig 4–15). Forty-nine patients had communications between the DRUJ and the RCJ through the triangular fibrocartilage (table, with 9 of these connections unidirectional (Fig 4–16). Eleven patients had all 3 compartments filled with medium. Forty-five patients had 50 capsular defects.

Conclusion.—When compared with results of other researchers, these findings indicate that communicatons between joints may rely on technical factors, such as which area receives the dye injection first. In addition, the delay time between the injections may also play a role in the final results.

▶ Communications between wrist compartments occur in asymptomatic older patients; however, this same finding in younger patients may indicate significantly posttraumatic ligamentous tears. This article presents the authors' vast experience with 3 compartment wrist arthrograms.—J.E. Madewell, M.D.

Plantar Fasciitis: MR Imaging
Berkowitz JF, Kier R, Rudicel S (Yale Univ, New Haven, Conn)
Radiology 179:665–667, 1991   4–24

Introduction.—Chronic heel pain with no known traumatic event characterizes the painful heel syndrome that often is caused by plantar

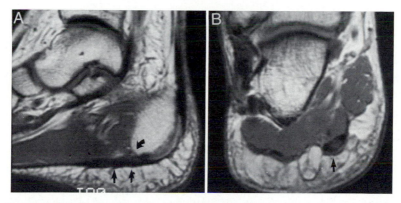

Fig 4–17.—Plantar fasciitis. **A,** a sagittal T_1-weighted (600/20) image shows thickened plantar fascia (*arrows*) and calcaneal spur (*curved arrow*). **B,** coronal intermediate (2,200/20) image demonstrates thickened plantar fascia (*arrow*) with intrasubstance increased signal intensity on 2,000/20 images. (Courtesy of Berkowitz JF; Kier R, Rudicel S: *Radiology* 179:665–667, 1991.)

fasciitis. The diagnostic results of MRI in patients with suspected plantar fasciitis were compared with those for matched controls and unmatched asymptomatic volunteers.

Methods.—Eight patients, 6 with unilateral and 2 with bilateral heel pain, were studied. The 7 women and 1 man had a mean age of 43 years. Plantar fasciitis was suspected if tenderness occurred under the calcaneus, along the plantar fascia, or along both the calcaneus and the plantar fascia. Magnetic resonance imaging included sagittal T_1-weighted spin-echo and coronal dual-echo spin-echo sequences.

Results.—Both control groups demonstrated a homogeneous low signal intensity and a uniform thickness on MRI. Patients with symptoms of the painful heel had significantly expanded plantar fascia areas compared with the 2 control groups. Sagittal images showed a 7.40-mm thick plantar fascia and coronal plane images demonstrated a 7.56-mm thick site (Fig 4–17). Nine of the 10 heels had an increased signal intensity within the fascia itself, especially within the area of thickening of the tissue. The marrow of the calcaneus showed no abnormalities and subcutaneous edema occurred in only 1 patient.

Conclusion.—Magnetic resonance imaging may be helpful in diagnosing morphologic alterations in the plantar fascia or uncovering the real cause of a patient's heel pain. The outcome of the MR studies are encouraging, particularly because the control subjects showed no changes in the plantar fascia. More MRI studies of patients with heel pain are needed to confirm these results.

▶ The painful heel syndrome may be caused by many conditions, 1 of which is plantar fasciitis. This article studies the MRI and morphologic criteria to establish the diagnosis.—J.E. Madewell, M.D.

Miscellaneous

Glenoid Hypoplasia: Assessment by Computed Tomographic Arthrography

Manns RA, Davies AM (Royal Orthopaedic Hospital, Birmingham, England)
Clin Radiol 43:316–320, 1991   4–25

Objective.—Since its first description in 1927, only 45 cases of isolated congenital dysplasia of the glenoid fossa and neck of the scapula have been reported in the literature. Glenoid hypoplasia ranges from mild to severe. The radiographic and CT arthrographic findings in 4 new cases of glenoid hypoplasia were studied.

Patients.—Scapular glenoid dysplasia was found by plain radiography in all 4 patients; in 1 patient, it was an incidental finding during chest radiography. Family history was unknown in all patients, and there were no other skeletal abnormalities. Radiographic findings included bilateral shallow glenoid cavities with shortening of the scapular neck and acromial overgrowth (Fig 4–18). Two patients could posteriorly sublux 1 of their humeral heads; this was visible on the axial shoulder view. Both conventional and arthrographic CT demonstrated that the cartilage was intact and thickened, despite the hypoplastic bony element of the inferior glenoid (Fig 4–19).

Discussion.—The radiographic and CT appearance of glenoid hypoplasia was examined. The incidence of this condition may be underesti-

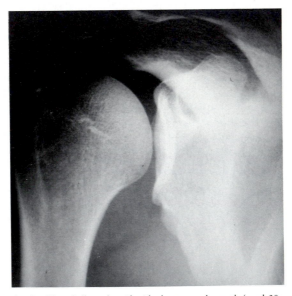

Fig 4–18.—Right shoulder, shallow glenoid with short scapular neck (aged 30 years). (Courtesy of Manns RA, Davies AM: *Clin Radiol* 43:316–320, 1991.)

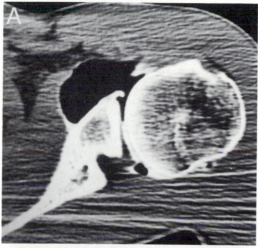

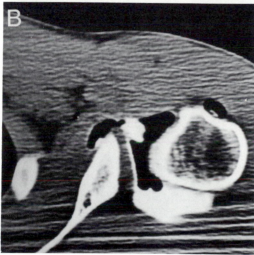

Fig 4–19.—Computed tomographic arthrogram of the left shoulder showing a flattened glenoid with thinning of the anterior glenoid cartilage and hypoplasia of the anterior labrum (**A**). Thickening of the inferior cartilage with a bulbous anterior labrum inferiorly (**B**). (Courtesy of Manns RA, Davies AM: *Clin Radiol* 43:316–320, 1991.)

mated because it is commonly asymptomatic. It appears to result from failure of the precartilage of the inferior aphophysis to develop, that accounts for the distinctive finding of a notch at the junction of the middle and lower thirds of the glenoid fossa. Computed tomographic arthrography is useful in assessing the condition, and MR would probably be useful as well. Glenoid hypoplasia has only limited clinical significance, although affected patients may wish to avoid activities that place undue loading on the shoulder joint.

▶ An uncommon congenital skeletal anomaly with characteristic plain film findings. Arthrographic and CT/arthrographic features are also demonstrated.—J.E. Madewell, M.D.

Clinically Occult Avascular Necrosis of the Hip: Prevalence in an Asymptomatic Population at Risk
Tervonen O, Mueller DM, Matteson EL, Velosa JA, Ginsburg WW, Ehman RL (Mayo Clinic and Found, Rochester, Minn)
Radiology 182:845–847, 1992   4–26

Introduction.—Avascular necrosis (AVN) may complicate a variety of disorders or occur as a complication of corticosteroid treatment. Many patients at risk may have clinically occult AVN contralateral to a symptomatic hip, but the prevalence of this problem is unknown. Magnetic resonance imaging was used to study the prevalence of occult AVN in patients treated with corticosteroids.

Methods.—The subjects were 100 sequential renal transplant patients who had been treated with corticosteroids for at least 6 months. There were 61 women and 39 men, mean age 48 years; the mean time since renal transplantation was 8.1 years, and the mean cumulative dose of prednisone was 32.1 g. All patients underwent an abbreviated screening MRI examination to detect occult AVN; none was symptomatic at the time.

Findings.—There were 6 patients with occult AVN. These patients tended to have a longer time of exposure and higher cumulative dose of steroids, but the differences were not significant. The cause of renal failure was not associated with AVN. Only 1 of the 6 patients had abnormal radiographic findings.

Conclusion.—There was a 6% incidence of clinically occult AVN in renal transplant patients treated with corticosteroids. Magnetic resonance imaging is a safe and effective screening procedure for this disabling complication; reported sensitivities have ranged from 93% to 100%.

▶ The frequency of AVN of the hip in an asymptomatic population at risk was studied and found to be 6 of 100 patients. The authors consider the potential of low-cost screening MRI.—J.E. Madewell, M.D.

Fat Intensity Within the Hypointense Zone on MR Imaging of Avascular Necrosis of the Femoral Head
Kokubo T, Takatori Y, Ninomiya S, Nakamura T, Itai Y (University of Tokyo,

Tokyo, Japan)
J Comput Assist Tomogr 15:470–473, 1991

Objective.—Although MRI is quite sensitive in detecting avascular necrosis of the femoral head (ANFH), it is not specific. The femoral head may show abnormal signal intensity in a variety of hip diseases. The finding of an area within the hypointense zone that has the signal intensity of subcutaneous fat on spin-echo (SE) images—referred to as the fat-intensity sign—was evaluated as a reliable clue to the diagnosis of ANFH.

Methods.—Two groups of patients were selected retrospectively. Group I consisted of 96 patients, mean age 45 years, with a proved diagnosis of ANFH. Group II included 41 patients, mean age 51 years, with a variety of other hip disorders. All underwent MRI using a 1.5-T unit with image reconstruction using the 2-dimensional Fourier transformation technique and a matrix size of 256 × 256. A section thickness of 10 mm, 2 excitations, and no interslice gap were used to obtain multislice SE images.

Results.—Magnetic resonance findings were abnormal, with an area of decreased signal intensity in all 133 femoral heads in group I. Forty-seven percent had a positive fat-intensity sign in this group in contrast to none of group II (Fig 4–20).

Conclusion.—The fat-intensity sign is a reliable MRI finding of ANFH. The area of fat intensity may reflect necrotic bone marrow with-

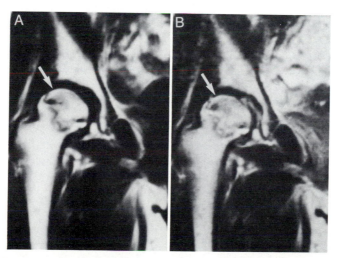

Fig 4–20.—Magnetic resonance images of avascular necrosis of the femoral head. Short TR/short TE (600/23) (**A**) and long TR/long TE (1,600/75) (**B**) images. In both imaging sequences, the area in which the signal intensity is the same as that of subcutaneous fat tissue is present within the hypointense zone (*arrows*). (Courtesy of Kokubo T, Takatori Y, Ninomiya S, et al: *J Comput Assist Tomogr* 15:470–473, 1991.)

out revascularization, which contains fat. No fat is found in revascularized tissue, such as granulation or bone sclerosis.

▶ There are many MRI findings in AVN of the hip. Abnormal signal intensity is a frequent pattern. The authors report their experience with an area of signal intensity that is the same as subcutaneous fat within the hypointense zone of AVN. They conclude that this fat intensity may represent necrotic bone marrow without revascularization and is one of the reliable MRI findings of AVN.—J.E. Madewell, M.D.

Freiberg's Disease in Diabetes Mellitus
Nguyen VD, Keh RA, Daehler RW (Univ of Texas, San Antonio, Tex)
Skeletal Radiol 20:425–428, 1991   4–28

Introduction.—Ischemic necrosis of the metatarsal head, or Freiberg's disease, is a rare condition. It mainly affects women, usually beginning during late childhood or adolescence. Seven cases of Freiberg's disease occurring in patients with diabetes were studied.

Patients.—On examination of 11 patients with Freiberg's disease, 5 were found to have diabetes mellitus. Two more patients were discovered on evaluation of foot radiographs of 120 patients with diabetes (table). Three of these patients had symptoms of foot neuropathy.

Observations.—Previous radiographic studies of patients with diabetes have found the incidence of exostoses to be 36%; osteoporosis was 12.2%; articular lesions was 5.1%; sclerosis was 4%; geodes was 3.7%; and destructive lesions was 3.9%. None of these studies have mentioned Freiberg's disease. This condition is 3 to 4 times more common in women than men and rarely involves both feet. Sixty-eight percent of cases involve the second metatarsal, 27% involve the third metatarsal, and 3% involve the fourth metatarsal. Local pain, tenderness, and swell-

Characteristics of Patients Studied				
Case	Age (years)	Sex	Duration of disease (years)	Neuropathy
1	61	F	13	+
2	72	M	15	−
3	77	F	9	−
4	48	F	18	+
5	53	M	10	−
6	61	M	12	−
7	51	F	10	+

(Courtesy of Nguyen VD, Keh RA, Daehler RW: *Skeletal Radiol* 20:425–428, 1991.)

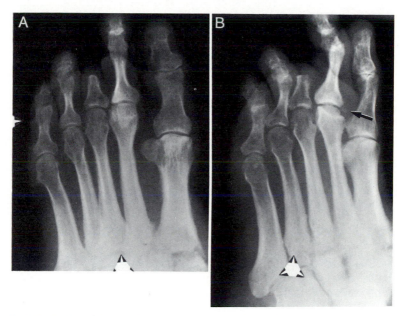

Fig 4–21.—Sinking of the central articular portion into a lesser deformed metatarsal head is evident, probably secondary to bony remodeling and healing. Note the formation of an intra-articular osseous body (*arrow*). (Courtesy of Nguyen VD, Keh RA, Daehler RW: *Skeletal Radiol* 20:425-428, 1991.)

ing are the acute symptoms, whereas many patients are asymptomatic during osteonecrosis and repair. Early in the course of the disease, radiography may show subtle flattening, areas of increased radio-density, and cystic lesions of the metatarsal head. Widening of the joint space may result from infraction of the subchondral trabeculae with collapse of the articular surface. Progressive osteochondral fragmentation with flattening and sclerosis of the metatarsal head and increased cortical thickening of the adjacent metaphysis and diaphysis of the bone may be seen (Fig 4-21). In the later stages, premature closure of the growth plate, intra-articular osseous formations, and enlargement of the metatarsal head with secondary degenerative joint disease may occur. The condition begins with a superficial fissure of the dorsal aspect of the metatarsal head, which disrupts the epiphyseal vascular supply, leading to necrosis and repair. Neuropathy is a concomitant finding in many patients with diabetes and may increase in incidence as the duration of disease increases.

Conclusion.—A variety of musculoskeletal disorders may result from neurotrophic, vascular, and metabolic changes in patients with diabetes. Any of these changes may predispose patients with diabetes to the development of Freiberg's disease.

▶ Thirteen cases of Freiberg's disease are presented. The high association with diabetic patients is reported.—J.E. Madewell, M.D.

Long-Term Reaction of the Osseous Bed Around Silicone Implants

Wanivenhaus A, Lintner F, Wurnig C, Missaghi-Schinzl M (Univ of Vienna, Austria)

Arch Orthop Trauma Surg 110:146–150, 1991   4–29

Introduction.—Physicians have used silicone in orthopedic surgery for 3 decades to fill in where needed at implant sites. With silicon, the implant-bone interface maintains its mobility. Good functional outcome rests on the buildup of a fibrous capsule around this interface. The results of silicone implants used in a series of patients over nearly 20 years, are investigated.

Methods.—Ninety-four individuals received 208 implants, with follow-up data available on 63% of the implants. More than 91% of patients received a joint replacement, and 77% had rheumatoid arthritis as the cause for the surgery. Follow-up examination included radiographs of the osseous bed.

Results.—Radiographic follow-up showed a total intact osseous bed in 52 of the 208 implants (41%). Seventy-four implants demonstrated degrees of implant bed problems. The radiographs depicting limited areas of lysis verified the existence of multiple cysts even on bones located far from the implant joint (Fig 4–22). Eleven patients had the implant exchanged or removed because of pain or increasing osteolysis. Histologic examination of the implant bed tissue from these 11 patients revealed silicone particles in each sample, surrounded by foreign body giant cells. The number and diameter of these giant cells attested to the aggressive reaction of the tissue.

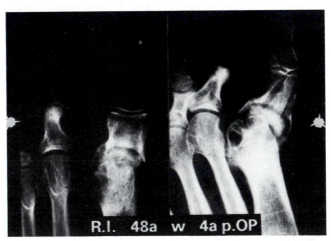

Fig 4–22.—Woman, 48, 4 years after insertion of single-stemmed great toe metatarsophalangeal joint implant. Massive lysis around the pedicle in proximal phalanges. Development of cysts in the metatarsal head. (Courtesy of Wanivenhaus A, Lintner F, Wurnig C: *Arch Orthop Trauma Surg* 110:146–150, 1991.)

Conclusion.—Although histologic and radiographic results from these patients indicate a serious histiocyte reaction to silicone particles, some 89% of the patients continued to claim subjective well-being, and 81% had functional improvement after the implant. It is recommended that physicians use silicone implants only when no other material or surgical alternative exists. New materials for implants need to be developed to avoid any implant effects in the patients.

▶ Silicone implants, since 1947, have been used as an implant material in orthopedic surgery. This article reports the long-term reaction of the osseous bed around the silicone implants.—J.E. Madewell, M.D.

Bone Scans in the Diagnosis of Bone Crisis in Patients Who Have Gaucher Disease
Katz K, Mechlis-Frish S, Cohen IJ, Horev G, Zaizov R, Lubin E (Beilinson Medical Center, Petah Tiqva, Israel; Tel Aviv University, Tel Aviv, Israel)
J Bone Joint Surg [Am] 73-A:513–517, 1991   4–30

Introduction.—Patients with Gaucher's disease, which is characterized by deposits of glucocerebroside in reticuloendothelial cells, may have nonspecific dull bone pain; severe pain ("bone crisis"); or pain from pyogenic osteomyelitis.

Methods.—A prospective assessment of bone scanning was carried out in 47 children and young adults with Gaucher's disease who were followed from 1978 to 1988. The average age was 13 years. Scans were made after injection of technetium 99m–methylene diphosphonate (MDP). A large-field analogue gamma camera and a parallel-hole low-energy collimator were used.

Findings.—Negative bone scans were obtained in patients reporting dull aching that lasted a few days. Most others with severe pain, swelling, and tenderness exhibited decreased uptake. Radiographs showed no new bone lesions. Subsequent scans showed a ring of increased nuclide uptake surrounding a photopenic area. Radiographs made at this time, 6 weeks after the onset of pain, showed periosteal elevation along the involved bone. After 6 months, there frequently was evidence of osteonecrosis with areas of mixed low and high bone density. Pathologic fracture sometimes developed in the initially photopenic area of bone. Bone crises were characterized by decreased uptake in all scan phases and persistently decreased uptake on delayed imaging 6 weeks later.

Conclusion.—Bone scanning is apparently a simple and sensitive means of demonstrating bone crisis in patients with Gaucher's disease.

▶ Bone pain is a common complaint in patients with Gaucher's disease. This may be caused by bone crises, and the authors demonstrate the value of bone scan with ^{99m}Tc-MDP in correctly diagnosing the bone crisis.—J.E. Madewell, M.D.

Is the Coned Lateral Lumbosacral Junction Radiograph Necessary for Radiological Diagnosis?
Lipton ME, Pellegrini V, Harris I (Royal Liverpool Hospital, Liverpool, England)
Br J Radiol 64:420–421, 1991   4–31

Background.—To potentially reduce the number of radiographic studies ordered, the usefulness of plain radiographic examination of the lumbar spine was reviewed. A study was done to determine the diagnostic necessity of the coned lateral lumbosacral junction (LSJ) radiograph.

Methods.—Lumbar spine radiographs of 400 unscreened orthopedic outpatients were reviewed. All underwent anteroposterior (AP), lateral, and coned lateral LSJ radiographs. One report was issued considering all 3 radiographs; a second report considered only the AP and lateral radiographs.

Results.—With only the AP and lateral radiographs, the LSJ was inadequately seen in 21% of patients. In these patients, the coned lateral LSJ radiograph aided 17 diagnoses (11 of spondylosis) that would otherwise have been missed.

Conclusion.—In a large population, significant diagnostic accuracy may be lost when the coned lateral LSJ radiograph is omitted.

▶ The authors present their experience from reviewing 400 lumbar spine radiographs and the positive value of the coned-down lateral LSJ radiograph.—J.E. Madewell, M.D.

5　Abdomen

Introduction

This past year saw continuation of many of the trends and "hot topics" that we identified last year, as well as a couple of new ones. I was pleased to include several excellent radiologic-pathologic correlation studies. Too many investigations reported in the radiology literature rely on poor standards of proof. We are finally seeing reports of imaging studies correlated with actual findings at liver resection, for instance, or at least surgical exploration and intraoperative ultrasound. The results, not surprisingly, suggest that we are not nearly as accurate in our routine imaging interpretations as we had believed. Dynamic bolus-enhanced CT and T_2-weighted MR (for high-field MR systems) have emerged as fairly comparable noninvasive studies of the liver. As more aggressive and innovative therapeutic options emerge, however (including resection, percutaneous ethanol injection, and transplantation), our clinical colleagues will demand even greater precision.

Large-scale population screening for major diseases was a hot topic this year. Although clinical, laboratory, and genetic screenings are important, imaging may play a crucial role for certain diseases. I have included provocative articles on screening for Barrett esophagus, abdominal aortic aneurysm, and prostate and ovarian carcinoma. All of these remain controversial topics, in part because of the issue of cost vs. likely benefit.

Endoscopic ultrasound remains of interest, with encouraging results reported for staging esophageal cancer and detecting and staging pancreatic tumors.

Laparoscopic cholecystectomy is on everyone's mind. As surgeons gain skill in the techniques, they are beginning to apply them to all sorts of "minimally invasive surgery," including appendectomy, hysterectomy, and even nephrectomy. Of course, we are now seeing reports of complications of laproscopic cholecystectomy. Several of our manuscripts indicate an important role for radiologists in preventing and detecting bile duct injuries during the procedure.

My colleagues Gerald (Chip) Dodd and Peter Davis have again provided valuable assistance in evaluating the ultrasonography and MR literature. Dr. Dodd has identified several new trends and observations, as well as a controversy or 2, in fetal sonography and lends his expert commentary. Dr. Davis predicts that breath-holding MR techniques will soon replace standard T_1-weighted spin-echo techniques and that organ-specific MR contrast agents will play an important role in the more distant future.

It has been my pleasure to review the exciting developments in abdominal imaging and to share the authors' collective wisdom with you. I hope the selections and my own modest insights prove useful to you.

Michael P. Federle, M.D.

General Abdomen

Upper Abdominal Lymph Nodes: Criteria for Normal Size Determined With CT
Dorfman RE, Alpern MB, Gross BH, Sandler MA (Henry Ford Hosp, Detroit)
Radiology 180:319–322, 1991   5–1

Background.—The diagnosis of abdominal lymph node abnormality with CT is based on size criteria, but published threshold criteria vary widely, with upper limits of normal sizes ranging from 6 to 20 mm. Different methods of scanning, node location, and axis of measurement limit the possible application of these criteria. This study was undertaken to establish standardized short-axis diameters and threshold estimates for the upper size limits of normal abdominal lymph nodes at 7 defined anatomic locations.

Methods.—The short-axis diameter of the lymph nodes was measured in 130 patients who were not likely to have enlarged abdominal lymph nodes. Seven anatomical locations were defined, and the largest nodal measurement for each was recorded. Threshold values for the maximum node size in each region were determined by histographic analysis and nonparametric statistical methods.

Findings.—The upper limit of normal-sized upper abdominal lymph nodes were 6 mm at the retrocrural space, 8 mm at the paracardiac space, 8 mm at the gastrohepatic ligament, 9 mm at the upper para-aortic region, 10 mm at the portacaval space, 7 mm at the porta hepatis, and 11 mm at the lower para-aortic region (table). Lower para-aortic lymph nodes larger than 11 mm by short-axis measurement are abnormal. Nodes in other locations smaller than 1 cm may be abnormal if the determined thresholds are exceeded.

Conclusions.—The normal upper sized limits of upper abdominal lymph nodes on CT was dependent on location. Short-axis nodal diameters exceeding the threshold values should be regarded as suspicious for lymph node abnormality, especially if several nodes are present.

▶ The authors have provided a valuable service to practicing radiologists with this painstaking analysis of abdominal lymph node size. One of the authors, Barry Gross, participated in a similar review of mediastinal lymph nodes, which should also be available in everyone's reference file (1).—M.P. Federle, M.D.

Threshold Estimates for the Upper Limit of Normal Short-Axis Node Size

Region	No. of Patients with Nodes Identified (n = 130)*	Short-Axis Nodal Diameter (mm)†	Tolerance Interval Estimate for Upper Limit of Normal (mm)‡	Histographic Estimate for Upper Limit of Normal (mm)
Paracardiac	33 (25.4)	3.9 ± 0.2	6.8 (5.0, 8.0)	8.0
Retrocrural space	64 (49.2)	3.0 ± 0.1	5.0 (5.0, 6.0)	6.0
Gastrohepatic ligament	25 (19.2)	4.1 ± 0.3	6.8 (6.0, 9.0)	8.0
Upper paraaortic (celiac to renal)	58 (44.6)	3.7 ± 0.2	7.0 (6.0, 9.0)	9.0
Lower paraaortic (renal to bifurcation)	130 (100)	3.4 ± 0.1	10.0 (10.0, 11.0)	11.0
Porta hepatis	13 (10.0)	3.2 ± 0.4	6.0 (5.0, 8.0)	7.0
Portacaval space	30 (23.1)	5.3 ± 0.4	8.0 (7.0, 10.0)	10.0

* Numbers in parentheses are percentages.
† Mean ± SD.
‡ Confidence interval is 90% and is given in mm in parentheses.
(Courtesy of Dorfman RE, Alpern MB, Gross BH, et al: *Radiology* 180:319–322, 1991.)

Reference

1. Glazer GM, et al: *AJR* 144:261, 1985.

Intraperitoneal Contrast Material Improves the CT Detection of Peritoneal Metastases
Halvorsen RA Jr, Panushka C, Oakley GJ, Letourneau JG, Adcock LL (Univ of Minnesota, Minneapolis; San Francisco Gen Hosp, San Francisco)
AJR 157:37–40, 1991   5–2

Background.—Standard CT of the abdomen is not reliable for detecting peritoneal metastatic disease from gynecological malignancy. The value of administering intraperitoneal contrast material before CT scanning was investigated.

Methods.—Both standard and intraperitoneal contrast-enhanced CT studies of the pelvis and abdomen were done prospectively in 16 patients with suspected gynecological tumors. All patients then underwent operative staging, and the location and number of metastases were recorded.

Findings.—The contrast-enhanced CT studies were more sensitive than standard CT studies in detecting peritoneal metastases. Routine CT detected peritoneal metastases in 64% of the 11 patients with surgically proved implants, whereas contrast-enhanced CT found them in all 11 patients. Enhanced CT had a sensitivity twofold to fourfold greater than that of standard CT studies, depending on the specific intraperitoneal compartments involved.

Conclusions.—Intraperitoneal enhanced CT appears to be superior to standard CT in the detection of peritoneal metastases. Enhanced CT may be useful in sparing some patients with ovarian cancer a second-look surgical procedure.

▶ I would like to see this study repeated with a larger group of patients. Intraperitoneal injection of contrast material is somewhat invasive and may be difficult to coordinate with the CT schedule. If the results are corroborated and if many patients can be spared surgery based on confident identification of peritoneal metastases, the time and effort would be warranted.—M.P. Federle, M.D.

Blunt Splenic Injuries: Nonsurgical Treatment With CT, Arteriography, and Transcatheter Arterial Embolization of the Splenic Artery
Sclafani SJA, Weisberg A, Scalea TM, Phillips TF, Duncan AO (State Univ of New York, Brooklyn)
Radiology 181:189–196, 1991   5–3

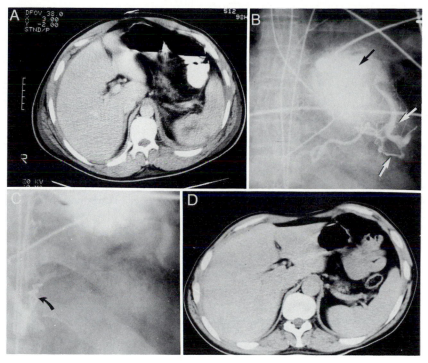

Fig 5–1.—Group 2 splenic injury. Man, 30, was involved in a high-speed automobile collision. In stable condition on admission, he had positive findings at DPL (RBC count of more than 200,000/mL [200 × 10⁶/L]). **A,** CT scan shows a hemoperitoneum, perisplenic hemorrhage, and an intrasplenic hematoma. **B,** arterial extravasation of contrast material (*arrows*) was seen extending out of the spleen into the left subphrenic space. His vital signs deteriorated at that time. **C,** coil occlusion of the proximal splenic artery was immediately performed with occlusion of the splenic artery (*arrow*). The patient received 2 units of transfused blood at the end of the procedure, his condition stabilized, and he had an uneventful recovery. **D,** follow-up CT scan obtained 7 weeks after admission appears normal. (Courtesy of Sclafani SJA, Weisberg A, Scalea TM, et al: *Radiology* 181:189–196, 1991.)

Background.—A method is needed for reliably differentiating splenic injuries that can be managed conservatively from those requiring definitive hemostasis. The management and outcome of blunt splenic injury diagnosed with CT were studied.

Methods.—In all, 44 consecutive patients who were hemodynamically stable or whose condition stabilized quickly with resuscitation were included in the study. Triage for nonsurgical treatment or hemostasis included celiac and splenic arteriography. Of the patients, 19 did not have arterial extravasation of contrast material at arteriography; they were treated with bed rest only. Seventeen had such extravasation and were treated with bed rest after percutaneous transcatheter coil occlusion of the proximal splenic artery. In 8 cases, the patient or attending surgeon did not abide by the treatment protocol; abdominal exploration without angiography or embolotherapy was begun in this patient group.

Outcomes.—Bed rest alone was successful in 18 of 19 patients. Hemorrhage was controlled clinically in all patients in the group treated with bed rest after splenic artery embolization. Exploratory laparotomy was therefore avoided in 94% of the patients in whom nonsurgical management was attempted. The spleen was salvaged in 97% (Fig 5–1).

Conclusions.—Computed tomography is a reliable, accurate method for detecting splenic injury. The angiographical findings in splenic injury are more predictive of the results of nonoperative treatment than CT alone. Nonoperative management seems likely to succeed when arteriography does not show arterial extravasation.

▶ This manuscript offers a real challenge to radiologists and surgeons: splenic lacerations in adults do not require surgery, assuming they have been triaged properly and treated, if necessary, by splenic artery embolization. Dr. Sclafani and his colleagues are experienced and excellent traumatologists and they certainly offer an exciting prospect of salvaging a functional spleen without surgery. I would like to see others confirm their results, because several investigations in the pre-CT era had concluded that arteriography had little predictive value in evaluating splenic trauma. The effort, time, and expense of their approach cannot be minimized, however. The typical patient with a splenic laceration that was actively bleeding would have, by their protocol, a diagnostic peritoneal lavage, CT scan, arteriography, embolization, repeat angiography (same sitting), and repeat CT scan and nuclear medicine scans for 5 to 7 days of hospitalization and for several weeks until complete healing was demonstrated. In most trauma centers, such a patient would have initial CT evaluation and surgery for any demonstrated splenic laceration.

I believe there will be more acceptance for this approach in patients who require angiography for other purposes (suspected traumatic aortic injury, pelvic fractures with exsanguination, etc.). The ability to evaluate and stop ongoing hemorrhage from multiple possible sources is a powerful option.—M.P. Federle, M.D.

Computed Tomography and Diagnostic Peritoneal Lavage: Complementary Roles in Blunt Trauma
Meredith JW, Ditesheim JA, Stonehouse S, Wolfman N (Wake Forest Univ)
Am Surg 58:44–48, 1992   5–4

Background.—There is disagreement on the use of CT and diagnostic peritoneal lavage (DPL) in assessing stable patients with blunt abdominal trauma. A study was done to further clarify their independent and combined value.

Methods.—One hundred sixteen patients were enrolled in the prospective study. All were adults satisfying the entry criteria of major blunt torso trauma, hemodynamic stability, equivocal or unreliable abdominal

TABLE 1.—Injuries by Organ Type

	Number	Injury Detected By CT	CT Recommended Surgery For Patient	DPL +	Initially Operated For Any Reason	Needed Surgery For Injury
Spleen	16	16	7	16	7	9
Liver	19	19	3	13	3	5
Kidney	7	7	0	3	0	3
Pancreas	1	1	1	1	1	1
Duodenum	2	2	2	1	1	2
Small bowel	5	0	0	5	5	4
Colon	2	0	0	2	2	2
Stomach	0					
Bladder	1	1	1	1	1	1
Diaphragm	1	0	0	0	1	0

(Courtesy of Meredith JW, Ditesheim JA, Stonehouse S, et al: *Am Surg* 58:44–48, 1992.)

examination, and absence of prior abdominal surgery and unstable pelvic fractures. The patients were admitted during an 11-month period and underwent CT scanning with a 9800 series GE scanner. The surgeon examined the results with a CT radiologist and determined whether laparotomy was needed. Patients then underwent DPL. Recommendations for laparotomy after this procedure were based on finding aspiration of more than 10 mL of blood or 100,000 red blood cells or more/mm^3, more than 500 white blood cells/mm^3, or positive Gram's stain. A final decision was made on the basis of data from both studies.

Findings.—Twenty-two patients underwent initial laparotomy, yet only 17 had injuries needing repair. Unnecessary laparotomy resulted from DPL findings in 15.5% of the patients compared with .8% from CT findings. Inappropriate observation was recommended by DPL in 1.7% of the patients and by CT in 6.9%. Computed tomography failed to identify

TABLE 2.—Validity and Predictive Value Based on Correctly Predicting Need for Laparotomy

	Sensitivity	Specificity	Positive Predictive Value	Negative Predictive Value	Accuracy (%)
CT	.53	.99	.90	.92	91
DPL	.88	.82	.45	.98	83
Both	.88	.94	.71	.98	93

(Courtesy of Meredith JW, Ditesheim JA, Stonehouse S, et al: *Am Surg* 58:44–48, 1992.)

5 bowel injuries. Half of the patients with positive DPL did not need surgery (Tables 1 and 2).

Conclusions.—These findings underscore the complimentary nature of CT and DPL. These modalities are not equivalent tests or substitutes for one another. Further research should focus not on establishing the superiority of 1 test over the other but on identifying which patients need which tests.

▶ As these authors note, the warring factions of CT fans and DPL fans are still at odds, although they have come closer over the past decade. Almost everyone agrees that patients with multiple potential sources of blood loss or an urgent need for extra-abdominal surgery should have DPL for fast evaluation of gross hemoperitoneum requiring laparotomy. This investigation helps to focus on advantages and disadvantages of CT and DPL in properly selected patients. One could argue over specific details of the results. Is a liver laceration shown by CT with minimal perihepatic blood to be considered a false negative when subsequent exploratory lapartomy reveals a liver laceration "easily controlled with topical hemostatic agents?" The major source of concern is the apparent failure of CT to depict bowel injuries. We have had much greater success, and I am not quite ready to acknowledge this as "an inherent inadequacy" of CT, although bowel injuries are often subtle. The authors seemed to have atypically good results of DPL in detecting bowel injuries; many authors report false negative results of DPL on the immediate posttrauma period. Perhaps the slight delay between CT and DPL contributed to the discordant results. Of note is the 54% rate of nontherapeutic laparotomies that would have resulted if DPL results alone had been used to select patients for surgery. With the growing trend toward nonoperative management of liver and spleen injuries, documentation of the source of hemorrhage (by CT) will remain essential. One should never hesitate to use DPL, repeat CT, or even laparotomy if the condition of the patient warrants it.—M.P. Federle, M.D.

Abdominal Aortic Aneurysm as an Incidental Finding in Abdominal Ultrasonography
Akkersdijk GJM, Puylaert JBCM, de Vries AC (Westeinde Hospital, The Hague, The Netherlands)
Br J Surg 78:1261–1263, 1991   5–5

Introduction.—Potentially fatal abdominal aortic aneurysm affects 1% to 4% of people who are older than age 50. The mortality rate from a ruptured aneurysm ranges from 85% to 95%. Prospective screening of the older population for this type of aneurysm appears to be helpful. A group of patients over age 50 underwent ultrasound study for nonvascular reasons.

Methods.—During 1 year, 3,055 consecutive individuals over age 50 underwent abdominal ultrasonography. This examination was the first

TABLE 1.—Mean Diameters of Incidental Abdominal Aortic
Aneurysms and Patient Ages

Patients	*n*	Abdominal aortic aneurysm		Diameter (mm) *	Age (years)
		n	%		
Men	693	61	8·8	36 (21–65)	71·8 (54–88)
Women	994	21	2·1	31 (19–45)	75·9 (51–88)
All	1687	82	4·9	35	72·9

* Values in parentheses are ranges.
(Courtesy of Akkersdijk GJM, Puylaert JBCM, de Vries AC: *Br J Surg* 78:1261–1263, 1991.)

such screening for 1,800 persons, 113 of whom had the test because of suspected abdominal aortic aneurysm or general vascular assessment and were therefore excluded. An abdominal aortic aneurysm was defined as an aortic local dilatation with an anterioposterior diameter greater than 30 mm or more than 1.5 times the anteroposterior diameter of the proximal aorta.

Results.—Of the 1,687 patients studied (994 women, 693 men), 82 had an abdominal aortic aneurysm. Of these 82, 21 were women and 61 were men, all with a mean age of 72.9 years (Table 1). As the patients aged, the prevalence of this disorder increased (Table 2). The mean aneurysm diameter for all patients was 35 mm, 36 mm for men and 31 mm for women. There was no significant association between abdominal aortic aneurysm diameter and patient age (Fig 5–2).

Conclusions.—The prevalence of incidental abdominal aortic aneurysm was 2.1% for women and 8.8% for men more than age 50. It is recommended that physicians screen for abdominal aortic aneurysm in ev-

TABLE 2.—Prevalence of Abdominal Aortic Aneurysm as an
Incidental Finding in Abdominal Ultrasonography

Patients	Age (years) *				
	50–59	60–69	70–79	80–89	All
Men	2·5	9·7	11·8	14·3	8·8
Women	0·8	0·6	2·7	6·4	2·1
All	1·5	4·2	6·6	9·2	4·9

* Values are percentages.
(Courtesy of Akkersdijk GJM, Puylaert JBCM, de Vries AC: *Br J Surg* 78:1261–1263, 1991.)

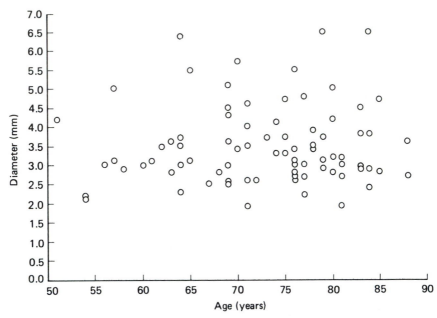

Fig 5–2.—Aneurysm diameter according to age. (Courtesy of Akkersdijk GJM, Puylaert JBCM, de Vries AC: *Br J Surg* 78:1261–1263, 1991.)

ery person older than age 50 who is undergoing abdominal sonography for the first time.

▶ The prevalence of abdominal aortic aneurysm appears to be increasing. Because of both the extreme morbidity and mortality of ruptured aneurysms and the relatively benign course of electively repaired aneurysms, effective screening programs are needed. Other studies have identified increased risk of abdominal aortic aneurysm in men, individuals more than 50 years of age, relatives of patients with abdominal aortic aneurysm, and those with other evidence of atherosclerotic disease. The incidence in patients in any of the last 3 risk groups is about 15% to 20%, clearly suggesting a role for noninvasive screening by ultrasound. The authors of the current study suggest routine imaging of the aorta in patients having their first abdominal ultrasound for any reason, and this is good advice. The yield will be at least as great as the routine testing of stool guiac or blood pressure that physicians perform during routine medical encounters.—M.P. Federle, M.D.

Biopsy

Tumor Seeding Occurring After Fine-Needle Biopsy of Abdominal Malignancies

Lundstedt C, Stridbeck H, Andersson R, Tranberg K-G, Andrén-Sandberg Å

(University Hospital, Lund, Sweden)
Acta Radiologica 32:518–520, 1991   5–6

Introduction.—Physicians often use fine-needle biopsy, with its low complication rate and somewhat high (85%) accuracy, in assessing tumors. Tumor seeding after fine-needle biopsy has been reported, however. The occurrence of implantation metastases after fine-needle biopsy was studied in 5 patients with abdominal malignancies.

Methods.—Of about 5,000 abdominal biopsies performed with 20- to 22-gauge needles over 1 decade, 5 resulted in implantation metastases. Three of these patients underwent only 1 biopsy each with 3, 3, and 4 needle passes.

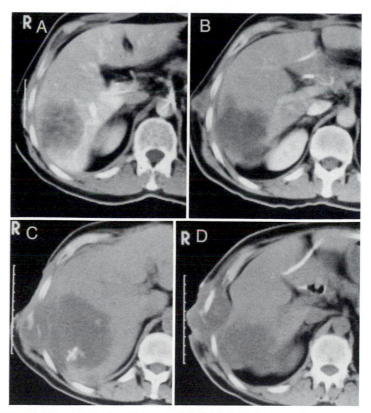

Fig 5–3.—**A,** CT scan of the liver during injection of contrast medium into the superior mesenteric artery, showing a tumor of the right liver lobe; **B,** 3 months later, the liver is about the same size, but a tumor is seen in the soft tissues of the flank; **C,** 1 year later, there is only a small difference in the size of the now partially calcified liver tumor, but the tumor in the flank is progressive, **D,** after another 6 months, the liver tumor is still stationary in size, but the tumor in the abdominal wall is growing, and bone destruction is seen. (Courtesy of Lundstedt C, Stridbeck H, Andersson R, et al: *Acta Radiologica* 32:518–520, 1991.)

Results.—The 5 implantation metastases were documented 1 to 6 months after the initial biopsy. In all patients, the lesions occurred away from the laparotomy scar. Three of the 5 patients underwent radical removal of the tumor.

Case Report.—Man, 51, previously had liver metastases and had undergone repeated resections for this and other cancers (Fig 5-3). He had laser coagulation of the liver tumor because he refused blood transfusion on principle. He underwent 3 separate needle passes after the laser surgery. Three months later, a soft tissue lesion, which corresponded to the needle tract in the abdominal wall and showed both cutaneous and subcutaneous metastatic growth, developed. The patient received local irradiation therapy, and the liver tumor remained unchanged but the abdominal wall tumor grew during 18 months of follow-up.

Conclusions.—Although fine-needle biopsy remains a useful diagnostic tool, it does pose some risk to the patient for the development of metastatic tumor implantations. If a fine-needle biopsy appears necessary to decide on the appropriate treatment of a tumor, the physician should use as fine a needle as possible and make the minimum number of needle passes. Fine-needle biopsy should not be used in patients who must undergo radical tumor resection.

▶ Experimental studies have detected tumor cells in the needle tract after fine-needle biopsy in up to 90% of cases. The authors report a rate of 1 in 1,000 clinically detectable implantation metastases in human beings, similar to other reported experiences. One reason for the discrepancy might be that many patients are lost to follow-up or die of their disease before implantation metastases become evident. Another explanation might be that a large "bolus" of tumor cells is needed to induce metastatic growth, usually far exceeding the small number left in biopsy tracts. I would not alter our aggressive approach to necessary biopsies after reading this report. I will continue to use the smallest needle and fewest passes necessary to provide the diagnosis and will resist performing biopsies on patients who will almost certainly require radical surgery (e.g., patients with solid renal masses).—M.P. Federle, M.D.

Transjugular Liver Biopsy
McAfee JH, Keeffe EB, Lee RG, Rösch J (Oregon Health Sciences Univ, Portland)
Hepatology 15:726–732, 1992   5-7

Introduction.—Percutaneous liver biopsy is a simple, quick, safe, and relatively inexpensive procedure; however, a transjugular or other approach may be used in patients with advanced liver disease complicated by a major coagulation disorder or major ascites. The technique of trans-

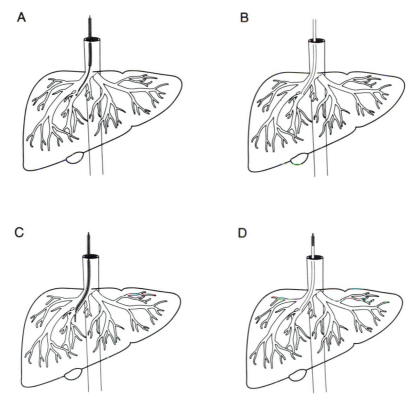

Fig 5–4.—**A,** a J-shaped guide wire is placed inside a 5F coaxial catheter within a larger 9F catheter. The tip of the guidewire is positioned into the appropriate hepatic vein. **B,** the 9F catheter is advanced into position in the hepatic vein, and the smaller guidewire and catheter are removed. **C,** the transjugular needle is advanced through the 9F catheter and hepatic vein wall into the hepatic parenchyma while suction is maintained. **D,** the needle and specimen are withdrawn. The 9F catheter is temporarily left in place for additional biopsies, if required. (Courtesy of McAfee JH, Keeffe EB, Lee RG, et al: *Hepatology* 15:726–732, 1992.)

jugular liver biopsy and a 21-year experience with this procedure were examined.

Technique.—Light sedation may be used to relieve anxiety and discomfort. Prophylactic antibiotics are not routinely used, but ECG monitoring is essential. Using local anesthesia, a no. 9 French catheter and a no. 5 French coaxial catheter are inserted by a Seldinger technique into the right internal jugular vein. The catheters and guidewire are passed to the inferior vena cava and into the right hepatic vein under fluoroscopic guidance. The right liver lobe is the best biopsy site. With the no. 9 French catheter positioned a safe distance from the liver capsule, the needle is inserted. The needle is passed through the wall of the hepatic vein to obtain a specimen (Fig 5–4). The procedure has been modified by mounting a Tru-Cut needle on a flexible coaxial cable. Failure usually results from anatomical factors.

Indications for Transjugular Approach to Liver Biopsy

Major
　Coagulation disorder
　　Prothrombin time > 3 sec over control value
　　Platelet count < 60,000/cm³
　Massive ascites
　Desire for ancillary procedures
　　Measurement of hepatic vein and inferior vena cava
　　　pressures
　　Opacification of hepatic veins and inferior vena cava
Minor
　Failed percutaneous liver biopsy
　Massive obesity
　Small, cirrhotic liver (increased risk; lower yield)
　Suspected vascular tumor or peliosis hepatis

(Courtesy of McAfee JH, Keeffe EB, Lee RG, et al: *Hepatology* 15:726–732, 1992.)

Experience.—One hundred forty-six attempts at transjugular liver biopsy in 140 patients were made during a 21-year period. The mean patient age was 51 years. Many patients underwent concurrent procedures, most often hepatic venograms. Cannulation was unsuccessful in 3.4% of the cases; use of the cutting needle appeared to improve the adequacy of specimens. The indication for the procedure was coagulopathy with or without ascites in 65.5% of the cases. There was only 1 infectious complication, and the patient was receiving antibiotics. Technical success was achieved in 91.8% of the attempts; adequate tissue for diagnosis was achieved in 78.8%. The rate of complications was 16.4%, but the rate of major complications was only 2.7%, with no deaths. A specific change in treatment resulted in 21.8% of the cases.

Discussion.—In certain situations, transjugular liver biopsy is a safe alternative for obtaining liver biopsy specimens. The procedure requires trained personnel and is time-consuming and moderately expensive, but its complication rate and mortality are low. Transjugular liver biopsy may be useful in patients with coagulopathy or ascites and in those with fulminant hepatic failure (table).

▶ The authors helped to pioneer the technique of transjugular liver biopsy more than 20 years ago. Even with their skill and enthusiasm, it remains an infrequently performed study, and most major centers for hepatic disease probably perform no more than 6 transjugular biopsies per year. Nevertheless, when indicated in high-risk patients, it is a very valuable procedure.—M.P. Federle, M.D.

Esophagus

Preoperative Staging of Esophageal Cancer: Comparison of Endoscopic US and Dynamic CT

Botet JF, Lightdale CJ, Zauber AG, Gerdes H, Urmacher C, Brennan MF (Mem Sloan-Kettering Cancer Ctr; Cornell Univ, New York)
Radiology 181:419–425, 1991   5–8

Background.—Esophageal carcinoma is relatively uncommon in the United States. Most patients have advanced disease at initial diagnosis. After surgical resection, the prognosis is closely related to pathologic stage. The accuracy of endoscopic ultrasonography (EUS) in the preoperative clinical staging of esophageal cancer was compared with that of dynamic CT.

Methods.—A group of 50 patients with esophageal cancer underwent preoperative staging with endoscopic US. Dynamic CT of the chest and abdomen was also done in 42. The results were compared with findings of pathologic assessment of the resected specimens.

Findings.—Endoscopic US was significantly more accurate (46 of 50 tumors [92%]) than CT (25 of 42 tumors [60%]) in staging the depth of tumor growth. It was also more accurate than CT (88% and 74% respectively) in staging the regional lymph nodes; however, this was not significant. Computed tomography was more accurate in staging distant metastases (90% and 70% for CT and EUS respectively). The highest concordance with surgical and pathologic results in overall stage oc-

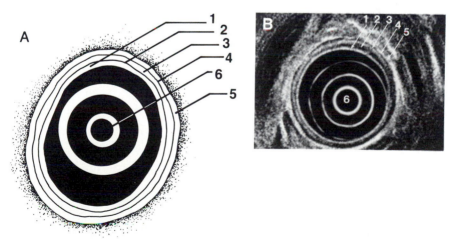

Fig 5–5.—A diagram **(A)** and ultrasound scan **(B)** depicting the 5-layered structure of the wall of the normal esophagus. The mucosa (hyperechoic) is indicated by *1*; *2* indicates the deep mucosa (hypoechoic); *3*, the submucosa (hyperechoic); *4*, the muscularis propria (hypoechoic); *5*, adventitial interface (hyperechoic); and *6*, transducer. (Courtesy of Botet JF, Lightdale CJ, Zauber AG, et al: *Radiology* 181:419–425, 1991.)

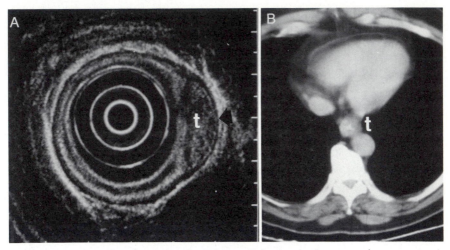

Fig 5–6.—A, an endosonogram showing a T2 tumor (*t*) that invades the mucosa, deep mucosa, and submucosa but does not extend through the muscularis propria (*arrow*). **B,** a CT scan of a T1-T2 tumor (*t*) shows circumferential thickening of the esophageal wall but no definite extension beyond the adventitial interface. (Courtesy of Botet JF, Lightdale CJ, Zauber AG, et al: *Radiology* 181:419–425, 1991.)

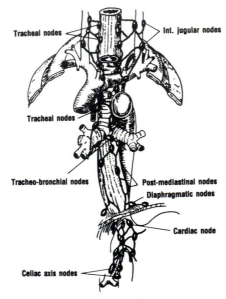

Fig 5–7.—Lymphatic drainage of the esophagus. Endoscopic ultrasound can enable evaluation of all the nodes depicted. *Int* indicates international. (Courtesy of Botet BF, Lightdale CJ, Zauber AG, et al: *Radiology* 181:419–425, 1991.)

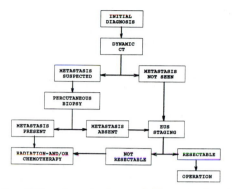

Fig 5–8.—*Abbreviation:* EUS, endoscopic ultrasound. Diagnostic algorithm for the preoperative staging of esophageal cancer. (Courtesy of Botet JF, Lightdale CJ, Zauber AG, et al: *Radiology* 181:419–425, 1991.).

curred with combined CT and EUS; this was significantly more accurate than using CT alone (86% and 64% respectively) (Figs 5–5 through 5–8).

Conclusions.—Dynamic CT of the chest and abdomen should be used to screen for distant metastases. When metastasis is suggested, percutaneous biopsy should be done for confirmation. If distant metastases are not confirmed, then EUS should be done to assess depth of tumor invasion and regional lymph node metastasis.

▶ Prior attempts at CT staging of esophageal cancer relied on indirect and fairly subjective findings, such as indentation of the tracheobronchial tree and loss of the fat plane between the esophagus and the aorta. The layers of the esophageal wall could not be visualized, and tumors might completely escape detection, particularly near the gastroesophageal junction. (Adenocarcinomas of this area appear to be increasing in prevalence.) The modern staging of esophageal cancer stresses depth of tumor invasion as the criterion for the "T" component; the ability of EUS to display reliably the layers of the normal and abnormal wall is an obvious advantage over CT, confirmed in this report by greater accuracy of EUS in determining local tumor invasion and spread. Endoscopic ultrasound is also excellent in depicting regional lymph tumor strictures and to depict distant (especially lung and liver) metastases, retaining an important role for dynamic CT scanning. The authors have done a commendable job of proving their premise and present a logical and cost-effective approach.—M.P. Federle, M.D.

Esophageal Ultrasound and the Preoperative Staging of Carcinoma of the Esophagus
Rice TW, Boyce GA, Sivak MV (Cleveland Clinic Found, Cleveland)
J Thorac Cardiovasc Surg 101:536–544, 1991   5–9

Introduction.—The International Union Against Cancer and the American Joint Committee on Cancer issued new guidelines for the staging of esophageal cancer in 1987 and 1988. The new guidelines are still based on the TNM classification, but evaluation of the primary tumor now involves assessing the depth of wall invasion, rather than anatomical location, tumor length, or percentage of wall circumference involved. Because the traditionally used methods for clinical staging are not useful for determining tumor invasion depth, the usefulness of esophageal ultrasound (US) in preoperative staging was evaluated.

Methods.—The normal esophageal wall consists of 5 distinct layers. If the tumor has involved the first 3 echo layers but is confined by the third echo layer, it is called T1. If the tumor has invaded the fifth echo layer and adjacent structures, it is called T4. Previous studies have shown that these 5 layers, as well as regional lymph nodes, can be visualized with esophageal US. Periesophageal tissue is also well visualized by esophageal US. Lymph node shape, margin, and internal structure can also be assessed.

Patients.—Preoperative staging by esophageal US was attempted in 6 women and 22 men aged 46 to 83 years less than 2 weeks before operation. All patients had carcinomas that involved the thoracic esophagus by AJCC definition. The esophageal US probe could not be passed through the malignant stricture in 6 patients (21%). The studies in the remaining 22 patients were evaluable. All studies were performed with a flexible endoscope and were videotaped. Depth of tumor invasion was confirmed by pathologic review.

Results.—Depth of tumor invasion was correctly identified in 13 of the 22 patients (59% accuracy). Tumor depth was overstaged in 4 patients (18%) and understaged in 5 patients (23%). Twenty patients had adequate lymph node staging at operation to allow comparison with the esophageal US findings. The disease was correctly identified by esophageal US as node negative in 7 patients and as node positive in 7 patients (70% accuracy). There were 3 false positive and 3 false negative assessments.

Conclusions.—Esophageal ultrasound provides a useful alternative method for clinical staging of esophageal cancer. It is anticipated that refinements of technique and increasing experience will improve the diagnostic accuracy of esophageal US.

▶ This article provides a nice background for the theory of esophageal cancer staging and the technique of endoscopic US. The results of this small study should be regarded as preliminary. Note the preceding article (Abstract 5–8) by Botet and colleagues for a larger study group and some meaningful trends that are discussed.—M.P. Federle, M.D.

The Radiologic Diagnosis of Barrett Esophagus: Importance of Mucosal Surface Abnormalities on Air-Contrast Barium Studies

Glick SN, Teplick SK, Amenta PS (Hahnemann Univ Hosp, Philadelphia; Univ of Arkansas, Little Rock, Ark; Robert Wood Johnson Univ–Univ of Medicine and Dentistry of New Jersey, New Brunswick, NJ)
AJR 157:951–954, 1991   5–10

Background.—Identifying patients with Barrett esophagus before esophageal adenocarcinoma develops is essential. The radiologic diagnosis of Barrett esophagus was reviewed.

Methods and Findings.—Barrett esophagus was diagnosed prospectively on routine biphasic upper gastrointestinal series in 9 patients. In these patients, a mucosal surface pattern change was the only radiological abnormality seen on the esophagogram. The diagnoses were confirmed surgically in 1 patient and by biopsy in 8. Only one third of the patients reported esophageal symptoms. There were 2 types of surface changes: a reticular pattern in 6 cases and a villous pattern in 5 (Figs 5–9 and 5–10). Two of the patients displayed both patterns. An additional 15 patients with Barrett esophagus and corresponding esophagograms were seen during the 5-year study period. All 15 had radiologic evidence of esophagitis, middle or distal esophageal strictures, or a combination thereof.

Conclusions.—The detection of Barrett esophagus may be improved by recognizing the subtle surface patterns, especially when other reflux-

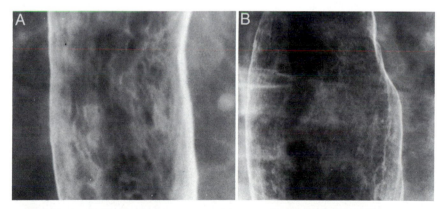

Fig 5–9.—A, reticular pattern. Air-contrast esophagogram of a man, 48, with discomfort in the right upper quadrant shows a network of intersecting lines of barium in mid-esophagus, producing an angular and round mosaic pattern. These changes extended to the gastroesophageal junction. A biopsy specimen showed columnar epithelium of the cardia type. **B,** villous pattern. Woman, 68, with anemia. Air-contrast esophagogram at the level of the main bronchus shows diffusely distributed, tiny, confluent, round lucencies resembling villi of the small intestine. Both specialized and cardia types of Barrett mucosa were noted on biopsy. (Courtesy of Glick SN, Teplick SK, Amenta PS: *AJR* 157:951–954, 1991.)

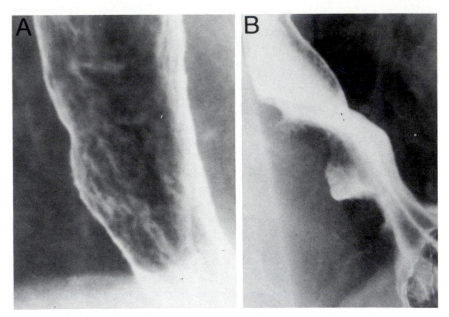

Fig 5–10.—A, man, 65, with hiccups and vague discomfort in the chest. A fine villous pattern was noted in the distal esophagus on air-contrast study. Barrett esophagus was suggested, and endoscopy was recommended but not performed. **B,** the patient returned 9 months later with dysphagia, and an esophagogram showed an ulcerating mass just proximal to the gastroesophageal junction. A resected specimen showed an infiltrating adenocarcinoma with adjacent fundal-type columnar mucosa. Superficial carcinoma was most likely present when the first study was done. (Courtesy of Glick SN, Teplick SK, Amenta PS: *AJR* 157:951-954, 1991.)

induced abnormalities are absent. The recognition of these patterns may also aid in selecting patients for surveillance.

▶ Barrett esophagus (columnar metaplasia of the mucosa) is a sequela of reflux esophagitis and predisposes to esophageal adenocarcinoma. The prevalence of the disorder in the general population may be 20 times greater than expected based on clinical reflux symptoms. Endoscopy is accurate in diagnosis but too expensive and invasive to be recommended as a screening test, especially because 20% to 40% of patients with Barrett esophagus do not report reflux or other esophageal symptoms. Barium esophagography would be an attractive alternative. Past reports have been pessimistic about the sensitivity of esophagrams to diagnose Barrett esophagus, with only 25% to 45% of patients having "suggestive criteria" (midesophageal strictures and ulcers). More recent articles have focused attention on earlier and potentially more sensitive and specific signs such as the reticular pattern of mucosa. These authors add another sign, the villous mucosal pattern.

I remain uncertain of the indications for screening (because only a minority of patients have esophageal symptoms) or the true sensitivity and specificity of radiographic findings. Several groups of superb gastrointestial radiologists have to date failed to identify reliable findings, but Glick and colleagues estimate that 95% of patients with Barrett esophagus will have at least nonspecific abnormalities on barium esophagrams, such as reflux, erosions, and strictures. Endoscopy should be reserved (and probably recommended) for follow-up in these patients.—M.P. Federle, M.D.

Small Intestine

Duodenitis: A Reliable Radiologic Diagnosis?
Levine MS, Turner D, Ekberg O, Rubesin SE, Katzka DA (Univ of Pennsylvania, Philadelphia)
Gastrointest Radiol 16:99–103, 1991   5–11

Purpose.—Duodenitis is generally diagnosed by endoscopic inspection of the duodenal bulb or by the results of endoscopic biopsy. Some reports suggest that upper gastrointestinal (GI) radiographic examination is of limited use in diagnosing duodenitis, but 1 study reported a diagnostic sensitivity and specificity of nearly 80%. The accuracy of diagnosing duodenitis by upper GI radiography was reviewed.

Methods.—The study sample comprised 50 patients with endoscopically diagnosed duodenitis who had also undergone double-contrast upper GI examination. The patients were 29 men and 21 women, average age 59 years. On endoscopy, the disease was rated as mild to moderate in 37 cases and severe in 13. All radiographic examinations were done as biphasic studies, including double-contrast duodenal views with high-density barium and prone compression duodenal views with low-density barium. Original radiographic diagnoses were reviewed, as well as the presence of 4 previously described radiographic signs of duodenitis. Another 20 patients with radiographically diagnosed duodenitis who later had endoscopy were also reviewed.

Findings.—Overall rate of diagnosis in the original radiographic report was 22%, including 16% of the patients with mild to moderate duodenitis and 38% of those with severe duodenitis. One or more of the radiographic signs was present in 52% of the patients overall (table); thus, use of these criteria improved radiographic sensitivity from 22% to 52%. The most common sign was folds more than 4 mm thick (Fig 5–11), followed by bulbar deformity, mucosal nodularity, and erosions (Fig 5–12). Of the patients who had the diagnosis made on radiographic examination, 45% had duodenitis on endoscopy. Seventeen of these 20 patients had 1 or more of the radiographic signs, and 9 of the 17 had duodenitis on endoscopy.

Conclusions.—Double-contrast upper GI radiography is not a reliable technique for diagnosing duodenitis. Even with the use of established criteria, the rate of false positive and false negative diagnosis is still about 50%.

Endoscopic-Radiologic Correlation in 50 Patients With Duodenitis

Endoscopic grade	No. patients	Thick folds	Nodularity	Deformity	Erosions	One or more signs
Mild-to-moderate	37	15 (41)	2 (5)	4 (11)	1 (3)	18 (49)
Severe	13	7 (54)	2 (15)	2 (15)	1 (8)	8 (62)
All grades	50	22 (44)	4 (8)	6 (12)	2 (4)	26 (52)

Note: percentages are presented in parentheses.
(Courtesy of Levine MS, Turner D, Ekberg O, et al: *Gastrointest Radiol* 16:99–103, 1991.)

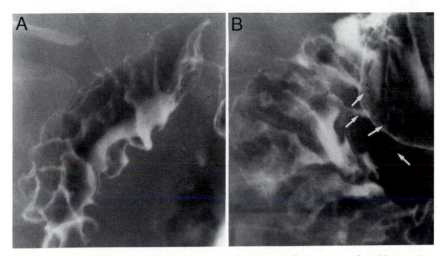

Fig 5–11.—Two patients (**A, B**) with radiographically diagnosed duodenitis manifested by irregular, thickened folds (more than 4 mm in thickness) in the proximal descending duodenum. However, only 1 patient (**A**) had endoscopic evidence of duodenitis. (Courtesy of Levine MS, Turner D, Ekberg O, et al: *Gastrointest Radiol* 16:99–103, 1991.)

▶ Duodenitis is believed to be an important cause of dyspepsia in the adult population, although much debate and confusion persists about its diagnosis and treatment. This article, from an excellent group of GI radiologists, confirms that the barium upper GI series is unreliable in diagnosing duodenitis. Some even question whether endoscopy alone can diagnose duodenitis or whether biopsy is necessary. However, many investigators and clinicians use

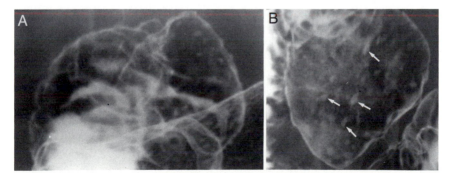

Fig 5–12.—Two patients with radiographically diagnosed erosive duodenitis. **A,** varioliform erosions with central barium collections surrounded by halos of edematous mucosa. **B,** tiny barium collections in bulbs (*arrows*) have no surrounding mounds of edema. Only 1 patient (**A**) had endoscopic evidence of duodenal erosions. (Courtesy of Levine MS, Turner D, Ekberg O, et al: *Gastrointest Radiol* 16:99–103, 1991.)

the endoscopic appearance of the duodenum as the standard for diagnosis, as in this study. Several studies have now confirmed the unreliability of the upper GI series in diagnosing duodenitis, being neither sensitive nor specific.—M.P. Federle, M.D.

Radiographic Evaluation of Suspected Small Bowel Obstruction
Shrake PD, Rex DK, Lappas JC, Maglinte DDT (Indiana Univ, Methodist Hosp of Indiana, Indianapolis)
Am J Gastroenterol 86:175–178, 1991   5–12

Background.—Although plain abdominal radiographs are usually used to investigate suspected small bowel obstruction, they may sometimes be misleading. Enteroclysis may be recommended for uncertain cases. The clinical utility of these studies was evaluated in 117 consecutive patients who underwent enteroclysis.

Methods.—All plain abdominal radiographs and all abnormal enteroclysis studies were examined by 2 reviewers in a blind fashion. History, surgical results, and follow-up data were obtained by chart review. All radiologic studies were done in standardized fashion.

Findings.—In 53 patients, radiographic interpretation was "abnormal nonspecific." The percentage and severity of obstruction on enteroclysis generally increased with the degree of abnormality on radiographs. However, 34% of patients with obstruction on enteroclysis had normal or nonspecific radiographs, and 42% of patients with obstruction on radiographs had normal findings or only minor, nonobstructive adhesions on enteroclysis. Radiography predicted the level of obstruction in 79% of surgical cases compared with 89% for enteroclysis (table). The predictive ability of enteroclysis was 100% for presence of obstruction, 88% for absence of obstruction, and 86% for cause of obstruction.

Level of Obstruction as Estimated by Plain
Abdominal Radiographs and Enteroclysis

	Determined by Surgery	
	Proximal	Distal
Plain radiograph		
Proximal	5	1
Distal	3	10
Enteroclysis		
Proximal	10	3
Distal	1	14

(Courtesy of Shrake PD, Rex DK, Lappas JC, et al: *Am J Gastroenterol* 86:175–178, 1991.)

Conclusions.—Enteroclysis appears to be the more accurate procedure for the evaluation of suspected small bowel obstruction. Plain abdominal radiographs may be misleading in this situation. Enteroclysis can predict not only the presence but also the level and cause of the obstruction.

▶ Is nothing sacred in plain film radiology? Can't we even diagnose bowel obstruction on abdominal radiographs? Unfortunately, the message of the article is that we cannot. Although 74% of patients with high-grade or complete intestinal obstructions had significantly abnormal plain radiographs, 36% had normal or nonspecific findings. Conversely, many patients with strongly suggestive plain films had no obstruction on enteroclysis. There are many possible explanations for the poor results of plain radiographs, including proximal obstruction, vomiting, or nasogastric tube decompression of obstructed loops, and early obstruction. However, this series of patients seems similar to those encountered in everyday practice, and the results are sobering. We too have found enteroclysis to optimally show the presence, level, and nature of the obstruction. This is largely because of the ability to bypass physiology and to distend the bowel maximally to detect partial obstructions and to deliver the head of the barium column distally within a short time frame (usually < 30 minutes). Having the patient drink barium or administering the barium into the stomach via a nasogastric tube is ineffective, in my experience, except for very proximal obstructions. Fluid in dilated bowel loops and sluggish peristalsis generally render delayed films useless, except to document some passage of barium into the colon in cases of incomplete obstruction. I know enteroclysis ("entero crisis" to many) is tedious, but I think we need to use it more often in cases of suspected bowel obstruction.—M.P. Federle, M.D.

Colorectal

Ultrasonography in the Diagnosis of Acute Appendicitis

Ooms HWA, Koumans RKJ, Ho Kang You PJ, Puylaert JBCM (Westeinde Hospital, The Hague, The Netherlands)
Br J Surg 78:315–318, 1991   5–13

Background.—Ultrasonography with graded compression markedly enhances accuracy in the diagnosis of acute appendicitis. Ultrasonography with graded compression was performed in 525 patients with clinical signs of acute appendicitis.

Patients.—Five hundred and twenty-five patients with clinical signs of acute appendicitis underwent ultrasonography. The appendix was considered inflamed if its diameter from the periphery of the muscularis to the opposite side was 6 mm or greater.

Results.—Two hundred and seven patients had surgically proved appendicitis. The inflamed appendix had been visualized sonographically in 86% of these patients (Fig 5–13). The rate of sonographic visualization

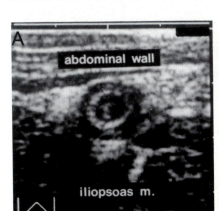 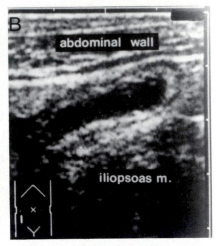

Fig 5–13.—Ultrasonographic image of an inflamed appendix during graded compression. The appendix is identified compressed between the abdominal wall and iliopsoas muscle. **A,** axial section of the appendix, clearly showing its concentrically layered structure. Its alternately hyperechoic and hypoechoic rings represent (from inside out): mucosal surface outlining the collapsed lumen; lamina propria; submucosa; muscularis; and the serosa, merging with the surrounding fatty tissue. The diameter is 10 mm. **B,** a longitudinal section shows the tubular nature of the appendix and its blind end. (Courtesy of Ooms HWA, Koumans RKJ, Ho Kang Yo PJ, et al: *Br J Surg* 78:315–318, 1991.)

for nonperforated appendicitis was 91% compared with 55% for perforated appendicitis. Of 38 patients who had abortive appendicitis, 22 did not undergo surgery. Four of these patients had recurrent appendicitis, and 18 had no recurrences. Ultrasonography made the correct diagnosis in 140 of 155 patients with a confirmed alternative condition, showed no abnormalities in 12, and made a false positive diagnosis of appendicitis in 3 patients. Of the 3 patients with a false positive diagnosis, 2 had perforated peptic ulcer and 1 had primary pneumococcal peritonitis. Bacterial ileocecitis was diagnosed in 69 patients, mesenteric lymphadenitis in 8, gynecologic conditions in 34, urologic conditions in 8, cecal diverticulitis in 6, perforated peptic ulcer in 6, Crohn's disease in 2, and miscellaneous conditions in 7. Ultrasonography showed no abnormalities in 138 of 139 patients with no definitive diagnosis. In the last 3 years of the study, the negative appendectomy rate decreased to 7%, and delay beyond 6 hours after admission decreased to only 2% of patients with surgically proved appendicitis.

Conclusions.—Ultrasonography with graded compression enhanced diagnostic accuracy of acute appendicitis. During the study in this institution, both the negative appendectomy rate and delay to surgery beyond 6 hours after admission decreased.

▶ Dr. Puylaert and his colleagues have done the original and best work on sonographic diagnosis of acute appendicitis, and this article is another valuable contribution. In most hospitals, the "negative appendectomy" rate ranges from 22% to 28% (35%–45% in young women), and a delay between hospital admission and surgery exceeding 6 hours because of diagnostic uncertainty occurs in 20% to 28%. This 3-year study reports a decrease in the negative appendectomy rate to 7% and a decrease in the delayed surgery rate to 2%. Although the sensitivity of sonographic diagnosis of perforated appendicitis was low (55%) compared with the rate for nonperforated appendicitis (91%), most of these patients have obvious clinical indications for surgery. When ultrasound demonstrates no appendiceal or other abnormality, there is still a 16% chance of appendicitis (28 of 178 in the study). However, when ultrasound indicates an alternative diagnosis, the chance of appendicitis decreases to 1%. By far the most common alternative condition detected by ultrasound was bacterial ileocolitis (*Yersinia, Campylobacter,* or *Salmonella*), with characteristic ultrasonographic features of mural thickening of the ileum and cecum with enlarged mesenteric nodes. In young women, demonstration of adnexal abnormalities suggested the gynecologic nature of the right lower quadrant symptoms.

Dr. Puylaert's excellent results have been corroborated by others (1). I hope that more radiologists will add this important examination to their practice.—M.P. Federle, M.D.

Reference

1. Jeffrey RB, et al: *Radiology* 163:11, 1987.

Pseudo-Obstruction Associated With Colonic Ischemia: Successful Management With Colonoscopic Decompression
Fiorito JJ, Schoen RE, Brandt LJ (Albert Einstein College of Medicine, Bronx, NY)
Am J Gastroenterol 86:1472–1476, 1991   5–14

Background.—Patients with colonic pseudo-obstruction have the signs and symptoms of colonic obstruction but no evidence of mechanical obstruction. In up to 10% of cases it occurs in association with colonic ischemia. Three patients with colonic ischemia associated with pseudo-obstruction had colonoscopic decompression and tube placement.

Case Report.—Man, 60, underwent successful cadaveric renal transplant for end-stage renal disease. Treatment included antithymocyte globulin and prednisone. He had a painless abdominal distention on the third postoperative day. An abdominal plain film showed dilation of the colon from the splenic flexure to the cecum, which measured 12 cm in its transverse diameter. Colonic decompression was performed with carbon dioxide as the insufflating agent and a no. 10 French decompression tube was positioned in the cecum. The presence of fecal material obscured visualization of the cecal and ascending colon mucosa. Rectal bleeding that required transfusion with 3 units of packed red blood cells occurred on the seventh postoperative day. The patient was given a balanced electrolyte solution before colonoscopy was repeated. At this time mucosal ulcerations, submucosal hemorrhage, and edema were noted in the ascending colon, all typical changes of colonic ischemia. The patient was treated with antibiotics and discharged on the 12th hospital day.

Discussion.—For patients with pseudo-obstruction and associated colonic ischemia, colonoscopic decompression and tube placement may obviate the need for laparotomy. This treatment is recommended if the cecum is larger than 12 cm and if a brief trial of conservative treatment fails.

▶ In 1948, Ogilvie described massive dilation of the colon without a mechanical cause. It has since been recognized as a common phenomenon, particularly in bedridden patients with a variety of systemic illnesses. Perforation of the colon occurs in up to 10% of the patients with pseudo-obstruction because of ischemia resulting from the dilated bowel and increased intraluminal pressure. Controversy exists over exact size criteria and clinical indications for interventions, but if cecal size is greater than 12 cm and a brief trial of conservative management is unsuccessful, decompression probably is indicated. Prior investigators have advocated laparotomy or percutaneous trocar catheter decompression. Fiorito and colleagues have demonstrated that colonoscopy with CO_2 as the insufflating agent and tube decompression can be effective in relieving both the obstruction and the mucosal ischemia.—M.P. Federle, M.D.

Colonoscopically Detected Colorectal Cancer Missed on Barium Enema
Anderson N, Cook HB, Coates R (Christchurch Hospital, Christchurch, New Zealand)
Gastrointest Radiol 16:123–127, 1991   5–15

Objective.—Cancer of the large intestine is the commonest malignancy in New Zealand and the barium enema examination remains the chief diagnostic method. The findings in 26 patients whose colorectal cancers were missed on the barium enema study and later detected at colonoscopy were reviewed. The patients were among 89 who had colorectal cancer confirmed pathologically in a 3-year period.

Findings.—The findings of rectal blood and anemia often were underreported to the radiologist. More than half of the missed cancers were in the sigmoid colon, but diverticula contributed to diagnostic failure in only 2 instances. The mean tumor size was 43 mm; 15 were polyps and 11 were annular lesions. Eighteen of 23 missed tumors were detected in retrospect, and in 10 instances the tumor was obvious. The main reasons for perceptive errors were failing to see a lesion in the barium pool, not seeing it en face, and missing it through overlapping loops. There were 3 interpretive misses. Treatment delay exceeded 6 months in 7 cases.

Implications.—Because most of the colorectal cancers were missed as a result of perceptive error by the observers, including some who were experienced, it seems wise to recommend double reporting of all barium enema examinations.

▶ The authors are to be commended for sharing candidly their disturbing experience in missing colon cancers on barium enema. Their data are drawn from real clinical experience reflecting the variations in expertise, technique, and lack of clinical information that plague us all. Kelvin and colleagues (1) reported a similar experience and also concluded that perceptual errors were the most common and might best be avoided by double reading of barium enemas. Unlike the Kelvin experience, where most missed lesions were small polyps, the Anderson et al. paper reports many larger polypoid and annular constricting tumors. Because the sigmoid colon is the most common site of missed cancers, special attention is warranted, including angled views to reduce overlapped segments. We favor reviewing the sigmoid in single contrast, as well as double contrast, taking spot films while filling the sigmoid with the thick barium. In cases of diverticulosis, it is also useful to refill the sigmoid with very diluted barium (some even use the CT barium preparations) after evacuation of the colon from the double-contrast exam. See also the paper by Ott et al. (2).—M.P. Federle, M.D.

References

1. Kelvin FM, et al: *AJR* 137:307, 1981.
2. Ott DJ, et al: *Gastrointest Radiol* 5:99, 1980.

Predictive Value of a Negative Computed Tomographic Scan in 100 Patients With Rectal Carcinoma
Cance WG, Cohen AM, Enker WE, Sigurdson ER (Memorial Sloan-Kettering Cancer Ctr, New York)
Dis Colon Rectum 34:748–751, 1991   5–16

Background.—Preoperative adjuvant treatment of patients with rectal carcinoma is becoming more common. It is therefore essential to have a reliable way to identify patients with disease localized to the pelvis. The ability of a CT scan to predict accurately the absence of periaortic nodal metastases or liver metastases in patients with rectal carcinoma was assessed.

Methods.—In 100 patients, operative findings and pathologic stages were correlated with preoperative CT scan findings. The predictive value of a negative CT scan was determined by making these correlations in patients without evidence of extrapelvic metastases on the scan before surgery.

Findings.—Sixty-four percent of the patients had stage T3 or T4 tumors. Ten patients had unsuspected distant metastases, yielding an over-

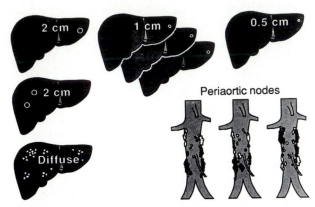

Fig 5–14.—The locations and sizes of the distant metastatic disease in the 7 patients with liver metastases and the 3 patients with periaortic nodal metastases. (Courtesy of Cance WG, Cohen AM, Enker WE, et al: *Dis Colon Rectum* 34:748–751, 1991.)

all negative predictive value of 90%. Seven patients had small liver metastases; 3 had periaortic nodal metastases. Six patients in the former group had their liver metastases completely resected at initial laparotomy. Computed tomography's predictive value decreased in patients selected to receive full-dose preoperative radiation therapy who had a mean delay of 12 weeks between CT scan and laparotomy. Preoperative carcinoembryonic antigen levels had no value in predicting the presence of distant metastases (Fig 5–14 and table).

Conclusions.—Computed tomography is a sensitive screening test for predicting whether a patient with rectal carcinoma has disease limited to the pelvis. A negative CT scan will not detect 10% of those with positive periaortic nodes or small liver metastases.

The Predictive Value of the CT Scan Based on T
Stages and the Interval Between CT Scan
and Laparotomy

	Predictive Value	
T Stage*	1-week Interval	12-week Interval
T2	100% (17/17)	100% (8/8)
T3/T4	91% (40/44)†	70% (14/20)†
Total	93% (57/61)†	79% (22/28)†

* Excludes 8 patients with T1 tumors and 3 patients with Tx tumors.
† *P* = .03 for T3/T4 tumors, 1 week vs. 12 weeks, and *P* = .04 for the entire group, 1 week vs. 12 weeks.
(Courtesy of Cance WG, Cohen AM, Enker WE, et al: *Dis Colon Rectum* 34:748–751. 1991.)

▶ The details of the CT techniques used in the study are not reported, except that 10-mm thick sections were used. I believe that optimal technique (5-mm thick sections with bolus infusion of contrast medium and dynamic scanning) might have allowed detection of a few more hepatic and nodal metastases, but the results are consistent with other reports. The poor predictive value of carcinoembryonic antigen was an important observation.—M.P. Federle, M.D.

Liver

Increased Lymphatic Flow From the Liver in Different Intra- and Extrahepatic Diseases Demonstrated by CT

Aspestrand F, Schrumpf E, Jacobsen M, Hanssen L, Endresen K (National Hospital; University of Oslo, Oslo, Norway)

J Comp Assist Tomogr 15:550–554, 1991   5–17

Background.—An increase in the production of hepatic lymph is a compensatory mechanism that occurs in cirrhosis, liver neoplasia, biliary obstruction, and right-sided cardiac decompensation with elevated hepatic venous pressure. In hepatic lymphostasis, dilated hepatic lymphatics appear on CT as low attenuation rims, or perivascular lucencies (PVLs), that surround the portal veins and intrahepatic vena cava. The prevalence of PVLs as a marker of increased lymph flow from the liver was studied.

Methods.—Computed tomography liver scans of healthy controls and patients with the 4 diseases named were assessed for the presence of

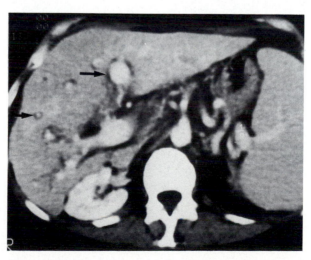

Fig 5–15.—Biliary cirrhosis. Lucent rims surrounding peripheral and central portal veins (*arrows*). (Courtesy of Aspestrand F, Schrumpf E, Jacobsen M, et al: *J Comp Assist Tomogr* 15:550–554, 1991.)

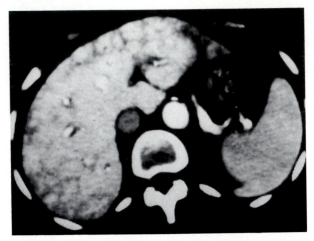

Fig 5–16.—Tricuspid incompetence. Lucent areas surrounding peripheral veins and partly embedded inferior vena cava. Mottled enhancement of liver parenchyma is seen. (Courtesy of Aspestrand F, Schrumpf E, Jacobsen M, et al: *J Comp Assist Tomogr* 15:550–554, 1991.)

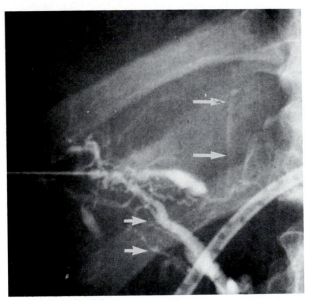

Fig 5–17.—Same patient as in Figure 5-15. Accidental hepatography during percutaneous cholangiography reveals filling of the dilated lymphatic vessels following the central portal vein (*short arrows*) and along course of inferior vena cava (*long arrows*). (Courtesy of Aspestrand F, Schrumpf E, Jacobsen M, et al: *J Comp Assist Tomogr* 15:550–554, 1991.)

PVLs. The presence or absence of PVLs was correlated with other CT findings and various biochemical and pathophysiologic parameters.

Findings.—Perivascular lucencies occurred at a frequency of 12% to 52% in patients in each of the 4 disease categories, but none of the normal control subjects had PVLs. Seven of 30 patients with biliary cirrhosis had PVLs (Fig 5–15). The presence of PVLs in patients with tricuspid incompetence correlated perfectly with the presence of mottled enhancement of the hepatic parenchyma (Fig 5–16). The presence of PVLs was also associated with increases in certain biochemical parameters, but there was no common biochemical marker across the disease categories. In 3 patients the findings at accidental hepatography during percutaneous cholangiography supported the interpretation of the CT findings (Fig 5–17).

Conclusions.—Perivascular lucencies on CT reflect changes in hepatic lymphatic dynamics. In the absence of impaired efferent lymph drainage, PVLs reflect increased lymphatic flow. The sensitivity of this finding, however, has not yet been assessed.

▶ For years, I had wondered about the origin of the PVLs described in this article. The University of Alabama–Birmingham group (1) first alerted me to the likely nature of the lesion, namely, dilated lymphatics. The Aspestrand et al. article provides a better understanding of the shared etiology of dilated lymphatics by seemingly unrelated process such as congestive heart failure and metastatic tumor. The most dramatic PVLs to be seen are in patients with liver transplantation where the increased production of lymph and the severed lymphatics draining the liver may produce perivascular lucent bands measuring in excess of 1 cm. Somewhat similar appearing lucencies may be seen in patients with hepatic trauma, when blood, not lymph, tracks along the portal and hepatic veins.—M.P. Federle, M.D.

Reference

1. Koslin DB, et al: *AJR* 150:111, 1988.

Focal Hepatic Lesions: Differentiation With MR Imaging at 0.5 T
Brown JJ, Lee JM, Lee JKT, Van Lom KJ, Malchow SC (Washington Univ, St Louis; Catholic University, Seoul, Korea; Scripps Mem Hosp, Chula Vista, Calif)
Radiology 179:675–679, 1991   5–18

Background.—Quantitative methods of MRI have been used to differentiate between benign and malignant hepatic lesions but the methods are impractical for daily radiologic use. Characterizing lesions by qualitative methods has usually involved lesion shape, internal architecture, and signal intensity characteristics relative to those of the liver on T_1- and T_2-weighted images. A qualitative analysis of focal hepatic lesions was re-

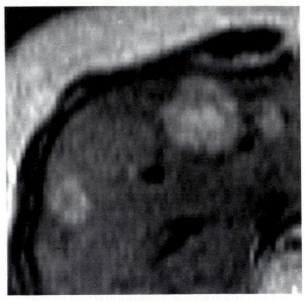

Fig 5–18.—Transaxial T2-weighted (2,100/90) image of the right upper quadrant in a patient with metastatic breast carcinoma. Note the heterogeneous appearance of the metastatic lesions. (Courtesy of Brown JJ, Lee JM, Lee JKT, et al: *Radiology* 179:675–679, 1991.)

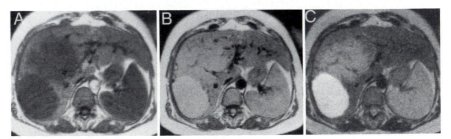

Fig 5–19.—Transaxial MR images of the liver in a patient with hepatocellular carcinoma and a cavernous hemangioma. The cavernous hemangioma is located in the right hepatic lobe. The hepatocellular carcinoma is located just anterior to the cavernous hemangioma, involving the anterior segment of the right hepatic lobe and the medial segment of the left hepatic lobe. **A,** on the T1-weighted (500/15) image, both lesions are hypointense relative to the liver. The cavernous hemangioma has smooth borders; the hepatocellular carcinoma has irregular margins. **B,** on the balanced (2,100/35) image, the cavernous hemangioma is hyperintense relative to liver parenchyma and the spleen. The hepatocellular carcinoma is slightly hyperintense relative to the liver and isointense compared with the spleen. **C,** on the T2-weighted (2,100/90) image, the cavernous hemangioma is markedly hyperintense relative to liver parenchyma. The hepatocellular carcinoma is hyperintense relative to the liver and isointense relative to the spleen. (Courtesy of Brown JJ, Lee JM, Lee JKT, et al: *Radiology* 179:675–679, 1991.)

Likelihood of Malignancy Predicted by Means of Logistic Regression Model

T2 Liver*	Internal Architecture	Balanced Spleen†	Predicted Likelihood of Malignancy	Standard Error
Iso/hyperintense	Inhomogeneous	Isointense	0.9998	0.0004
Iso/hyperintense	Inhomogeneous	Hyperintense	0.9991	0.0014
Iso/hyperintense	Homogeneous	Isointense	0.9880	0.0150
Iso/hyperintense	Homogeneous	Hyperintense	0.9530	0.0510
Markedly hyperintense	Inhomogeneous	Hyperintense	0.7470	0.1550
Iso/hyperintense	Homogeneous	Hypointense	0.1880	0.1160
Markedly hyperintense	Homogeneous	Isointense	0.1760	0.1820
Markedly hyperintense	Homogeneous	Hyperintense	0.0490	0.0590

* Lesion signal intensity relative to liver on T$_2$-weighted images.
† Lesion signal intensity relative to spleen on balanced images.
(Courtesy of Brown JJ, Lee JM, Lee JKT, et al: *Radiology* 179:675–679, 1991.)

fined by comparing signal intensity of lesions with that of structures outside the liver and by analyzing balanced images in addition to T$_1$- and T$_2$-weighted images.

Methods.—The MRI examinations of 43 patients with 95 focal hepatic lesions were analyzed retrospectively for lesion shape, homogeneity, and relative signal intensity compared with normal liver parenchyma, spleen, and skeletal muscle.

Findings.—Of the 95 focal hepatic lesions evaluated, most metastases, cavernous hemangiomas, and cysts were smooth and round or oval, and 70% of metastatic lesions, 85% of cavernous hemangiomas, and 100% of simple hepatic cysts were of homogeneous signal intensity (Fig 5–18). All lesions with irregular borders were malignant (Fig 5–19). Logistic regression analysis showed that heterogeneous lesions had a high likelihood of malignancy, whereas markedly hyperintense lesions had a very low probability of being malignant (table). Other lesions with a high likelihood of malignancy were homogeneous lesions that were isointense or hyperintense compared with the spleen on balanced images but were not markedly hyperintense in T$_2$-weighted images.

Conclusions.—Logistic regression analysis showed that marked hyperintensity of lesions on T$_2$-weighted images and homogeneous internal structure have a low risk of malignancy, whereas heterogeneous internal architecture and lesion isointensity relative to spleen on balanced images strongly favor malignancy.

▶ This article provides a simple and very useful approach to MR of liver lesions that should appeal to radiologists and the way we reason. Most of us approach lesion characterization by qualitative rather than quantitative methods. We are good at recognizing shape, architecture, and "density," and we develop a feel for the reliability of these characteristics for indicating certain pathologies. These authors have reviewed almost 100 focal lesions and found that 73% had a predicted likelihood of malignancy of greater than 95% or less than 5%.

I hope that similar study will be performed using higher-field magnets and including a larger variety of malignant lesions. I am concerned that hypervascular metastases (e.g., renal cell and endocrine tumors) will prove more difficult to distinguish from benign disease using only these authors' simple criteria.—M.P. Federle, M.D.

Computed Tomography Attenuation Measurements for the Characterization of Hepatic Haemangiomas

Whitehouse RW (Manchester University, Manchester, England)
Br J Radiol 64:1019–1022, 1991   5–19

Introduction.—Computed tomography has documented the characteristics of hepatic cavernous hemangiomas during the past 10 years. These characteristics can have a 100% positive predictive value, but only 55% of known lesions meet the CT criteria. Quantitative observations were made of CT images in patients with hepatic hemangiomas.

Methods.—Nineteen patients (13 women and 6 men with a mean age of 52 years) with 21 hepatic hemangiomas underwent CT imaging. The nonenhanced CT scans showed a lesion with lower attenuation than the

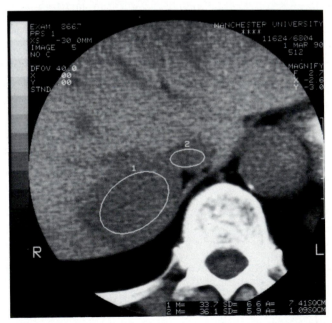

Fig 5–20.—Typical precontrast CT scan of hepatic hemangioma demonstrating ROI choice for hemangioma (*1*) and IVC (*2*). (Courtesy of Whitehouse RW: *Br J Radiol* 64:1019–1022, 1991.)

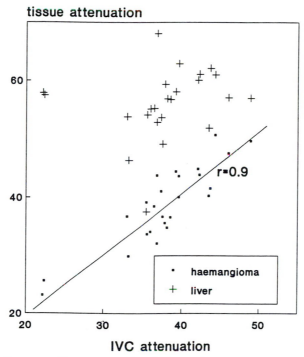

tissue attenuation

IVC attenuation

Fig 5–21.—Precontrast CT attenuation values for liver and hepatic hemangiomas plotted against attenuation values for the inferior vena cava content on the same section. (Courtesy of Whitehouse RW: *Br J Radiol* 64:1019–1022, 1991.)

surrounding liver tissue. These images became isodense with the liver upon delayed postcontrast CT scanning. Fifteen of the 19 patients also underwent ultrasound imaging, which showed defined hyperechoic areas. Five patients had biopsies that confirmed the diagnosis. The oval CT scan region of interest (ROI) included the largest possible area within the lesion (Fig 5–20).

Results.—The hemangiomas ranged from .61 to 15 cm². The results of general attenuation or blood attenuation did not differ significantly between the small and large lesions, so the results for both sizes were combined. The hemangiomas did demonstrate a significantly lower mean precontrast attenuation than that of the nearby liver tissue, but this did not relate to the attenuation in the rest of the liver. The attenuation of the hemangiomas significantly correlated with that of blood measured in the inferior vena cava (IVC), and all hemangiomas fell within 7 HU of blood attenuation (Fig 5–21). The liver lesions in patients with malignant cancer were hypodense in comparison to liver tissue but did not correlate with liver or IVC attenuation.

Conclusions.—Clinical requirements often dictate the type of CT scanning of the liver needed. Comparing the attenuation characteristics of liver lesions and of blood in the IVC can aid in deciding whether further enhanced CT studies are necessary.

▶ You may be weary of reading articles about hepatic hemangiomas, but this manuscript emphasizes a simple important observation that is otherwise likely to be confused. Most articles about hemangiomas compare the attenuation of the mass to the surrounding liver on precontrast and postcontrast scans. To be considered typical, the hemangioma is supposed to be hypodense on the precontrast scans and isodense or hyperdense after contrast. This relationship is unreliable, given the potentially wide variations in liver attenuation (from fatty liver to hemosiderosis) and the attenuation of blood (varying with hematocrit, circulating contrast media, etc.). The sensible basis for comparison is the lesion and the IVC. These authors have proved a straight line correlation of attenuation of hemangiomas and the IVC. Lesions that vary considerably from this correlation were never hemangiomas, and dynamic enhanced scans or delayed scans may be superfluous in this setting.—M.P. Federle, M.D.

Hepatic Metastases: CT Versus MR Imaging at 1.5T
Vassiliades VG, Foley WD, Alarcon J, Lawson T, Erickson S, Kneeland JB, Steinberg HV, Bernardino ME (Emory Univ, Atlanta, Ga; Medical College of Wisconsin, Milwaukee)
Gastrointest Radiol 16:159–163, 1991   5–20

Background.—The most effective imaging modality for detecting focal hepatic lesions is debated. A multicenter study was done to prospectively compare state-of-the-art CT with high-field-strength MR imaging for the detection of hepatic metastases in patients with cancer.

Methods.—Sixty-nine patients known to have malignancies were selected randomly from patients referred for CT studies because of suspected metastatic disease. T_1-weighted and T_2-weighted spin-echo (SE) MRI were compared with CT.

Findings.—Noncontrast CT had an overall sensitivity of 57%; dynamic CT had an overall sensitivity of 71%; and delayed CT had an overall sensitivity of 72%. T_1-weighted SE MRI had an overall sensitivity of 47%, and T_2-weighted SE MRI had an overall sensitivity of 78%. There was no significant difference among dynamic CT, delayed CT, and T_2-weighted SE MRI, but these methods were significantly more sensitive than noncontrast CT and T_1-weighted SE MRI. T_2-weighted SE MRI was significantly more sensitive than CT or T_1-weighted SE MRI in detecting lesions less than 1 cm. Computed tomography was more sensitive in detecting extrahepatic lesions.

Conclusions.—A T_2-weighted SE MRI is superior to T_1-weighted SE pulse sequences at 1.5 T. With improvements in motion artifact-reduction methods, the sensitivity of MRI is likely to improve and may surpass that of CT. Currently, CT is still more reliable in detecting extrahepatic metastatic disease.

▶ This study further confirms the superiority of T_2-weighted sequences over T_1-weighted for scanning at 1.5 T. T_2-weighted MRI and good-quality CT were equivalent for detecting most hepatic lesions, whereas CT remained superior for extrahepatic disease detection. These authors have found MRI superior to CT detection of hepatic lesions less than 1 cm, whereas others (see following abstracts) have reached the opposite conclusion. This may be, in part, because of the inclusion of certain hypervascular primary tumors (carcinoma, renal, etc.) whose metastatic hepatic deposits are known to be difficult to detect on dynamic bolus-enhanced CT. The other major difference in protocol is the absence of pathologic correlation. We know the most small (< 1.5 cm) hepatic lesions are benign, even in patients with a known primary malignancy (Abstract 5–17) and that up to 20% of the general population have hemangiomas in the liver. Magnetic resonance imaging will detect these much more readily than CT, and this would clearly influence the results.—M.P. Federle, M.D.

Detection of Hepatic Metastases: Comparison of Contrast-Enhanced CT, Unenhanced MR Imaging, and Iron Oxide-Enhanced MR Imaging

Fretz CJ, Stark DD, Metz CE, Elizondo G, Weissleder R, Shen J-H, Wittenberg J, Simeone J, Ferrucci JT (Massachusetts Gen Hosp, Harvard Med School, Boston; Univ of Chicago, Chicago)
AJR 155:763–770, 1990   5–21

Objective.—For evaluation of hepatic metastases, unenhanced MRI has been shown to equal or surpass the accuracy of contrast-enhanced CT. Superparamagnetic iron oxide-enhanced MRI may improve detection of hepatic lesions. The diagnostic accuracy of these 3 techniques was compared in 10 patients with histologically proved hepatic metastases.

Methods.—The 6 women and 4 men had a mean age of 57 years and underwent all 3 diagnostic studies. The ability of radiologists to recognize the presence or absence of hepatic metastases was measured by using receiver-operating characteristic (ROC) analysis of single images; the total number of lesions detected by both CT and MR imaging on matching anatomical sections was counted; and lesion-liver contrast/noise ratios (CNR) were measured in all MR images. The dose of contrast material was 20 μmol of iron oxide/kg in 9 patients.

Findings.—Contrast-enhanced CT had a mean area under the ROC curve of .67, compared with .81 for the unenhanced SE 260/14 MRI sequence and .92 for the enhanced SE 1,500/40 MRI sequence. Accuracy was significantly greater with the enhanced SE 1,500/40 sequence than with contrast-enhanced CT. Nineteen percent more lesions were found with the enhanced 1,500/40 sequence than with the best unenhanced

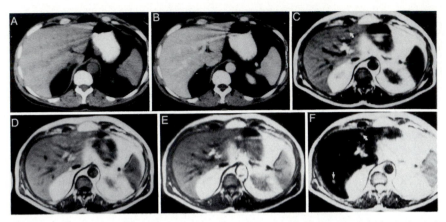

Fig 5–22.—Metastatic colon cancer. **A,** unenhanced CT scan; no lesion visible. **B,** iodine-enhanced CT scan; good opacification of the hepatic vessels; streaklike artifacts partially obscure the left lobe of the liver; no lesion is visible. **C,** SE 260/14 MR image obtained before injection of iron oxide shows 1 lesion (*arrow*) in the left lobe of the liver. **D** and **E,** 500/30 (**D**) and SE 1,500/40 (**E**) MR images obtained before injection of iron oxide; lesion in the left lobe of the liver is not visible. **F,** SE 1,500/40 MR image obtained after injection of 20 µmol of FE/kg of AMI-25; lesion in the left lobe (*curved arrow*) is confirmed; an additional lesion (*straight arrow*) is visible in the right lobe. (Courtesy of Fretz CJ Stark DD, Metz CE, et al: AJR 155:763-770, 1990.)

MRI sequence (Fig 5-22) and 36% more were found than with enhanced CT. The CNR of this sequence was 19.5, the best of all MRI sequences.

Conclusions.—On our .6T MR system, detection of hepatic metastases appears to be best with iron oxide–enhanced MRI. The results justify prospective studies of this technique for screening purposes.

▶ These data, if corroborated in larger series, would have important implications and would likely cause much greater interest in MRI of the liver. Unfortunately, it has been difficult for other groups to duplicate the consistently positive results that the MGH group reports for liver MRI. This may be largely because of the unique capabilities of the .6-T Technicare scanner that has been optimized for body imaging. This machine is no longer in production, and we have learned that imaging sequences that are optimal on this equipment are not optimal on others, particularly 1.5-T systems. For instance, heavily T_1-weighted images show liver masses best on the MGH Technicare scanner, whereas high-field systems routinely show liver lesions best on T_2-weighted images. Similarly, others (1) have not shown any increased detectibility of liver lesions at 1.5 T when comparing superparamagnetic iron oxide–enhanced with nonenhanced scans.—M.P. Federle, M.D.

Reference

1. Marchal G, et al: AJR 152:771, 1989.

Comparison Between High-Field-Strength MR Imaging and CT for Screening of Hepatic Metastases: A Receiver Operating Characteristic Analysis

Rummeny EJ, Wernecke K, Saini S, Vassallo P, Wiesmann W, Oestmann JW, Kivelitz D, Reers B, Reiser MF, Peters PE (Westfaelische Wilhelms-University, Münster, Germany; Massachusetts Gen Hosp, Boston)
Radiology 182:879–886, 1992   5–22

Background.—The presence of hepatic metastases in patients with malignancies has important treatment implications. The diagnostic performance of high-field-strength MRI 1.5 T, and CT for detecting liver metastases was compared.

Methods and Findings.—Fifty-two patients had preoperative screening with MRI with T_1-weighted, proton density–weighted, and T_2-weighted pulse sequences. They also had CT scanning with unenhanced, incremental dynamic bolus-enhanced, and delayed contrast medium-enhanced methods. Receiver operating characteristic analysis was done to assess diagnostic performance. Eight hundred images—half with and half without lesions—and 5 readers were used. Images were obtained from 39 patients in whom the same anatomical levels were available for all MR and CT studies. Direct comparison of the best MRI technique and the best CT technique showed a strong trend of superiority of T_2-weighted MRI over incremental dynamic bolus CT. However, these 2 techniques did not differ very significantly (Figs 5–23 and 5–24).

Conclusions.—Hepatic metastases screening should be done using T_2-weighted pulse sequences at high-field-strength MRI and the incremental dynamic bolus method at CT scanning. The MR method seems to be better than the CT.

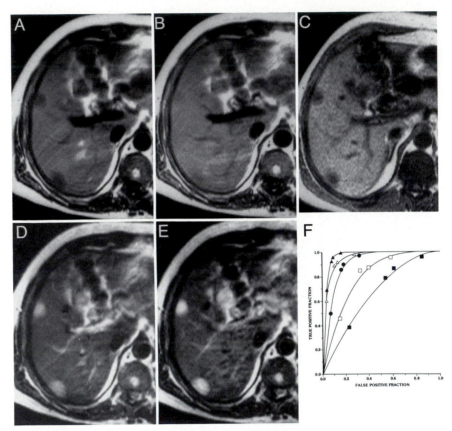

Fig 5–23.—A–E, magnetic resonance images of hepatic metastases from colon cancer. **A,** T1-weighted spin-echo (SE) 800/15 image shows metastases that are hypointense relative to the liver. **B,** proton-density-weighted SE 2,000/15 image displays lesions as nearly isointense to liver. **C,** T1-weighted gradient echo 100/6 image (1 signal average, 60-degree flip angle). Note the improved contrast of hypointense lesions relative to uninvolved liver compared with that in **A,** and **B. D,** T2-weighted SE 800/70 image shows lesions as hyperintense relative to liver. **E,** lesion contrast on heavily T2-weighted SE 2,000/70 image is maximal compared with that in other pulse sequences. **F,** composite receiver operating characteristic curves display relative accuracies with which liver metastases are detected by means of different pulse sequences at 1.5 tesla. Receiver operating characteristic points of all readers for SE 2,000/70 (*filled triangle*), SE 800/70 (*open triangle*), gradient echo 100/6 (*circle*), SE 800/15 (*open square*), and SE 2,000/15 (*filled square*) are plotted. (Courtesy of Rummeny EJ, Wernecke K, Saini S, et al: *Radiology* 182:879–886, 1992.)

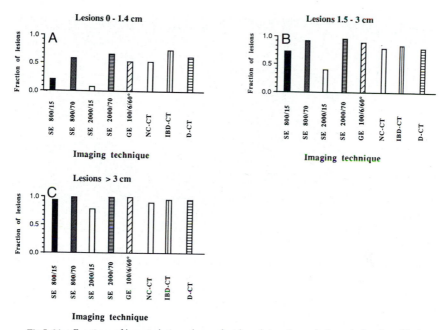

Fig 5–24.—Fractions of hepatic lesions detected with each imaging technique. **A,** fraction of lesions smaller than 1.4 cm in diameter. **B,** fraction of lesions 1.5–3 cm in diameter. **C,** fraction of lesions larger than 3 cm in diameter. *Abbreviations:* NC-CT, nonenhanced CT; IBD-CT, incremental dynamic bolus CT; D-CT, delayed CT. (Courtesy of Rummeny EJ, Wernecke K, Saini S, et al: *Radiology* 182:879–886, 1992.)

Detection of Hepatic Masses in Patients With Carcinoma: Comparative Sensitivities of Sonography, CT, and MR Imaging

Wernecke K, Rummeny E, Bongartz G, Vassallo P, Kivelitz D, Wiesmann W, Peters PE, Reers B, Reiser M, Pircher W (Univ of Münster, Münster, Germany)
AJR 157:731–739, 1991   5–23

Background.—The use of imaging techniques to detect hepatic masses from colorectal metastases can aid in preoperative determination of the number, size, and location of the metastases. The sensitivity of sonography, CT, and MRI in the detection of focal hepatic masses was evaluated.

Methods.—In a prospective study, 75 patients with gastrointestinal tumors who were admitted for surgical resection of the primary tumor were examined with sonography, CT, and MRI. The emphasis was on detection, not characterization, of hepatic lesions. Sonography was performed with convex transducers of 3.5 and 5.0 MHz. The CT scanning included unenhanced CT scans first, followed by the incremental bolus dynamic scanning technique, and delayed scanning 4 to 6 hours after bolus injection of iodine. T_1- and T_2-weighted spin-echo MR sequences and breath-holding fast low-angle shot sequences were obtained. The

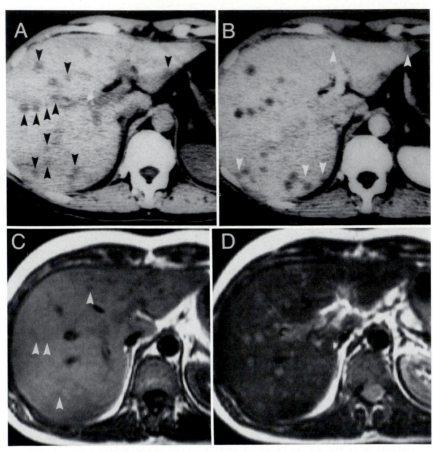

Fig 5–25.—Visualization of small hepatic metastases (adenocarcinoma of pancreas) by various CT and MRI techniques. **A,** unenhanced CT scan shows multiple metastases (*arrowheads*) 1 cm in diameter in both hepatic lobes. **B,** on incremental bolus dynamic CT scan, additional small lesions (*arrowheads*) can be detected in the left lobe and posterior segment of the right lobe. **C,** on T1-weighted SE 800/15 MRI, only a few metastatic lesions (*arrowheads*) are faintly visible. **D,** on T2-weighted SE 800/70 MRI, multiple small metastases are shown in the right lobe and medial segment of the left lobe. Three lesions in the lateral segment of the left lobe, shown on incremental bolus dynamic CT scan (**B**) were not detected. (Courtesy of Wernecke K, Rummeny E, Bongartz G, et al: AJR 157:731–739, 1991.)

results of the examinations were interpreted blindly and compared with the gold standard of surgical examination, intraoperative sonography, and biopsy of the liver. To overcome factors leading to inconsistent results among many comparative studies, rules for this study included the examination of a comparatively large number of patients with a gold standard adapted to a clinical study, inclusion of no more than 5 foci per patient in the lesion-by-lesion analysis, and additional patient-by-patient analysis with reference to therapeutic consequences.

TABLE 1.—Lesion Detection by Sonography, CT, and MRI

Imaging Technique	No. of Patients	No. of Lesions	True Positive	False Negative	False Positive	% Sensitivity
Sonography	34	95 [21]	50 [10]	45 [11]	0	53 [48]
Unenhanced CT	33	90	46	44	1	51
Incremental bolus dynamic CT	30	91	61	30	1	67
Delayed CT	33	94	50	44	2	53
CT (overall)	34	95 [21]	65 [12]	30 [9]	2	68 [57]
SE 800/15	34	95	32	63	1	34
SE 800/70	34	95	48	47	0	50
SE 2000/15	31	80	13	67	0	16
SE 2000/70	31	80	41	39	0	51
FLASH 15°	25	57	3	54	0	5
FLASH 60°	34	94	48	46	0	51
MR (overall)	34	95 [21]	60 [6]	35 [15]	1	63 [29]

Abbreviations: SE, spin echo; FLASH, fast low-angle shot.
Numbers in brackets represent benign lesions; 74 of the 95 hepatic lesions were metastases, and 21 were benign.
Significance of difference between CT (overall) and sonography: $P < .008$; between CT (overall) and MRI (overall): $P > .168$.
(Courtesy of Wernecke K, Rummeny E, Bongartz G, et al: AJR 157:731–739, 1991.)

Findings.—Computed tomography detected 68% of the focal hepatic masses compared with 63% detected by MRI and 53% detected by sonography. All imaging techniques had 100% sensitivity for lesions greater than 2 cm. With lesions 1 to 2 cm in diameter, the detection rate was 74% for CT, 77% for MRI, and 61% for sonography (Fig 5–25 and Table 1). The detection rate of lesions measuring less than 1.0 cm decreased more drastically with MRI (31%) than with CT (49%) and was

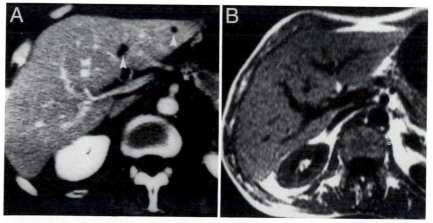

Fig 5–26.—Small metastases (adenocarcinoma of the stomach) in the left hepatic lobe shown by CT, but not by MRI. **A,** incremental bolus dynamic CT scan shows 2 small metastases (1.5 and 1 cm in diameter, *arrowheads*) in the left hepatic lobe. **B,** on T1-weighted fast low-angle shot 60-degree image and on other MRI sequences (*not shown*), these lesions were not detected. (Courtesy of Wernecke K, Rummeny E, Bongartz G, et al: AJR 157:731–739, 1991.)

TABLE 2.—Patient-by-Patient Analysis: Correlation of Presurgical Sonography, CT, and MRI With Intraoperative Findings

Imaging Study/Finding	Operative Finding		
	No Lesions	Resectable Hepatic Lesions	Unresectable Hepatic Lesions
Sonography			
No lesions	43 TN	8 FN	3 FN
Resectable hepatic lesions	0 FP	6 TP	5 FN
Unresectable hepatic lesions	0 FP	0 FP	10 TP
CT			
No lesions	41 TN	5 FN	3 FN
Resectable hepatic lesions	2 FP	9 TP	1 FN
Unresectable hepatic lesions	0 FP	0 FP	14 TP
MR			
No lesions	43 TN	8 FN	4 FN
Resectable hepatic lesions	0 FP	5 TP	2 FN
Unresectable hepatic lesions	0 FP	1 FP	12 TP

Abbreviations: TN, true negative; FN, false negative; FP, false positive; TP, true positive.
(Courtesy of Wernecke K, Rummeny E, Bongartz G, et al: AJR 157:731–739, 1991.)

the lowest with sonography (20%) (Fig 5–26). Combining all 3 imaging techniques yielded a sensitivity of only 77%.

Conclusions.—Computed tomography offered the highest sensitivity in determining the precise number, size, and location of focal hepatic lesions before hepatic resection and sonography produced the poorest results (Table 2). The combined sensitivity of CT, MRI, and sonography, 77%, is still low because CT and MRI have a size threshold of about 1.0 cm and are relatively unreliable for the detection of smaller lesions.

▶ These are 2 excellent studies from the same group of investigators, and many of the same patients or subjects were likely used. I read these articles in different journals many months apart, initially did not realize they were the same authors, and my impression was that the studies came to quite different conclusions. How can this be?

The protocol of both studies included excellent-quality CT, ultrasound, and MRI performed in close-time sequence to laparotomy with intraoperative ultrasound and palpation of the liver. Partial hepatic resection and pathologic sections carefully correlated with the imaging tests were performed in patients who met the surgical criteria of fewer than 5 metastases limited to 1 lobe. Analysis of results by ROC curves suggests that T_2-weighted spin-echo imaging is slightly better than CT using incremental bolus dynamic technique. This is a very useful and practical way of analyzing imaging test performance, because it incorporates measures of confidence, sensitivity, and specificity. The other study concludes that dynamic CT substantially outperformed MRI and ultrasound, particularly in detecting lesions smaller than 1.5 cm. In fact, CT, MRI, and ultrasound detected *all* lesions greater than 2 cm, and all imaging tests did poorly (< 50% sensitivity) in detecting lesions less than 1 cm. The ROC study seems to have excluded some patients with very small lesions. There was no way of predicting which type of patient or tumor would be depicted best by MRI, CT, or ultrasound, but at high-field-strength, T_2-weighted images and dynamic bolus CT scanning clearly out performed other MRI or CT techniques.

I am not prepared to analyze the statistical methods that were used in these studies. I think I know a reasonable approach to patients with gastrointestinal malignancy who are to be evaluated for liver metastases and possible resection. Because of the lower cost of CT, its wider availability, and its superiority in detecting extrahepatic tumor spread, dynamic-enhanced CT should be employed routinely. Most patients with metastases will be detected, and unresectability can often be established. If partial hepatic resection is still being considered after CT, MRI is indicated, especially if CT shows only 1 or 2 lesions. Although not addressed in these papers, we have found CT arterial portography to be more sensitive (but not specific) in detecting smaller liver metastases, but the technique is invasive and expensive. I would predict that MRI techniques emphasizing artifact reduction and liver-specific contrast agents will supplant the more elaborate CT techniques soon but may not displace routine CT screening of patients with gastrointestinal malignancies.—M.P. Federle, M.D.

The Frequency and Significance of Small (≤ 15 mm) Hepatic Lesions Detected by CT

Jones EC, Chezmar JL, Nelson RC, Bernardino ME (Emory Univ, Atlanta)
AJR 158:535–539, 1992   5–24

Background.—Advances in hepatic imaging have led to an increased detection of small liver lesions. When such lesions are found in patients with known malignancy, further diagnostic studies may be needed. The frequency and significance of small hepatic lesions found during routine CT scanning were studied.

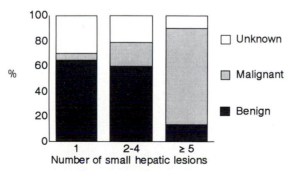

Fig 5–27.—Graph shows percentage of patients with benign, malignant, or unknown small hepatic lesions, categorized according to the number of small hepatic lesions detected. (Courtesy of Jones EC, Chezmar JL, Nelson RC, et al: *AJR* 158:535–539, 1992.)

Classification of Hepatic Lesions

Lesion Classification	No. of Patients (%)		
	With Small Lesions (n = 254)	With Known Malignant Neoplasm (n = 209)	With No Known Malignant Neoplasm (n = 45)
Benign			
Histologic or imaging findings (MR, sonography, ^{99m}Tc-labeled RBC SPECT)	16 (6)	8 (4)	8 (18)
Stability on follow-up (mo)			
6–12	33 (13)	29 (14)	4 (9)
≥12	80 (32)	70 (33)	10 (22)
Total	129 (51)	107 (51)	22 (49)
Malignant			
Histology or progression as shown on CT	55 (22)	55 (26)	0
Indeterminate			
No follow-up or follow-up <6 mo	70 (27)	47 (23)	23 (51)

Abbreviation: SPECT, single-photon emission CT.
(Courtesy of Jones EC, Chezmar JL, Nelson RC, et al: AJR 158:535–539, 1992.)

Methods and Findings.—The contrast-enhanced abdominal CT images of 1,454 patients were assessed. Hepatic lesions 15 mm or smaller were found in 17%. In 51% of these patients, the lesions were considered benign based on other imaging studies, biopsy findings, or CT-demonstrated stability for 6 months or more. Lesions were considered malignant if they progressed radiologically or if biopsy suggested it. Twenty-two percent of lesions were thought to be malignancies. In the remaining 27%, the lesions could not be classified. Eighty-two percent of the patients with small hepatic lesions were known to have a malignant extrahepatic tumor. In 51% of these patients, the hepatic lesions were judged to be benign. None of the patients without known malignancies had a small liver lesion judged to be malignant. The presence of multiple small lesions was more likely to indicate malignancy than that of small single lesions (Fig 5–27, table).

Conclusions.—Small lesions in the liver appear to be common. Lesions smaller than 15 mm are most likely benign, even in patients with known extrahepatic malignancy.

► What are we to do with all the small hepatic lesions we detect each day? This important study, even with some flaws candidly acknowledged by the authors, helps put the issue into perspective. We know that benign hepatic lesions are very common in the general population (hepatic cysts in 2.5%–7%; hemangiomas in 7.3%–20%), so we should expect to find small lesions frequently. The authors have shown that a single small hepatic lesion in a patient with no known extrahepatic malignancy is almost surely benign. Even patients with 2 to 4 small lesions were judged to be benign in 59% of cases. When the number of lesions increased, or in the presence of an additional large lesion, the chance of malignancy increased. But even though the larger lesion was likely to be malignant, a single accompanying small lesion was still likely to be benign. This has important implications for possible surgical resection of limited hepatic metastases. Characterization of lesions by ultrasound, MRI, or SPECT is very useful. Biopsy is also valuable but difficult for small lesions and should be reserved for cases in which malignancy is a substantial possibility (e.g., known extrahepatic primary tumor, multiple or larger lesions).—M.P. Federle, M.D.

Focal Fatty Infiltration of the Liver Appearing as a Defect on a Liver-Spleen Scintigram: Case Report

Marmolya GA, Miron SD, Eckhauser M, McCullough A (MetroHealth Med Ctr/Case Western Reserve Univ, Cleveland, Ohio)
Clin Nucl Med 17:300–302, 1992   5–25

Introduction.—A discrete area of photopenia on a technetium-99m sulfur colloid liver/spleen scintigram usually signifies that the lesion is not focal fatty infiltration of the liver. A patient with such a defect who was subsequently found to have focal fatty infiltration of the liver was studied.

Case Report.—Woman, 41, was referred for evaluation of an enlarged liver. Liver function studies were normal. On nonenhanced CT, a low-density area was seen in the right lobe of the liver along the falciform ligament and anterior liver edge (Fig 5–28). Contrast CT showed no significant enhancement or portal vein displacement. A matching area of increased echogenicity was seen on ul-

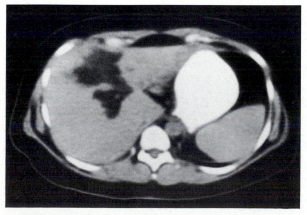

Fig 5–28.—Nonenhanced CT scan with a geographic area of low attenuation. There is no mass effect. (Courtesy of Marmolya GA, Miron SD, Eckhauser M, et al: *Clin Nucl Med* 17:300–302, 1992.)

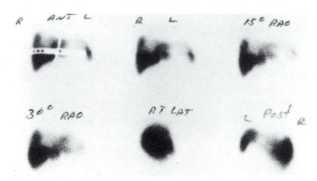

Fig 5–29.—Technetium-99m sulfur-colloid liver/spleen scintigram with a defect matching the area of low attenuation seen in Figure 5-28. (Courtesy of Marmolya GA, Miron SD, Eckhauser M, et al: *Clin Nucl Med* 17:300-302, 1992.)

trasonography. A liver/spleen scintigram showed a focal area of photopenia matching the previously imaged lesion in location and size (Fig 5-29); this suggested a space-occupying lesion, despite the classic CT findings of focal fatty infiltration of the liver. The biopsy specimen confirmed the diagnosis of focal fatty infiltration of the liver. The patient was asymptomatic 1 year later; on CT, the original lesion had resolved but new ones had developed.

Discussion.—A defect on a liver/spleen scintigram may indicate focal fatty infiltration of the liver in some cases, contrary to a previously reported guideline. Although the case appears to be isolated, it should be borne in mind when planning the diagnostic work-up.

▶ I rarely include case reports in the YEAR BOOK, but this one makes an interesting and important point. As the authors point out, sulfur-colloid scans are usually reliable in identifying a focal "mass" as fatty infiltration by demonstrating normal uptake in the area identified by CT or sonography. In such cases, biopsy may be obviated. Even in the case reported here, the CT and ultrasound findings were perhaps characteristic enough to delay biopsy, particularly if a changing pattern of density or echogenicity is demonstrated by CT or ultrasound.—M.P. Federle, M.D.

Intrahepatic Recurrence After Resection of Hepatocellular Carcinoma Complicating Cirrhosis
Belghiti J, Panis Y, Farges O, Benhamou JP, Fekete F (Hôpital Beaujon, Clichy, France)
Ann Surg 214:114–117, 1991   5–26

Background.—There is a high rate of recurrence after resection for hepatocellular carcinoma (HCC) that is caused in part by undetected tumorous tissue. Whether this outcome could be improved by the use of preoperative CT and intraoperative ultrasound examination was determined.

Methods.—A group of 47 adult patients who underwent hepatic resection for HCC between 1984 and 1989 was evaluated. All had cirrhosis and a single tumor. The size of the tumor was less than 5 cm in 59% of the patients, capsule was present in 63%, and the α-fetoprotein level was less than 100 ng/mL in 55%. All the patients were followed for 6 months or more.

Results.—Of the 47 patients, 17 were alive as of August 1990—8 without apparent recurrence. Tumor recurrence was the cause of death in 21 patients; the remaining 9 died of liver failure without evidence of recurrence. Reoperation and chemotherapy increased the survival times of those with recurrence. The cumulative intrahepatic recurrence rate was significantly higher in patients with tumors ≥5 cm and in those with preoperative α-fetoprotein levels ≥ 100 ng/mL. At 5 years, the cumulative intrahepatic recurrence rate reached 100%. Tumor recurrence was predominantly in the liver and away from the resected margin.

Conclusions.—Even a careful evaluation of tumor extension using CT and ultrasound does not prevent recurrence in cirrhotic patients with resectable HCC. The high rate of recurrence suggests that liver transplantation should be considered for these patients.

▶ The best imaging tests available at this time for detection of HCC are CT after intra-arterial injection of lipiodol and intraoperative ultrasound. These authors have used these tests in an excellent prospective study of a large group of patients and then followed them for a sufficiently long period (up to 6 years) for verification. They proved that even optimal preoperative imaging and adequate resection margins will not prevent the recurrence of HCC in cirrhotic livers. In part this may be because of the difficulty in distinguishing tumor from regenerating nodules or other pathologic processes in the cirrhotic liver. (Detection of metastases to an otherwise normal liver is much easier, and prognosis after resection is much better.) The authors postulate that liver transplantation might be curative if all the tumor is confined to the liver. Unfortunately, our experience at the University of Pittsburgh with hundreds of liver transplants for HCC and cholangiocarcinoma proves that almost all of these patients develop recurrent tumors in the transplanted liver! Our surgeons have tried "cluster resections," removing not only liver but regional lymph nodes and essentially all the upper abdominal viscera. Still the tumors recurred. Our present protocol is preoperative chemotherapy for HCC and subsequent transplantation if stabilization or regression of disease and apparent limitation to the liver are demonstrated. Although our short-term survival rates have improved, I am dubious about long-term survival.—M.P. Federle, M.D.

Percutaneous Ethanol Injection Therapy for Hepatocellular Carcinoma: A Histopathologic Study

Shiina S, Tagawa K, Unuma T, Takanashi R, Yoshiura K, Komatsu Y, Hata Y, Niwa Y, Shiratori Y, Terano A, Sugimoto T (University of Tokyo; Mitsui Memorial Hospital, Tokyo, Japan)

Cancer 68:1524–1530, 1991   5–27

Background.—Hepatocellular carcinoma (HCC) is commonly treated with surgical resection, although some patients have been treated with transcatheter arterial embolization or chemotherapy when surgery is not a viable option. Recently, ultrasonographically guided percutaneous ethanol injection therapy (PEIT) has been used successfully with good long-term survival. Patients with HCC were histopathologically examined after PEIT to determine short-term efficacy of the therapy.

Methods.—In 18 patients, the diagnosis of hepatocellular carcinoma was confirmed by fine-needle biopsy before PEIT. The number of treatment sessions ranged from 1 to 9, depending on the size of the lesion, the volume of injected ethanol per session, the patient's compliance, the schedule of surgery or other treatments, the findings in imaging techniques and serum tumor marker levels, and other factors. Transcatheter arterial embolization was performed with PEIT in 10 of the 18 cases.

Findings.—Histopathologic examination after PEIT revealed a completely necrotic lesion in 13 patients, a 90% necrotic lesion in 4 patients,

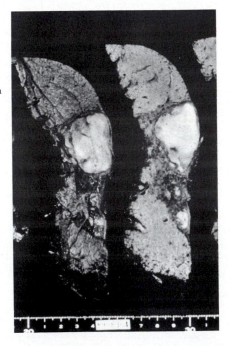

Fig 5–30.—Cut surfaces of the resected specimen after PEIT. Not only the tumor itself, but also the capsule and a certain amount of the surrounding liver parenchyma are degenerative in response to ethanol. (Courtesy of Shiina S, Tagawa K, Unuma T, et al: *Cancer* 68:1524–1530, 1991.)

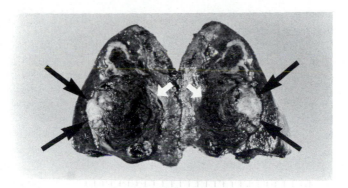

Fig 5–31.—Cut surfaces of the resected specimen after PEIT. Viable cancer tissue is found in the tumor nodule adjacent to the main tumor (*black arrows*) and in some portions along the edge of the main tumor (*white arrows*). Original magnification, ×.45. (Courtesy of Shiina S, Tagawa K, Unuma T, et al: *Cancer* 68:1524–1530, 1991.)

and a 70% necrotic lesion in the remaining patient. The optimal tumor size for PEIT is considered to be less than 3 cm in diameter, but a 5-cm lesion was completely necrotic and destruction of an 8-cm lesion has been reported. Serum α-fetoprotein levels were elevated to more than 100 ng/mL in 7 cases but dropped after PEIT. Levels remained elevated in 2 cases in which the lesion was not completely necrotic. Percutaneous ethanol injection therapy was effective against intercapsular, extracapsular, and vascular invasions (Fig 5–30). To ensure complete necrosis, ethanol should be injected in different portions of the tumor (Fig 5–31). There was no ethanol damage to noncancerous liver parenchyma distant from injected sites and no local dissemination of the cancer cells.

Conclusions.—Lesion response was not obviously better with the combined therapy of PEIT and transcatheter arterial embolization. Complete necrosis of the lesion appeared to be linked to a greater quantity of injected ethanol and accuracy of the injection. Injecting ethanol into different portions of the lesion is recommended so that viable cancer tissue does not remain in isolated portions. As an alternative to surgery for small HCCs, PEIT appears to be a valuable therapy.

▶ Hepatocellular carcinoma is 1 of the most common malignant neoplasms in the world, and few effective treatment options are available. Surgical resection of small tumors is only theoretically curative; most HCC occurs in cirrhotic livers, and the severe liver dysfunction does not allow even partial resection. Hepatic arterial chemoembolization is currently under trial, but evaluation is extremely costly and tedious, involving multiple angiograms and CT scans typically. Orthotopic liver transplantation has been tried, only to find nearly 100% recurrence of HCC in the transplanted liver or elsewhere. Clearly we are dealing with a deadly disease, and our best hope is prolonging disease-free comfortable life. (Actually, HCC incidence and mortality would probably decrease if we took all the money spent on high-tech care of hospitalized patients with HCC and spent it on aggressive hepatitis immunization programs and better sewers in developing countries.)

For patients with small HCC masses, PEIT seems an attractive alternative treatment. Necrosis appears to be achieved reliably, and the procedure is not unduly complex or invasive. It can be repeated when the HCC recurs (and it usually will) in other parts of the liver. Unlike cryosurgery (freezing the tumor with a liquid nitrogen–containing probe), PEIT does not require surgical exposure of the liver. One last major limitation, however, is that we rarely diagnose the small HCC masses (1–5 cm) that the Japanese treat with PEIT. Perhaps we need more aggressive screening with α-fetoprotein and ultrasound in high-risk groups, as practiced in Japan.—M.P. Federle, M.D.

Biliary Tract

Laparoscopic Cholecystectomy: Treatment of Choice for Symptomatic Cholelithiasis
Schirmer BD, Edge SB, Dix J, Hyser MJ, Hanks JB, Jones RS (Univ of Virginia Health Sciences Ctr, Charlottesville, Va)
Ann Surg 213:665–677, 1991   5–28

Introduction.—Laparoscopic cholecystectomy (LC), a recently introduced technique, has generated much controversy and attention. Some reports have attested to the efficacy and safety of LC. The LC results at the University of Virginia Health Sciences Center are presented.

Methods.—After a training course in the performance of LC, 2 of the authors attempted the procedure on 152 patients with symptomatic cholelithiasis, biliary dyskinesia, or cholecystitis. The procedure was performed with the patients under general anesthesia.

Technique.—After careful establishment of the pneumoperitoneum, the surgeon places the secondary trocars. Gallbladder exposure occurred through use of 2 5-mm grasping forceps to pull back the gallbladder fundus up toward the diaphragm. The second grasping forceps raises the infundibulum to expose the triangle of Callot. After dissection of the peritoneum, the cystic artery and duct, and the porta hepatis are defined and located. After completion of intraoperative cholangiography, the gallbladder is removed and a finger inserted through the umbilical trocar location to maintain the pneumoperitoneum to locate and remove the other 2 trocars. Cardiac monitoring and measuring end-tidal carbon dioxide ensure the safety of the procedure.

Results.—The 152 patients included 118 females and 34 males with an average age of 43.2 years and an average weight of 170.3 lb. Of the 152, 143 had cholelithiasis based on ultrasonography. The operation required an average of 138 minutes. The procedures that included a completed cholangiogram took significantly longer than operations that did not. Thirteen of the 152 procedures became open surgeries. Intraoperative cholangiography was tried in 78% of patients, achieving success in 66%.

No deaths occurred, and complications remained low. Major complications numbered 6 (3.95%), including an isolated common duct laceration; minor complications (mostly wound infections) occurred in 7.2%. The LC was performed successfully in 139 of the 152, for a success rate of 91.5%. Most patients left the hospital on the first day after surgery.

Conclusions.—Laparoscopic cholecystectomy provides the safety of conventional cholecystectomy but without the pain and lengthy recovery period that accompanies the traditional procedure.

▶ Perhaps no other surgical procedure, save organ transplantation, has galvanized the surgical community as much as LC. Some have estimated that 80% of the hundreds of thousands of cholecystectomies done annually will be via the laparoscope. Once general surgeons become facile with the use of laparoscopic instruments and techniques, these will undoubtedly be applied to other surgical procedures. An entire field of "minimal access surgery" opens up, promising shorter recovery times and less pain for patients and, less assuredly, less expense. I believed that radiologists would be interested in learning some details of the procedure. If you have the opportunity, I recommend viewing actual procedures or videotapes of operations to develop a feel for the formidable challenge faced by the surgeon using this technique. Among other impressions will be the utility of intraoperative cholangiography in helping to recognize ductal anomalies and avoid injury. Note that use of cholangiography added about 30 minutes to each case in this series, and see the article by Handy et al. (Abstract 5–29) for an innovative way to reduce this time expenditure.—M.P. Federle, M.D.

Intraoperative Cholangiography: Use of Portable Fluoroscopy and Transmitted Images
Handy JE, Rose SC, Nieves AS, Johnson RL, Hunter JG, Miller FJ (Univ of Utah Med Ctr, Salt Lake City)
Radiology 181:205–207, 1991   5–29

Introduction.—The place of intraoperative cholangiography in laparoscopic cholecystectomy remains to be defined. The use of intraoperative cholangiography done with a portable fluoroscope and transmitted to the radiology department during the procedure was assessed.

Methods.—Intraoperative cholangiograms were obtained in this way in 53 consecutive patients over a 7-month period. The image transmittal system was used with pre-existing equipment and cost about $4,000 to install (Fig 5–32). Images were evaluated for diagnostic quality and bile duct abnormalities.

Results.—Overall rate of aberrancies observed in the region of surgical dissection was 5.7%, which compared well with results of reported large series. Seven intraluminal filling defects were seen, 4 of which were identified as air bubbles. Three patients had cystic duct and common bile

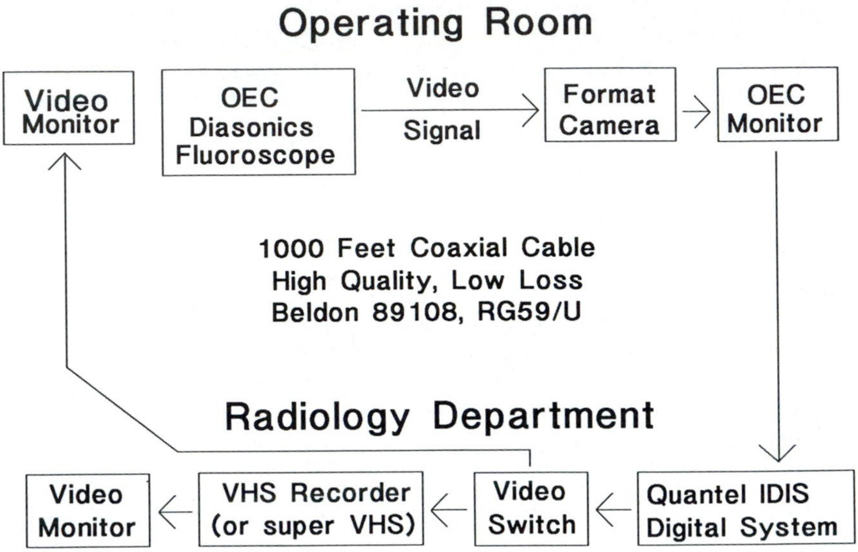

Operating Room

```
┌──────────┐   ┌──────────────┐   Video    ┌──────────┐   ┌──────────┐
│  Video   │   │  OEC         │           →│  Format  │  →│   OEC    │
│ Monitor  │   │  Diasonics   │   Signal   │  Camera  │   │ Monitor  │
└──────────┘   │  Fluoroscope │            └──────────┘   └──────────┘
               └──────────────┘
```

**1000 Feet Coaxial Cable
High Quality, Low Loss
Beldon 89108, RG59/U**

Radiology Department

```
┌──────────┐   ┌──────────────┐   ┌──────────┐   ┌──────────────┐
│  Video   │ ← │ VHS Recorder │ ← │  Video   │ ← │ Quantel IDIS │
│ Monitor  │   │ (or super VHS)│   │  Switch  │   │ Digital System│
└──────────┘   └──────────────┘   └──────────┘   └──────────────┘
```

Fig 5–32.—Diagram of system for transmitting images. The video signal can be taken directly from the fluoroscope with some systems; however, it may be necessary to take the signal from the fluoroscope monitor (there is less signal degradation if taken directly from the fluoroscope). High-quality, low-loss coaxial cable is necessary to transmit the signal over long distances. Interface with a digital imaging system is optional. (Courtesy of Handy JE, Rose SC, Nieves AS, et al: *Radiology* 181:205–207, 1991.)

duct stones (Fig 5–33). Surgical course was altered by the intraoperative cholangiogram in 7 cases. Mean fluoroscopic time was 1.8 minutes and estimated radiologist time less than 5 minutes.

Conclusions.—Intraoperative cholangiography using portable fluoroscopy can provide diagnostic images with real-time visualization, immediate communication with the surgeon, and the potential to decrease risk of bile duct injury. Image quality is not as good as with radiography, but it is adequate for diagnostic purposes.

▶ The remote TV monitor linked by cable that many of us use to monitor fluoroscopic or sonographic studies within the radiology department has been adapted for use in the operating room during laparoscopic cholecystectomy. The system is inexpensive and seems to provide adequate images. When interpretation of the transmitted fluoroscopic image is provided, real time as opposed to waiting for static radiographs to be exposed and developed, average savings of 30 minutes of anesthesia time have been reported. This, along with reduction of potential injury to aberrant ducts or the common bile duct and recognition of biliary calculi, makes a strong case for the technique.—M.P. Federle, M.D.

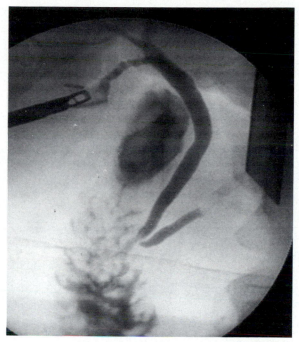

Fig 5–33.—Fluoroscopic cholangiogram of extrahepatic ducts demonstrates retained stone in cystic duct, retrograde filling of distal pancreatic duct, and normal common bile duct. (Courtesy of Handy JE, Rose SC, Nieves AS, et al: *Radiology* 181:205–207, 1991.)

Bile Duct Disruption and Biloma After Laparoscopic Cholecystomy: Imaging Evaluation

Walker AT, Shapiro AW, Brooks DC, Braver JM, Tumeh SS (Harvard Med School, Boston)
AJR 158:785–789, 1992   5–30

Background.—Biliary tree disruption occurs after laparoscopic cholecystectomy in up to 7% of the patients. It probably is the most significant postoperative complication. The presence and extent of a bile leak are often hard to document. Bile duct disruptions and biloma formations in patients undergoing laparoscopic cholecystectomy were studied.

Methods and Findings.—Seven cases of bile extravasation or biloma formation occurred in the first 264 laparoscopic cholecystectomies done at Brigham and Women's Hospital in Boston. The prevalence was, therefore, 2.7%. All patients were seen initially in the early postoperative period and had abdominal pain and low-grade fever. Sonography was done in 5 cases, CT in 5, hepatobiliary scintigraphy with diisopropyliminodiacetic acid (DISIDA) in 5, and endoscopic retrograde cholangiopancreatography (ERCP) in 4. Sonography and CT were helpful at first in

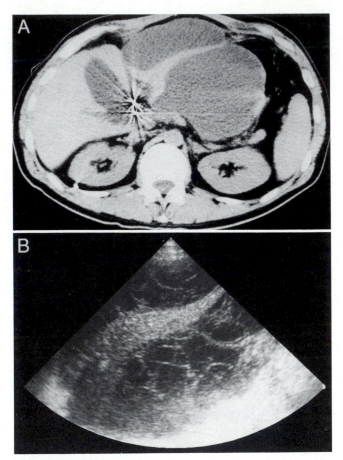

Fig 5–34.—Postoperative biloma. Man, 44, with right upper quadrant pain and jaundice 9 days after laparoscopic cholecystectomy. **A,** CT scan of the abdomen shows large, bilobed, low-attenuation collection surrounding, and to some degree compressing, the left lobe of the liver. **B,** a sonogram of the same region shows a large anechoic area with multiple fine septa. Septation may be seen in infected bilomas, as here, making differentiation from postoperative hematoma difficult. At surgery, a tear in the right hepatic duct was found, and a T-tube was placed across the disruption. (Courtesy of Walker AT, Shapiro AW, Brooks DC, et al: *AJR* 158:785–789, 1992.)

determining the presence of abdominal fluid collections, but they did not differentiate between postoperative seroma, lymphocele, hematoma, and bile leak. Hepatobiliary scintigraphy was useful in showing continuity of these fluid collections with the biliary tree and in guiding future treatment. Endoscopic biliary decompression was performed in 4 patients using sphincterotomy or nasobiliary stent placement. The clinical result was good. The remaining 3 patients had surgery with T-tube or external drainage. All did well clinically, with no signs of bile reaccumulation (Figs 5–34 through 5–36).

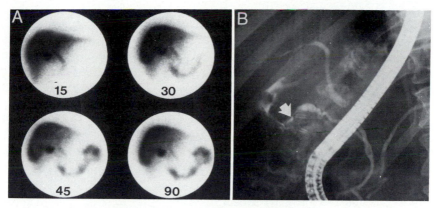

Fig 5–35.—Postoperative bile leak. A man, 64, with abdominal pain and nausea 6 days after laparoscopic cholecystectomy. **A,** scintigrams 15, 30, 60, and 90 minutes after administration of ^{99m}Tc-DISIDA show extrabiliary accumulation of radiopharmaceutical in the gallbladder fossa, with extension over the dome of the liver. Extravasation surrounding the liver can be mistaken for normal hepatic uptake on early images, but delayed images show persistent perihepatic activity as normal liver activity decreases. **B,** ERCP shows contrast extravasation from a distal cystic duct remnant (*arrow*). (Courtesy of Walker AT, Shapiro AW, Brooks DC, et al: *AJR* 158:785–789, 1992.)

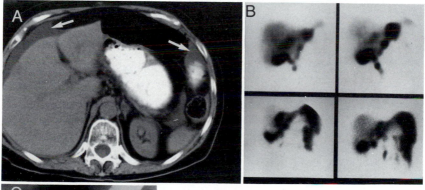

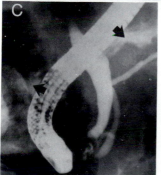

Fig 5–36.—Bile leak seen only with hepatobiliary scintigraphy. A woman, 67, with abdominal pain, jaundice, and mild leukocytosis 3 days after laparoscopic cholecystectomy. **A,** CT scan of the abdomen shows free peritoneal fluid surrounding the liver and extending into the left paracolic gutter (*arrows*). **B,** scintigrams 15, 30, 60, and 90 minutes after administration of ^{99m}Tc-DISIDA show abnormal uptake in the gallbladder fossa, with extension into the left upper quadrant surrounding the spleen, lesser sac, and left paracolic gutter. **C,** ERCP does not show evidence of bile leak. However, the study was limited by difficulty in cannulating and maintaining position within the common bile duct, so that much of the injected contrast material escaped into the duodenum (*arrows*). Evaluation was also limited by residual barium within the colon from previous CT. Although no bile leak was demonstrated, the patient was treated with sphincterotomy. (Courtesy of Walker AT, Shapiro AW, Brooks DC, et al: *AJR* 158:785–789, 1992.)

Conclusions.—Sonography and CT seem useful in detecting postoperative fluid collections but do not differentiate bile from other fluids. Hepatobiliary scintigraphy is a valuable noninvasive way to study possible bile leaks and guide treatment.

▶ Bile extravasation after open or laparoscopic cholecystectomy is predominantly attributed to anatomical variations of bile ducts, including small biliary radicles entering directly into the biliary bed. Injury to larger bile ducts or surgical mishaps, such as clips slipped off the cystic duct remnant, also occur. Clinically insignificant bile leaks are common after cholecystectomy, demonstrated in 44% of patients who had DISIDA scanning 2 to 4 hours after open cholecystectomy. Most of these bile leaks are small, asymptomatic, and resolve spontaneously. Imaging should be reserved for symptomatic patients exhibiting pain, fever, jaundice, or bilious drainage from surgical drains. We have used ultrasound or CT with guided-needle aspiration as the first line of diagnosis but agree with the authors about the value of DISIDA scans to confirm *continued* bile leak, the only situation requiring biliary decompression or surgical repair. Patients scheduled for intervention or repair should probably have direct cholangiography (percutaneous transhepatic cholangiography or ERCP) for more precise anatomical resolution and planning.—M.P. Federle, M.D.

Scintigraphic Evaluation of Postoperative Complications of Laparoscopic Cholecystectomy

Estrada WN, Zanzi I, Ward R, Negrin JA, Margouleff D (Cornell Univ Med College, Manhasset, NY)
J Nucl Med 32:1910–1911, 1991   5–31

Introduction.—Surgeons use laparoscopic cholecystectomy as an alternate operation to open cholecystectomy. The former surgery has shown lower morbidity and mortality and a reduced hospital stay than the latter standard procedure. Postsurgical complications occurred in 3 of about 400 patients who underwent (DISIDA) technetium 99m–diisopropyliminodiacetic acid cholescintigraphy.

Case Report 1.—Woman, 40, developed recurrent pain in the right upper section of her abdomen. After elective laparoscopic cholecystectomy, the pain resolved. Five days after surgery, the patient had severe abdominal and right shoulder discomfort. A Tc-DISIDA study demonstrated localization of medium along the right lobe of the liver, caused by a transected common bile duct. After repair of this defect, the patient recovered.

Case Report 2.—Woman, 59, had right shoulder and abdominal discomfort along with hyperbilirubinemia 2 days after elective laparoscopic cholecystectomy. The DISDA procedure showed a biliary leak based on radiotracer accumulation around the gallbladder soon after injection of the medium (Fig 5–37). The pa-

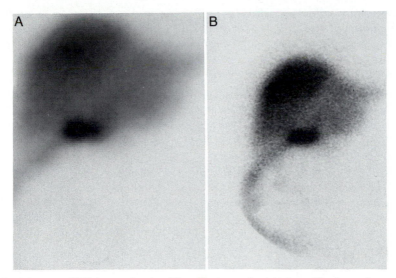

Fig 5–37.—A, a DISIDA scan of patient RR at 30 minutes after injection, with a focus of tracer localization in the gallbladder fossa. **B,** the 60-minute image demonstrates persistent activity in the gallbladder fossa and also along the inferolateral portion of the peritoneal cavity. (Courtesy of Estrada WN, Zanzi I, Ward R, et al: *J Nucl Med* 32:1910–1911, 1991.)

tient then had a laparotomy to confirm the biliary leak, which resolved after reoperation.

Case Report 3.—Man, 37, had elective laparoscopic cholecystectomy for chronic cholecystitis but 2 days later developed nausea and had a raised bilirubin level. The ^{99m}Tc-DISIDA study showed retention of medium around the hepatic parenchyma. On further surgery, a stone was removed from the common bile duct, and the patient recovered.

Conclusions.—The ^{99m}Tc-DISIDA scintigram offers a better detection procedure for biliary leaks. The DISIDA scan is the procedure of choice to assess abdominal pain or hyperbilirubinemia in patients who had recently undergone laparoscopic cholecystectomy.

▶ Biliary tract injury, retained stones, and dislodged cystic duct surgical clips are more common after laparoscopic surgery as opposed to open cholecystectomy. This will likely remain true, although reduced by more liberal use of intraoperative cholangiography. Ultrasound can detect fluid collections and dilated ducts, but DISIDA scans allow definitive recognition of bile leaks and should help in recognition of obstructing common duct–retained stones.—M.P. Federle, M.D.

Sonography of the Gallbladder: Significance of Striated (Layered) Thickening of the Gallbladder Wall

Teefey SA, Baron RL, Bigler SA (Univ of Washington)
AJR 156:945–947, 1991   5–32

Background.—Gallbladder wall thickening has been reported as not being directly related to gallbladder disease. Sonographic findings of thickening of the gallbladder wall consisting of multiple striations (alternate hypoechoic and hyperechoic layers) has been considered evidence of acute cholecystitis. Twenty-seven patients with striated thickening of the gallbladder wall on sonograms were studied to determine the diagnostic significance and specificity of this finding.

Methods.—Striations seen on sonography were classified as focal or diffuse. The sonograms were correlated with pathologic findings in 16 patients and with clinical diagnoses and laboratory findings in 11 patients. The patients were categorized as having cholecystitis with or without gangrene or edema of the gallbladder wall unrelated to gallbladder disease.

Findings.—In 10 patients, striated thickening of the gallbladder wall was caused by cholecystitis, and all 10 had gangrenous changes at surgery or at pathologic examination. Striated thickening of the gallbladder wall was focal in 8 of the patients and diffuse in 2 (Figs 5–38 and 5–39). Focal striations in 11 patients and diffuse striations in 6 patients were

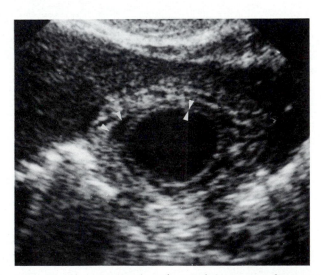

Fig 5–38.—A man, 75, with pancreatitis who underwent cholecystectomy. Sonogram shows diffuse striations as multiple hypoechoic layers (*arrowheads*) separated by echogenic zones. Histologic examination of gallbladder showed a well-preserved mucosa and no evidence of wall inflammation; however, serosa was thickened and had the appearance of granulation tissue. Striations were thought to be caused by reactive changes in serosa from pancreatitis. (Courtesy of Teefey SA, Baron RL, Bigler SA: AJR 156:945–947, 1991.)

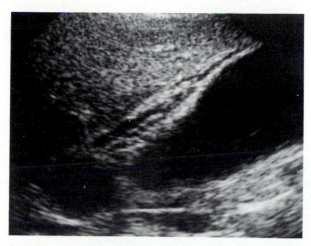

Fig 5–39.—A man, 41, who underwent cholecystectomy. Histologic examination of the gallbladder revealed gangrenous changes. Sonogram shows focal, striated thickening of the gallbladder wall adjacent to the hepatic surface. (Courtesy of Teefey SA, Baron RL, Bigler SA: *AJR* 156:945–947, 1991.)

caused by edema of the wall unrelated to gallbladder disease. The most frequent finding in this group was hepatitis.

Conclusions.—The sonographic finding of striated gallbladder wall thickening is no more specific for cholecystitis than the observation of gallbladder wall thickening by itself. Striated thickening of the gallbladder wall is seen in a variety of abnormalities. However, if there is clinical evidence of acute cholecystitis, the presence of striations suggests gangrenous changes in the gallbladder. The focal or diffuse extent of striations was not helpful in determining the cause of the striated gallbladder wall thickening.

▶ Uniform thickening of the gallbladder wall has long been recognized as nonspecific for gallbladder disease, occurring frequently in patients with a variety of other causes, including hepatic and renal disease. Other authors have suggested that the striated or layered thickening of the gallbladder wall might be more specific (1). Teefey and colleagues confirmed the frequent association with gangrenous cholecystitis but found many other causes unrelated to gallbladder disease. The reason for the discrepancy is not apparent, but their observations are nonetheless important.—M.P. Federle, M.D.

Reference

1. Cohan RH, et al: *Radiology* 164:31, 1987.

Primary Sclerosing Cholangitis: Value of Cholangiography in Determining the Prognosis

Craig DA, MacCarty RL, Wiesner RH, Grambsch PM, LaRusso NF (Mayo Clinic and Foundation, Rochester, Minn)
AJR 157:959–964, 1991   5–33

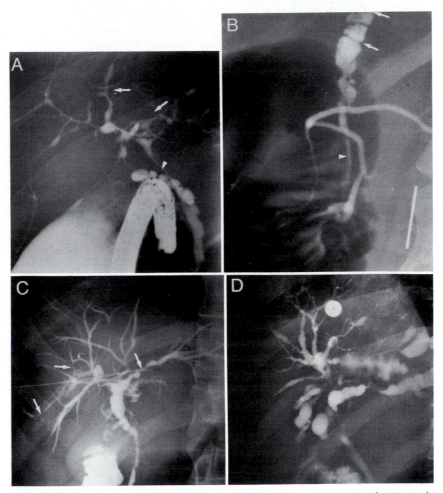

Fig 5–40.—Cholangiograms show characteristics of bile duct strictures in patients with primary sclerosing cholangitis. **A,** multiple segmental (*arrows*) and confluent (*arrowheads*) strictures. **B,** multiple band strictures (*arrows*) and confluent stricture (*arrowheads*) of extrahepatic ducts. **C,** localized involvement of intrahepatic ducts (*arrows*) and diffuse involvement of extrahepatic ducts. **D,** marked dilation of segments of intrahepatic ducts. (Courtesy of Craig DA, MacCarty RL, Weisner RH, et al: *AJR* 157:959–964, 1991. **A** and **B** from MacCarty RL, La Russo NF, Wiesner RH, et al: *Radiology* 149:39–44, 1983; Courtesy of the Radiological Society of North America, Inc.)

Prognostic Predictors of a Poor Outcome in Patients With Primary
Sclerosing Cholangitis

Duct Location	Predictors	
	Statistically Significant (p)	Trend Indicated* (p)
Intrahepatic	Grade 4 strictures (.050)	Confluent strictures (.140)
	Diffuse strictures (.012)	Marked dilatation (.069)
Extrahepatic	None	Grade 4 strictures (.088) Confluent strictures (.170) Diffuse strictures (.128)

* Decreased survival observed, but $p > .05$.
(Courtesy of Craig DA, MacCarty RL, Wiesner RH, et al: AJR 157:959–964, 1991.)

Background.—The course of primary sclerosing cholangitis (PSC) is unpredictable and insidious. The condition is diagnosed by cholangiography. The initial cholangiograms of 129 patients with well-established PSC were assessed to determine the usefulness of cholangiography in predicting clinical outcome in PSC.

Patients.—Seventy-nine of the patients were still alive without liver transplant, 36 were dead, and 14 had received a liver transplant; mean follow-up was 3.8 years. Cholangiograms were reviewed in blinded fashion to determine whether grade, length, and extent of strictures; degree of bile duct dilatation; and distribution of lesions were related to prognosis (Fig 5–40).

Findings.—Patients with high- vs. low-grade intrahepatic strictures had a 19% decrease in 3-year survival. Patients with diffuse versus localized intrahepatic strictures had a 16% decrease in 3-year survival. Nonsignificant decreases in survival were noted with high-grade extrahepatic strictures, diffuse extrahepatic involvement, long confluent strictures at any location, and marked intrahepatic duct dilatation (table).

Conclusions.—In patients with PSC, high-grade strictures and diffuse intrahepatic strictures may indicate a poor prognosis. Intrahepatic disease appears to have greater prognostic significance than extrahepatic disease.

▶ This paper takes on more importance as therapeutic options become more available and effective for patients with PSC. The fact that intrahepatic ductal disease has greater impact on survival than does extrahepatic disease suggests that aggressive attempts at relieving extrahepatic obstruction may not be warranted in patients with co-existing intrahepatic disease. Isolated or dominant strictures in the extrahepatic ducts may be relieved by transhepatic or endoscopic balloon dilatation, which is preferable to surgery (choledochojejunostomy), because the latter makes subsequent hepatic transplantation technically more difficult. Liver transplantation offers the only substantial hope for patients with advanced PSC, and the timing of transplantation and the triaging of patients for other therapies can be better judged using information in this article.—M.P. Federle, M.D.

Pancreas

Localization of Endocrine Tumors of the Pancreas With Endoscopic Ultrasonography

Lightdale CJ, Botet JF, Woodruff JM, Brennan MF (Mem Sloan-Kettering Cancer Ctr, Cornell Univ, New York)
Cancer 68:1815–1820, 1991
5–34

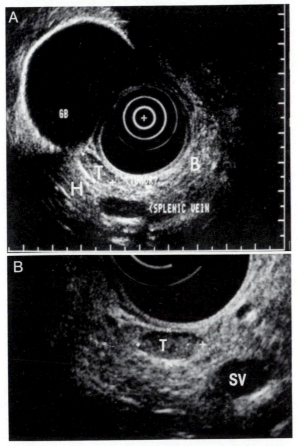

Fig 5–41.—A, endocrine tumor in the head of the pancreas in a woman, 28. The transducer (+) is in the second portion of the duodenum. *Abbreviations: GB,* gallbladder; *H,* head of pancreas; *T,* tumor; *B,* body of pancreas. **B,** a closer view of the same tumor (*T*) demonstrates it to be 1.3 × .7 cm in size, with decreased echogenicity compared with the surrounding pancreas. *Abbreviation: SV,* splenic vein. (Courtesy of Lightdale CJ, Botet JF, Woodruff JM: et al: *Cancer* 68:1815–1820, 1991.)

Background.—In patients with endocrine tumors of the pancreas preoperative localization can be a major factor in successful surgery. Existing imaging techniques are variably successful; a more sensitive technique is desirable. Endoscopic ultrasonography (EUS) was used in 13 patients with suspected endocrine tumors of the pancreas or duodenum.

Methods.—Twelve patients with suspected endocrine tumors of the pancreas and 1 with a suspected duodenal tumor were examined. The 8 women and 5 men had an average age of 40 years. All underwent EUS and dynamic CT, and 8 had selective angiography. Eight patients underwent laparotomy. Endoscopic ultrasonography was performed with a sector scan system that included a switchable 7.5- and 12.0-MHz transducer and conscious sedation.

Findings.—Endocrine tumors were detected by EUS in 10 patients (Fig 5–41). Five patients had more than 1 tumor, including 1 of 2 patients with multiple endocrine neoplasia syndrome type I. One of the laparotomy patients had a false positive finding because of hypertrophic peripancreatic lymph nodes and another had a false negative finding that, in retrospect, should have been interpreted correctly. Tumors as small as .5 to 2.0 cm were found at EUS in 5 cases that were missed by CT and selective angiography.

Conclusions.—Endoscopic ultrasonography appears to be an important new test for preoperative localization of endocrine pancreatic tumors. It is especially useful in detecting small tumors, but it cannot replace US, CT, or MRI in evaluating the liver for metastases.

▶ Preoperative localization of pancreatic endocrine tumors is difficult. Both noninvasive (CT, MRI, transabdominal US) and invasive (angiography, selective venous sampling) have detected fewer than half of these tumors. Placing the ultrasound transducer on the end of a fiberoptic endoscope allows application of a high-frequency, high-resolution transducer essentially onto the surface of the pancreas, separated only by the wall of duodenum or stomach. In most cases, the entire pancreas can be visualized. Others (1, 2) have reported success in visualizing the more common pancreatic ductal carcinoma, including cases of small tumors missed by CT. Preoperative assessment of resectability by evaluating vascular invasion and local node metastases may also be improved. Standard sonography, CT, or MRI will remain necessary to evaluate the liver for metastases, because the field of view and depth of penetration of EUS are too limited.—M.P. Federle, M.D.

References

1. Yasuda K, et al: *Gastrointest Endosc* 34:1, 1988.
2. Tio TL, et al: *Scand J Gastroenterol* 21:135, 1986.

Staging of Pancreatic and Ampullary Carcinoma by Endoscopic Ultrasonography: Comparison With Conventional Sonography, Computed Tomography, and Angiography

Rösch T, Braig C, Gain T, Feuerbach S, Siewert JR, Schusdziarra V, Classen M (Technical Univ of Munich, Germany)
Gastroenterology 102:188–199, 1992   5–35

Background.—In pancreatic and ampullary cancer, imaging can determine the primary diagnosis of the lesion and provide tumor staging to assess resectability. Assessment criteria for local tumor resectability include tumor size, invasion beyond the border of the organ, and the presence of multiple lymph node metastases. The performance of endoscopic ultrasonography (EUS), transabdominal ultrasonography (US), CT, and angiography in local tumor staging were compared in a prospective study.

Methods.—Forty-six patients with pancreatic cancer and 14 patients with ampullary cancer considered to be candidates for surgery were evaluated with EUS, transabdominal US, CT, and angiography for diagnosis and tumor staging. The study protocol included assessment of tumor size and the presence or absence of lymph node metastases. A malignant lymph node was diagnosed only by size and tumor involvement of major extrapancreatic vessels was examined.

Results.—The diagnosis of ampullopancreatic malignancy was made by operation in 40 patients and by needle biopsy in 20 patients. Endoscopic US was significantly superior to abdominal US and CT in determining tumor size and extent and lymph node metastases of pancreatic and ampullary cancer. Endoscopic US correctly assessed involvement of the portal venous system with 95% sensitivity compared with 85% assessed by angiography, 75% by CT, and 55% by abdominal US. Endo-

Sensitivity, Specificity, and Predictive Values in Assessing
Involvement of the Portal Vein in 28 Patients With Pancreatic
Cancer and 12 Patients With Ampullary Cancer Who
Underwent Surgery

Involvement of portal vein	EUS	US	CT	Angiography
Sensitivity	91%	9%*	36%*	45%*
Specificity	97%	72%ᵃ	85%	100%
Positive predictive value	91%	11%*	50%*	100%
Negative predictive value	97%	68%*	78%*	83%*

* P < .05 vs. EUS.
(Courtesy of Rösch T, Braig C, Gain T, et al: *Gastroenterology* 102:188–199, 1992.)

scopic US also had a higher predictive value for portal venous infiltration found at surgery compared with the other modalities (table). In the 20 patients who did not undergo surgery, EUS detected portal venous invasion but was less reliable in detecting arterial encasement.

Conclusions.—Tumor staging results with parameters of tumor size, involvement of different major vessels, infiltration depth (in ampullary cancer), and lymph node metastases were compared for EUS, US, CT, and angiography. Endoscopic US was the single most accurate diagnostic method for local tumor staging and was superior to CT and angiography, particularly in the assessment of the portal venous system. The high sensitivity of EUS for primary diagnosis of tumors may decrease the need for exploratory laparotomy.

▶ This is a well-designed study that confirms the potential advantages of EUS. The ability to place a high-frequency, high-resolution US transducer "on" the pancreas via endoscopy allows greater spatial resolution at the expense of a small field of view. Still, I doubt that EUS will be needed very often, and my projected estimate of its limited indications and formidable demands of operator expertise suggests that it may be limited to large academic medical centers. Most patients with symptomatic pancreatic or ampullary carcinomas are incurable by any means, and our goal as radiologists should be to prevent unnecessary surgery. Good-quality CT (small field of view, thin contiguous sections, dynamic scanning, mechanically injected constrast medium at 2.5–3 mL/sec) will demonstrate distant metastases or local invasion of vessels or bowel in the majority of cases. I don't believe the CT or transabdominal US results reported here are representative of the best that can be achieved, although they may be closer to those in common practice if radiologists are not personally monitoring the examinations.—M.P. Federle, M.D.

Pancreatic Disease: Prospective Comparison of CT, ERCP, and 1.5-T MR Imaging With Dynamic Gadolinium Enhancement and Fat Suppression
Semelka RC, Kroeker MA, Shoenut JP, Kroeker R, Yaffe CS, Micflikier AB (University of Manitoba, Winnipeg, Man, Canada; Siemens Electric, Toronto, Ont, Canada)
Radiology 181:785–791, 1991   5–36

Objective.—Because the only effective approach to pancreatic cancer is resection, lesions are best detected when small and potentially curable. Computed tomography has not substantially improved survival because it does not reliably detect small lesions. The value of MRI was studied in 35 patients, 23 of whom were investigated for neoplastic disease and 12 for inflammatory disease of the pancreas.

Methods.—Endoscopic retrograde cholangiopancreatography (ERCP), CT examination, and MRI were carried out within a 4-week period in all

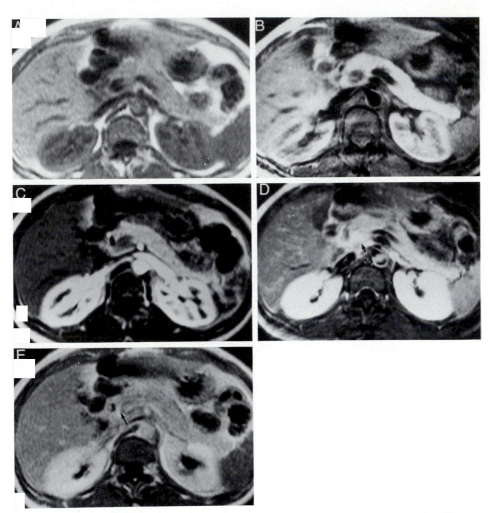

Fig 5–42.—Normal pancreas seen on (**A**) FLASH (130/4.5, 80-degree flip angle); (**B**) FSSE (500/15, 90-degree flip angle); (**C**) 1-second postcontrast FLASH; (**D**) Gd-enhanced FSSE; and (**E**) 10-minute postcontrast FLASH MR images obtained in a woman, 46. The SI of pancreas is minimally higher than that of the surrounding tissue on FLASH images and considerably higher on FSSE images. *Arrows* mark the superior mesenteric vein, in which variable-flow SI is apparent. (Courtesy of Semelka RC, Kroeker MA, Shoenut JP, et al: *Radiology* 181:785–791, 1991.)

cases, and usually within 2 weeks. The MR studies included breath-hold fast low-angle shot imaging and fat-suppressed spin-echo (FSSE) imaging. The studies were interpreted in a prospective blinded manner by individual investigators.

Findings.—Six patients were proved to have pancreatic cancer, and 4 had neoplasms at other sites. Pancreatography helped define 4 of the 6 pancreatic cancers. Computed tomography was helpful in detecting all

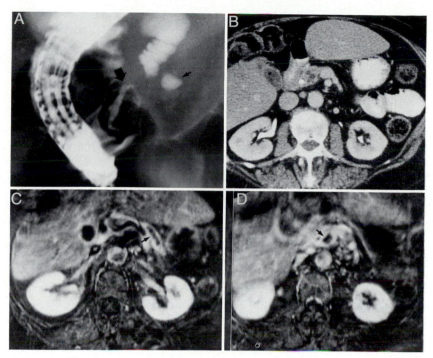

Fig 5–43.—Chronic pancreatitis with pseudocysts in the head of the pancreas seen on (**A**) ERCP, showing irregularity of the common bile duct in the head of the pancreas (*large arrow*) and high-grade obstruction of the pancreatic duct (*small arrow*). (**B**) contrast-enhanced 5-mm CT and (**C,D**) Gd-enhanced FSSE (500/15) images, showing atrophy of the body and tail of the pancreas with dilatation of the pancreatic duct (*arrow* in **C**) and multiple cysts in the head of the pancreas (*arrow* in **D**). The results were considered to have been caused by chronic pancreatitis with pseudocysts in the pancreatic head. (Courtesy of Semelka RC, Kroeker MA, Shoenut JP, et al: *Radiology* 181:785–791, 1991.)

but 1 of these neoplasms. All the pancreatic tumors were identified by MRI, which accurately demonstrated the size and shape of the pancreas (Fig 5–42). Done before and after Gd enhancement, FSSE imaging showed the tumors most distinctly. Magnetic resonance imaging also detected all cases of chronic pancreatitis (Fig 5–43). Both pseudocysts were well visualized on postcontrast images. Receiver operating characteristic analysis showed MRI to have higher observer confidence in detecting and excluding pancreatic disease than did the other modalities.

Discussion.—Although MRI is useful in evaluating patients for neoplastic or inflammatory disease of the pancreas, its high cost suggests that it be used as a problem-solving modality when the results of other studies are indefinite or discordant.

▶ This is a scholarly manuscript that at least hints at some problem-solving role for MRI of the pancreas, although certainly not proving it. I am bothered by the apparent assumption that any imaging study is going to have an impact on survival of patients with *symptomatic* pancreatic carcinoma. In fact, I believe we detect these tumors very well (by CT, sonography, and ERCP), even when small. The problem is that symptomatic patients are usually incurable because of local vascular or neural invasion or distant metastases. The only hope for substantial increase in survival is screening large groups of asymptomatic individuals with a sensitive, inexpensive test, and neither MRI nor CT fits that description.—M.P. Federle, M.D.

Kidney

Cystic Renal Masses: Usefulness of the Bosniak Classification
Aronson S, Frazier HA, Baluch JD, Hartman DS, Christenson PJ (Natl Naval Med Ctr, Uniformed Services Univ of the Health Sciences, Bethesda, Md)
Urol Radiol 13:83–90, 1991   5–37

Introduction.—In 1986 Bosniak proposed a classification scheme for cystic renal masses that distinguished between classic simple cysts (category I), minimally complicated cysts (category II), "more complicated cystic lesions" (category III), and probable malignancies (category IV). The implication was that category III lesions should be explored surgically but often could be adequately managed by parenchyma-sparing surgery.

Validation.—Data on 16 patients with pathologically proved cystic renal masses were reviewed. The mean age of the 16 was 53 years. None of the patients had a classic simple cyst. All 4 category II lesions were benign, but all 5 category IV masses were malignant. Three of 7 category III masses were benign and 4 were malignant.

Application.—The Bosniak classification is quite useful in planning the management of cystic renal masses. Category II cysts must be closely scrutinized to ensure that the calcium is thin, that no associated soft tissue mass is present, and that no part of the mass enhances. A cyst cannot be taken as benign if thick, irregular, extensive calcification is present or if noncalcified areas of the cyst wall are thickened. Irregular septa suggest that a lesion may be malignant. Multiloculated renal masses most often represent renal cell carcinoma or multilocular cystic nephroma. Although a thick-walled cystic mass may be seen in cases of benign nonneoplastic cysts, such as an infected cyst, abscess, or organizing hematoma, it may be the only manifestation of a cystic renal cell carcinoma.

▶ Mort Bosniak and his colleagues have contributed consistently to our understanding of imaging characteristics of renal pathology, including the classic article that formed the basis for this study (1). Aronson and his colleagues have confirmed that renal cysts that are classic, simple, thinly septated, minimally calcified infected or high density (nonenhancing and small) need not be operated on. More complicated (category III) lesions should be surgically explored, though nephrectomy may not be necessary. The Bosniak et al. article belongs in every radiologist's reference file.—M.P. Federle, M.D.

Reference

1. Bosniak MA: *Radiology* 158:1–10, 1986

Renal Lesion Characterization With Gadolinium-Enhanced MR Imaging: Efficacy and Safety in Patients With Renal Insufficiency
Rofsky NM, Weinreb JC, Bosniak MA, Libes RB, Birnbaum BA (New York Univ Med Ctr)
Radiology 180:85–89, 1991   5–38

Background.—The use of iodinated contrast material in characterizing renal lesions with CT is a key element in a diagnostic work-up. Magnetic resonance imaging of the kidneys without contrast material has not been completely successful in detecting renal tumors. On MRI, kidney tumors may be homogeneous with no specific signal intensities of measurements that are diagnostic of renal cell carcinoma. However, for patients with renal insufficiency who may be at risk for nephrotoxic reactions to the contrast material used in CT, Gd-enhanced MRI has been an effective alternative. Five representative cases using Gd-enhanced MRI in patients with renal insufficiency are presented.

Methods.—The 5 patients with renal insufficiency had renal lesions detected with nonenhanced CT that were considered indeterminate. The patients were studied with T$_1$-weighted MRI before and after intravenous administration of Gd-DTPA.

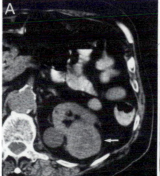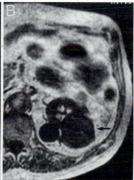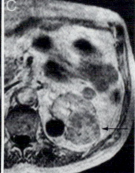

Fig 5–44.—Renal cell carcinoma and a simple cyst. **A,** a nonenhanced CT scan. A 5-cm heterogeneous renal mass (*arrow*) extends off the posterior aspect of the upper pole of the left kidney. Medially, a smaller lesion measuring 5 HU is also seen, consistent with a simple cyst. **B,** a nonenhanced axial MR image (300/23). The larger lesion (*arrow*) is isotense to the renal parenchyma. Also note the relatively low signal intensity of the adjacent cyst. **C,** Gd-enhanced MRI (300/20). Enhancement of the mass is seen (*arrow*). Note that there is no enhancement of the adjacent cyst. A left nephrectomy revealed renal cell carcinoma and a simple cyst. An additional, unsuspected mass in the right kidney (not shown) also demonstrated enhancement and was proved to be renal cell carcinoma after partial nephrectomy. (Courtesy of Rofsky NM, Weinreb JC, Bosniak MA, et al: *Radiology* 180:85–89, 1991.)

Findings.—In 4 patients who had enhanced renal lesions after Gd administration, 5 lesions were surgically resected. All 5 were determined to be renal cell carcinoma at pathologic examination. In 2 of the patients, benign cysts not enhanced with Gd with MRI were removed during nephrectomy (Fig 5–44). In the fifth patient, a hyperattenuated lesion found on unenhanced CT was determined to be a benign cyst because it did not enhance with intravenous Gd. The serial serum creatinine levels obtained before and after Gd administration showed no changes, and there were no nephrotoxic reactions in any of the patients.

Conclusions.—Gadolinium-enhanced MRI is an effective method for characterizing renal lesions, even in patients with renal insufficiency. Serum creatinine levels did not change during Gd administration, and there were no nephrotoxic reactions.

▶ Gadopenetate dimeglumine appears to be a safe and effective means of characterizing renal masses in patients with renal insufficiency and would likely be useful in patients with a history of adverse reaction to iodinated contrast media. Both CT and sonography provide adequate or even superior information in most cases and probably will remain the primary means of identifying and characterizing renal lesions. Magnetic resonance imaging of the kidney without Gd-DTPA enhancement is markedly inferior to contrast-enhanced CT. Gadolinium-enhanced MRI should prove useful in evaluation of other renal conditions that require contrast material for characterization, such as infection and infarction.—M.P. Federle, M.D.

Asymmetry of the Renal Nephrograms on CT: Significance of the Unilateral Prolonged Cortical Nephrogram
Birnbaum BA, Bosniak MA, Megibow AJ (New York Univ Med Ctr, New York)
Urol Radiol 12:173–177, 1991   5–39

Introduction.—Valuable diagnostic information on renal function can be obtained by assessment of the progression of renal enhancement on dynamic contrast-enhanced CT studies. Subtle asymmetries, reflected by a prolonged cortical nephrogram in 1 kidney, can provide important clues to the presence of abnormalities.

Normal Nephrograms.—Normally the nephrogram evolves through 4 stages: cortical arteriorgram, glomerulogram, cortical nephrogram, and tubular nephrogram. The first 2 stages are transient, the second 2 routinely imaged. In the cortical nephrogram, corticomedullary differentiation normally lasts about 67 seconds; this parameter is prolonged in patients with impaired renal function.

Asymmetric Cortical Nephrograms.—Unilateral prolonged corticomedullary differentiation can reflect any process that alters the normal hemodynamics of renal parenchymal perfusion or tubular transit. One such abnormality is renal artery stenosis, which may result from

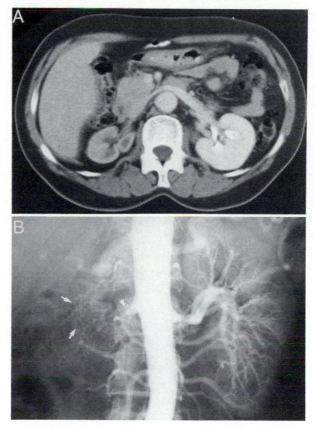

Fig 5–45.—Renal artery occlusion with intrarenal collateral circulation. **A,** contrast-enhanced CT reveals a small right kidney exhibiting markedly prolonged corticomedullary differentiation. **B,** aortogram: arterial phase depicts total occlusion of the right renal artery (*arrowhead*). Multiple collateral vessels are seen extending into the renal hilum (*white arrows*). (Courtesy of Birnbaum BA, Bosniak MA, Megibow AJ: *Urol Radiol* 12:173–177, 1991.)

mild stenosis or complete occlusion (Fig 5–45). Prolonged cortical nephrogram must not be confused with the "cortical rim" sign, which refers to a thin margin of peripheral enhancement of the outer renal cortex and is seen in acute renal artery occlusion. Other causes may include compression by a subcapsular hematoma or other pararenal mass. In renal vein thrombosis, CT depiction of a thrombus within the vein allows definitive diagnosis (Fig 5–46). Sometimes delayed progression of the nephrogram may be the only indication of urinary obstruction, particularly in cases of subtle obstruction before hydronephrosis develops.

Discussion.—Asymmetric renal nephrograms on dynamic contrast-enhanced CT can lead to differential diagnoses of stenosis or occlusion of

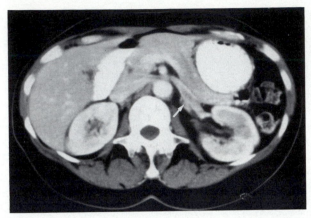

Fig 5–46.—Renal vein thrombosis. Dynamic sequential bolus-enhanced CT reveals the presence of a low-attenuation clot within a partially thrombosed left renal vein (*arrow*). A prolonged cortical nephrogram is evident. (Courtesy of Birnbaum BA, Bosniak MA, Megibow AJ: *Urol Radiol* 12:173–177, 1991.)

the renal artery, thrombosis of the renal vein, or obstruction of the urinary tract.

▶ Here is a nice, simple, and useful paper. A prolonged cortical nephrogram generally indicates obstruction (partial or complete) of the renal artery, vein, or ureter. Ancillary findings, including collateral vessels, vascular filling defects, or visualized calculi, can allow definitive diagnosis.—M.P. Federle, M.D.

Renal Lesions: Controlled Comparison Between CT and 1.5-T MR Imaging With Nonenhanced and Gadolinium-Enhanced Fat-Suppressed Spin-Echo and Breath-Hold FLASH Techniques
Semelka RC, Shoenut JP, Kroeker MA, MacMahon RG, Greenberg HM (St Boniface Gen Hospital, Winnipeg, Man, Canada)
Radiology 182:425–430, 1992   5–40

Background.—Magnetic resonance imaging has only recently been shown to detect renal lesions that are less than 2 cm in diameter. The effectiveness of breath-hold, gradient-echo MRI, fat-suppressed spin-echo MRI, and contrast-enhanced CT was compared in the detection and characterization of renal lesions.

Methods.—The subjects were 38 patients with signs of renal lesions. Twenty-four had solid renal masses and 14 had renal cysts; the lesions were less than 8 mm in diameter. Patients underwent T_1-weighted fat-suppressed spin-echo (T1FS) and gradient-echo fast low-angle shot (FLASH) MRI. These were followed by rapid injection of gadopenetate dimeglumine and another FLASH image at 1 second, another T1FS im-

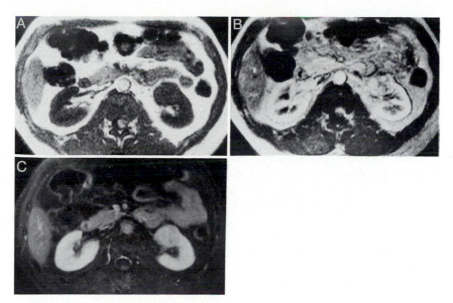

Fig 5–47.—Renal cell cancer seen on (**A**) nonenhanced gradient-echo fast low-angle shot (FLASH); (**B**) immediate postcontrast FLASH; and (**C**) postcontrast T1-weighted fat-suppressed spin-echo (T1FS) MR images obtained in a man, 47, with a stage I 3.5-cm renal cell tumor in the left kidney. The homogeneous, slightly hypointense mass on the nonenhanced image (**A**) is enhanced in an inhomogeneous fashion after contrast enhancement (**B**) and is hypointense relative to renal cortex on the postcontrast T1FS image (**C**). Although the tumor is well demonstrated on the postcontrast FLASH image (**B**), the tumor margins are not as well defined as on the postcontrast T1FS image (**C**). (Courtesy of Semelka RC, Shoenut JP, Kroeker MA, et al: *Radiology* 182:425–430, 1992.)

age at 30 seconds, and another FLASH image at 10 minutes. Computed tomography was done with, without contrast enhancement, or both.

Results.—Solid tumors were seen in 18 patients; renal cysts occurred in 17; cortical scarring was seen in 2; and hypertrophied column of Ber-

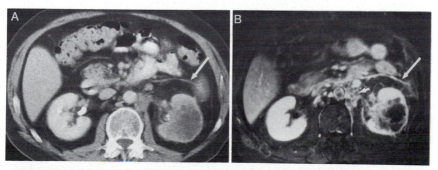

Fig 5–48.—**A**, contrast-enhanced CT scan and (**B**) contrast-enhanced T1FS MR image obtained in a man, 63, with stage IVb renal cell cancer. **A**, enlarged nodes are apparent in a paraaortic location on the CT scan. On the contrast-enhanced T1FS image (**B**), the nodes are enhanced in an inhomogeneous fashion with central low signal intensity (*short arrow*), an appearance similar to that of the primary tumor. Thickening of the Gerota fascia is shown on both the CT (**A**) and MR (**B**) images (*arrow* in **A** and *long arrow* in **B**). (Courtesy of Semelka RC, Shoenut JP, Kroeker MA, et al: *Radiology* 182:425–430, 1992.)

tin occurred in 1. Contrast-enhanced T1FS detected 114 lesions; contrast-enhanced FLASH detected 110 lesions; and CT detected 109 lesions (Figs 5–47 and 5–48). Lesions smaller than 5 mm and tumors as small as 1 cm in diameter were detected with MRI and CT. Use of combined contrast-enhanced FLASH and T1FS improved characterization of lesions as cystic or solid.

Conclusions.—Breath-hold imaging and fat suppression appear to greatly improve the ability of MRI to detect renal mass lesions. Compared with CT, MRI allows higher contrast resolution, better determination of hemorrhage into a cyst, and enhancement of tumor thrombus and adenopathy.

▶ I am still inclined to view MRI of the kidneys as rarely indicated (on a clinical basis) except to evaluate a renal lesion in a patient who cannot tolerate intravenous iodinated contrast material. If intravenous contrast can be used, CT can almost always answer all clinically relevant questions, including differentiating neoplastic from benign, and characterizing and staging tumors. In 1 very fast study, CT can image the thorax, abdomen, and pelvis, including lung parenchyma, soft tissues, and bones. The authors' protocol calls for at least 4, often 5, different MR sequences just for the kidney themselves, to overcome the substantial drawbacks of any 1 sequence (including inability to even see the renal tumor). It is useful to have these recent MRI adaptations in your diagnostic weaponry when the need arises.—M.P. Federle, M.D.

Radiographic Assessment of Blunt Renal Trauma
Eastham JA, Wilson TG, Ahlering TE (Univ of Southern California, Los Angeles; City of Hope Natl Med Ctr, Duarte, Calif)
J Trauma 31:1527–1528, 1991   5–41

Background.—Radiographic evaluation of patients with blunt abdominal trauma and microscopic hematuria but no shock was routine until 1985. To determine the safety of of managing such cases without radiographic studies, the charts of 337 patients were reviewed retrospectively.

Methods.—These patients were seen at the Los Angeles County-University of Southern California Medical Center between May 1986 and December 1989. Most (268) were involved in some type of vehicular accident. All had microscopic hematuria (but no shock) and underwent an intravenous pyelogram (IVP). Abnormal IVP findings were followed up by CT scans, angiography, or retrograde pyelography, depending upon the nature of the suspected problem.

Results.—Thirty patients had abnormal IVP findings. Fourteen had CT scans that confirmed renal contusions, 1 had angiography that revealed a congenitally absent kidney, and retrograde pyelography confirmed 1 case of disruption of the uteropelvic junction (UPJ). Patients with contusions were managed without operation, and the UPJ disruption was successfully repaired.

Conclusions.—Only 1 of these 337 patients (.3%) would have had a missed injury without IVP. Radiographic assessment should be necessary only in patients involved in major accidents; those with shock, gross hematuria, or both; and those with suspected intra-abdominal injuries.

▶ This study confirms the findings of several other large investigations that routine radiographic assessment of urologic injuries in normotensive blunt trauma patients with microscopic hematuria is not indicated. The combined results reported in several studies totaling more than 2,000 patients suggest that only .1% of significant urologic injuries would be missed. Nevertheless, I suspect that most physicians will continue to practice defensive medicine out of fear of malpractice claims.—M.P. Federle, M.D.

Laparoscopic Nephrectomy: Initial Case Report
Clayman RV, Kavoussi LR, Soper NJ, Dierks SM, Meretyk S, Darcy MD, Roemer FD, Pingleton ED, Thomson PG, Long SR (Washington Univ, St Louis; Cook Urological Inc, Spencer, Ind)
J Urol 146:278–282, 1991

5–42

Background.—Although small lesions and small hollow organs can be removed laparoscopically, there are 3 deterrents to the use of laparoscopy in other areas of abdominal surgery: the need for extensive tissue dissection and vascular control, the need for proper organ isolation to preclude abdominal contamination with bacteria or cancerous cells from

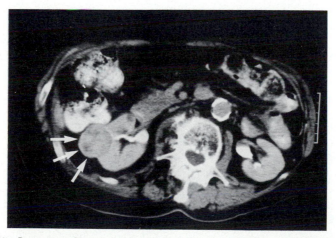

Fig 5–49.—Preoperative CT scan reveals a 3-cm renal mass (*arrows*) that occupies the lateral border of the midportion of right kidney. The right kidney measures 6.5 × 8.5 × 6.5 cm. (Courtesy of Clayman RV, Kavoussi LR, Soper NJ, et al: *J Urol* 146:278–282, 1991.)

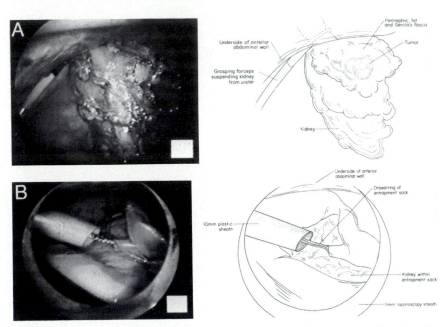

Fig 5–50.—A, intraoperative view of the kidney, completely freed from its retroperitoneal attachments and vascular supply. The kidney is suspended from the renal hilus via 5-mm grasper passed through 1 abdominal sheath. **B,** an intraoperative view of the kidney placed into a nylon surgical sack. (Courtesy of Clayman RV, Kavoussi LR, Soper NJ, et al: *J Urol* 146:278–282, 1991.)

the diseased organ, and the development of an instrument to safely and rapidly remove tissue through an 11-mm laparoscopic port. In 1 case, an electric tissue morcellator made laparoscopic nephrectomy possible.

Case Report.—Woman, 85, underwent CT after suffering a fall. Although no intra-abdominal injury was found, an asymptomatic 3-cm solid mass was visualized on the lateral border of the midportion of the right kidney (Fig 5–49). A newly developed method for intra-abdominal organ entrapment and a recently designed laparoscopic tissue morcellator made it possible to completely excise the right tumor-bearing kidney (Fig 5–50). The 190-g kidney was delivered through an 11-mm incision.

Conclusions.—This new method for organ entrapment and the new laparoscopic tissue morcellator enabled laparoscopic removal of this tumor-bearing kidney. The report has implications that go well beyond the urologic realm.

▶ As a rule, I do not select case reports for inclusion in the YEAR BOOK. I was so struck by the originality and future implications that this manuscript seemed to warrant exemption. The authors have developed a means of isolating, fragmenting, and evacuating a large solid organ through a minimally invasive laparoscopic procedure. One can argue that the kidney could have been surgically excised through a standard operative procedure even more quickly, but this 85-year-old patient did make a remarkably fast recovery from this pioneering laparoscopic procedure. Similarly, the necessary fragmentation of the tissue limits applicability of this technique for malignancies where depth of tumor invasion is a key consideration.

The ability to entrap abdominal or retroperitoneal organs with an impermeable tough nylon sac makes possible the subsequent fragmentation of large masses without excessive concern for spread of malignancy or infection. Already, laparoscopic surgery has been extended to pelvic lymph node dissection, appendectomy, cholecystectomy, and hysterectomy. Other novel applications are sure to follow.—M.P. Federle, M.D.

Potential Role of PFOB Enhanced Sonography of the Kidney: I. Detection of Renal Function and Acute Tubular Necrosis
Munzing D, Mattrey RF, Reznik VM, Mitten RM, Peterson T (Univ of California, San Diego)
Kidney Int 39:733–739, 1991   5–43

Background.—Sonography has been unable to detect renal function. Whether sonography aided by perfluorooctylbromide (PFOB) could detect and distinguish normal from abnormal osmotic gradient was investigated.

Methods.—Both kidneys in 17 rabbits were imaged both before and 24 hours after 1 renal artery was temporarily occluded and again after as much as 5 mL of PFOB or saline solution per kg was infused. Two normal rabbits were also imaged before and after PFOB infusion and after intravenous furosemide.

Results.—The normal and impaired kidneys were indistinguishable without PFOB. After PFOB administration, the echogenicity of the medulla, which was darker than the cortex in normal kidneys, became brighter than the cortex. The contrast agent was visible in the renal medulla on real-time sonography, and it produced an echogenic gradient that intensified in brightness toward the papillary tip. The acute tubular necrotic (ATN) kidneys were distinguishable from the normal kidneys in all 10 rabbits after 2.5 mL of PFOB per kg was administered. This occurred because the medulla of the kidneys with ATN increased mildly in brightness after PFOB infusion and also because the echogenic gradient produced by PFOB was reversed. In normal kidneys, the medullary echogenicity produced by PFOB was lost after furosemide.

Conclusions.—When aided by a blood pool contrast agent, sonography can reliably distinguish a normally functioning kidney from a kidney with an impaired osmotic gradient. This important physiologic information has previously been unattainable.

Potential Role of PFOB Enhanced Sonography of the Kidney: II. Detection of Partial Infarction

Coley BD, Mattrey RF, Roberts A, Keane S (Univ of California, San Diego)
Kidney Int 39:740–745, 1991   5–44

Background.—Although color Doppler and gray-scale sonography can identify flow velocity within vessels, it cannot distinguish perfused from nonperfused tissues. Whether perfluorooctylbromide (PFOB), a sonographic contrast agent given intravenously, could aid with this recognition was determined.

Methods.—In 20 normal rabbits, partial renal infarction was produced by a 1-mm bead embolized in the right, the left, or both renal arteries. A sonographer who was unaware of the group assignment of the rabbits attempted to diagnose the infarct 24 hours later. All the rabbits were studied with gray-scale and color Doppler sonography. Of these, 10 were studied before and after PFOB, and 10 were studied only after PFOB administration.

Results.—The sonographer was unable to diagnose the 10 partial infarctions in the 20 kidneys assessed before PFOB administration. Color Doppler sonography identified 50% of the infarcted kidneys; however, it localized the infarction accurately in only 2. All 20 partial infarctions were diagnosed accurately with both gray-scale and color Doppler sonography after PFOB was infused. The contrast agent enhanced the echogenicity of the perfused renal tissue, thereby permitting easy detection of the unenhanced infarct. Because the signal from vessels was increased after PFOB, color Doppler displayed the entire vascular tree, allowing the truncated embolized branch to be identified.

Conclusions.—When aided by PFOB, sonography provided accurate and detailed anatomical visualization of the renal parenchyma and vascular tree. This contrast agent promises to improve the ease and timeliness of diagnosing segmental renal infarctions. This may hasten the institution of treatment and result in better preservation and recovery of functional renal tissue.

▶ Sonography was once regarded as a purely morphologic or anatomical imaging test, lacking the ability of contrast-enhanced radiographic, CT, or MRI studies to determine the physiologic status of organs. Doppler assessment of the vascular system was a major advancement, with vascular velocity used as a direct or indirect indicator of various disease states. These authors have introduced an additional ultrasound contrast agent that enhances the Doppler signal from vessels and enhances the perfused tissue to a degree commensurate with their blood content. Their models of ATN and renal infarction support the theoretical basis for PFOB as an ultrasound contrast agent. If further studies confirm these exciting early results, much wider application of contrast-enhanced sonography can easily be anticipated. Interestingly, PFOB has also shown promise (by the same researchers) as a CT and MR contrast agent because of its radiopacity and other qualities while remaining an inert and apparent safe agent for intravascular and oral use.—M.P. Federle, M.D.

Prostate

Early Detection Program for Prostate Cancer: Results and Identification of High-Risk Patient Population

Babaian RJ, von Eschenbach AC, Miyashita H, Ramirez EI, Evans RB (MD Anderson Cancer Ctr, Houston)
Urology 37:193–197, 1991   5–45

Background.—One strategy for the early detection of prostate cancer involves a 3-pronged assessment: digital rectal examination (DRE), transrectal ultrasound (TRUS), and determination of prostate-specific antigen (PSA). Two years' experience with this policy was reviewed to determine the value of each approach and the interaction.

Patients and Findings.—Three hundred sixty-two men underwent prostate TRUS, DRE, and PSA determination. Thirty-seven cancers were detected, for an incidence of 10%. The DRE had the highest sensitivity and specificity at 89% and 84%, respectively. Transrectal ultrasound had a sensitivity of 84% and a specificity of 82%; PSA had a sensitivity of 81% and a specificity of 82%. The positive predictive value of DRE was 39%; of TRUS, 35%; and of PSA determination, 33%. The cancer detection rate among patients with symptoms of bladder outlet obstruction was

TABLE 1.—Correlation of Clinical Findings With Presence or Absence of Cancer

Clinical Examination	Cancer (N = 37)	No Cancer (N = 325)	Total (N = 362)
TRUS			
Positive	31	57	88†
Negative	6	268	274
DRE			
Positive	33	52	85‡
Negative	4	273	277
PSA			
>4 ng/mL	30	60	90
≤4 ng/mL	7	265	272

Note: Presence of cancer defined by positive biopsy specimen; absence of cancer defined by negative biopsy specimen, refusal of biopsy, or no recommendation of biopsy.
† Five patients refused biopsy.
‡ Six patients refused biopsy.
(Courtesy of Babaian RJ, von Eschenbach AC, Miyashita H, et al: *Urology* 37:193–197, 1991.)

TABLE 2.—Cancer Detection by Positive Clinical
Examination Results

Examination Results*	No.	No. With Cancer (%)
TRUS (+), DRE (−), PSA (−)	17	0 (0)
TRUS (−), DRE (+), PSA (−)	14	0 (0)
TRUS (−), DRE (−), PSA (+)	4	1 (25)
TRUS (+), DRE (+), PSA (−)	28	7 (25)
TRUS (+), DRE (−), PSA (+)	9	3 (33)
TRUS (−), DRE (+), PSA (+)	8	5 (62)
TRUS (+), DRE (+), PSA (+)	29	21 (72)
TOTALS	109	37 (34)

(Courtesy of Babaian RJ, von Eschenbach AC, Miyashita H, et al: *Urology* 37:193–197, 1991.)

16%. In patients without these symptoms, it was 5%. Physician-referred patients had a detection rate of 36%, whereas self-referred patients had a rate of 3% (Tables 1 and 2).

Conclusions.—The best use of medical resources to increase detection of prostate cancer would be to educate men to have yearly medical examinations by primary care physicians who are encouraged to incorporate risk assessment and screening DRE in their routine practice. Men with abnormal findings on examination or with an increased risk should be referred to a urologist for further assessment.

▶ I like the common sense approach to this common and important problem of prostate cancer, which has become the second leading cause of cancer death in American men. Clinical assessment of advanced age, urinary outlet obstruction, black race, or close family history of prostate cancer constitutes relatively higher risk. All men past age 50 years should have an annual DRE of the prostate. Use of TRU5 and serum PSA as screening tests, especially in higher-risk groups is also warranted. No one test found all the patients with cancer, and they had remarkably similar sensitivity and predictive value. The cancer detection rate improved as the number of abnormal test results increased. Cancer was found in only 1 of 35 patients with only 1 positive test result; in 15 (33%) of patients with 2 positive test results; and in 21 of 29 (72%) of patients who had positive TRUS, DRE, and PSA determinations. Even though the positive predictive value of any one test is not high, biopsy of the gland is relatively noninvasive and should be practiced more frequently.—M.P. Federle, M.D.

Stage B Adenocarcinoma of the Prostate: Transrectal US and Pathologic Correlation of Nonmalignant Hypoechoic Peripheral Zone Lesions

Hamper UM, Sheth S, Walsh PC, Holtz PM, Epstein JI (Johns Hopkins Med Insts, Baltimore)
Radiology 180:101–104, 1991   5–46

Introduction.—Various benign disorders can produce hypoechoic lesions in the prostate, mimicking early prostatic cancer. Pathologic correlates of hypoechoic lesions of the peripheral prostate were examined in 160 men with biopsy-proved prostatic cancer. All had clinically localized stage B lesions.

Methods.—Biplane transrectal ultrasonography was performed with a high-resolution endorectal probe and a 5-MHz or 7.5-MHz transducer. Radical prostatectomy was carried out within 48 hours of sonography.

Findings.—Hypoechoic peripheral zone lesions that did not correspond to areas of cancer on step sections of the prostate were found in 25 patients. In 8 patients the lesions correlated with areas of dilated acinar glands lined by atrophic epithelium. Other patients had dilated glands with dysplasia, chronic inflammation, dysplasia alone, or nodules of benign prostatic hypertrophy.

Conclusions.—A contralateral hypoechoic lesion in a patient with prostatic cancer does not necessarily represent further tumor. Biopsy is necessary to rule out cancer when hypoechoic areas are observed.

▶ This manuscript is another sobering reminder of the limitations of imaging alone, in this case ultrasound, in diagnosing or staging prostatic carcinoma. Others have reported similarly poor differentiation of benign from malignant processes. The compelling nature of this study from Johns Hopkins is due to the correlation of transrectal US with pathologic step sections of the whole prostate gland obtained within 48 hours of the ultrasound study. Biopsy of hypoechoic lesions remains necessary in patients with known tumor (staging) or as part of screening by sonography. Digital palpation and serum assays for prostate-specific antigen remain attractive means of screening the general population.—M.P. Federle, M.D.

Preoperative Prediction of Pathological Tumor Volume and Stage in Clinically Localized Prostate Cancer: Comparison of Digital Rectal Examination, Transrectal Ultrasonography and Magnetic Resonance Imaging
McSherry SA, Levy F, Schiebler ML, Keefe B, Dent GA, Mohler JL (Univ of North Carolina, Chapel Hill, NC)
J Urol 146:85–89, 1991   5–47

Background.—Accurate preoperative staging, which is necessary for the appropriate selection of patients for surgical cure of prostate cancer, cannot be reliably obtained by digital rectal examination, CT, transrectal ultrasound, or MRI. Because none of these methods can determine the microscopic extent of disease, various indirect means, such as prostate specific antigen (PSA) and Gleason grade, have been tried. The power of each modality was compared to predict pathologic stage, tumor volume, and the percentage of the gland involved with tumor.

Methods.—The patient group included 25 patients (median age, 66 years) who underwent radical retropubic prostatectomy with obdurator fossa lymph node dissection. All patients underwent a digital rectal examination, transrectal ultrasound, MRI, PSA, prostatic acid phosphatase (PAP) by α-naphthyl phosphate enzymatic assay after tartrate inhibition, and a bone scan. Both PSA and PAP were obtained before prostate biopsy.

Results.—Pathologically, 12 patients had tumor that did not penetrate through the prostatic capsule. The predictive value for tumor confinement was 36% by rectal examination, 37% by ultrasound, and 30% by MRI. The predictive value for extracapsular disease was 100% by rectal examination, 83% by ultrasound, and 66% by MRI. There was no correlation between tumor volume measured by any modality and pathologic volume. The majority of patients (67%) had an intermediate Gleason grade; the prognosis of patients with such a grade is uncertain.

Conclusions.—There is clearly a need for further improvement in preoperative staging to arrive at an accurate clinical decision. Although digital rectal examination, ultrasound, and MRI can predict extracapsular disease, these modalities clinically understage the disease in most patients.

▶ In the 1992 YEAR BOOK, we reviewed several reports of screening methods for detecting prostate cancer and concluded that digital rectal examinations and serum assays for PSA were preferred. In this report of 25 patients and encyclopedic review of the literature on *staging* prostate cancer, imaging studies are also disappointingly unreliable, routinely understaging neoplasms. Transrectal ultrasound and MRI have reasonable (70%–80%) predictive value when they predict extracapsular extension. Others report even poorer results (Abstract 5–48).—M.P. Federle, M.D.

MR Imaging in Adenocarcinoma of the Prostate: Interobserver Variation and Efficacy for Determining Stage C Disease
Schiebler ML, Yankaskas BC, Tempany C, Spritzer CE, Rifkin MD, Pollack MD, Holtz P, Zerhouni EA (Univ of Pennsylvania, Philadelphia; Univ of North Carolina, Chapel Hill, NC; Johns Hopkins Univ, Baltimore; Duke Univ, Durham, NC; Thomas Jefferson Univ, Philadelphia)
AJR 158:559–562, 1992   5–48

Introduction.—Patients with stage C adenocarcinoma of the prostate, in which the cancer penetrates the capsule or invades the seminal vesi-

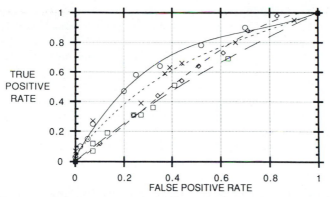

Fig 5–51.—Receiver-operating-characteristic curves for 4 experienced radiologists evaluating 100 MR images of the prostate for the presence of extracapsular extension of tumor (X = reader 1, *diamond* = reader 2, *circle* = reader 3, and *square* = reader 4). This evaluation included all 61 cases of capsular penetration and/or seminal vesicle invasion (.5–10 mm). (Courtesy of Schiebler ML, Yankaskas BC, Tempany C, et al: *AJR* 158:559–562, 1992.)

cles, are not good candidates for surgical cure. The ability of 4 radiologists to detect stage C disease on MRI scans was compared.

Methods.—The 4 radiologists evaluated 100 consecutive MRI studies of the prostate. Each patient underwent radical prostatectomy, and the prostate capsule and seminal vesicles were carefully inspected for any sign of stage C disease. For each radiologist, sensitivity, specificity, and accuracy in detecting stage C disease were calculated. Five specific anatomical areas were used to calculate percentage agreement; variability was assessed by comparing the observations of the best reader with those of the other 3.

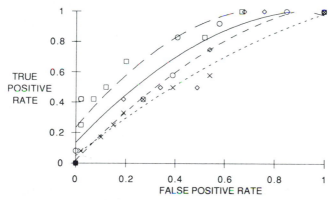

Fig 5–52.—Receiver-operating-characteristic curves for the same 4 radiologists charted in previous figure plot MR evaluations of only those 12 lesions with pathologically proved extracapsular extension of more than 3mm (X = reader 1, *diamond* = reader 2, *circle* = reader 3, and *square* = reader 4). (Courtesy of Schiebler ML, Yankaskas BC, Tempany C, et al: *AJR* 158:559–562, 1992.)

Findings.—Sensitivity ranged from 24% to 61%, and specificity ranged from 49% to 79%. One of the readers differed significantly from the other 3 (Fig 5–51), even when cases with more than 3 mm of capsular penetration were included (Fig 5–52). For the 5 anatomical regions, the average percentage agreement among the 3 interpreters compared with the fourth interpreter was 70%.

Conclusions.—Interpretation of MRI studies for staging prostate cancer is prone to considerable interobserver variation. In the current study, the average accuracy was 55%, only slightly better than a chance guess. Microscopic disease cannot be identified by MRI in patients with prostate adenocarcinoma.

▶ This sobering article addresses a common and important clinical entity. Prostatic cancer limited to the gland is optimally treated by radical prostatectomy. Many patients who are judged to have such limited tumor by clinical means (digital rectal exam plus laboratory tests) and bone scan are later found at surgery to have stage C, extraprostatic spread. An imaging study that would accurately predict extraprostatic disease would have an important influence on management. Good-quality body coil MR as practiced by university-based radiologists with special interest in the subject has proved to be of little value in this setting, with results barely exceeding that of random chance. These results cannot be dismissed casually; the studies were done carefully on state-of-the-art (for 1991) equipment and software. Hope persists that endorectal-coil MRI will be a marked improvement. I hope that similar research protocols are in place, allowing careful pathologic correlation, as was provided in this excellent publication.—M.P. Federle, M.D.

Other Genitourinary

CT and Pathologic Predictive Features of Residual Mass Histologic Findings After Chemotherapy for Nonseminomatous Germ Cell Tumors: Can Residual Malignancy or Teratoma Be Excluded?
Stomper PC, Kalsih LA, Garnick MB, Richie JP, Kantoff PW (Dana-Farber Cancer Inst, Boston; Brigham and Women's Hosp, Boston)
Radiology 180:711–714, 1991   5–49

Background.—Residual masses in patients who have undergone chemotherapy for disseminated nonseminomatous germ cell tumors may prove to be teratoma, necrosis and fibrosis, or malignancy. Forty-eight patients were studied to determine factors that might exclude malignancy or teratoma in these masses.

Methods.—The patients, median age 25 years, all received 3–6 cycles of chemotherapy for treatment of primary testicular tumors. Available for review were prechemotherapy and postchemotherapy abdominal-pelvic CT scans, pathology reports, and all histologic evaluations of initial orchiectomy specimens and postchemotherapy retroperitoneal lymph node dissection tissue.

Results.—Twenty-seven patients had teratoma, 15 had necrosis, and 6 had residual malignancy. Neither the type of primary testicular tumor cell nor CT findings, such as residual mass size and degree of shrinkage during chemotherapy, was significantly correlated with malignancy or teratoma vs. necrosis in residual masses. Patient age and size of the primary tumor were not predictive of risk for malignancy or teratoma, nor were preoperative serum α-fetoprotein and human chorionic gonadotropin levels.

Conclusions.—Neither radiographic nor pathologic features can be used to characterize residual masses after chemotherapy for nonseminomatous testicular cancer. Excision will continue to be necessary for histologic confirmation and treatment decisions.

▶ I suspect the results of this investigation come as a surprise to radiologists who are accustomed to interpreting any residual or enlarging mass in a cancer patient undergoing therapy as residual or recurrent malignancy. In this group of patients with residual masses, only 13% had residual malignancy; 31% had necrosis and 56% had teratoma. Although these results are slightly different than those reported by other investigators, the central teaching point is well established. Combined cisplatin-based chemotherapy, followed by surgical excision of residual masses in patients whose serum tumor markers have returned to normal, has resulted in long-term survival of more than 80% of patients.—M.P. Federle, M.D.

Ureteral Pseudodiverticula: Frequent Association With Uroepithelial Malignancy

Wasserman NF, Zhang G, Posalaky IP, Reddy PK (VA Med Ctr, Minneapolis)
AJR 157:69–72, 1991   5–50

Background.—Ureteral pseudodiverticula (UPD) are small cut pouchings of the ureter usually found incidentally in patients undergoing retrograde urography. Previous reports have suggested that UPD are associated with uroepithelial neoplasm.

Patients.—Thirty-seven patients, mean age 69 years, had UPD recognized on excretory or retrograde urography, most commonly on evaluation for hematuria (Fig 5–53). Assessment included urinalysis, urine culture, cystoscopy, and ureteroscopy as needed. An associated uroepithelial malignancy was present in 17 of these patients (46%). The diagnosis was transitional cell carcinoma in 16 cases and squamous cell carcinoma in the remaining case; 65% of the tumors were in the urinary bladder, 25% in the renal calyces, and 10% in the ureter. Seven of 9 patients with UPD and a urinary tract filling defect proved to have malignancy. Fifty-three percent of patients with tumors had a single ureteral pseudodiverticulum. The UPD were recognized as long as 4 years before the tumor.

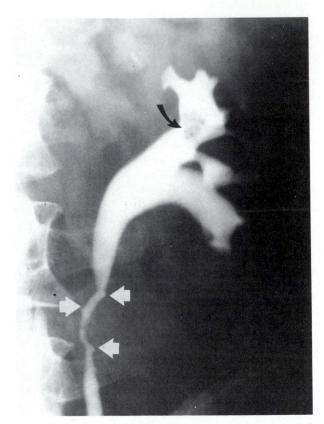

Fig 5–53.—A man, 74, with hematuria. Retrograde urogram shows ureteral pseudodiverticula (*white arrows*) and associated filing defect in the left upper calix (*black arrow*). Histologic examination of the surgical specimen showed the filing defect was transitional cell carcinoma. (Courtesy of Wasserman NF, Zhang G, Posalaky IP, et al: AJR 157:69–72, 1991.)

Conclusions.—Nearly half of patients with UPD may have uroepithelial malignancy. The pseudodiverticula may be a serious marker for malignancy and may predate the diagnosis of the tumor by several years. A patient with both UPD and a stricture or filling defect is likely to have a tumor.

▶ Chronic proliferative epithelial changes should be considered a risk factor for development of carcinoma. Barrett esophagus and chronic ulcerative colitis come to mind in the gastrointestinal tract. A radiographic sign of chronic epithelial changes in the urinary tract is ureteral pseudodiverticulosis. These authors have added a substantial number of new observations and reviewed the literature, allowing useful guidelines to be suggested. Patients with UPD have nearly a 50% likelihood of developing uroepithelial malignancy, 70% of such cases involving the urinary bladder. Repetitive home screening by hematuria "dipsticks," semiannual urinalysis and cytology, and annual cytoscopy are recommended.—M.P. Federle, M.D.

Accuracy of Adrenal Biopsy Guided by Ultrasound and CT

Tikkakoski T, Taavitsainen M, Päivänsalo M, Lähde S, Apaja-Sarkkinen M (University Central Hospital, Oulu, Finland; University Central Hospital, Helsinki, Finland)
Acta Radiologica 32:371–374, 1991   5–51

Introduction.—Imaging studies alone can rarely diagnose primary adrenal malignancy; short of surgery, the only way to obtain tissue for microscopic analysis is needle biopsy. The effectiveness of fine-needle biopsy of adrenal masses was evaluated.

Patients.—Over a 5-year period, 30 men and 28 women with a mean age of 54.3 years were referred for adrenal fine-needle biopsy. Ultrasound guidance was used in 45 patients and CT guidance in 11 (2 patients did not have biopsy). Ten patients had bilateral adrenal masses. The indication for biopsy was suspected metastasis in 27 cases, confirmation of an incidentally found expansion in 17, sampling of widespread malignancy from the easiest accessible place in 9, large symptomatic mass in 2, and suspected recurrent adrenal carcinoma in 1.

Technique.—A 3- or 5-MHz transducer with freehand technique is used with ultrasound-guided procedures. A local cutaneous anesthetic is given and the shortest possible route is chosen for biopsy, usually a right-sided transhepatic approach and a left-sided retroperitoneal or transintestinal approach. Computed tomography examinations are done with and without contrast enhancement.

Final diagnosis	No.	Cytologic class			
		0	1–2	3	4–5
Metastasis	22		2	2	18
Adenoma	21	1	19		1
Adrenal cyst	6	1	5		
Hematoma	3		3		
Amyloid	1		1		
Lymphoma	1			1	
Pheochromocytoma	1		1		
Lymph node	1		1		
Total	56	2	32	3	19

True Diagnoses and Cytologic Findings of Adrenal Masses at Fine-Needle Biopsy in 56 Patients

(Courtesy of Tikkakoski T, Taavitsainen M, Päivänsalo M, et al: *Acta Radiologica* 32:371–374, 1991.)

Findings.—Final diagnoses included metastasis in 22 patients, adenoma in 21, adrenal cyst in 6, and hematoma in 3 (table). Adequate material for cytologic analysis was obtained in 96.4% of cases, and the overall accuracy in differentiating benign from malignant disease was 85.7%. There were 2 false negative and 1 false positive diagnoses. Results of 3 biopsies were inconclusive, and 2 of these patients had an additional cutting needle biopsy. There were no complications.

Discussion.—Guided fine-needle biopsy is a useful diagnostic method for disseminated malignant disease with suspected adrenal masses. The technique is also useful in primary adrenal lesions, particularly if the aspirate consists of something other than adrenal cells. Both CT and ultrasound guidance are accurate.

▶ To my knowledge, this is the largest published series of adrenal fine-needle biopsy. These authors confirm some important findings of other investigations but make some novel observations and suggestions. Only about half of patients with a known malignancy and half of patients with bilateral adrenal masses proved to have adrenal metastases. Computed tomography was seldom required for guided biopsy, and accuracy and adequacy of CT- or ultrasound-guided procedures were excellent. Bernardino and his colleagues (1) have noted that asymptomatic small adrenal masses discovered in patients with no known malignancy are rarely malignant and may not require biopsy. Tikkakoski and colleagues, however, confirmed adrenal metastases in 9 patients who had unknown primary tumors. Primary adrenal neoplasms and benign conditions also were confirmed histologically. Clearly, clinical judgment is required for patient selection, and this article provides more excellent guidelines.—M.P. Federle, M.D.

Reference

1. Bernardino ME, et al: *AJR* 144:67, 1985.

Female Genitourinary

Prevalence of Simple Adnexal Cysts in Postmenopausal Women
Wolf SI, Gosink BB, Feldesman MR, Lin MC, Stuenkel CA, Braly PS, Pretorius DH (Univ of California, San Diego; Portland State Univ, Portland, Ore)
Radiology 180:65–71, 1991   5–52

Background.—The presence of an ovarian cystic lesion in a postmenopausal woman raises suspicion of a neoplasm. However, there has been no systematic study to define the prevalence of simple cysts in asymptomatic postmenopausal women.

Study Design.—In a prospective study transabdominal and transvaginal ultrasound were performed on 149 unselected, asymptomatic women aged 50 years and older to assess the prevalence of unilocular,

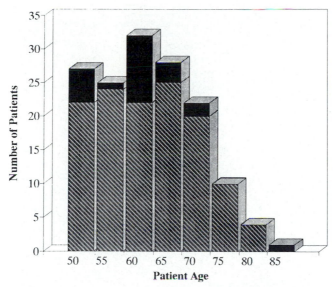

Fig 5–54.—Histogram of age and cyst distribution of postmenopausal patient sample. Bar height = the number of patients in appropriate age category. *Hatched areas,* number of patients with no cysts; *filled areas,* number of patients with cysts. (Courtesy of Wolf SI, Gosink BB, Feldesman MR, et al: *Radiology* 180:65-71, 1991.)

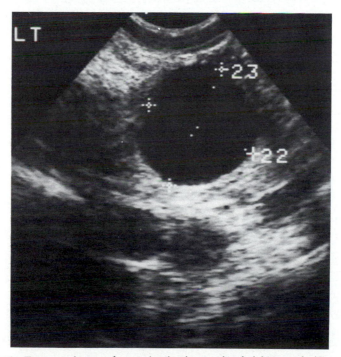

Fig 5–55.—Transvaginal image of a typical unilocular cyst identified during study. (Courtesy of Wolf SI, Gosink BB, Feldesman MR, et al: *Radiology* 180:65-71, 1991.)

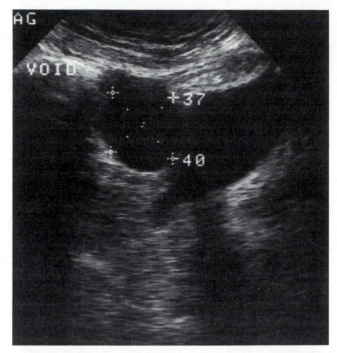

Fig 5–56.—Unilocular cyst 4 cm in diameter that was identified as a benign papillary cystadenoma at surgery. (Courtesy of Wolf SI, Gosink BB, Feldesman MR, et al: *Radiology* 180:65–71, 1991.)

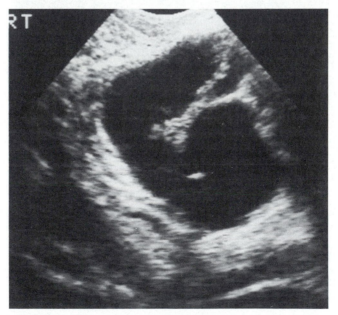

Fig 5–57.—A multiseptated adnexal mass identified as hydrosalpinx at surgery. (Courtesy of Wolf SI, Gosink BB, Feldesman MR, et al: *Radiology* 180:65–71, 1991.)

nonseptated adnexal cysts ("simple cysts") in postmenopausal women. The frequency of the cysts in relation to hormone replacement regimens (no hormones, unopposed estrogen, continuous daily estrogen and progesterone, and sequential estrogen and progesterone) and the time since onset of menopause (<5 years, 5–10 years, and >10 years) were also studied.

Results.—Figure 5–54 depicts the age and cyst distribution of the patients in 5-year intervals. Twenty-two women had simple adnexal cysts (Fig 5–55), for a relative frequency of 14.8% and a prevalence of 14,800 patients with cysts per 100,000 patients. One patient with a cyst 4 cm in diameter underwent surgery, and at pathologic examination the cyst was found to be a benign papillary cyst adenoma (Fig 5–56). Another patient had a multiseptated adnexal mass, which proved to be a hydrosalpinx (Fig 5–57). In combination, transabdominal and transvaginal ultrasound identified 68% of the ovaries, but neither transabdominal nor transvaginal ultrasound alone was optimal for identifying cysts. The occurrence of cysts was independent of the hormone replacement regimen and length of menopause.

Conclusions.—Ovarian cysts are remarkably common in postmenopausal women regardless of age, hormone replacement status, and duration of menopause. Whether they possess the potential to be malignant is unknown. Both transabdominal and transvaginal ultrasound are required to visualize these cysts.

▶ In an attempt to detect curable ovarian cancer, several large screening projects are underway using ultrasound (transabdominal or transvaginal) to screen for ovarian lesions in postmenopausal women. Because most ovarian neoplasms (85% to 90%) are of the cystic epithelial type, and because simple ovarian cysts are presumed to be rare in postmenopausal women, the occurrence of any ovarian cyst in a postmenopausal woman has been considered abnormal and an indication for surgery.

These authors have conducted an excellent investigation demonstrating that simple ovarian cysts can be shown in about 15% of postmenopausal women by a combination of transabdominal (best depicting high pelvic cysts) and transvaginal (best depicting small, deep lesions) sonography. They recommend Doppler study of the ovarian artery. A normal high-resistance pattern (resistive index > .7) is reassuring for benignity. Patients with unilocular cysts up to 3 cm in diameter with such a normal Doppler waveform generally are followed up with ultrasound examinations. (Many cysts seem to disappear spontaneously.) Surgical evaluation is still indicated for cysts greater than 3 cm in diameter, those with septations or solid elements, and those with low-resistance Doppler waveforms.—M.P. Federle, M.D.

Ovarian Cancer Screening in Asymptomatic Postmenopausal Women by Transvaginal Sonography

van Nagell JR Jr, DePriest PD, Puls LE, Donaldson ES, Gallion HH, Pavlik EJ, Powell DE, Kryscio RJ (Univ of Kentucky Med Ctr, Lexington, Ky)

Cancer 68:458–462, 1991   5–53

Objective.—Ovarian cancer remains the prime cause of death from gynecologic cancer in the United States. The value of transvaginal sonography (TVS) in screening for ovarian cancer was examined in a series of 1,300 postmenopausal women in 1987 to 1991. All were asymptomatic. Real-time ultrasonography was carried out using a 5-MHz vaginal transducer.

Findings.—Thirty-three women had abnormal ovarian morphologic conditions or size for longer than 1 month (Table 1). The mean diameter of the lesion was 4 cm. Ovarian enlargement was apparent clinically in 10 of the women. All 27 women who had exploratory surgery had tumors similar in size to that predicted sonographically. Fourteen patients had serous cystadenomas and 3 had ovarian cancer, which was primary in 2 cases and metastatic from colon carcinoma in 1 (Table 2). Women with a family history of ovarian cancer were at increased risk.

Conclusions.—Transvaginal sonography is an experimental method whose value in screening for ovarian cancer remains to be established. A multicenter trial is needed to compare TVS and serum CA-125 estimation with pelvic examination for the detection of ovarian cancer.

TABLE 1.—Sonographic Screening Data

Category	No.
Women screened	1300
Normal scans	1267
Abnormal scans	33
Clinically palpable	10
Surgery	27
TP	3
FP	24
TN	1267
FN	0
Specificity (TN/TN + FP)	0.981
Sensitivity (TP/TP + FN)	1.000

Abbreviations: TP, true positive; FP, false positive; TN, true negative; FN, false negative.

(Courtesy of van Nagell JR Jr, DePriest PD, Puls LE, et al: *Cancer* 68:458–462, 1991.)

TABLE 2.—Ovarian Histologic Condition in
27 Patients With Abnormalities on
Transvaginal Sonography

Category	No.
Adenocarcinoma	3
Serous cystadenoma	14
Epithelial cyst	3
Leiomyoma	3
Hydrosalpinx	2
Endometrioma	1
Thecoma	1

(Courtesy of van Nagell JR Jr, DePriest PD, Puls LE, et al:
Cancer 68:458–462, 1991.)

▶ Transvaginal sonography is unquestionably sensitive in diagnosing ovarian pathologic conditions in postmenopausal women. The key issues remain whether TVS is cost-effective, particularly given the relatively low prevalence of disease and lack of specificity of the TVS findings. Concerning the latter issue, we now know that adnexal cysts are much more common in postmenopausal women than previously thought (Abstract 5-52). Criteria for identifying these patients without requiring surgery is mandatory if TVS screening of large populations is to gain credibility. The second issue is always controversial: cost/benefit ratios. In this study, 1,300 women were screened and 2 primary ovarian carcinomas were detected. This is similar to the results of Campbell and colleagues, who detected 5 primary ovarian cancers in 5,000 women screened by abdominal ultrasound. All of the other pathologic conditions detected (metastatic tumors, benign cystadenomas, cysts) must be considered false positives for the purposes of finding curable ovarian cancer in asymptomatic women. I would favor identification of higher-risk groups, including those with a positive family history of ovarian cancer or a personal history of breast cancer (a link has been established) for aggressive screening.—M.P. Federle, M.D.

Ovarian Lesions: Detection and Characterization With Gadolinium-Enhanced MR Imaging at 1.5 T

Stevens SK, Hricak H, Stern JL (Univ of California, San Francisco)
Radiology 181:481–488, 1991   5–54

Introduction.—The efficacy of Gd-enhanced MRI for detecting ovarian masses has not been determined. In a prospective study, enhanced T_1-weighted and unenhanced T_1- and T_2-weighted spin-echo images were compared, and the MRI results were compared with surgical staging in 33 women with 60 lesions. The T_2-weighted and Gd-enhanced and unenhanced T_1-weighted MRIs were used to characterize the lesions

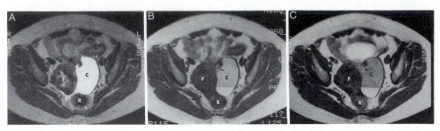

Fig 5–58.—Transaxial (**A**) T2-weighted (2,000/70), (**B**) T1-weighted (700/20) and (**C**) Gd-enhanced T1-weighted (700/20) images of bilateral adnexal masses: a right ovarian fibroma (*F*) and a left ovarian mucinous cystadenofibroma (*C*) in a woman, 60, with a history of breast carcinoma. The right ovarian fibroma demonstrates low signal intensity on T1-weighted image, heterogeneous higher signal intensity on the T2-weighted image, and slight enhancement after administration of gadopentetate dimeglumine. The left ovarian mucinous cystadenofibroma has fluid-fluid level and thin-wall mural nodularity, part of which (*arrow*) is enhanced on the Gd-enhanced image; a malignancy could not be excluded. At pathologic examination, a low-intensity mural nodule represented a focal region of wall thickening that contained extensive fibrosis and calcification, and the enhanced portion contained fibrosis. The lower (gravity-dependent) fluid level contained hemorrhage. R indicates rectum. (Courtesy of Stevens SK, Hricak H, Stern JL: *Radiology* 181:481–488, 1991.)

prospectively, and these findings were compared with those of staging laparotomy. Staging by MRI was performed if malignancy was suspected.

Results.—Of the 60 lesions, MRI demonstrated 57. All malignant lesions were correctly diagnosed (Fig 5–58), but 4 benign lesions were misdiagnosed as malignant. There were 5 significant primary criteria for malignancy: size larger than 4 cm, solid mass or large solid component (Fig 5–59), wall thicker than 3 mm, septa thicker than 3 mm and/or vegetations or nodularity, and necrosis, and 4 ancillary criteria. Using the primary criteria, characterization was correct in 84% of lesions for all pulse sequences combined (Table 1); adding the ancillary criteria, characterization was correct in 95% of lesions (Table 2). On Gd-enhanced images, correct characterization was 78% with the primary criteria and

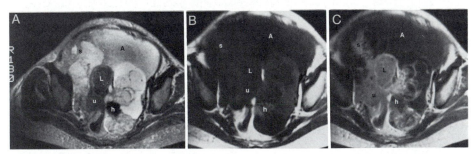

Fig 5–59.—Transaxial (**A**) T2-weighted (2,000/70), (**B**) T1-weighted (700/20) and (**C**) Gd-enhanced T1-weighted (700/20) images of poorly differentiated endometrioid carcinoma seen as bilateral complex pelvic masses in a woman, 55. The left ovarian tumor is a multiloculated lesion with a hemorrhagic component (*h*). The complex mass on the right has a solid (*s*) component that demonstrates enhancement. Differentiation between cystic and solid components or delineation of loculated ascites is best seen on the Gd-enhanced image. **A,** indicates ascites; *u,* uterus; *L,* leiomyoma. (Courtesy of Stevens SK, Hricak H, Stern JL: *Radiology* 181:481–488, 1991.)

TABLE 1.—Rates of Correct Classification of Ovarian Lesions With MRI Using 5 Primary Criteria for Malignancy

	Lesion		
Pulse Sequence Combination*	Benign (*n* = 34)	Malignant (*n* = 23)	Total (*n* = 57)
Unenhanced T1- and T2-weighted	30 (88)	13 (56)	43 (75)
Enhanced and unenhanced T1-weighted	30 (88)	18 (78)*	48 (84)
T2- and enhanced and unenhanced T1-weighted	30 (88)	18 (78)	48 (84)

Note: Numbers in parentheses are percentages.
* *P* = .0625.
(Courtesy of Stevens SK, Hricak H, Stern JL: *Radiology* 181:481–488, 1991.)

100% with both sets of criteria. Accuracy of staging was 63% with unenhanced and 75% with the addition of enhanced images.

Conclusions.—Magnetic resonance imaging is useful in detecting and characterizing adnexal masses. The differentiation of benign from malignant masses is improved with gadopentate enhancement. The technique may also be useful in surgical staging.

▶ The main role of imaging of pelvic masses is to characterize them as obviously benign or not. The former category includes simple cysts, some endometriomas and abscesses, leiomyomas, and intrauterine pregnancies. The "not" category included a wide variety of pathologic processes that share the common pathway of surgical exploration. Magnetic resonance imaging certainly can help characterize benign processes and lend confidence to conservative management. The authors note that MR staging of ovarian carcinoma compares favorably with that of CT (75%–90%), but clinicians rarely are influenced by CT in their management of ovarian carcinoma. Both CT

TABLE 2.—Rates of Correct Classification of Ovarian Lesions With MRI Using Primary and Ancillary Criteria

	Lesion		
Pulse Sequence Combination	Benign (*n* = 34)	Malignant (*n* = 23)	Total (*n* = 57)
Unenhanced T1- and T2-weighted	31 (91)	19 (83)	50 (88)
Unenhanced and enhanced T1-weighted	31 (91)	23 (100)*	54 (95)
T2-weighted and enhanced and un-enhanced T2-weighted	31 (91)	23 (100)	54 (95)

Note: Numbers in parentheses are percentages.
* *P* = .125.
(Courtesy of Stevens SK, Hricak H, Stern JL: *Radiology* 181:481–488, 1991.)

and MRI frequently miss peritoneal, omental, and bowel implants, and routine MRI does not even include sections through the liver. I doubt that we will have much influence on management except by demonstrating obvious bowel or bladder invasion (plan surgical assistance) or extensive retroperitoneal adenopathy or sidewall invasion (frozen pelvis).—M.P. Federle, M.D.

Value of Lipid- and Water-Suppression MR Images in Distinguishing Between Blood and Lipid Within Ovarian Masses

Kier R, Smith RC, McCarthy SM (Yale Univ, New Haven, Conn)

AJR 158:321–325, 1992   5–55

Background.—It may be difficult in routine MRI of ovarian masses to make the important differentiation between blood and lipid in ovarian

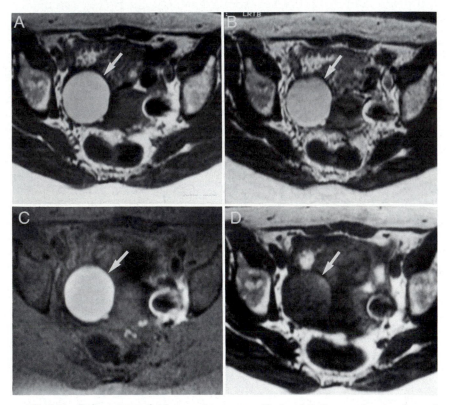

Fig 5–60.—Endometrioma of right ovary in a woman, 33. **A** and **B,** 5-cm ovarian mass (*arrows*) appears isointense compared with subcutaneous fat on both T1-weighted (500/20) **(A)** and T2-weighted (2,900/126) **(B)** axial MRI. **C** and **D,** lesion (*arrows*) becomes markedly hyperintense relative to subcutaneous fat on axial T1-weighted (600/20) MRI with lipid suppression **(C)** and hypointense relative to fat on axial T1-weighted (600/20) MRI with water suppression **(D).** (Courtesy of Kier R, Smith RC, McCarthy SM: *AJR* 158:321–325, 1992.)

masses. The usefulness of lipid- and water-suppression MRI in making this distinction was investigated.

Methods.—The study included 21 adnexal masses with the signal intensity of subcutaneous fat in 16 women. Ten patients underwent laparoscopy and 6 had surgery; 16 endometriomas, 4 lipid-containing mature cystic teratomas, and 1 hemorrhagic leiomyosarcoma were found. In addition to T_1-weighted spin-echo images, each patient underwent supplementary imaging with presaturation of fat protons for lipid suppression and presaturation of water protons for water suppression.

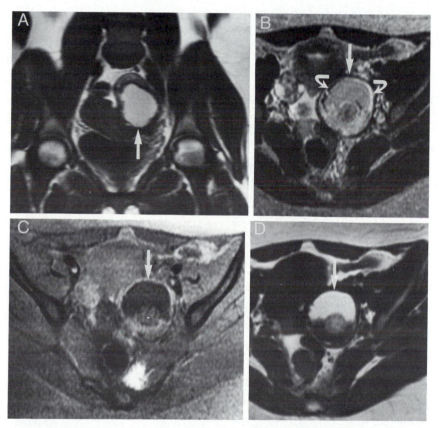

Fig 5–61.—Mature cystic teratoma in a woman, 28. **A,** 4-cm left adnexal mass (*arrow*) is isointense compared with subcutaneous fat on coronal T1-weighted (500/20) MRI. **B,** on axial T2-weighted (1,900/80) MRI, the left ovarian mass (*straight arrow*) appears isointense compared with subcutaneous fat, although slightly heterogeneous. Chemical-shift artifact may be seen along the superomedial and superolateral margins of the mass (*curved arrows*), suggesting cystic teratoma. **C,** anterior component (*arrow*) of the ovarian lesion becomes slightly hypointense relative to subcutaneous fat on axial T1-weighted (567/11) MRI with lipid suppression, indicating that lipid in this teratoma differs from lipid in subcutaneous fat. **D,** mass (*arrow*) remains isointense compared with subcutaneous fat on axial T1-weighted (567/11) MR image with water suppression. (Courtesy of Kier R, Smith RC, McCarthy SM: AJR 158:321–325, 1992.)

Findings.—All 17 hemorrhagic lesions had a greater signal intensity compared to subcutaneous fat on lipid-suppression images; on water-suppression images, intensity was less than that of fat (Fig 5–60). In the 4 lipid-containing lesions, signal intensity was comparable with that of subcutaneous fat on both lipid- and water-suppression images (Fig 5–61).

Conclusions.—The use of lipid- and water-suppression MRI permits accurate distinction between blood and lipid in ovarian masses. These 2 methods should become a useful part of the differential diagnosis of such lesions.

▶ Most ovarian masses appear hypointense relative to subcutaneous fat on T_1-weighted images and hyperintense to fat on T_2-weighted images. Exceptions to this include both hemorrhagic and lipid-containing lesions. The author's protocol of adding 2 extra series of T_1-weighted images after selective water or lipid signal suppression reportedly required only 10 extra minutes of exam time, including 2 minutes of imaging time. The results are convincing and add valuable, often definitive, information in the differential diagnosis of adnexal masses.—M.P. Federle, M.D.

MR Imaging Evaluation of Endometrial Carcinoma: Results of an NCI Cooperative Study
Hricak H, Rubinstein LV, Gherman GM, Karstaedt N (Univ of California, San Francisco; Natl Cancer Inst, Bethesda, Md; Bowman Gray School of Medicine, Winston-Salem, NC)
Radiology 179:829–832, 1991   5–56

Background.—The prognosis for patients with endometrial cancer depends on histologic tumor grade, tumor stage, depth of myometrial invasion, and presence of lymph node metastasis at the time of diagnosis. The National Cancer Institute sponsored a prospective cooperative study to assess the role of MRI in the evaluation of tumor extent in patients with endometrial carcinoma. Five institutions participated in the study.

Methods.—The 5 hospitals entered a total of 107 patients in the study, 88 of whom met the study's inclusion criteria. The mean age of the patients was 61.7 years. All 88 patients underwent hysterectomy. Sixty patients had stage I disease, of whom 43 had stage IA and 17 had stage IB; 11 had stage II; 4 had stage III; and 8 had stage IV disease. Twenty-two patients had no tumor invasion. Six different commercially available MR imagers were used, ranging in magnetic field strength from .15 to 1.5 T. The T_1- and T_2-weighted sequences in the transverse plane and T_2-weighted sequences in the sagittal plane appropriate for each unit were used for the study.

Outcome.—The overall image quality was rated poor in 18%, adequate in 75%, and excellent in 7%. Imaging was judged adequate for pelvic lymph node evaluation in 92%, but it was adequate for evaluation of the para-aortic nodes in only 8%. The abnormality within the endometrial cavity was correctly identified in 81% of cases. The overall staging accuracy with MRI was 85%. When staging analysis included separate evaluation of each stage, the accuracy decreased to 65%. In the evaluation of depth of myometrial invasion for stage I disease, the overall accuracy with MRI was 74%. The overall accuracy was 66% if all stages were analyzed. The sensitivity for detecting deep myometrial invasion with MRI was 54% and the specificity was 89%.

Conclusions.—Magnetic resonance imaging is useful in the preoperative staging of endometrial carcinoma. As image quality improves and techniques advance, the accuracy in evaluating patients with endometrial carcinoma will likely improve even further.

▶ This is another commendable effort to meet the demand for more vigorous, multi-institution trials of new technology to prove its worth before being introduced into general clinical practice. Strict statistical analysis of data similarly is demanded if the research presented in our radiology literature is to gain credibility. Unfortunately, the manuscript is a good example of the pitfalls of this approach. Given the complexity of gathering enough patient data to meet strict criteria, the data will likely be outdated by the time it reaches publication. This 5-institution study was conducted in 1985 through 1987 using various MR equipment, some of which is no longer in production. Image quality was often poor or suboptimal. Still, one could interpret the results as showing reasonable accuracy for MRI in staging endometrial carcinoma. I could interpret the data quite differently, noting that the accuracy is artificially high because of the prevalence of early cancer (77 of 88 patients had stage I disease; if the readers couldn't even see the cancer and called every case stage I, their accuracy would look good!). In fact, the sensitivity for detecting deep myometrial invasion with MRI was only 54% and the specificity 89%. Detection of lymph node metastases was similarly poor; many MR studies were judged inadequate to evaluate the nodes, and I see no correlation between the MR findings and the presence or absence of tumor in nodes dissected at surgery. I am sure that newer advances in MR hardware and software, along with MR contrast agents, can improve the performance, but these data should not serve as a convincing endorsement of MRI.—M.P. Federle, M.D.

Cancer of the Endometrium: Value of MR Imaging in Determining Depth of Invasion Into the Myometrium
Lien HH, Blomlie V, Tropé C, Kærn J, Abeler VM (Norwegian Radium Hospital, Oslo, Norway)
AJR 157:1221–1223, 1991   5–57

Introduction.—Depth of invasion into the myometrium is an important prognostic factor in patients with endometrial adenocarcinoma, particularly the distinction between less than or greater than 50% invasion.

Methods.—The ability of MRI in making this differentiation was investigated in 33 patients with stage I or II endometrial cancer. All patients underwent MRI before total abdominal hysterectomy without lymphadenectomy, and the pathologic findings were compared with those on MRI.

Results.—There was deep myometrial invasion in 22 patients, and all but 2 of these were correctly identified by MRI. In the 11 patients with only superficial invasion, MRI erroneously suggested deep invasion in 4. Thus, MRI had an accuracy of 82% in demonstrating deep invasion, a sensitivity of 91%, and a specificity of 64%. The positive predictive value was 83% and the negative predictive value 78%.

Conclusions.—In patients with endometrial cancer, MRI can differentiate between superficial and deep myometrial invasion. However, false positive results may occur with exophytic polypoid tumors that have significant intraluminal extension.

▶ Unlike the National Cancer Institute study (Abstract 5–56), this is a single institution investigation using a modern high-field MR system for all patients. I still have some difficulty accepting that their results demonstrate reliability of MRI in staging endometrial cancer. Both the normal postmenopausal uterus and endometrial cancer may have variable signal intensities. The authors state that "potential changes in MR appearances at various times during the menstrual cycle seldom pose a problem," but none of their postmenopausal women was on hormone replacement therapy (extremely popular in this country), which may cause uterine changes similar to a menstrual cycle. The variable signal characteristics of endometrial tumor, chemical shift and other artifacts, and post–dilatation and curettage changes all present challenges to proper MR interpretation. Further work seems warranted, perhaps with intravenous contrast material and special coils, before MRI can stage endometrial cancer reliably. Poor candidates for surgery and those with a high clinical suspicion of deep myometrial invasion might benefit from MRI; unequivocal evidence of deep invasion would help defer surgery in favor of whole-pelvis radiation.—M.P. Federle, M.D.

Diagnostic Imaging in Puerperal Febrile Morbidity
Lev-Toaff AS, Baka JJ, Toaff ME, Friedman AC, Radecki PD, Caroline DF (Temple Univ Hosp, Hahnemann Univ Hosp, Philadelphia)
Obstet Gynecol 78:50–55, 1991   5–58

Background.—Imaging studies have not been widely used in the management of postpartum febrile morbidity. The use of ultrasound, CT, and MRI in the diagnosis and management of patients with refractory puerperal febrile morbidity was evaluated in a prospective study.

Patients.—The medical records and imaging studies of 31 patients referred with puerperal febrile morbidity that did not respond to antibiotic treatment were reviewed; these cases accounted for .4% of all deliveries during the 3-year study period. Thirty of the patients were black, and 11 were adolescents. Forty-two percent of women delivered prematurely, and 74% delivered by cesarean section. Forty-five percent had bleeding that required blood transfusions.

Findings.—Eleven women had hematomas, 2 of which were broad ligament hematomas. Six of the 11 women were delivered by cesarean section and 5 were managed conservatively. A rectovaginal septum hematoma disclosed by ultrasound in 1 case was managed conservatively and followed by ultrasound. There were 7 abscesses, 2 cases of ovarian venous thrombosis, and 1 case of small bowel obstruction, 1 of vesicouterine fistula, and 1 of subcutaneous seroma. Endomyometritis was found in 21 patients, 13 of whom had other extrauterine abnormalities, including 6 cases of abscess, 4 of hematoma, 1 of ovarian venous thrombosis, 1 of vesicouterine fistula, and 1 of small bowel obstruction. Two patients had retained placental tissue. Imaging studies were negative in only 2 patients; in most patients they led to a specific diagnosis and allowed definitive therapy.

Conclusions.—Imaging studies can be useful in the evaluation of women with puerperal fever. Ultrasound is the first imaging study for most patients, although CT or MRI may be required for obese patients or if skilled personnel are unavailable.

▶ Puerperal fever persisting beyond 24 hours postpartum complicates 2% to 3% of vaginal deliveries and 29% to 95% of cesarean sections. Endometritis is the most common cause (about 50% of cases), is usually evident clinically, and usually responds to antibiotic therapy. Antibiotic resistant endometritis is the most common cause of persistent fever, and these authors have demonstrated the value of imaging in diagnosis of this and associated complications. Ultrasound was not very sensitive in diagnosing endometritis (11 of 21 cases), showing combinations of endometrial fluid, debris, and gas. However, many patients (13 of 21) have extrauterine abnormalities demonstrated well by sonography. For patients with fever persisting for more than 72 hours in spite of antibiotics or in situations where other complications such as internal blood loss are suspected, sonography is the initial imaging procedure of choice. Magnetic resonance imaging makes nice pictures but has shown few unique advantages in this setting. Computed tomography may be necessary in obese patients or those with excessive gas, particularly if percutaneous drainage of a deep fluid collection is planned.—M.P. Federle, M.D.

A Clinical Comparison of Sonographic Hydrotubation and Hysterosalpingography

Mitri FF, Andronikou AD, Perpinyal S, Hofmeyr GJ, Sonnendecker EWW
(Coronation and Johannesburg Hospitals, University of the Witwatersrand
Medical School, Johannesburg, South Africa)
Br J Obstet Gynaecol 98:1031–1036, 1991   5–59

Background.—The value of hysterosalpingography (HSG) in infertile women undergoing laparoscopy is limited to demonstrating intrauterine and intratubal abnormalities. In addition, HSG is time consuming, labor intensive, and associated with the risk of reaction to contrast media. The value of using vaginal sonographic hydrotubation instead was investigated.

Methods.—Sixty women undergoing routine infertility testing agreed to participate in the prospective, blind, comparison study of HSG and sonographic hydrotubation. Within the 4 weeks before or after HSG, sonographic hydrotubation was done. The uterus and tubes were identified using a 5-MHz vaginal ultrasound probe, and 10 to 20 mL of normal saline solution was injected into the uterine cavity through an endocervical catheter. The main outcome measures were the shape of the uterus and its cavity, the flow of saline solution through the tubes, the presence of hydrosalpinges before and after saline solution injection, and the presence of free fluid in the pouch of Douglas.

Results.—Sonographic and HSG uterine assessment findings were comparable in 82% of the women. Tubal findings were comparable in 72%. Twelve percent of the women had bipolar tubal disease on sonography and cornual block on HSG, with sonographic diagnosis confirmed at laparoscopy. Sonographic hydrotubation enabled a more certain diagnosis of septate uterus in 3 cases.

Conclusions.—Sonographic hydrotubation is a simple office procedure that should be used in the initial evaluation of the uterine cavity and fallopian tubes. The use of this technique will decrease the need for HSG and, in some cases, laparoscopy.

▶ Infertility is a major problem affecting at least 10% of couples and frequently is caused by a tuboperitoneal pathologic condition. Hysterosalpingography has been the standard imaging means of evaluating fallopian tube patency and uterine abnormalities that might impede fertilization or implantation. The authors believe that sonographic hydrotubation can largely replace HSG as a screening test for the tube and uterus. It seems logical that ultrasound can better depict uterine wall abnormalities than HSG. Newer studies in centers using fluoroscopic guided catheterization of the tubes in conjunction with dilatation of tubal strictures suggest that selective cannulation and injection are necessary to assess patency. I predict that sonographic hydrotubation will have appeal to obstetricians and gynecologists who can do the procedure in their office. Hysterosalpingography will likely be done more selectively in a subset of patients being considered for fallopian tube recanalization. For further discussion, see Thurmond and Rosch's paper (1).—M.P. Federle, M.D.

Reference

1. Thurmond AS, Rosch J: *Radiology* 174:371, 1990.

Obstetric/Fetal Sonography

Sonography of the Cervix During the Third Trimester of Pregnancy: Value of the Transperineal Approach

Hertzberg BS, Bowie JD, Weber TM, Carroll BA, Kliewer MA, Jordan SG (Duke Univ, Durham, NC)

AJR 157:73–76, 1991   5–60

Introduction.—It has proved difficult to accurately assess the cervix by transabdominal sonography in the third trimester of pregnancy. As an alternative, transperineal examination was performed in a prospective

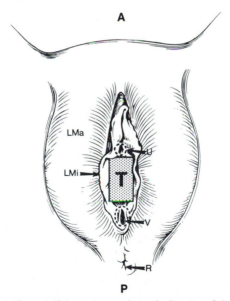

Fig 5–62.—Schematic diagram of the perineum shows the location of the transducer during transperineal sonography. The transducer is applied directly over the labia minora in a sagittal plan just posterior to the urethra. Transducer location and angle are adjusted under sonographic control to optimize visualization of the cervix. *Abbreviations:* T, transducer; A, anterior; LMa, labia majora; LMi, labia minora; U, urethra; V, vaginal orifice; R, rectal orifice; P, posterior. (Courtesy of Hertzberg BS, Bowie JD, Weber TM, et al: *AJR* 157:73-76, 1991.)

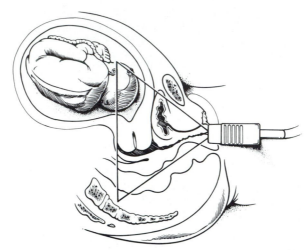

Fig 5–63.—Sagittal illustration of the gravid uterus in a supine patient (with the transducer positioned on perineum) reveals the typical scanning plane obtained during transperineal sonography. (Courtesy of Hertzberg BS, Bowie JD, Weber TM, et al: AJR 157:73-76, 1991.)

series of 158 third-trimester patients after transabdominal attempts had failed.

Methods.—The transducer was placed sagittally between the labia majora (Fig 5–62), with its center posterior to the urethra and anterior to the vagina. Mild perineal pressure was applied with the transducer. This approach depicts the vagina in a vertical plane with the cervix horizontal

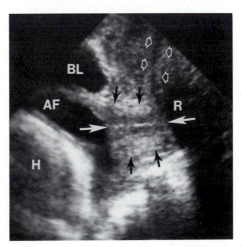

Fig 5–64.—Transperineal sonogram of third-trimester vervic (*black arrows*) reveals endocervical canal (*solid white arrows*) in a horizontal plane, approximately perpendicular to the ultrasound beam. The region of the canal is depicted as a central echogenic stripe surrounded by a hypoechoic region, similar to pattern seen during transabdominal sonography. Vagina is oriented in a nearly vertical plane (*open arrows*). *Abbreviations:* BL, maternal urinary bladder; AF, amniotic fluid; R, rectal gas; H, fetal head. (Courtesy of Hertzberg BS, Bowie JD, Weber TM, et al: AJR 157:73-76, 1991.)

and its long axis approximately perpendicular to the ultrasound beam (Fig 5–63).

Observations.—The cervix was better visualized transperineally than by the transabdominal method in all patients (Fig 5–64). In 14% of cases, the area of the external os was obscured by rectal gas. This problem sometimes was solved by scanning with the patient in the lateral decubitus position or by rotating the patient. No patient had significant discomfort during the study.

Conclusions.—Transperineal sonography is a safe, simple, and effective means of imaging the cervix in late pregnancy.

▶ Although transvaginal sonography is an excellent alternative imaging technique to transabdominal sonography for visualization of the cervix, some radiologists and obstetricians argue that it poses an unnecessary risk for patients with placenta previa, cervical incompetence, or ruptured membranes. In this article the authors have presented a new noninvasive sonographic technique for visualization of the cervix, transperineal sonography. Our own experience with this technique supports their claim that it is a very good alternative imaging technique for the patient with "nothing per vagina" orders.—G. Dodd, III, M.D.

Placenta Accreta: Additional Sonographic Observations
Hoffman-Tretin JC, Koenigsberg M, Rabin A, Anyaegbunam A (Albert Einstein College of Medicine, Bronx, NY)
J Ultrasound Med 11:29–34, 1992   5–61

Introduction.—Placenta accreta is a complication of pregnancy that is recognized more frequently. The antenatal sonographic diagnosis of pla-

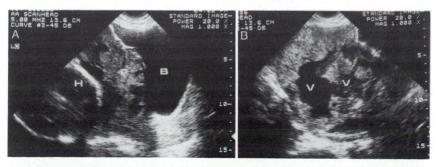

Fig 5–65.—Evolution of placenta percreta on sequential sonograms (patient 1). **A,** sagittal midline sonogram of the lower uterine segment at 35—37 weeks of fetal development reveals partial placental previa and absence of the hypoechoic zone peripheral to the placenta (P), which abuts on the dome of the bladder (B). Invasion of the bladder wall may be suspected from this view. **B,** section depicts the bizarre intraplacental vascular spaces (V) confirmed by Doppler interrogation. (Courtesy of Hoffman-Tretin JC, Koenigsberg M, Rabin A, et al: *J Ultrasound Med* 11:29-34, 1992.)

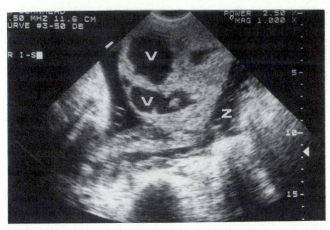

Fig 5–66.—Placenta previa and posterior increta (patient 2). Transverse sonogram. Note that prominent placental venous lakes (V) may be found in regions adjacent to the placenta accreta, where the peripheral hypoechoic zone (Z) is still present. This was confirmed by Doppler interrogation. (Courtesy of Hoffman-Tretin JC, Koenigsberg M, Rabin A, et al: *J Ultrasound Med* 11:29–34, 1992.)

centa accreta has been based on the nonvisualization of a hypoechoic zone next to the placenta.

Methods.—The histologic basis and differential diagnosis of placenta accreta in 7 patients, aged 27 to 35 years, were reviewed. The diagnosis was established sonographically on the basis of lack of hypoechoic zone peripheral to the placenta.

Results.—New observations included prominent large or multiple placental venous lakes and periuterine vascularity in 6 patients. In 2 patients, there was progressive thinning and disappearance of the retroplacental hypoechoic zone on sequential assessments. Also of diagnostic value was loss of normal venous flow pattern on Doppler interrogation of the peripheral placental margin in 2 patients. Histologic correlates were suggested on the basis of the primary histopathologic feature of placenta accreta, deficiency of the decidua basalis. Differential diagnostic considerations included abdominal pregnancy and trophoblastic disease (Figs 5–65 and 5–66).

Conclusions.—The progression of sonographic findings of placenta accreta in sequential studies supports the notion that placenta accreta is an acquired abnormality. There are at least 2 differential diagnoses to be considered when placenta accreta is suspected.

▶ The sonographic diagnosis of placenta accreta is difficult because it relies on the identification of the loss of the normal subplacental hypoechoic zone, a subtle sign at best. In this manuscript, the authors identified a new finding, large subplacental venous lakes, which they believe is highly suggestive of the diagnosis. Additional studies will be necessary to fully evaluate the usefulness of this sign.—G. Dodd, III, M.D.

Fetal Crown-Rump Length: Reevaluation of Relation to Menstrual Age (5–18 Weeks) With High-Resolution Real-Time US
Hadlock FP, Shah YP, Kanon DJ, Lindsey JV (Baylor College, Houston)
Radiology 182:501–505, 1992   5–62

Background.—Measurements of crown-rump length (CRL) long have been the standard of reference for ultrasound (US) fetal dating. Recently the validity of traditional data—developed with conventional static-image scanners—has been challenged.

Objective and Methods.—Crown-rump length was related to menstrual age in 416 patients, providing reliable menstrual dates. The goal was to construct a single CRL chart that could be applied to measurements from 2 mm to 12 cm. Various commercially available transabdominal and transvaginal real-time US probes were utilized.

Results.—A chart was successfully constructed for predicting the menstrual age of fetuses from CRL measurements taken at 5 to 18 weeks' gestation (table). Variability in predicting menstrual age was relatively constant at ±8% (2 SD) when expressed as a percentage of the predicted value. After 14 weeks, CRL measurements were as accurate as biparietal diameter and femur length in predicting menstrual age but not more so.

Conclusions.—Measurements of CRL acquired early in the middle trimester of gestation predict menstrual age as well as but not better than more frequently used predictors such as biparietal diameter. For studies in the first trimester, variability is ±8% of the estimate, not ±5 days as is presently thought.

▶ Current sonographic equipment depicts anatomy and pathologic conditions not visible with older equipment. Consequently, the validity of observations gleaned from images made on early generation equipment is rightfully subject to reanalysis and potential revision. In this article, Hadlock et al. have reaffirmed the fetal CRL measurement as the measurement of choice for dating first-trimester pregnancies. Furthermore, they have extended the CRL dating charts to include gestational weeks' 5 to 18 and suggest that confidence levels in dating accuracy are better reported as a percent variation than as a fixed number of days.—G. Dodd, III, M.D.

Predicted Menstrual Age, In Weeks, From CRL Measurements, in Centimeters

CRL (cm)	MA (wk)	CRL (cm)	MA (wk)	CRL (cm)	MA (wk)	CRL (cm)	MA (wk)	CRL (cm)	MA (wk)	CRL (cm)	MA (wk)
0.2	5.7	2.2	8.9	4.2	11.1	6.2	12.6	8.2	14.2	10.2	16.1
0.3	5.9	2.3	9.0	4.3	11.2	6.3	12.7	8.3	14.2	10.3	16.2
0.4	6.1	2.4	9.1	4.4	11.2	6.4	12.8	8.4	14.3	10.4	16.3
0.5	6.2	2.5	9.2	4.5	11.3	6.5	12.8	8.5	14.4	10.5	16.4
0.6	6.4	2.6	9.4	4.6	11.4	6.6	12.9	8.6	14.5	10.6	16.5
0.7	6.6	2.7	9.5	4.7	11.5	6.7	13.0	8.7	14.6	10.7	16.6
0.8	6.7	2.8	9.6	4.8	11.6	6.8	13.1	8.8	14.7	10.8	16.7
0.9	6.9	2.9	9.7	4.9	11.7	6.9	13.1	8.9	14.8	10.9	16.8
1.0	7.1	3.0	9.9	5.0	11.7	7.0	13.2	9.0	14.9	11.0	16.9
1.1	7.2	3.1	10.0	5.1	11.8	7.1	13.3	9.1	15.0	11.1	17.0
1.2	7.4	3.2	10.1	5.2	11.9	7.2	13.4	9.2	15.1	11.2	17.1
1.3	7.5	3.3	10.2	5.3	12.0	7.3	13.4	9.3	15.2	11.3	17.2
1.4	7.7	3.4	10.3	5.4	12.0	7.4	13.5	9.4	15.3	11.4	17.3
1.5	7.9	3.5	10.4	5.5	12.1	7.5	13.6	9.5	15.3	11.5	17.4
1.6	8.0	3.6	10.5	5.6	12.2	7.6	13.7	9.6	15.4	11.6	17.5
1.7	8.1	3.7	10.6	5.7	12.3	7.7	13.8	9.7	15.5	11.7	17.6
1.8	8.3	3.8	10.7	5.8	12.3	7.8	13.8	9.8	15.6	11.8	17.7
1.9	8.4	3.9	10.8	5.9	12.4	7.9	13.9	9.9	15.7	11.9	17.8
2.0	8.6	4.0	10.9	6.0	12.5	8.0	14.0	10.0	15.9	12.0	17.9
2.1	8.7	4.1	11.0	6.1	12.6	8.1	14.1	10.1	16.0	12.1	18.0

Abbreviation: MA, menstrual age.
Note: The 95% CI is ± 8% of the predicted age.
(Courtesy of Hadlock FP, Shah YP, Kanon DJ, et al: *Radiology* 182:501–505, 1991.)

Yolk Sac Diameter and Shape at Endovaginal US: Predictors of Pregnancy Outcome in the First Trimester
Lindsay DJ, Lovett IS, Lyons EA, Levi CS, Zheng X-H, Holt SC, Dashefsky SM
(Health Sciences Centre, Winnipeg, Man, Canada)
Radiology 183:115–118, 1992   5–63

Objective.—The normal size and shape of the secondary yolk sac (YS) were established in 486 consecutive women having endovaginal sonography before their fetuses were 10 weeks of menstrual age. In addition, the value of YS measurements in predicting pregnancy outcome was determined.

Observations.—Yolk-sac diameter increased rapidly up to 42 to 44 days' menstrual age. The YS size did not correlate closely with crown-rump length in cases with a normal outcome. In contrast, YS diameter correlated well with the mean gestational sac diameter (MSD), as shown in the table. A YS diameter more than 2 SD above the mean when compared with the MSD predicted an abnormal pregnancy outcome with a sensitivity of 15.6% and a specificity of 97.4%; its positive predictive value was 60%. A YS diameter more than 2 SDs below the mean had a positive predictive value of 44.4%. In no pregnancy with a normal outcome was the YS diameter more than 5.6 mm before 10 weeks' menstrual age. All 3 pregnancies with a persistently abnormal YS shape had an abnormal outcome. The normal appearance is shown in Figure 5–67.

Conclusions.—Abnormal YS size or shape is an early predictor of abnormal pregnancy outcome. The YS should be routinely evaluated in pregnancies less than 10 weeks of menstrual age. If it is abnormal and the pregnancy continues past the first trimester, sonography should be done before 20 weeks to rule out fetal anomaly.

Normal Values for YS Diameter
v. MSD

MSD (mm)	YS Diameter (mm)	
	Mean	95% CI*
2	0.4	0–1.8
3	0.6	0–2.1
4	0.9	0–2.4
5	1.2	0–2.7
6	1.5	0–2.9
7	1.7	0.3–3.2
8	1.9	0.5–3.4
9	2.1	0.7–3.6
10	2.3	0.8–3.7
11	2.4	1.0–3.9
12	2.6	1.1–4.0
13	2.7	1.2–4.1
14	2.8	1.3–4.2
15	2.8	1.4–4.3
16	2.9	1.5–4.3
17	3.0	1.5–4.4
18	3.0	1.6–4.4
19	3.0	1.6–4.5
20	3.1	1.6–4.5
21	3.1	1.6–4.5
22	3.1	1.6–4.5
23	3.1	1.6–4.5
24	3.1	1.6–4.5
25	3.1	1.6–4.5
26	3.1	1.6–4.5
27	3.1	1.6–4.5
28	3.1	1.6–4.5
29	3.1	1.6–4.5
30	3.1	1.7–4.6
31	3.1	1.7–4.6
32	3.1	1.7–4.6
33	3.2	1.7–4.6
34	3.2	1.8–4.7
35	3.3	1.8–4.7
36	3.3	1.9–4.8
37	3.4	1.9–4.9
38	3.5	2.0–5.0
39	3.6	2.1–5.1
40	3.7	2.2–5.2
41	3.9	2.3–5.4
42	4.1	2.5–5.6
43	4.2	2.6–5.8
44	4.4	2.7–6.0
45	4.5	2.8–6.1

Note: $r = 435$, $n = 327$, $P < .0001$, YS diameter $= .47 + .418(MSD) - .016(MSD)^2 + .0002(MSD^3)$.

* CI, confidence interval.

(Courtesy of Lindsay DJ, Lovett IS, Lyons EA, et al: *Radiology* 183:115–118, 1992.)

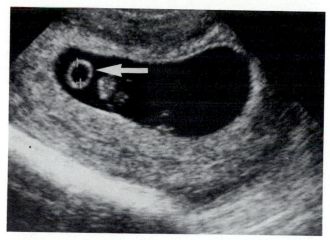

Fig 5–67.—Ultrasound scans of normal YS shape. (Courtesy of Lindsay DJ, Lovett IS, Lyons EA, et al: *Radiology* 183:115–118, 1992.)

Can Detection of the Yolk Sac in the First Trimester Be Used to Predict the Outcome of Pregnancy? A Prospective Sonographic Study

Kurtz AB, Needleman L, Pennell RG, Baltarowich O, Vilaro M, Goldberg BB
(Thomas Jefferson Univ Hosp, Philadelphia)
AJR 158:843–847, 1992

5–64

Objective.—Reports suggest that the failure to visualize a yolk sac (YS) on first-trimester sonography is a strong indicator of abnormal pregnancy. A prospective study included 163 normal and 49 abnormal singleton gestations in women examined both abdominally and transvaginally.

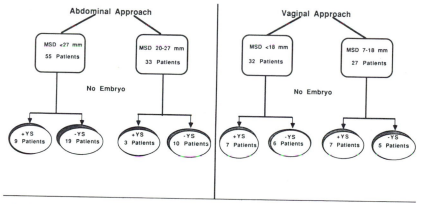

Fig 5–68.—Chart depicting first-trimester sonographic detection of the yolk sac in 163 patients with normal findings. *Abbreviations:* YS, yolk sac; *MSD,* mean sac diameter; +, present, −, absent. (Courtesy of Kurtz AB, Needleman L, Pennell RG, et al: *AJR* 158:843–847, 1992.)

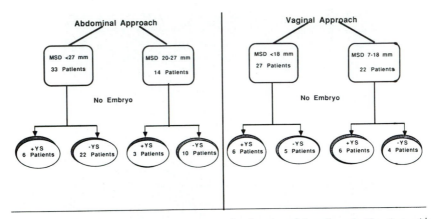

Fig 5–69.—Chart depicting first-trimester sonographic detection of the yolk sac in 49 patients with abnormal findings. *Abbreviations:* YS, yolk sac; MSD mean sac diameter; +, present; −, absent. (Courtesy of Kurtz AB, Needleman L, Pennell RG, et al: *AJR* 158:843–847, 1992.)

Findings.—The YS was visualized in 96% of cases of normal pregnancy. Among cases with a mean sac diameter below 27 mm on abdominal examination, there were 55 normal and 33 abnormal intrauterine pregnancies (Figs 5–68 and 5–69). The embryo was not seen in 28 normal and 28 abnormal pregnancies. In transvaginal studies as well, there was a fairly even distribution of visualization and lack of visualization of the YS in both normal and abnormal cases.

Conclusions.—The presence or absence of a YS in the first trimester cannot be used to determine whether a pregnancy is normal or abnormal.

▶ These 2 articles (Abstracts 5–63 and 5–64), both from reputable research groups, report nearly diametrically opposed results on the prognostic significance of visualization of the YS in early first-trimester pregnancies. What gives? A review of the materials and methods yields no significant flaws in protocol design in either study. However, a brief inspection of the example images in each paper reveals a marked difference in image quality. If we ascribe to the adage "one picture is worth a thousand words," then the study by Lindsay et al. appears to have used superior equipment or imaging technique and thus is the more accurate study. Unfortunately, we have only a few of the hundreds of images from the 2 studies to evaluate and must conclude that the determination of the prognostic significance of visualization of the YS in the first-trimester pregnancy will require at least 1 more study.—G. Dodd, III, M.D.

Correlation Between Omphalocele Contents and Karyotypic Abnormalities: Sonographic Study in 37 Cases

Getachew MM, Goldstein RB, Edge V, Goldberg JD, Filly RA (Univ of California, San Francisco)

AJR 158:133–136, 1991

5–65

Objective.—Previous findings suggest that fetuses whose omphaloceles contain only bowel and not liver have a particularly high proportion of karyotypic abnormalities. Thirty-seven fetuses found sonographically to have an omphalocele in 1984 to 1990 were reviewed.

Observations.—Nine fetuses had morphologic findings of amniotic band syndrome. In 22 of the other fetuses, the liver was exteriorized (Fig 5–70), whereas in 6 cases, the sac contained only bowel (Fig 5–71). Karyotyping was abnormal in 1 of the 16 fetuses tested with liver exteriorized. In contrast, 4 of the 6 fetuses whose sacs contained only bowel had abnormal karyotypic findings. The latter fetuses all had morphologic abnormalities other than omphalocele, whereas the 2 with normal karyotypes had no other abnormality.

Conclusions.—A small omphalocele or 1 containing only bowel should not be a source of reassurance. Karyotypic abnormalities are far more prevalent when liver is absent from the sac than when it is present.

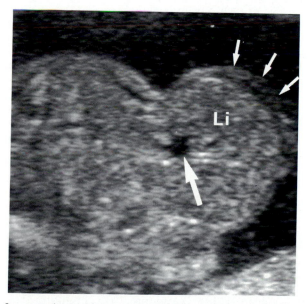

Fig 5–70.—Sonogram shows a liver-containing omphalocele. The lesion is covered by a membrane (*small arrows*). Portal vessel (*large arrow*) confirms that the mass within omphalocele is liver (Li). (Courtesy of Getachew MM, Goldstein RB, Edge V, et al: *AJR* 158:133–136, 1991.)

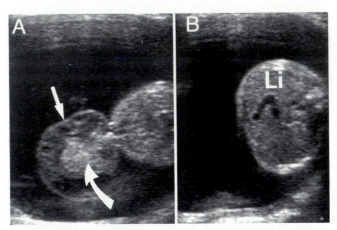

Fig 5–71.—Sonograms of a fetus with trisomy 18 show an omphalocele containing bowel only. **A,** ompalocele is covered by a membrane (*straight arrow*) and contains collapsed segments of bowel (*curved arrow*). **B,** liver (Li) is within fetal abdomen and is not exteriorized. This fetus also had a lumbosacral myelomeningocele (*not shown*). (Courtesy of Getachew MM, Goldstein RB, Edge V, et al: AJR 158:133–136, 1991.)

▶ Getachew et al. reinforce the significance of the contents over the size of omphaloceles as predictors of karyotypic abnormalities in fetuses. It is now well established that fetuses with omphaloceles that contain only bowel are much more likely to have a karyotypic abnormality than those with omphaloceles containing other abdominal viscera. Nonetheless, because all fetuses with omphaloceles (except those with obvious amniotic band syndrome or limb body wall complex) exhibit a high incidence of karyotypic abnormalities, karyotyping is recommended for all.—G. Dodd, III, M.D.

MR Techniques and Contrast Media

T1-Weighted Sequences for MR Imaging of the Liver: Comparison of Three Techniques for Single-Breath, Whole-Volume Acquisition at 1.0 and 1.5 T
Semelka RC, Simm FC, Recht M, Deimling M, Lenz G, Laub GA (Univ of Manitoba, St Boniface General Hospital, Winnipeg, Man, Canada; Medical Engineering Group, Siemens AG, Erlangen, Germany)
Radiology 180:629–635, 1991   5–66

Background.—Recently it has been suggested that standard short repetition time/echo time sequences do not achieve adequate T_1 weighting at high-field strength and that inversion recovery performs similarly to T_2-weighted sequences in lesion detection. However, inversion recovery is a lengthy sequence. Three T_1-weighted MRI techniques for acquiring images that encompass the entire liver in 1 breath hold were compared.

Methods and Results.—Twenty healthy volunteers were imaged at 1.0 or 1.5 T. Results were compared with those of regular short repetition time/echo time spin-echo imaging. Rapid acquisition spin echo was re-

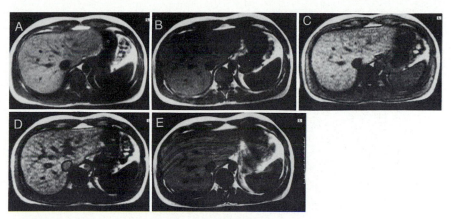

Fig 5–72.—Images of a healthy volunteer obtained at 1.5 tesla. **A**, FLASH; **B**, RASE; **C**, sequential single-section TurboFLASH; **D**, single-section TurboFLASH; **E**, spin echo. Saturation pulses were applied during FLASH, RASE, and spin-echo sequences, effectively removing flow artifacts. Higher S/N and SD/N of FLASH sequence compared with those of other sequences can be appreciated. (Courtesy of Semelka RC, Simm FC, Recht M, et al: *Radiology* 180:629–635, 1991.)

sistant to artifacts and had good image quality. However, it had the lowest liver signal/noise (S/N) and spleen-liver signal difference/noise (SD/N) values. Fast low-angle shot (FLASH) had the highest S/N and SD/N and unusually good image quality, with only mild artifacts. The Turbo-FLASH also had good S/N and SD/N. However, its reduced matrix size diminished image quality. All 3 sequences had better SD/N than regular spin echo; FLASH and TurboFLASH had greater S/N (Fig 5–72 and table).

Conclusions.—The FLASH sequence appears most attractive for T_1-weighted breath-hold imaging. In this series FLASH had the overall highest quantitative and qualitative ratings.

▶ Abdominal CT scanning improved considerably once the scan could be obtained during a single breath hold. This article reports similar findings for MRI. In the near future, these fast scan techniques will undoubtedly replace the standard T_1-weighted spin-echo sequence. In this series FLASH had the overall highest quantitative and qualitative ratings. However, the regular non–breath-hold spin-echo sequence was placed at a disadvantage by not using respiratory compensation techniques.—P.L. Davis, M.D.

Artifacts on Breath-Hold and Regular Spin-Echo Images

Severity of Artifacts	FLASH	RASE	Multisection TurboFLASH	Spin Echo
Severe	...	...	...	Ghosting (2, 1.5 T)
Moderate	Flow (8)	...	Pixel graininess (18) Phase cancellation (18)	Ghosting (10)
Mild	Truncation (10) Flow (10)	Flow (14)	Pixel graininess (2) Phase cancellation (2)	Ghosting (4)
Minimal	Truncation (10) Flow (2) Pixel graininess (20) Phase cancellation (10, 1.0 T)	Pixel graininess (20) Truncation (20) Flow (6)	...	Ghosting (3) Flow (6) Chemical shift (20)

Note: *Numbers in parentheses* represent the number of cases of artifacts in each category. (Courtesy of Semelka RC, Simm FC, Recht M, et al: *Radiology* 180:629–635, 1991.)

MR Imaging of the Portal Venous System: Value of Gradient-Echo Imaging as an Adjunct to Spin-Echo Imaging

Silverman PM, Patt RH, Garra BS, Horii SC, Cooper C, Hayes WS, Zeman RK
(Georgetown Univ Hosp, Washington, DC)

AJR 157:297–302, 1991   5–67

Introduction.—The portal venous system (PVS) has undergone successful noninvasive imaging, via CT, MRI, and sonography. Spin-echo (SE) MRI and gradient-recalled echo (GRE) pulse techniques have also proved useful in assessing the PVS. The GRE imaging outcomes of the portal vein in 16 patients with portal vein problems were reviewed and compared with GRE results in 15 volunteers.

Methods.—The 16 patients and 15 normal subjects all underwent PVS analysis of the portal vein at 1.5 T using fast imaging with steady-state free precision. Six volunteers and 15 patients underwent standard SE imaging also, whereas 13 of the 16 patients had CT examinations of the upper half of the abdomen.

Results.—The GRE images from the 15 volunteers demonstrated a high signal intensity in the PVS, but 9 of the 16 patients showed a decreased signal in the portal vein, which was isolated to the main portal vein in 4 and extended into the right or left branches in 5. Spin-echo imaging of this area in 6 volunteers confirmed it as an artifact. The GRE imaging demonstrated a thrombus or an occlusion with lower intensity in 8 of the 16 patients. Of 5 focal thrombi found by GRE imaging in patients, 3 were not confirmed by SE imaging. The SE and GRE images correlated with CT scans in 5 of 6 patients with extrinsic portal vein compression. One patient with an arteriovenous fistula found by GRE had this diagnosis confirmed by angiography. Nine patients had collateral vessels imaged by CT, sonography, or angiography, but only in 4 of these cases did GRE and SE techniques produce similar images. The linear or curvilinear low-intensity section seen on volunteers' GRE images was observed in patients but was found to be artifactual.

Conclusions.—These findings support the use of GRE MRI as an additional noninvasive method to assess problems with the PVS. The GRE technique produces a high contrast among the occlusion, the moving blood, and the tissues, and has the advantage of being a quick procedure for an often very sick patient.

▶ These findings support for the PVS what has been determined for vessels elsewhere in the body. Namely, GRE MRI usually provides the same or more vascular information than SE MRI. It has a particular advantage for the PVS in that images can be obtained in a single breath hold, substantially decreasing the motion artifact present with the SE techniques. It does not generate the slow-flow artifacts seen with the SE techniques. We have found it more sensitive to slow blood flow than the SE technique. It appears to have only 2 major limitations: (1) soft tissue contrast is absent, and (2) turbulence can cause false positive findings. The GRE technique should be used whenever blood flow and vascular morphology is being evaluated.—P.L. Davis, M.D.

Dynamic Gadolinium-Enhanced Rapid Acquisition Spin-Echo MR Imaging of the Liver

Mirowitz SA, Lee JKT, Gutierrez E, Brown JJ, Heiken JP, Eilenberg SS (Washington Univ, St Louis)
Radiology 179:371–376, 1991   5–68

Background.—Rapid acquisition spin-echo (RASE) MRI enables the whole liver to be covered with highly T_1-weighted SE images in a single 23-second breath-holding period. The RASE sequence was used with rapid intravenous injection of gadopentetate dimeglumine in the dynamic contrast material-enhanced MRI of the liver.

Methods and Findings.—Twenty-four patients with 62 liver lesions 1 cm or more in diameter were studied. The RASE images were devoid of respiratory-related ghost artifacts and blurring at the edges. Dynamic contrast-enhanced RASE was associated with contrast/noise and contrast/artifact values and time efficiency measures that were significantly better than those associated with the use of conventional T_1- and T_2-weighted pulse sequences. This indicated a greater likelihood for lesion detectability. Lesion conspicuity was highest during or just after bolus administration of gadopentetate dimeglumine. Lesions often became obscured at delayed postcontrast imaging.

Conclusions.—This method successfully eliminated respiratory-related ghost artifacts and edge blurring and was implemented effectively with a bolus injection of gadopentetate dimeglumine, resulting in dynamic SE liver imaging. It also considerably improved quantitative measures of hepatic lesion conspicuity over conventional T_1- and T_2-weighted sequences.

▶ Computed tomography detection of liver lesions improves substantially when a bolus of iodinated contrast agent is used. This article demonstrates a *quantitative* improvement of hepatic lesion conspicuity when a Gd bolus is given during rapid MRI compared with conventional T_1- and T_2-weighted MR sequences. However, the lack of respiratory motion compensation techniques and the differences in slice thickness and phasing encoding steps between the T_2-weighted series and the RASE technique favors the noise statistics for RASE. The authors themselves state that a large double-blind study using the more qualitative receiver operatior characteristic analysis is necessary. I agree that this is necessary before the recommendation of Gd-enhanced fast imaging should become part of the routine MR liver study. Differences in manufacturer supplied imaging techniques may even make the decision machine dependent.—P.L. Davis, M.D.

Dynamic MR Imaging of the Abdomen With Gadopentetate Dimeglumine: Normal Enhancement Patterns of the Liver, Spleen, Stomach, and Pancreas

Hamed MM, Hamm B, Ibrahim ME, Taupitz M, Mahfouz AE (Freie Universität Berlin, Berlin, Germany)
AJR 158:303–307, 1992   5–69

Background.—The contrast enhancement pattern on MR images can be used to differentiate normal or diseased organs. Intravenous injection of Gd-DTPA has been useful for dynamic contrast-enhanced MRI of the abdominal organs. Changes in signal intensity and the enhancement patterns of the liver, spleen, pancreas, and stomach on dynamic Gd-DTPA-enhanced MR images were described.

Methods.—Almost all of the patients, 26 women and 22 men, had originally been examined for focal liver lesions. None of them had diffuse parenchymal disease of any of the examined organs. The subjects underwent MRI with a heavily T_1-weighted gradient-echo sequence (100/5 [repetition time/echo time], 80-degree flip angle). Imaging was performed before and repeatedly for a period of 10 minutes after an intravenous bolus injection of Gd-DTPA. Signal enhancement in the liver, spleen, pancreas, and stomach was calculated by measuring the differences in unenhanced and enhanced signal intensity.

Results.—The pancreas, liver, stomach wall, spleen, and renal cortex showed a pronounced signal enhancement within the first 2 minutes and a subsequent continuous decline thereafter. The peak signal enhancement of all organs was seen at 45 seconds after injection of contrast medium. The liver and pancreas showed homogenous enhancement pattern throughout the examination, whereas the spleen appeared heterogenous during the first 60 seconds and homogenous thereafter. The gastric wall had a hyperintense inner zone and a hypointense outer zone. The renal cortex showed the highest enhancement peak of all organs examined.

Conclusions.—The characteristic normal pattern of Gd-DTPA enhancement was homogenous in the liver and pancreas, early heterogenous enhancement of the spleen, followed by homogenous enhancement, and hyperintense enhancement of the inner zone of the gastric wall.

▶ Gadopentetate dimeglumine is a paramagnetic agent with pharmacokinetic properties similar to those of iodinated contrast material. It is cleared mainly by renal excretion and rapidly equilibrates between the intravascular and interstitial compartments. It is well established as a nonspecific contrast medium that improves sensitivity but not specificity in brain imaging. Uses in body MRI have lagged behind because lesion/organ contrast is often decreased when using standard spin-echo sequences that last more than 2 minutes, when much of the contrast agent has reached tissue equilibrium. New studies with various fast MR pulse sequences make possible rapid dynamic scanning during and after bolus infusion of Gd-DTPA. These suggest improved sensitivity and specificity with liver and kidney imaging showing the greatest potential. This manuscript is a useful primer and reference for normal patterns of parenchymal enhancement with Gd-DTPA.—M.P. Federle, M.D.

Focal Liver Lesions: MR Imaging With Mn-DPDP: Initial Clinical Results in 40 Patients

Hamm B, Vogl TJ, Branding G, Schnell B, Taupitz M, Wolf K-J, Lissner J (Freie Universität Berlin, Germany; Ludwig-Maximilians-Universität, Munich, Germany)
Radiology 182:167–174, 1992   5–70

Background.—A number of different contrast agents have been used to improve MRI of focal liver lesions. Manganese (II) N,N′-dipyridoxyl-ethylenediamine-N,N′-diacetate-5,5′-bis(phosphate) (Mn-DPDP) is a new paramagnetic contrast agent that has demonstrated early signal enhancement of the liver and sustained signal intensity up to 30 minutes after intravenous injection. The clinical results with Mn-DPDP–enhanced MRI on patients with suspected liver neoplasms were described.

Methods.—Forty patients with suspected liver lesions on the basis of ultrasound (US) or CT examinations underwent MRI. The subjects received intravenous Mn-DPDP doses of 5 or 10 μmol/kg. The Mn-DPDP–enhanced T_1-weighted images were compared quantitatively and subjectively with standard T_1-and T_2-weighted nonenhanced images. Patient tolerance, based on tests of potential cardiovascular, hematologic, renal, and hepatobiliary effects, was also evaluated.

Results.—After doses of Mn-DPDP, 5 and 10 umol/kg, selective signal enhancement of the liver parenchyma improved the visualization of nonenhancing malignant lesions relative to precontrast images (Fig 5–73). The demarcation of the nonenhancing lesions and the distinction between sharply demarcated, lobulated, and diffusely infiltrating tumors was clearest in the Mn-DPDP-enhanced images. Benign lesions could also be classified as either enhancing or nonenhancing. The lesion/liver contrast in Mn-DPDP–enhanced gradient-recalled echo images was superior to precontrast images. The number of nonenhancing malignant liver lesions detected in spin-echo images was increased from 272 in T_2-weighted spin-echo images to 390 in T_1-weighted Mn-DPDP–enhanced spin-echo images (Fig 5–74).

Conclusions.—In these 40 patients, Mn-DPDP was well-tolerated and improved the ability to assess nonenhancing malignant liver lesions when compared with precontrast images. The finding of Mn-DPDP uptake in hepatocellular carcinomas may enable distinction of primary hepatocellular carcinomas from secondary malignant liver tumors.

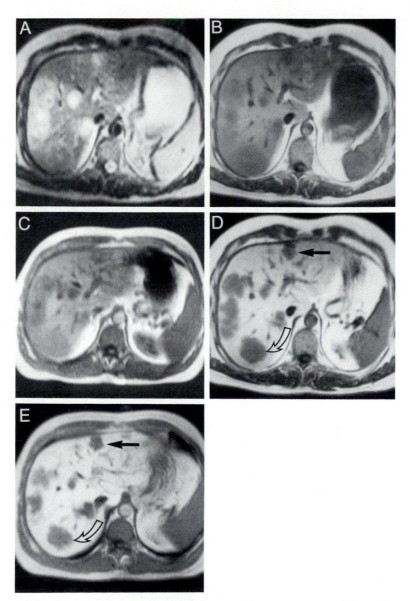

Fig 5–73.—Magnetic resonance images show metastatic colon carcinoma **(A–C)** before and **(D, E)** after administration of Mn-DPDP, 10 μmol/kg. There is a pronounced increase in signal intensity of liver parenchyma in the postcontrast images **(D, E)** compared with the T1-weighted precontrast images **(B, C)**. The metastases, which do not show signal enhancement, are more conspicuous in the postcontrast images than in all precontrast images. Note sharper demarcation of all lesions and better visualization of the larger metastasis in the right liver lobe (*curved arrow*) and of the metastasis in the left lobe (*straight arrow*) in Mn-DPDP–enhanced images. The signal enhancement of the liver and the lesion-to-liver contrast after administration of Mn-DPDP is most pronounced in the heavily T1-weighted GRE image **(E)**. **A,** spin echo 2,300/90 image. **B** and **D,** spin echo 500/15 images. **C** and **E,** gradient-recalled-echo 160/5 images, with a flip angle of 80 degrees. (Courtesy of Hamm B, Vogl TJ, Branding G, et al: *Radiology* 182:167–174, 1992.)

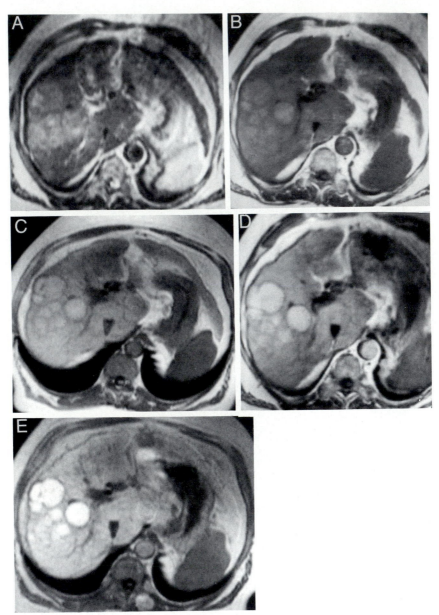

Fig 5–74.—Magnetic resonance images show liver cirrhosis and multiple lesion of hepatocellular carcinoma obtained **(A–C)** before and **(D, E)** after administration of Mn-DPDP, 10 μmol/kg. Compared with the T1-weighted precontrast images **(B, C)**, the masses in the tight hepatic lobe show a pronounced and homogeneous signal enhancement after administration of the contrast agent **(D, E)**, making the masses more conspicuous. Peritumor pseudocapsules remain as hypointense rims. Again, the signal enhancement is more pronounced in the T1-weighted gradient-recalled-echo image **(E)** than in the T1-weighted spin-echo image **(D)**. The paraspinous mass on the left in **E** corresponds to a pulsation artifact from the aorta. **A,** spin-echo 2,300/90 image. **B** and **D,** spin-echo 500/15 images. **C** and **E,** gradient-recalled-echo 160/5 images, with a flip angle of 80 degrees. (Courtesy of Hamm B, Vogl TJ, Branding G, et al: *Radiology* 182:167–174, 1992.)

▶ The paramagnetic contrast agent Mn-DPDP has several attractive features that suggest an important role in future MRI of the liver. It has relatively low toxicity, though requiring a slow drip infusion over 10 minutes. The liver enhancement it produces lasts several hours, extending the "imaging window" well beyond that which is practical for Gd-DTPA (1–2 minutes), the only commercially available MR contrast agent. Only T_1-weighted images need to be obtained after Mn-DPDP infusion because it is a predominantly T_1-relaxing agent. This allows excellent anatomical resolution and good demarcation of tumor margins and blood vessels.

Some problems remain with this agent, however. Overall toxicity remains undetermined because patients with an "allergic" history were excluded from the study. The uptake of Mn-DPDP in all hepatocytes, normal or abnormal, is a mixed blessing. Regenerating modules, focal nodular hyperplasia, and liver adenomas will enhance, presumably nearly rendering them isointense with the liver in many cases, but they can be differentiated reliably from most other tumors by this effect. However, hepatocellular carcinoma also takes up Mn-DPDP, and I would predict that detection of hepatoma in cirrhotic livers will remain extremely difficult. Distinguishing liver lesions from blood vessels will remain difficult on Mn-DPDP enhanced scans as well, because both will appear as hypointense areas.—M.P. Federle, M.D.

The Value of Barium as a Gastrointestinal Contrast Agent in MR Imaging: A Comparison Study in Normal Volunteers

Ros PR, Steinman RM, Torres GM, Burton SS, Panaccione JL, Rappaport DC, McGorray SP (Univ of Florida, Gainesville, Fla; Methodist Hosp, Jacksonville, Fla)

AJR 157:761–767, 1991   5–71

Background.—Barium sulfate suspension may be a useful negative gastrointestinal contrast agent for MRI. This hypothesis was tested in a controlled study.

Methods.—Abdominal and pelvic MR images were obtained in 10 healthy volunteers before and after oral and rectal administration of barium. Three observers interpreted the standard spin-echo coronal T_1-, axial T_1-, proton density–, and T_2-weighted images, obtained at 1.5 T. Several bowel segments and anatomical structures were examined.

Results.—There was a significant improvement in both bowel visualization and definition of normal anatomy after administration of barium, especially on the T_1-weighted images. Improvement in bowel visualization ranged from 59% to 123%, depending on the segment, and improvement in normal anatomy delineation ranged from 23% to 68%, depending on the structure. Barium was tolerated well and did not produce artifacts (Fig 5–75).

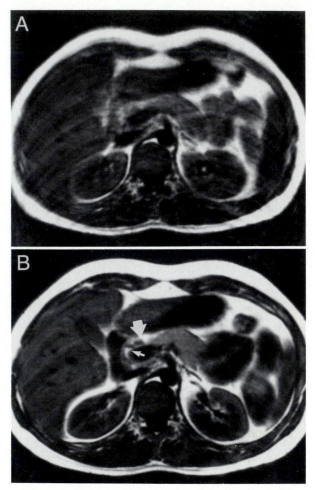

Fig 5–75.—Axial T1-weighted MR images of duodenum-pancreas. Compared with a prebarium MR image **(A)**, good marking of duodenal sweep and proximal jejunum is seen after administration of barium **(B)**. The duodenum and proximal bowel are also well delineated, with good visualization of the adjacent structures such as the portal vein, body of the pancreas, and the left adrenal gland. The hepatic artery (*long arrow*) and common bile duct (*short arrow*) can be identified. (Courtesy of Ros PR, Steinman RM, Torres GM, et al: *AJR* 157:761–767, 1991.)

Conclusions.—Barium sulfate is a useful negative gastrointestinal contrast agent for MRI. It improves bowel visualization and the delineation of abdominal anatomy, especially on T_1-weighted sequences.

▶ This report demonstrates that barium sulfate suspensions can improve the visualization of bowel and its differentiation from other abdominal and pelvic structures. This will become more important as attempts are made to extend MRI's usefulness from organ-contained disease to disease extending from the organ and in the specific case of the pancreas. Several agents are being studied as potential gastrointestinal MRI contrast agents. In addition to barium sulfate, these include water, iron particle suspensions, paramagnetic solutions, and emulsions. Barium sulfate has the advantage of being 1 of the simpler. However, better bowel demarcation has been seen with other agents, such as perfluoroctylbromide. Further studies will help determine which agents will be optimal under which situations.—P.L. Davis, M.D.

Experimental Hepatocellular Carcinoma: MR Receptor Imaging

Reimer P, Weissleder R, Brady TJ, Yeager AE, Baldwin BH, Tennant BC, Wittenberg J (Massachusetts Gen Hosp, Harvard Med School, Boston; Cornell Univ, Ithaca, NY)

Radiology 180:641–645, 1991   5–72

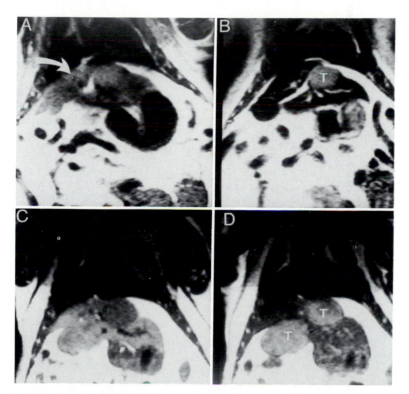

Fig 5–76.—Spin-echo MRI (500/30, 4 signals averaged) shows woodchuck hepatoma (T = tumor) imaged before (**A, C**) and after (**B, D**) intravenous administration of 10 μmol Fe/kg of arabinogalactan -stabilized, ultrasmall, super paramagnetic iron oxide (AG-USPIO) (**A, B**) or AMI-25 (**C, D**). The receptor agent decreases the liver signal intensity to a greater degree than does the reticuloendothelial system agent. As a result, the contrast between the liver and the HCC is higher in **B** than in **D**. A hyperintense area (*curved arrow* in **A**) was proved to correspond to a regenerating nodule. This area decreases homogeneously in signal intensity after intravenous administration of the receptor agent (**B**). (Courtesy of Reimer P, Weissleder R, Brady TJ, et al: *Radiology* 180:641–645, 1991.)

Background.—Hepatocellular carcinoma (HCC), the most common primary malignant liver tumor in the world, is often associated with the hepatitis B virus. Structural abnormalities of the liver are common, tumor detection is often obscured. Relaxation time measurements and MRI were done in 3 different animal models of HCC.

Methods and Findings.—After asialoglycoprotein-directed arabinoga-lactan-stabilized ultrasmall superparamagnetic iron oxide was administered intravenously to rats, the T_2 of normal liver declined from 41.6 msec to 19.4 msec. However, the T_2 of HCC implanted in normal liver or in liver with chronic hepatitis essentially did not change. Although these findings were comparable to those obtained by administration of a reticuloendothelial cell–directed conventional iron oxide, the required dose of receptor agent was lower. In a woodchuck model of virally induced HCC, MRI confirmed the hepatocyte-directed agent distribution to areas of functioning and differentiated hepatocytes but not malignant tumor tissue (Figs 5–76 and 5–77).

Conclusions.—Magnetic resonance receptor imaging improves the detection of HCC in normal and diseased liver because of the preferential biodistribution of the receptor agents. The increased relaxivity of receptor-specific agents can be used to reduce the dose or achieve greater contrast.

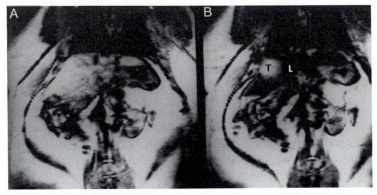

Fig 5–77.—Gradient-recalled-echo MRI (120/16, 70-degree flip angle, 4 signals averaged) shows woodchuck HCC before (**A**) and after (**B**) administration of the receptor agent (dose, 2 μmol Fe/kg) (L = liver). With this low dose, the carbon/nitrogen ratio (C/N) increased from − 3.9 ± 2.7 to 18.9± 3.7. The tumor (T) is readily detectable after administration of the receptor agent (**B**). (Courtesy of Reimer P, Weissleder R, Brady TJ, et al: *Radiology* 180:641-645, 1991.)

▶ This MR contrast agent consists of 2 components: (1) a very small iron oxide particle that causes T_2 relaxation time to decrease, and (2) a galactose-containing polysaccharide coating that causes the particle to be picked up by a unique liver cell receptor absent in hepatomas. Therefore, this agent is fundamentally different from the nonspecific Gd-base agents and closer to the organ specific agents used in nuclear medicine. The potential exists to coat the iron particle with other organ-specific compounds and even attach it to antibodies. Although these agents will not be available for human MRI soon, they have the potential of changing MRI applications in the future.—P.L. Davis, M.D.

6 Pediatric Radiology

Introduction

It seems that there were more pediatric radiology–related articles to choose from for this 1993 YEAR BOOK. I've not counted them or researched it, but I like to think that interest in pediatric radiology is up and a lot is being written. Whatever the reason, the effort of selecting, abstracting, and commenting is balanced by the satisfaction that the articles selected are informative and stimulating.

The samplings from the broad pool are arranged into 5 organ system categories: (1) neuroendocrine, (2) musculoskeletal, (3) cardiopulmonary, (4) gastrointestinal, and (5) genitourinary. The neuroendocrine category—modified from the neurologic category in the 1992 YEAR BOOK—combines topics on neural crest tissues and endocrine glands with those on CNS.

In this organ system format, I've attempted to place mainly technical or ancillary subject matter with the category to which it is more frequently associated or on which it has significant impact. For example, a pediatric radiation dose article is placed in the genitourinary category or a digital radiography article is placed in the cardiopulmonary category.

References to recent or pertinent articles of related interest are listed after each comment. Sometimes a reference might be as good as the indexed article, might offer another valid point of view, or might allow inclusion of a related topic that merits attention.

The 1993 pediatric radiology section features such appealing topics as flow-sensitive MRI of venipuncture shunts, intraoperative sonography of spinal cord lesions and soft tissue arteriovenous malformations, color Doppler waveforms in normal renal arteries, a recurrent and familial Caffey's disease, ifosfamide rickets, tonsillitis complicated by MRI-demonstrated pseudoaneurysm of the carotid artery, MRI findings of radiation recall supraglottitis, MRI distinctions of dysmyelinating leukodystrophies, the scourge of maternal cocaine shown on neonatal brain MRI, dynamic infant hip sonography, and radionuclide imaging of acute pyelonephritis.

In each category, abstracts and comments are sequenced in a consistent order beginning with technique, to normal variations, to congenital/develomental, to inflammatory/infectious, to neoplastic, to traumatic, to metabolic, and on to miscellaneous.

It should be abundantly clear that all diagnostic imaging modalities have application in pediatrics. More and more advances in pediatric radiology, especially with ultrasound, CT, and MRI, are coming from the hands of general pediatric radiologists but, fortunately, not exclusively. Others who work in the field of diagnostic radiology make major contributions. What is important in this process is that the best surfaces for the benefit of the pediatric patient.

This enjoyable endeavor could not be done without the gentle overseeing hand of Bernadette Buchholz, the help of her YEAR BOOK OF DIAGNOSTIC RADIOLOGY staff, and the invaluable secretarial and librarial assistance of Barbara Longo from my office—my thanks to them!

Lionel W. Young, M.D.

Neuroendocrine

Sedation for Pediatric Patients Undergoing CT and MRI
Hubbard AM, Markowitz RI, Kimmel B, Kroger M, Bartko MB (Children's Hosp of Philadelphia, Philadelphia)
J Comput Assist Tomogr 16:3–6, 1992   6–1

Background.—Sedation can be the most difficult part of performing CT and MRI in children. The effectiveness and safety of a standard sedation protocol for these patients was evaluated.

Methods.—A team of trained pediatric critical care nurses administered sedation to 1,158 children over an 11-month period. The protocol recommended chloral hydrate, 60 to 75 mg/kg orally, followed by a second dose as needed, for children less than age 18 months, and pentobarbital sodium (Nembutal), 2 to 6 mg/kg intravenously, for children older than age 18 months. Other regimens were sometimes used for children with previous sedation problems and some older children who needed some sedation but not intravenous sedation. Sedation records were reviewed on a monthly basis by a nurse and a physician.

Results.—A total of 407 outpatients were sedated for CT; inpatients were not included in the analysis. Two hundred sixty-five patients received chloral hydrate orally, average dose 80 mg/kg, and 25% required a second dose; 115 patients received pentobarbital intravenously, average dose 3.3 mg/kg. Sedation was successful in 97% of cases.

A total of 75 patients were sedated for MRI. Two hundred fifty-nine patients received chloral hydrate orally, average dose 82 mg/kg; 420 received pentobarbital intravenously, average dose 4.2 mg/kg. Sedation was successful in 96% of cases. For both CT and MRI, there was a 3% rate of transient hypoxia. Alternative sedation regimens were used for various indications in 108 patients, including intravenous morphine added to pentobarbital; oral pentobarbital and meperidine (Demerol), which has since been discontinued; intravenous midazolam (versed), and oral diazepam (Valium). Two serious complications occurred: a decrease in oxygen saturation to 70% in a patient who received oral pentobarbital and meperidine and wheezing in an asthmatic patient who received intravenous pentobarbital.

Discussion.—Chloral hydrate appears to be an effective sedative in most infants, and pentobarbital is effective in most older children. The safety of the sedation protocols has been enhanced by electronic monitoring and nursing observation.

▶ Sedation of infants and children for multiplanar imaging continues to be a subject of concern and discussion. These authors affirm the use of pentobarbital or chloral hydrate as the most reliable of agents for safety and effectiveness. With passage of each year there are improvements in regimens proposed and new or refined anesthetic agents. Based on a double-blind study of rectal midazolam as sedation for CT, Coventry et al. (1) determined that it is not a reliable agent for CT sedation. Recent articles of related interest on sedation for diagnostic imaging in children are listed (2–4).—L.W. Young, M.D.

References

1. Coventry DM, et al: *Eur J Anaesthesiol* 8:29, 1991.
2. Neuman GG, et al: *Anesth Analg* 74:931, 1992.
3. Bissett GS III, et al: *Semin Ultrasound CT MR* 12:376, 1991.
4. 1992 YEAR BOOK OF DIAGNOSTIC RADIOLOGY, p 371.

Cerebellar Dimensions in Assessment of Gestational Age in Neonates
Co E, Raju TNK, Aldana O (Univ of Illinois, Chicago)
Radiology 181:581–585, 1991   6–2

Background.—Neonates at high risk routinely undergo cranial ultrasound (US). It would be useful if cerebellar dimensions obtained with US could be used to assess gestational age. However, normative data for various cerebellar dimensions have not been published, and their clinical value in predicting gestational age has not been determined.

Methods.—Authors measured the computed area and circumference, and vertical length of the vermis and the computed area and circumference, and maximum transverse width of the cerebellar body in 80 healthy neonates (Fig 6–1). They then correlated these dimensions with clinical assessments of gestational age (table). A color Doppler flow scanner with a 5-MHz short-focus transducer was used for US.

Results.—There was a strong relationship between gestational age and all cerebellar measurements; however, the area and circumference of the vermis were better than the maximum transverse cerebellar width in predicting gestational age. Dimensions increased as a linear function of gestation between 25 and 41 weeks. Multiple regression models using a single vermis measurement and either the cerebellar area or circumference further improved predictability of gestational age. No nonlinear models

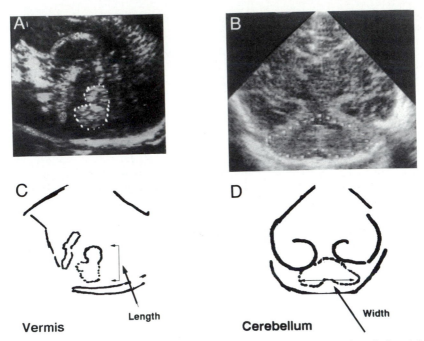

Fig 6–1.—The vermis measurements were made with the midline sagittal view (**A** and **B**), and the cerebellar measurements were made with the coronal view via the quadrigeminal cistern (**C** and **D**). When the electronic caliper markings are placed around the vermis and cerebellar body (*dotted areas* in **A** and **C**), the area and circumference values are displayed by the built-in computer. The method of measurement of the vertical length of vermis (**B**) and the maximum transverse width of the cerebellum (**D**), respectively, is shown. (Courtesy of Co E, Raju TNK, Aldana O: *Radiology* 181:581–585, 1991.)

corresponded to the cerebellar growth data better than linear models. Cerebellar measurements also correlated strongly with clinically determined gestational age in subgroups of premature neonates, neonates small for their gestational age, and neonates in whom clinical and obstetric assessments of gestational age varied by more than 2 weeks.

Conclusions.—The vermis can be measured during the course of routine neonatal cranial US, and its dimensions can be used to assess gestational age. The result can corroborate clinical estimations. Changes in the vermis "area" during gestation are roughly 1 cm at 25 weeks, 2 cm at 30 weeks, 3 cm at 35 weeks, and 4 cm at term. Further studies—especially those that focus on extreme prematurity—may clarify the clinical value of this method and provide more narrow gestational-age prediction bands based on these dimensions.

▶ Vermian measurements can be used with cerebellar dimensions obtained by US in assessing gestational age. Sonographic vermian measurements alone may be better than the sonographic cerebellar measurements alone, but they are even more accurate together. In utero, the vermian measurement might be used in conjunction with the standard biparietal diameter and

Gestational Age and Cerebellar Measures

Gestational Age (wk)	Vermis Area (cm)		Cerebellar Circumference (cm)	
	Mean	95% CI	Mean	95% CI
25	1.07	0.8–1.3	6.88	6.4–7.3
26	1.27	1.0–1.5	7.21	6.8–7.6
27	1.46	1.3–1.7	7.53	7.2–7.9
28	1.66	1.5–1.8	7.87	7.5–8.2
29	1.86	1.7–2.0	8.19	7.9–8.5
30	2.05	1.9–2.2	8.52	8.3–8.8
31	2.25	2.1–2.4	8.85	8.6–9.1
32	2.45	2.3–2.6	9.18	8.9–9.4
33	2.64	2.5–2.8	9.50	9.3–9.7
34	2.84	2.7–3.0	9.83	9.6–10.1
35	3.03	2.9–3.2	10.16	9.9–10.4
36	3.23	3.1–3.4	10.49	10.2–10.8
37	3.43	3.2–3.6	10.82	10.5–11.1
38	3.62	3.4–3.8	11.14	10.8–11.5
39	3.82	3.6–4.0	11.47	11.1–11.9
40	4.02	3.8–4.3	11.80	11.4–12.2
41	4.21	3.9–4.5	12.12	11.7–12.6

Abbreviation: CI, confidence interval.
(Courtesy of Co E, Raju TNK, Aldana O: *Radiology* 181:581–585, 1991.)

length of femur sonographic measurements to arrive at gestational age. Recent articles of related interest are listed (1, 2).—L.W. Young, M.D.

References

1. Segura-Roldan MA, et al: *Ginecol Obstet Mex* 60:33, 1992.
2. Lee W, et al: *Am J Obstet Gynecol* 165:1044, 1991.

Intramedullary Lesions of the Pediatric Spinal Cord: Correlation of Findings From MR Imaging, Intraoperative Sonography, Surgery, and Histologic Study
Brunberg JA, DiPietro MA, Venes JL, Dauser RC, Muraszko KM, Berkey GS, D'Amato CJ, Rubin JM (Univ of Michigan, Ann Arbor, Mich)
Radiology 181:573–579, 1991   6–3

Background.—Preoperative MRI displays detailed anatomy, but it does not show internal cord anatomy. Intraoperative sonography (IOS) does provide this capability. Many surgeons use IOS to localize intraspinal masses, but previous studies have not directly compared MRI with IOS.

Methods.—Eleven patients, aged 2 to 15 years, who had intramedullary spinal cord mass lesions underwent preoperative MRI and radiologist-directed IOS. Radiologists performed IOS after laminectomy and

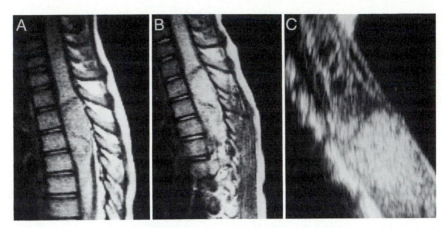

Fig 6–2.—Spinal cord venous angioma. **A** and **B**, magnetic resonance images (600/20 and 2,500/60) at .35 tesla. Sagittal T2-weighted image (**B**) is off axis relative to **A** because of movement between sequences. **C**, intraoperative sonography performed before the dura mater is opened demonstrates increased echogenicity of the venous angioma, with linear regions of echogenicity within the cord at the rostral extent of the angioma, possibly representing venous pathways. (Courtesy of Brunberg JA, DiPietro MA, Venes JL, et al: *Radiology* 181:573–579, 1991.)

before the surgeon opened the dura mater. Findings from MRI were correlated with those from IOS.

Results.—Both modalities demonstrated internal architecture and cord contour well; however, neither MRI nor IOS provided specific solid tissue characterization. Tumors, gliosis, and edema were more echogenic than normal cord parenchyma, but in some cases, edema and gliosis could not be differentiated from tumor margins. However, with IOS, the surgeon could assess the completeness of tumor evacuation, the re-expansion of subarachnoid spaces, the effectiveness of drainage, or the position of an implanted shunt device. In 1 patient with spinal cord venous angioma, the mass was isointense on both T_1- and T_2-weighted images (Fig 6–2). Before the dura mater was opened, IOS demonstrated fusiform cord enlargement with diffusely increased echogenicity at the site of enlargement. When the dura mater was opened, there were enlarged veins on the cord surface.

Conclusions.—Magnetic resonance imaging and IOS are complementary techniques for imaging intramedullary cord lesions. Cord contour and structural intramedullary abnormalities seen on MRI can be quickly correlated with IOS images, allowing rapid intraoperative localization of lesions and correlation with MRI findings before the dura mater is opened. Combined IOS and preoperative MRI provided precise localization for determining the extent of the laminectomy and for defining the location and extent of myelotomy. In patients with intramedullary spinal cord lesions, surgeons can use a more specific surgical approach, accomplish a more complete resection, and reduce long-term morbidity by using a combined technique of preoperative MRI and IOS.

▶ The clear preoperative definition of gross CNS anatomy and pathology by MRI is wonderfully balanced by the facility of intraoperative sonography to refine in real-time delicate internal CNS morphopathology. Color Doppler ultrasound for intraoperative CNS imaging also is considerably useful (1). Intraoperative sonography has also been used with success in a musculoskeletal soft tissue tumor surgery (2).—L.W. Young, M.D.

References

1. Barr LL, et al: *Radiology* 181:567, 1991.
2. Bober SE, et al: *Orthopedics* 14:1007, 1991.

Flow-Sensitive MR Imaging of Ventriculoperitoneal Shunts: In Vitro Findings, Clinical Applications, and Pitfalls

Castillo M, Hudgins PA, Malko JA, Burrow BK, Hoffman JC Jr (Emory Univ, Atlanta, Ga)
AJNR 12:667–671, 1991   6–4

Background.—Partial flip angle imaging is extremely sensitive to flow, particularly when the radiologist uses large flip angles. However, the technique has not been used to assess ventriculoperitoneal shunt patency. Use of fast-field-echo (FFE) T_1-weighted sequences was studied to evaluate CSF shunt patency in 23 patients.

Methods.—Fourteen male and 9 female patients had ventriculoperitoneal shunts placed for hydrocephalus resulting from intracranial neoplasia, Chiari malformation, neonatal meningitis, or idiopathic causes. Shunts had been in place for 3 months to 10 years before the study. To determine the sensitivity of the FFE sequences in identifying CSF flow in the shunt, a phantom was constructed. Patients' studies

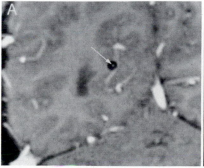 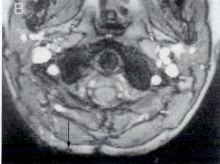

Fig 6–3.—A, oblique coronal T1-weighted flow-sensitive image (130/11/2, with 90-degree flip angle) through intraparenchymal portion of a shunt (medium-pressure valve system). Note the bright signal intensity within the shunt (*arrow*), indicating active CSF flow. **B,** an axial image (130/11/2, with 90-degree flip angle) of the neck of the same patient as in **A** shows bright signal intensity (*arrow*). (Courtesy of Castillo M, Hudgins PA, Malko JA, et al: *AJNR* 12:667–671, 1991.)

were compared with previous MRI or CT, paying particular attention to ventricular size. Current clinical histories were also examined for symptoms indicative of shunt malfunction. The FFE studies were divided into 2 groups: those with high-signal intensity and those with no signal.

Results.—Eighteen FFE studies showed shunt flow (Fig 6-3), and 5 showed no flow. In 17 cases with high signal intensity consistent with CSF flow, the patients had medium-pressure valve shunts; 1 patient had a high-pressure valve shunt. All 5 patients in whom no signal was seen had high-pressure valve shunts. Three of these 5 patients also had clinical evidence of probable shunt malfunction; however, 2 had patent shunts at surgery, and 1 had true shunt malfunction. The 2 patients with patent shunts at surgery might have had temporary shunt obstruction at the time of MRI and clinical evaluation. The remaining 2 patients had no clinical evidence of shunt malfunction. The MRI findings probably reflected periodic CSF flow. One patient who showed no flow on MRI had an unconnected intracranial segment. There were no false positive FFE findings, (e.g., apparent flow in a nonfunctioning shunt). A phantom confirmed clinical observations.

Conclusions.—Imaging with FFE T_1-weighted sequences may be a practical and noninvasive method of determining the patency of medium-pressure shunt systems in patients undergoing routine MRI of the head. At present, the method cannot be recommended for patients with high-pressure shunt systems.

▶ Fast-field-echo or flow-sensitive MRI is a promising new method for determining CSF shunt malfunction. The authors beautifully combine inventive bench research with clinical observations. The technique may be used either as an alternative to or in conjunction with continuous pressure monitoring, radionuclide imaging, and thermography in selected and difficult diagnostic cases. Recent articles of related interest are listed (1–5).—L.W. Young, M.D.

References

1. McLone DG: *AJNR* 12:673, 1991.
2. Frank E, et al: *Childs Nerv Syst* 8:73, 1992.
3. Drake JM, et al: *J Neurosurg* 75:535, 1991.
4. Hennig J, et al: *Magn Reson Imaging* 8:543, 1990.
5. Bradley WG Jr, et al: *Radiology* 178:459, 1991.

The Dandy-Walker Syndrome
Hutterer C, Baierl P, Ring-Mrozik E, Muller M (Univ Munich, Munich, Germany)
Z Kinderchir 34:14–15, 1990   6–5

Introduction.—The Dandy-Walker syndrome is marked by cystic dilatation of the fourth ventricle, severe hydrocephalus, cerebellar hemi-

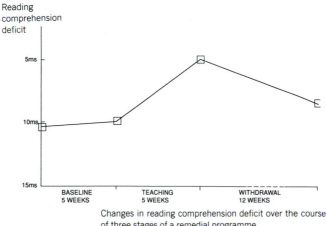

Changes in reading comprehension deficit over the course of three stages of a remedial programme

Fig 6–4.—Midline sagittal spin-echo MR image showing elevated tentorium and hypoplastic cerebellar vermis. (Courtesy of Hutterer C, Baierl P, Ring-Mrozik E, et al: *Z Kinderchir* 34:14–15, 1991.)

spheric separation, and absence of the Luschka and Magendie foraminae. Ten patients with the Dandy-Walker syndrome underwent MRI, and the studies were reviewed to determine the cranial characteristics of this disorder.

Methods.—The records of 10 young patients with Dandy-Walker syndrome were reviewed for initial signs and symptoms and for the presence of related abnormalities. The patients also underwent MRI studies.

Results.—The chief initial symptoms were an obvious growth in head circumference during the first 12 months of life and motor development delay, found in 3 patients. Another patient had microcephaly and multiple dysmorphia. One patient had unexplained seizures and a normal head size, but MR images showed a Dandy-Walker malformation. In 3 children aged 2 to 5 years, the Dandy-Walker syndrome symptoms included severe hydrocephalus and hemiparesis. More than three fourths of the children had congenital anomalies, including spina bifida, hypertelorism, aqueductal stenosis, craniofacial dysmorphia, syndactyly, and mitochondrial myopathia. Magnetic resonance imaging proved more useful than CT for radiographic diagnosis of the syndrome (Fig 6–4). The MRI findings included cystic dilatation of the fourth ventricle, agenesis of the vermis, hypoplasia of the cerebellar hemispheres, and a high position of the tentorium.

Conclusion.—Definitive diagnosis of the Dandy-Walker syndrome is dependent on thorough radiologic evaluation. Information gained from MRI is particularly valuable.

▶ Magnetic resonance imaging is particularly valuable in the imaging of Dandy-Walker malformation and its spectrum of associated anomalies. However, the Dandy-Walker complex (the term introduced by Barkovich et al. [1]

to include the Dandy-Walker malformation, the Dandy-Walker variant, and mega-cisterna magna) might be better differentiated by CT. Associated recent articles of related interest concerning imaging and other aspects of the Dandy-Walker complex are listed (2–5).—L.W. Young, M.D.

References

1. Barkovich AJ, et al: *AJR* 153:1289, 1989.
2. Bindal AK, et al: *Neurosurgery* 28:844, 1991.
3. Kadonaga JN, et al: *Pediatr Dermatol* 9:37, 1992.
4. Pillay P, et al: *Pediatr Neurosci* 15:74, 1989.
5. Asai A, et al: *Pediatr Neurosci* 15:66, 1989.

Giant Interhemispheric Cysts Associated With Agenesis of the Corpus Callosum

Mori K (Kochi Med School, Nankoku City, Japan)
J Neurosurg 76:224–230, 1992   6–6

Background.—Giant interhemispheric cysts, now diagnosed mainly by MRI, are often associated with agenesis of the corpus callosum. The pathogenesis of these cysts varies, as do the prognostic and therapeutic implications. Four large interhemispheric cystic lesions were seen at 4 different institutions. The differential diagnosis and therapeutic considerations of such lesions were reviewed.

Classification.—Most interhemispheric cysts cause symptoms during childhood, although 1 of the 4 patients was an adult. Various names have been given to agenesis of the corpus callosum with a midline cyst in the supratentorial compartment; common radiographic features besides agenesis are midline location and ventricular dilation. In the interhemispheric area, cysts may be extra-axial or intra-axial (table). The differential diagnosis has important prognostic and therapeutic implications. Classification of intra-axial cysts includes "congenital midline porencephaly," holoprosencephaly, and simple agenesis of the corpus callosum. Extra-axial cysts may be bilateral midline cysts or unilateral parasagittal cysts. Interhemispheric cysts may be unusually large with no communication and are often associated with agenesis of the corpus callosum (Fig 6–5).

Histopathology.—Two of the 4 patients underwent surgical fenestration, and the pathologic diagnosis was arachnoid cyst. This is a rather unusual site for arachnoid cyst, so pathologic findings may vary. With agenesis of the corpus callosum, cysts diagnosed as neuroepithelial or glioependymal have been reported; the prognosis is better with arachnoid cysts. Neuroepithelial cysts may show associated anomalies, which may be helpful in making the preoperative diagnosis.

Therapeutic Considerations.—Surgery is not indicated if the mass effect is minimal and there are no neurologic effects. Arachnoid cysts may

Differential Diagnosis of Interhemispheric or Parasagittal Cysts

Factor	Interhemispheric Cyst	Porencephalic Cyst	Holoprosencephaly	Agenesis of Corpus Callosum
nature of cyst	extra-axial	intra-axial	dorsal	cystic dilatation of 3rd ventricle
location of cyst	midline or parasagittal	midline or parasagittal	midline	midline
size of cyst	large	variable	small	small
mass effect	+	−	−	−
communication with ventricle	−	+	+	+
corpus callosum	±	+	−	−
falx	+	+	−	+
hydrocephalus	+	−	±	±
asymmetry of lateral ventricle	+	±	monoventricle	−
anterior cerebral artery	separation, abnormal course	abnormal course	azygous	abnormal course
deep cerebral vein	abnormal course	abnormal course	dysgenesis	abnormal course
frequently associated anomalies	gyral abnormality, neuronal heterotopia	nonspecific	facial anomaly	Aicardi syndrome, Dandy-Walker syndrome, Chiari II malformation
onset of symptoms	early or late	early	early	early, if present
neurological deficits	minimal	severe	severe	subclinical or severe

Abbreviations: +, feature present; −, feature absent; ±, presence or absence of feature equivocal.
(Courtesy of Mori K: *J Neurosurg* 76:224–230, 1992.)

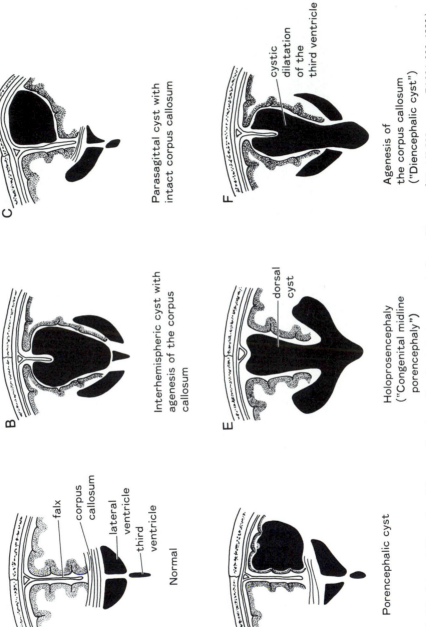

Fig 6–5.—Schematic illustration of the coronal sections of interhemispheric or parasagittal cysts. (Courtesy of Mori K: *J Neurosurg* 76:224–230, 1992.)

be treated by membranectomy and cystoperitoneal shunt insertion; each procedure has its advantages. Cyst fenestration is indicated for patients without hydrocephalus, which required a shunt in this series. Shunting may be the initial preferred treatment for patients with interhemispheric arachnoid cysts.

Conclusions.—Interhemispheric cysts are often associated with agenesis of the corpus callosum and have little uniformity of pathogenesis. Magnetic resonance imaging is the diagnostic method of choice for such cysts and is helpful in the differential diagnosis.

▶ Recognition of the different types of interhemispheric cysts is clinically significant because of differences in their potential treatability. The detection of the cyst in association with agenesis of the corpus callosum may indicate that the 2 conditions are causally related and, perhaps, are manifestations of heterotopia. Various types of interhemispheric cysts are well shown by MRI and CT. Findings from each modality are useful in the differential diagnosis. Other recent related articles of interest are listed (1, 2).—L.W. Young, M.D.

References

1. Schwartz AM, et al: *Clin Neuropathol* 9:177, 1990.
2. Byrd SE, et al: *Eur J Radiol* 10:65, 1990.

Chiari III Malformation: Imaging Features
Castillo M, Quencer RM, Dominguez R (Univ of Texas Med School at Houston; Univ of Miami School of Medicine)
AJNR 13:107–113, 1992   6–7

Background.—The finding of cervical spina bifida with multiple cerebellar and brain stem anomalies traditionally has been classified as a Chiara III malformation. Now this definition has been expanded to include herniation of the hindbrain into a low occipital or high cervical encephalocele (or both), along with features of the Chiari II malformation. The MRI and CT findings in 9 infants with Chiari III malformations were reviewed.

Patients and Findings.—The patients were 6 girls and 3 boys, all born at term. Sonography showed encephalocele before birth in 5 cases. All had plain skull radiographs, 7 had MRI, and 2 had CT. All had high cervical to low occipital encephaloceles (Fig 6–6), and 4 had low and middle hypoplasia of the parietal bones. Varying amounts of brain tissue were found in the encephaloceles; 6 contained cerebellum and occipital lobes and 3 contained cerebellum only. The fourth ventricle was included in 6 cases, and the lateral in 3. Other findings included the cisterns, medulla, and pons. There were 5 cases of petrous and clivus scalloping, 2 of overgrown cerebellar hemisphere, and 3 of cerebellar tonsillar herniation. All patients had deformation of the midbrain. Two

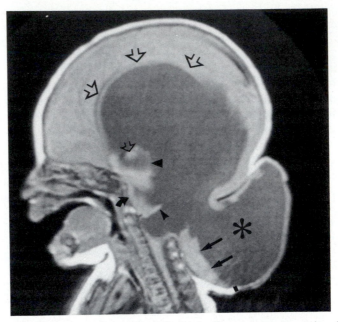

Fig 6–6.—Case 7: A sagittal spin echo (750/20), slightly off-center image shows a large low occipital/high cervical encephalocele. The CSF density (*asterisk*) inside the cephalocele is believed to be a markedly dilated 4th ventricle, with the roof of the 4th ventricle displaced superiorly (*small arrowhead*). The 3rd ventricle (*large arrowhead*) and massa intermedia (*small open arrow*) are mildly prominent. The corpus callosum (*large open arrows*) is thin, and the splenium is absent. Residual cerebellar tissue (*small arrows*) are present inside the encephalocele. Note that there is absence of the posterior elements of C1, C2, and C3. Scalloping (*curved arrow*) of the clivus is present. There is marked dilatation of the lateral ventricles. (Courtesy of Castillo M, Quencer RM, Dominguez R: *AJNR* 13:107–113, 1992.)

patients had hydrocephalus, 6 had corpus callosum dysgenesis, 3 had agenesis of the posterior cervical vertebra, and 2 had spinal cord syrinxes. Aberrant deep draining veins and ectopic venous sinuses were found within the encephaloceles in 4 patients who underwent resection and closure. On pathologic examination of 4 encephaloceles, numerous abnormalities were found that could not be seen on imaging studies. These included necrosis, gliosis, heterotopias, and meningeal fibrosis.

Conclusions.—In newborns with Chiari III malformation, MRI can be used to determine displacement of the medulla and sometimes the pons before surgery. The surgeon must remember that venous anomalies are common. Although it demonstrates the major features of Chiari III, MRI has not facilitated the detection of markedly disorganized tissue abnormalities within the cephalocele. Magnetic resonance imaging clearly displays the position of the cephalocele and its gross morphology.

▶ Magnetic resonance imaging is ideal for demonstrating all types of Chiari malformation. The distinctions of the rare Chiari III malformation in 9 cases are reported in this article. Recent articles of related interest on Chiari malformations, mostly types I and II, are listed (1–5).—L.W. Young, M.D.

References

1. Azimullah PC, et al: *Childs Nerv Syst* 7:63, 1991.
2. Yamanaka M, et al: *Neurol Med Chir* 30:246, 1990.
3. Pollack IF, et al: *Neurosurgery* 30:709, 1992.
4. Nohria V, et al: *Pediatr Neurosurg* 16:222, 1990–1991.
5. Elster AD, et al: *Radiology* 183:347, 1992.

Cranial CT and MR in the Klippel-Trenaunay-Weber Syndrome
Williams DW III, Elster AD (Bowman Gray School of Medicine of Wake Forest Univ, Winston-Salem, NC)
AJNR 13:291–294, 1992   6–8

Background.—Klippel-Trenaunay-Weber syndrome (KTWS) is a rare congenital condition. Affected patients have cutaneous port wine hemangiomas, venous varicosities, and osseous and soft tissue hypertrophy of the affected body part, along with a variety of central nervous system abnormalities. Unusual CT and MRI intracranial findings in 2 patients with KTWS are reported.

Case Report.—Male infant had glaucoma and cutaneous hemangiomas of both sides of the face, head, and neck, in the $V_{1,2,3}$ distribution of cranial nerve 5. He also had hemangiomas of the left shoulder, arm, upper half of the chest, buttock, backs of legs, and lateral sides of feet. At 4 months old he had seizures,

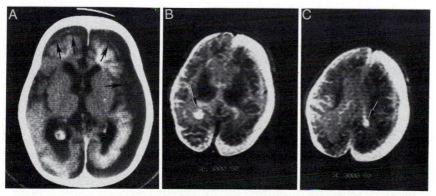

Fig 6–7.—Patient 2; 18-month-old male with KTWS. **A and B,** unenhanced (A) and enhanced (B) CT scan shows severe, bilateral cerebral atrophy, extensive cerebral calcifications, a prominently enhancing choroid plexus, and diffuse, angiomatous leptomeningeal enhancement (*arrows*). **C and D,** axial T2-weighted (3,000/80/1) MR images obtained the same day as the CT scan demonstrate bilateral asymmetric cerebral atrophy, extensive parenchymal low signal corresponding to cerebral calcifications on CT scan, and increased signal intensity of choroid plexuses (*arrows*). (Courtesy of Williams DW III, Elster AD: *AJNR* 13:291–294, 1992.)

involving mainly the face and extremities. At 18 months old, he had phenytoin toxicity, developmental delay, and enlarging left arm. Cranial CT findings included marked bilateral cerebral atrophy, extensive calcifications on both sides of the cortex, and mild angiomatous leptomeningeal enhancement. On MRI, the child was found to have prominent choroid plexi with high signal on T_2-weighted images, asymmetric cerebral atrophy, and large areas of decreased signal, which corresponded to the parenchymal calcifications seen with CT (Fig 6–7).

Discussion.—Unusual intracranial findings have been described in 2 patients with KTWS. The findings include marked enhancement of the choroid plexuses, severe cerebral atrophy, cerebral calcifications, and angiomatous leptomeningeal enhancement. Such cases could be confused with bilateral Sturge-Weber syndrome, though the external marks should allow the distinction. These angiodysplasias may represent a spectrum of involvement with considerable overlap.

▶ Klippel-Trenaunay-Weber syndrome includes lesions of the CNS that are well shown by CT and MRI. Bilateral CNS lesions of Sturge-Weber syndrome may overlap with CNS findings of KTWS. Clinical distinctions can be made by external stigmata. A rare complication of KTWS is arteriovenous fistulization. Intracranial or intraspinal arteriovenous fistulization may be shown by arteriography. Several recent articles of related interest on angiodysplasia and phacomatosis are listed (1–4).—L.W. Young, M.D.

References

1. Marti-Bonmati L, et al: *AJR* 158:867, 1992.
2. Burke JP, et al: *J Pediatr Ophthalmol Strabismus* 28:41, 1991.
3. Good WV, et al: *J Pediatr Ophthalmol Strabismus* 26:288, 1989.
4. Terdjman P, et al: *Neuropediatrics* 22:115, 1990.

Neuroimaging in Lissencephaly Type I

de Rijk-van Andel JF, van der Knaap MS, Valk J, Arts WFM (Westeinde Hospital, The Hague, The Netherlands; Wilhelmina Children's Hosp, Utrecht, The Netherlands; Free University Hospital of Amsterdam, Amsterdam, The Netherlands)
Neuroradiology 33:230–233, 1991   6–9

Background.—Lissencephaly is a developmental disorder of the cerebral cortex in which sulci are either not formed or are only partially formed. In type I lissencephaly, the disturbance mainly concerns the cerebral cortex, but in type II lissencephaly, the cerebellum, eyes, and muscles are disturbed as well. Quantitative criteria for the diagnosis of lissencephaly type I were obtained by measuring a number of cerebral structures. The relationship between the number of sulci and the cortical thickness was examined.

Methods. —Computed tomography scans of 22 patients with lissencephaly were studied. Magnetic resonance imaging examinations were also performed in 6 patients. These CT and MRI scans were compared with those of a control group of 49 patients who had normal CT or MR scans. Patients were divided into 2 groups: those younger and those older than age 3 years to account for differences in maturation of the brain, myelination, and changes in cellular components.

Findings. —In lissencephaly patients, the absolute value of the cortical thickness was always more than 10 mm on CT and MR scans compared with the control group, which always had values of less than 5 mm on the CT scan and less than 7 mm on the MR scan. The lissencephaly patients always had a width/depth index of the sylvian fissure (WSF/DSF index) larger than .29, but that of the control group measured less than .25. A number of measurements were completed on axial slices and sagittal images (when present).

Conclusions. —With CT scanning it was possible to diagnose lissencephaly reliably by measuring the cortical thickness and using the WSF/DSF index in addition to the criteria of Dobyns and McGluggage. In difficult cases, MRI had advantages over CT scanning in visualizing the cortical surface and detecting heterotopias.

▶ The sensitivity of MRI in increasing recognition of neuronal migrational abnormalities has led to more detailed study of such anomalies. Such is the case with lissencephaly type I. It can be diagnosed by CT, but MRI provides so much more information. The diagnostic challenge of these lesions is exciting. Other noteworthy recent articles on neuronal migration anomalies are listed (1–5).—L.W. Young, M.D.

References

1. Barkovich AJ, et al: *AJNR* 13:85, 1992.
2. Barkovich AJ, et al: *AJNR* 13:95, 1992.
3. Barkovich AJ, et al: *Ann Neurol* 30:139, 1991.
4. Hayward JC, et al: *J Child Neurol* 6:109, 1991.
5. Byrd SE, et al: *Eur J Radiol* 12:53, 1991.

Dysmyelinating Leukodystrophies: "LACK Proper Myelin"
Hatten HP Jr (Radiology Associates of Birmingham, Birmingham, Ala)
Pediatr Radiol 21:477–482, 1991   6–10

Introduction. —The dysmyelinating leukodystrophies are a heterogeneous group of disorders that feature deficient or defective synthesis of myelin. Several reports have presented the imaging findings of children with these conditions. A mnemonic that serves as a helpful framework for differential diagnosis of the dysmyelinating leukodystrophies has been developed.

TABLE 1.—Mnemonic Providing
Differential Diagnostic Framework

Dysmyelinating leukodystrophies
"LACK Proper Myelin"

L = Leigh's disease

A $<$ Alexander's disease
Adrenoleukodystrophy

C = Canavan's disease

K = Krabbe's disease

P = Pelizaeus-Merzbacher disease

M = Metachromatic leukodystrophy

(Courtesy of Hatten HP Jr: *Pediatr Radiol*
21:477–482, 1991.)

Discussion.—Leigh's disease is an inherited disorder featuring progressive generalized dystonia, including facial and bulbar involvement. On MRI there is a striking signal increase in the putamen on T_2-weighted images. Alexander's disease may occur in an infantile form, which is the most severe; a juvenile form; and an adult form. The diagnosis is dependent on pathologic identification of Rosenthal fibers in brain biopsy specimens. Adrenoleukodystrophy, seen almost exclusively in boys, is diagnosed by abnormalities in adrenal function and increased very-long-chain fatty acids in serum and cultured skin fibroblasts. Neuroradiologic studies show abnormalities beginning bilaterally in the posterior parts of the brain and proceeding anteriorly. Canavan's disease is a rare, fatal disorder that manifests in the first few months of life. Imaging studies show megalencephaly with diffuse hypodensity on CT and increased T_2 signal

---

TABLE 2.—Clinical Information

Laboratory diagnosis

– Adrenoleukodystrophy
  • adrenal gland dysfunction
  • very-long-chain fatty acids in serum and cultured skin fibroblasts

– Canavan's disease
  • increased urine and serum levels N-acetylaspartic acid

– Krabbe's disease
  • assay of β-galactosidase from WBC's or skin fibroblasts

– Metachromatic Leukodystrophy
  • decreased levels arylsulfatase A in urine and WBC's

(Courtesy of Hatten HP Jr: *Pediatr Radiol* 21:477–482, 1991.)

TABLE 3.—Alexander's Disease
and Canavan's Disease

Macrocephaly

– Alexander's disease
(initially frontal dysmyelination)

– Canavan's disease

(Courtesy of Hatten HP Jr: *Pediatr Radiol*
21:477–482, 1992.)

of the deep white matter of both cerebral hemispheres on MRI. Krabbe's disease shows a relatively low total lipid content and increased density in the thalami, caudate nucleus, and corona radiata on CT.

Pelizaeus-Merzbacher disease is a rare familial disorder featuring progressive neurologic deficits; MRI shows arrested myelination without evidence of white matter destruction. In metachromatic leukodystrophy, pathologic accumulation of metachromatic granules occurs with myelin loss in the central and peripheral nervous system. Diffuse low density scattered throughout the white matter is seen on CT.

The Mnemonic.—"LACK Proper Myelin" is helpful in dealing with this confusing range of abnormalities (Table 1). Adrenal leukodystrophy, Canavan's disease, Krabbe's disease, and metachromatic leukodystrophy all have characteristic laboratory findings (Table 2). Macrocephaly is a feature of Alexander's disease and Canavan's disease: the former typically has initial frontal dysmyelination that proceeds posteriorly, but the latter has a more diffuse dysmyelinating process (Table 3). Adrenoleukodystrophy and Pelizaeus-Merzbacher disease are usually inherited in an X-linked recessive fashion and thus are seen in male subjects only; however, both can occur in female subjects (Table 4).

Conclusions.—The "LACK Proper Myelin" mnemonic can help the radiologist in the differential diagnosis of a child with an extensive dys-

TABLE 4.—Adrenoleukodystrophy
and Pelizaeus-Merzbacher Disease

X-linked recessive inheritance
(males only)

– Adrenoleukodystrophy
(rare autosomal recessive from)

– Pelizaeus-Merzbacher disease
(rare females)

(Courtesy of Hatten HP Jr: *Pediatr Radiol*
21:477–482, 1991.)

myelinating process. The specific diagnosis is made by using laboratory and clinical information.

▶ This clever mnemonic helps in remembering the dysmyelinating leukodystrophies. By combining clinical, laboratory, and MRI data, the specific disease might be identified more easily from the differential diagnostic mnemonic. Current articles of related interest on dysmyelinating and demyelinating white matter disease are listed (1–7).—L.W. Young, M.D.

References

1. Arend AO, et al: *Clin Neuropathol* 10:122, 1991.
2. Low PS: *J Singapore Paediatr Soc* 33:1, 1991.
3. Aubourg P, et al: *Neurology* 42:85, 1992.
4. van der Knaap MS, et al: *Neuroradiology* 33:478, 1991.
5. Curless RG, et al: *Pediatr Neurol* 7:223, 1991.
6. Qualman SJ, et al: *Pediatr Pathol* 11:171, 1991.
7. Grodd W, et al: *Radiology* 181:173, 1991.

Surgical Indications for Infantile Subdural Effusion
Sakai N, Nokura H, Deguchi K, Decarlini E, Futamura A, Yamada H (Gifu University, Gifu, Japan)
Childs Nerv Syst 6:447–450, 1990   6–11

Background.—There is no clearly accepted definition, diagnosis, or treatment of infantile subdural effusion (ISE). Infantile subdural effusion is characterized clinically by the onset of symptoms of a large head and convulsive attacks in some cases, without induction by head trauma or infection. A series of 34 cases of ISE reviewed retrospectively is reported.

Patients.—The initial symptoms were a large head in 23 cases and convulsive attacks in 11 cases. Surgical indications were assessed by the size of the ISE on CT scans and metrizamide CT cisternography (MCTC). Axial-view CT scans were graded as grade 1 if maximum thickness of ISE (ISE t) was equivalent to or less than that of the corresponding frontal

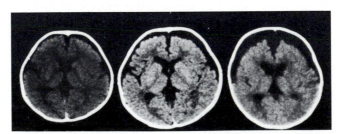

Fig 6–8.—Typical CT scans demonstrating ISE CT grading: grade 1 ≤ 1 time **(left)**; grade 2 ≤ 2 times **(middle)**; grade 3 > 3 times **(right)**. (Courtesy of Sakai N, Nokura H, Deguchi K, et al: *Childs Nerv Syst* 6:447–450, 1990.)

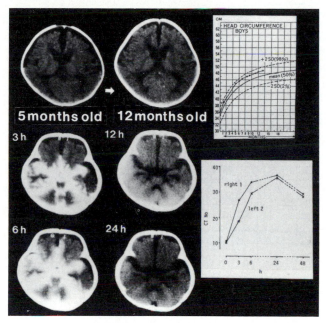

Fig 6–9.—A typical group A case (male patient; birth: June 17, 1988). This case resulted in excellent development with clinical observation only. Photograph, showing the first CT scan of initial diagnosis **(upper left)**, follow-up CT scan (7 months later, **upper center**), MCTC **(middle and lower CT scans)**, head circumference measurements **(upper right)**, and CT number changes of ISE in MCTC **(lower right)**. (Courtesy of Sakai N, Nokura H, Deguchi K, et al: *Childs Nerv Syst* 6:447–450, 1990.)

skull (front T), grade 2 if the ISE t was 1 to 2 times that of the front t, and grade 3 if the ISE t was more than 2 times that of the front t (Fig 6–8). The MCTC was classified as type A for influx into ISE 3 to 24 hours after intrathecal metrizamide injection, type B for slow influx (more than 24 hours) or scant influx, and type C for dynamics similar to type B but complicated with subdural hematoma.

Findings.—Eighteen cases were categorized as MCTC type A, including 61.1% of ISE CT grade 1. A nontreatment regimen for type A cases yielded excellent results in 83.3% of the cases (Fig 6–9). The 10 cases of MCTC type B included 50% of cases of ISE CT grade 3. Surgery yielded excellent results in 80% of cases. Of 6 cases categorized as MCTC type C and ISE CT grade 3, 66.7% responded excellently to surgery. Antiepileptic drugs were given to 27.3% of the 11 patients who had convulsive attacks (table).

Conclusions.—The surgical indications for ISE were based mainly on MCTC and the clinical course. In the early stages, surgery is needed if

Summary of Treatment of ISE

MCTC \ CT grade	1	2	3
Type A	Observed	Closely observed *	More closely observed *
Type B	Observed	Observed * or SP shunt	SP shunt
Type C	Observed (for 1 to 2 months)	Trepanation (or closely observed[a])	Trepanation ↓ (SP shunt, craniotomy)

* *Abbreviations:* MCTC, metrizamide CT cisternography; SP, subdural peritoneal.
[a] Surgical treatment is indicated if head circumference increases by more than the mean ± 2 SD, or if development retards.
(Courtesy of Sakai N, Nokura H, Deguchi N, et al: *Childs Nerv Syst* 6:447–450, 1990.)

the head circumference increases by more than the critical level plus 2 SD or developmental impairment is noticed.

▶ The subject of subdural effusion in infancy is fascinating because of its occasional complete benignity. In many instances, it lacks a relationship to either trauma or infection, even when shunting is required. The authors use a grading system—derived retrospectively from axial CT images and metrizamide CT cisternography—that helps to determine when surgical intervention is needed as contrasted with observation without treatment. High-resolution ultrasonography combined with MRI allows a distinction between benign subdural effusion ("external hydrocephalus") and progressing subdural effusion (1). Radionuclide and CT medrizamide cisternography can be used to assess the pattern of CSF flow (1). Radionuclide brain scintigraphy also may be used. It is unclear whether this liquid is subdural, subarachnoid, or in both locations. Other recent articles of related interest on subdural effusion are listed (2–4).—L.W. Young, M.D.

References

1. DeVries LS, et al: *Neuropediatrics* 21:72, 1990.
2. Gordin SJ, et al: *South Med J* 84:644, 1991.
3. Odita JC: *Childs Nerv Syst* 8:36, 1992.
4. Laubscher B, et al: *Eur J Pediatr* 149:502, 1990.

Cervical Neurenteric Fistula Causing Recurrent Meningitis in Klippel-Feil Sequence: Case Report and Literature Review

Gumerlock MK, Spollen LE, Nelson MJ, Bishop RC, Cooperstock MS (Univ of

Missouri-Columbia Health Sciences Ctr, Columbia, Mo)
Pediatr Infect Dis J 10:532–535, 1991

Background.—Establishing the cause of meningitis can be difficult in patients with Klippel-Feil sequence. Such patients have a spectrum of associated musculoskeletal and neurologic abnormalities. The causes of meningitis can be varied. The ordering of differential diagnoses is often based on the patient's age, type of organisms cultured, and related struc-

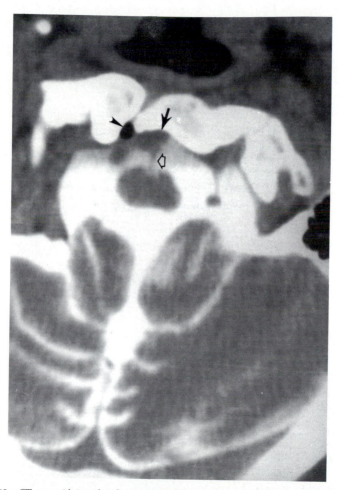

Fig 6–10.—CT scan with intrathecal contrast medium reveals a ventral intradural/extradural nodule at the C1–C2 level (*closed arrow*), associated with a defect in the vertebrae. A small bubble of gas is present in the soft tissue (*arrowhead*). The adjacent nasopharyngeal mucosa appears to be atrophic; however, no tract was identified, and no definite leakage of contrast medium is seen. The spinal cord is abnormal in shape and appears to be tethered to the nodule (*open arrow*). (Courtesy of Gumerlock MK, Spollen LE, Nelson MJ, et al: *Pediatr Infect Dis J* 10:532–535, 1991.)

tural problems. A patient with Klippel-Feil sequence had many episodes of meningitis that defied etiologic determination for 10 years.

Case Report.—Girl, 10 years, with Klippel-Feil sequence had her first episode of meningitis 1 month after birth. No organisms could be cultured, and the patient improved with ampicillin and gentamicin treatment. Two months later she was again seen with meningitis. It was *Streptococcus pneumoniae* meningitis, which responded to penicillin. The clinical triad of Klippel-Feil sequence—low hairline, short neck, and limited neck movement—was evident. Cervical spine radiography showed bony changes consistent with type I disease, involving all cervical vertebrae, including T1. By age 10, the patient had had 59 episodes of

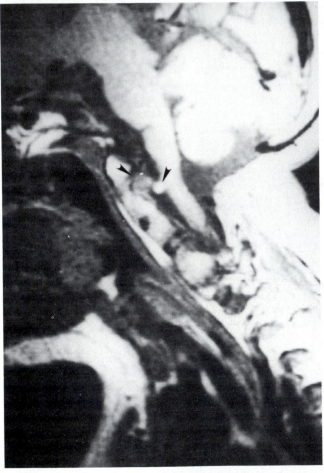

Fig 6–11.—Nodule (*arrowheads*) demonstrated on MRI scan, with areas of high and low signal intensity on T1-weighted images. (Courtesy of Gumerlock MK, Spollen LE, Nelson MJ, et al: *Pediatr Infect Dis J* 10:532–535, 1991.)

meningitis. Bacterial pathogens were recovered in 32 and included *S. pneumoniae, Haemophilus influenzae,* and *Staphylococcus aureus,* all upper respiratory tract flora. During this time she was assessed extensively and surgically treated for possible CSF leaks in various regions of the skull base. Despite surgery, she continued to have recurrent meningitis. In the 59th episode of meningitis, she complained of neck pain with transient leg pain and paresthesias. Severe right neck pain without meningismus was found on physical examination. Computed tomography with intrathecal iodinated contrast medium showed a mass extending on both sides of the dura ventrally at the C1–C2 level in association with an anterior bifid defect of the vertebral body (Fig 6–10). Although there was no definitive sign of contrast leakage, a small collection of gas was seen posterior to the vertebral body. Magnetic resonance imaging confirmed a mass ventral to the spinal cord at C1–C2 associated with the vertebral cleft (Fig 6–11). On laminectomy and intradural exploration, a mass extending across a dural defect was found. This mass indented the cord and pushed it posteriorly. The mass was removed, and the patient has remained free of meningitis for 16 months.

Conclusions.—Multiple sources of potential CSF leakage have been reported in patients with Klippel-Feil sequence. Each of these sources needs to be explored when meningitis develops in such patients.

▶ A presumed cervical neurenteric fistula in Klippel-Feil sequence causing meningitis is difficult or, as in this case, was not possible to demonstrate preoperatively. Multiple imaging modalities were used to help find the suspected fistula, but to no avail. The 2 methods, radionuclide scintigraphy and CT with intrathecal contrast medium, which should have been more likely to succeed in demonstrating a fistula did not show a frank CSF leak. Computed tomography showed a gas bubble, and MRI showed a mass—findings that helped in operative planning. Pertinent articles of related interest on this topic are noteworthy (1, 2).—L.W. Young, M.D.

References

1. Barcz DV, et al: *Am J Otol* 6:157, 1985.
2. Nagib MG, et al: *Childs Nerv Syst* 1:255, 1985.

Hamartomas of the Tuber Cinereum: CT, MR, and Pathologic Findings
Boyko OB, Curnes JT, Oakes WJ, Burger PC (Duke Univ, Durham, NC; Greensboro Radiology Associates, Greensboro, NC)
AJR 156:1053–1058, 1991   6–13

Background.—Hamartoma of the tuber cinereum is a congenital, non-neoplastic heterotopia. The association of congenital anomalies with this midline hamartoma is indicative that it may result from an insult around the first month of gestation. Histologically, the hamartoma closely resembles normal gray matter, with some hypothalmic-like neurons and some myelinated axons. The tuber cinereum is the name of the region that includes the middle hypothalmic nuclei (small bilateral protuberances of gray matter) and is located between the infundibular stalk and the large, prominent mamillary bodies. The CT and MRI findings in 5 cases of biopsy-proved hamartoma were reviewed.

Methods.—Neuroimaging studies, clinical evaluations, and surgical and pathologic findings in 3 girls and 2 boys with hamartomas were examined. The 3 patients with pedunculated hamartomas had precocious puberty, and the 2 patients with sessile lesions had seizures.

Findings.—None of these 5 patients had associated congenital anomalies, although this has been reported elsewhere. All 3 preoperative MRI studies showed lesions isointense with gray matter in T_1-weighted images and hyperintense relative to gray matter in the second echo of the T_2-weighted images. These MRI findings may be more indicative of hamartomas than of gliomas. In every case, the bright MRI signal of the posterior pituitary on T_1-weighted images was preserved. This could mean that gonadotropin–releasing factor neurons are more resistant to compression than are vasopressin neurons; that only complete transection of the stalk results in loss of posterior pituicyte signal; that the tumor does not affect the pituitary stalk, but the mechanism for precocious puberty is neurosecretion from the hamartoma; or that the posterior pituitary bright signal has no relationship with the hypothalamic gonadotropin-releasing factor neurons. There was no contrast enhancement on MRI or CT in the 1 case in which contrast medium was administered.

Conclusions.—In children who have precocious puberty or seizures, the finding at MRI of masses below the floor of the third ventricle with signal characteristics suggestive of gray matter should lead to a confident preoperative diagnosis of tuber cinereum hamartoma.

▶ Hamartoma of the tuber cinereum at the hypothalamic base of the brain is a relatively rare but distinctive lesion. Characteristically, it is associated with precocious puberty and gelastic epilepsy. Magnetic resonance imaging, which is superior to plain CT or CT cisternography in showing the lesion's exact size and anatomical location, is the procedure of choice for its detection. Recent articles of related interest to hypothalamic hamartomas are listed (1–3).—L.W. Young, M.D.

References

1. Burton EM, et al: *AJNR* 10:497, 1989.
2. Marliani AF, et al: *Can Assoc Radiol J* 42:335, 1991.
3. Lona-Soto A, et al: *Comput Med Imaging Graph* 15:415, 1991.

Bilateral Arachnoid Cysts of the Temporal Fossa in Four Children With Glutaric Aciduria Type I

Hald JK, Nakstad PH, Skjeldal OH, Strømme P (University of Oslo, Rikshospitalet, Oslo, Norway)

AJNR 12:407–409, 1991   6–14

Background and Methods.—Type I glutaric aciduria is a rare inborn metabolic anomaly that is often fatal. Here, CT scans were retrospectively evaluated in 5 children (from 3 families) with type I glutaric aciduria. Two children were also examined with MRI.

Results.—In 1 patient, the CT scan demonstrated diffusely reduced attenuation of white matter in both cerebral hemispheres. The other 4 patients had normal attenuation. All patients had slight ventricular enlargement without evidence of loss of the caudate nuclei. One patient

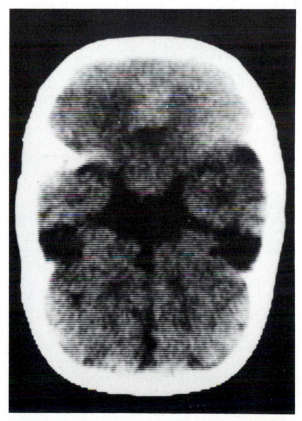

Fig 6–12.—An axial CT scan of a boy, 2 years, shows fluid collections of the temporal regions, consistent with arachnoid cysts. (Courtesy of Hald JK, Nakstad PH, Skjeldal OH, et al: *AJNR* 12:407–409, 1991.)

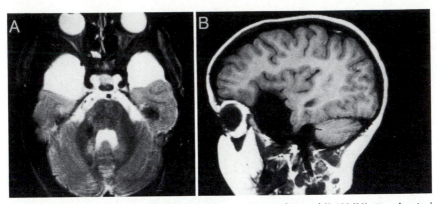

Fig 6–13.—Brother, 5 years, of the patient in Figure 6-12. **A** and **B,** axial (3,100/90) **(A)** and sagittal (600/15) **(B)** MR images show fluid collections of the temporal regions, consistent with arachnoid cysts. (Courtesy of Hald JK, Nakstad PH, Skjeldal OH, et al: *AJNR* 12:407-409, 1991.)

had otherwise normal CT and MRI scans. The other 4 children had variously sized bilateral fluid collections in the middle cranial fossa at the tips of the temporal lobes (Figs 6-12 and 6-13). Fluid collections ranged from 2 to 4 cm in largest diameter, and in all but 1 patient, they were symmetric in size and shape. One patient had a slightly larger fluid collection on the right than on the left. In 2 patients, bilateral frontoparietal subdural hematomas were shunted and evacuated by trephination, respectively. These patients later had hydrocephalus and were shunted to their lateral ventricles. Evacuation of the hematomas had no apparent effect upon the size or shape of the temporal fluid collections in 1 patient who underwent CT scanning before and after surgery.

Conclusions.—The association between bilateral temporal fluid collections and type I glutaric aciduria is as yet unexplained. The metabolic disorder may go unnoticed among children with developmental retardation, cerebral palsy, or acute idiopathic encephalopathy. This enzyme deficiency should be considered in patients with bilateral arachnoid cysts. Although CT and MRI are comparable in detecting arachnoid cysts, MRI is superior in defining cysts in several planes and in tissue discrimination, which makes it possible to differentiate arachnoid cysts from other lesions that appear hypodense on CT.

▶ When associated with metabolic defects, morphologic abnormalities and their phenotypes can be better classified. Example in point is the association of arachnoid cysts of the temporal fossa with glutaric aciduria. The discovery of either should lead to examination for the other, earlier discovery and, in turn, expeditious treatment. Other recent articles on CNS lesions associated with biochemical abnormalities are listed (1–4).—L.W. Young, M.D.

References

1. Sawada H, et al: *Acta Neurol Scand* 84:70, 1991.
2. Altman NR, et al: *AJNR* 12:966, 1991.
3. Naidu S, et al: *AJNR* 12:413, 1991.
4. Shaw DWW, et al: *AJNR* 12:403, 1991.

MR Imaging of Pituitary Hypertrophy Due to Juvenile Primary Hypothyroidism: A Case Report

Kuroiwa T, Okabe Y, Hasuo K, Yasumori K, Mizushima A, Masuda K (Kyushu University, Fukuoka, Japan)
Clin Imaging 15:202–205, 1991   6–15

Background.—Magnetic resonance imaging has been useful in diagnosing pituitary adenomas, but its use in hypothyroidism with associated enlargement of the pituitary has not been widely reported. In 1 case, Gd-DTPA–enhanced MRI was used to distinguish pituitary hypertrophy from pituitary adenoma.

Case Report.—Girl, 5 years, had anemia and was of short stature. She had no history of cretinism, but her small stature and inactivity were recognized when she was age 3 years. Laboratory results showed excessive secretion of both thyrotropin-stimulating hormore (TSH) and prolactin. The Gd-DTPA–enhanced images showed homogeneous enhancement of an enlarged gland with the intensity of a normal pituitary gland (Fig 6–14). After supplemental therapy with dried thyroid gland, there was clinical improvement and serum levels of triiodothyronine, thyroxine, and TSH became normal. After 3 months of therapy, MRI showed a normal-appearing pituitary gland on T_1-weighted images. The MRI findings suggested that the enlarged pituitary gland was not a tumorous change, but was caused by hypertrophy or hyperplasia.

Conclusions.—It was not possible to distinguish pituitary hypertrophy from pituitary macroadenoma with suprasellar extension on plain T_1-weighted images alone, but Gd-DTPA–enhanced sagittal and coronal images were useful in the differential diagnosis of pituitary hypertrophy and pituitary adenoma.

▶ Pituitary hypertrophy caused by juvenile primary hypothyroidism can be distinguished from pituitary adenoma by the use of Gd-DTPA–enhanced MRI. With hypertrophy, the entire gland showed uniform increased signal intensity vs. less signal intensity increase by adenoma. This finding has been duplicated in other cases contained in recent articles (1–3).—L.W. Young, M.D.

References

1. Hutchins WW, et al: *AJNR* 11:410, 1990.
2. van Nesselrooij JH, et al: *Magn Reson Imaging* 8:525, 1990.
3. Koyama T, et al: *No To Shinkei* 43:187, 1991.

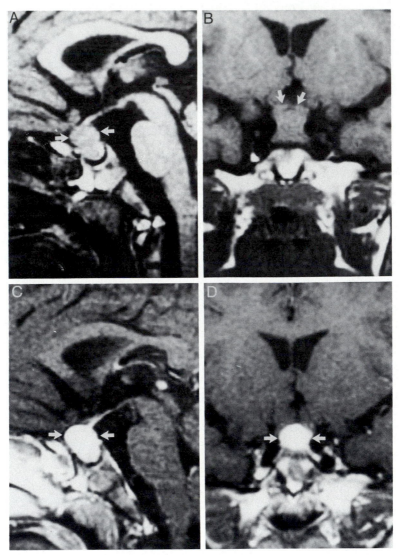

Fig 6–14.—Pituitary hypertrophy caused by primary hypothyroidism. **A,** sagittal T1-weighted image shows enlargement of the anterior lobe of the pituitary gland with suprasellar extension (*arrows*). The posterior pituitary lobe is normally located (*arrowhead*). **B,** coronal T1-weighted image shows compression of the optic chiasm (*arrows*). **C,** Gd-DTPA–enhanced sagittal and (**D**) coronal images show homogenous enhancement of an enlarged gland with the intensity of a normal pituitary gland (*arrows*). (Courtesy of Kuroiwa T, Okabe Y, Hasuo K, et al: *Clin Imaging* 15:202–205, 1991.)

View From Within: Radiology in Focus: CT and MR Imaging in Lateral Sinus Thrombosis

Irving RM, Jones NS, Hall-Craggs MA, Kendall B (Hospital for Sick Children, London, England)

J Laryngol Otol 105:693–695, 1991   6–16

Background.—Early recognition and treatment of lateral sinus thrombosis secondary to otologic disease are essential for favorable outcome, but establishing a preoperative diagnosis can be difficult. Computed tomography and MRI are the preferred diagnostic techniques. Cerebral arteriography and retrograde jugulography are both invasive procedures that risk complications from stroke and dislodgement of thrombus, respectively. Intravenous digital subtraction angiography is less invasive and may provide diagnostic images in cooperative patients.

Case Report.—Girl, 15 years, was seen with 1-week history of right-sided otorrhea, headache, vomiting, diplopia, and lower-limb weakness. Contrast-enhanced CT (Fig 6–15) demonstrated poorly developed mastoid air cells on the right side and complete opacification of the right middle-ear cavity and mastoid. Erosion of the malleus and incus suggested chronic infection and cholesteatoma formation. Localized gas in the sinodural angle suggested a bone defect between the mastoid and posterior fossa or an epidural abscess (or both). Preoperative cranial MRI showed high signal in the right transverse sigmoid sinuses and upper jugular vein (Fig 6–16). An MR venogram showed high signal in the left sigmoid sinus and proximal jugular vein but no corresponding flow on the right (Fig 6–17). This combination—abnormal signal and absent flow—suggested a diagnosis of lateral sinus thrombosis. The patient underwent a modified radical mastoidectomy. The internal jugular vein was not ligated because there were no signs

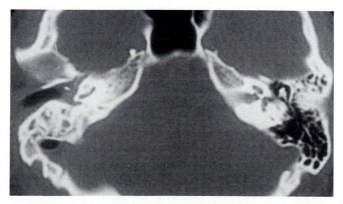

Fig 6–15.—High-resolution CT made through temporal bones with wide window. The right middle ear and mastoid air cells are opaque. There is erosion of bone around the mastoid antrum and of the auditory ossicles. Gas in the right sinodural angle indicates either an abscess caused by a gas forming organism or a fistula caused by erosion into the angle from the mastoid. (Courtesy of Irving RM, Jones NS, Hall-Craggs MA, et al: *J Laryngol Otol* 105:693–695, 1991.)

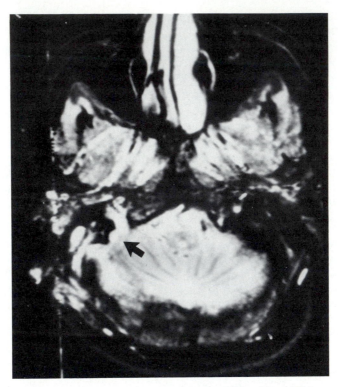

Fig 6–16.—Transverse STIR (TI = 145 ms, TR = 3,000 ms, TE = 85 ms) MR images at the level of the sigmoid venous sinus and the jugular foramen. Abnormal signal (*arrowhead*) is present in the right-sided venous sinuses (compare with the flow void in the left venous sinuses). (Courtesy of Irving RM, Jones NS, Hall-Craggs MA, et al: *J Laryngol Otol* 105:693–695, 1991.)

or symptoms of emboli. The patient received a 2-week course of parenteral antibiotics, followed by oral antibiotics. Headache and vomiting resolved within 8 hours of surgery. Abducens nerve palsy resolved after 3 days.

Conclusions.—In this case, CT provided valuable information, but it was nondiagnostic, whereas MRI was highly suggestive of thrombosis. If MRI shows an abnormal signal from the sinus, it is likely indicative of venous sinus occlusion by thrombus. As with any other angiographic technique, MR venography does not delineate the extent of thrombus as signal loss distal to the obstruction. This may be because of higher orders of motion or to saturation of slowly moving blood. Magnetic resonance imaging is the preferred diagnostic technique. It is noninvasive, and it accurately delineates the thrombus; MRI should be performed in conjunction with CT to fully evaluate associated otologic and cerebral pathologic conditions.

▶ This well-written and succinct article on lateral sinus thrombosis is highly recommended. Lateral sinus thrombosis is a dreaded complication of oto-

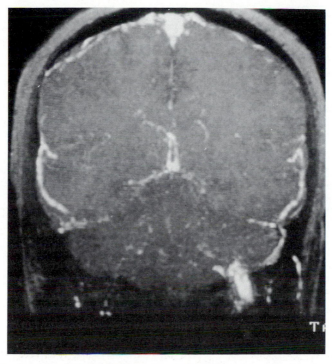

Fig 6–17.—A maximum intensity projection image of an MR venogram (flip angle, 40 degrees; TR = 40 ms, TE = 12 ms) showing flow (high signal) in the left sigmoid sinus and proximal jugular vein. No corresponding flow is seen on the right. A combination of abnormal signal with absence of flow is highly suggestive of venous sinus occlusion by thrombus. (Courtesy of Irving RM, Jones NS, Hall-Craggs MA, et al: *J Laryngol Otol* 105:693–695, 1991.)

logic disease. Magnetic resonance imaging, MR angiography, CT and, if necessary, digital subtraction angiography may be used individually or in combination to make the diagnosis. They are the modalities preferred over the much more invasive imaging procedures of cerebral arteriography and retrograde jugulography. Another useful procedure for assessing this disease is radionuclide brain flow imaging (1). Other recent articles of related interest concerning cranial sinus thrombosis and venous thrombosis are listed (2–4).—L.W. Young, M.D.

References

1. Stein EH, et al: *Ann Otol Rhinol Laryngol* 101:363, 1992.
2. Tovi F, et al: *Ann Otol Rhinol Laryngol* 100:682, 1991.
3. Voutsinas L, et al: *Clin Imaging* 15:273, 1991.
4. Fritsch MH, et al: *Otolaryngol Head Neck Surg* 103:451, 1990.

Magnetic Resonance Imaging of the Brain in Congenital Rubella Virus and Cytomegalovirus Infections

Sugita K, Ando M, Makino M, Takanashi J, Fujimoto N, Niimi H (Chiba University, Chiba, Japan)
Neuroradiology 33:239–242, 1991   6–17

Background.—Children with congenital rubella virus and cytomegalovirus (CMV) infections sometimes have long-term secondary neurologic impairment. Because MRI is well-suited to detect white matter abnor-

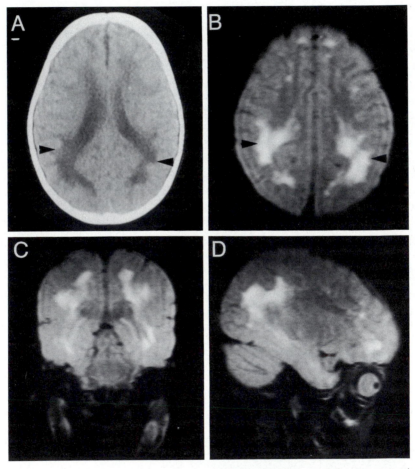

Fig 6–18.—A, an unenhanced CT scan shows a bilateral low-density area of the white matter (*arrowheads*). **B,** a transverse T2-weighted image (2,080/80) at the same level shows more remarkable white matter lesions, such as periventricular hyperintensity and subcortical hyperintensity (*arrowheads*). **C** and **D,** periventricular hyperintensity and subcortical hyperintensity on coronal (**C**) and parasagittal (**D**) T2-weighted images, respectively. (Courtesy of Sugita K, Ando M, Makino M, et al: *Neuroradiology* 33:239–242, 1991.)

malities or changes in the water content of neural tissues, cranial MRI might be clinically useful in examining patients with congenital CMV and rubella virus infections.

Methods.—Cranial MRI was used to examine 8 patients, aged $2\frac{1}{2}$ to 6 years. Two children had congenital rubella virus and 6 had CMV infections. Subsequently, the children had symptoms of neurologic damage, including mental retardation, cerebral palsy, sensorineural hearing defect, and epilepsy. Patients also underwent CT scanning.

Results.—The MRI defined abnormalities of the brain parenchyma, anatomical details, and gray white matter differentiation better than CT (Fig 6–18), but CT and MRI were about equally effective in demonstrating cerebellar hypoplasia and oligo/pachygyria. For showing calcifications, CT was better; MRI showed no calcifications, whereas CT demonstrated calcifications in 4 children.

Discussion.—Infection with CMV and rubella virus causes inflammatory and destructive changes and tissue damage that may result in malformations. Congenital CMV infection can cause microcephaly, patchy spongiosis or encephalomalacia, microcephalia, periventricular and arterial calcifications, cystic degeneration, areas of persistent cerebral cortical immaturity related to inhibited growth, and focal cerebral or cerebellar hypoplasia. Congenital rubella virus infection can cause brain malformation, microcephaly, and vasculitis.

Conclusions.—Magnetic resonance imaging is a useful diagnostic tool in children with congenital rubella virus and CMV infections. It is consistently more sensitive than CT in defining the extent of parenchymal lesions and identifying delayed myelination; however, CT is better at visualizing intracranial calcification. The extent of parenchymal lesions is apparently related to neurologic sequelae. In children with congenital infection involving the CNS, MRI is probably the preferred neuroimaging technique.

▶ The sensitivity of MRI for postinfectious intracranial parenchymal lesions is unparalleled for white matter disease affecting changes in water content. However, CT better demonstrates intracranial calcification and can corroborate findings of other parenchymal lesions as demonstrated by MRI. Ultrasound and SPECT are also valuable modalities for examining the CNS for postinfectious parenchymal lesions (1). Recent articles of related interest are listed (2, 3).—L.W. Young, M.D.

References

1. Kugler SL, et al: *Pediatr Neurol* 7:207, 1991.
2. Bazan C III, et al: *Neurology* 41:1522, 1991.
3. Yamashita Y, et al: *Pediatr Radiol* 21:547, 1991.

Multiple Intracranial Calcifications After Western Equine Encephalitis

Somekh E, Glode MP, Reiley TT, Tsai TF (Univ of Colorado, Denver; Ctrs for Disease Control, Ft Collins, Colo)
Pediatr Infect Dis J 10:408–409, 1991   6–18

Background.—Western equine encephalitis is usually self-limiting, but severe encephalitis can occur in young children. In 1 infant infection early in life led to multiple intracranial calcifications.

Case Report.—Infant girl, with a birth weight of 3 kg, was born to healthy parents after an uncomplicated 37-week pregnancy. At 4 weeks of age, the infant was seen at a local hospital with a temperature of 40°C and seizures that included back arching, nystagmus, and tonic-clonic movements of both arms. Cerebrospinal fluid was clear and without blood cells; glucose level was 65 mg/dL, and protein level was 65 mg/dL. The patient was given antibiotics and transferred to Children's Hospital of Denver. The child was irritable and had a high-pitched cry. Extremities were hypertonic, but there were no focal neurologic signs. Hemoglobin level was 12 g/dL, platelet count was 210,000/μL, and white blood cell count was 9,400/μL. Cerebrospinal fluid contained 20 white blood cells and 3,500 red blood cells. Blood, urine, and CSF cultures were sterile. Lactic and pyruvic acids were elevated. An electroencephalogram (ECG) showed diffuse cerebral dysfunction with multifocal irritable epileptiform areas. A CT scan of the head revealed diffuse, slightly low-density white matter. The patient was treated with antibiotics, acyclovir, and anticonvulsants for 10 days and then was discharged on valproic acid and thiamine therapy. When readmitted 4 months later, the patient had bilateral vertical nystagmus, increased tonus of the extremities with brisk tendon reflexes, and positive ankle clonus. She had no head or neck control. She also had nonspecific mild chorioretinitis. Serologic test results were indicative of recent infection with western equine encephalitis. The ECG revealed severe diffuse seizure activity, and CT scan showed enlarged lateral and third ventricles with numerous intracranial calcifications in symmetric distribution within both hemispheres, the insular cortex, and thalamus bilaterally. There were also patchy areas of decreased attenuation in the cortex that were consistent with encephalomalacia.

Discussion.—The pattern of CT findings in this case was unique. Other accounts of patients with arbovirus infections have reported CT scans showing nonspecific signs (e.g., cerebral ventricular dilatation and slight atrophy), whereas in this case, initial CT scan showed diffuse low-density signals in the white matter. Four months later, there were extensive and numerous bilateral intracranial calcifications. Infection with western equine encephalitis should be included in the differential diagnosis of intracranial calcifications.

▶ This is the first report of western equine encephalitis as yet another cause of multiple intracranial calcifications. Plain CT scanning has the excellent contrast resolution to show intracranial calcification better than any other modality. Recent articles of related interest concerning intracranial calcification are listed (1–4).—L.W. Young, M.D.

References

1. Koga Y, et al: *Am J Obstet Gynecol* 163:1543, 1990.
2. Ruiz ME, et al: *Neuroradiology* 33:79, 1991.
3. Kugler SL, et al: *Pediatr Neurol* 7:207, 1991.
4. Parisot S, et al: *Pediatr Radiol* 21:229, 1991.

Pseudoaneurysm of the Internal Carotid Artery: A Forgotten Complication of Tonsillitis?

Watson MG, Robertson AS, Colquhoun IR (Freeman Hospital, Newcastle upon Tyne, England)
J Laryngol Otol 105:588–590, 1991   6–19

Background.—A rare life-threatening complication of tonsillitis was studied.

Case Report.—Boy, 7 years, who was previously well was seen with a 2-week history of tonsillitis that had failed to respond to antibiotics. Just before admission, the patient had sudden severe epistaxis. There were no obvious signs of

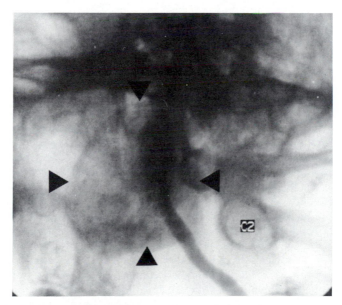

Fig 6–19.—Unsubtracted image from a carotid angiogram demonstrating the relationship of the pseudoaneurysm (*arrowheads*) to the skull base. (Courtesy of Watson MG, Robertson AS, Colquhoun IR: *J Laryngol Otol* 105:588–590, 1991.)

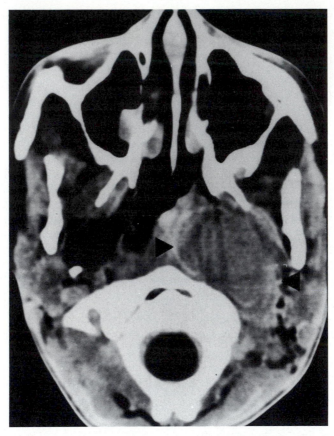

Fig 6–20.—A CT scan showing an internal carotid pseudoaneurysm (*arrowheads*) displacing the left tonsil into the pharyngeal lumen. (Courtesy of Watson MG, Robertson AS, Colquhoun IR: *J Laryngol Otol* 105:588–590, 1991.)

peritonsillar abscess or recent hemorrhage within either nasal cavity. Hemoglobin concentration was 10.2 g/dL and white blood cell count was 31×10^9/L. The patient had a tentative diagnosis of peritonsillar cellulitis and was begun on intravenously administered benzylpenicillin therapy. In the next 24 hours, the patient had 2 sudden, severe episodes of bleeding from the nose and mouth with 500 mL of blood loss each time. The patient was given a blood transfusion and examined under anesthesia. The left tonsil was displaced anteriorly by a large mass lying outside the lateral pharyngeal wall. The mass, which was believed to be a tumor arising in the parapharyngeal space, extended from the nasopharynx to just below the lower pole of the tonsil. Overlying mucosa was normal, except for a small ulcerated area in the nasopharynx, from which a biopsy specimen was taken. Histologic examination of the specimen revealed only nonspecific granulation tissue. After another severe hemorrhage, the patient underwent further examination that revealed the mass consisted of firm blood clot. Carotid angiography showed a 4-cm pseudoaneurysm arising from the left internal carotid artery just below the skull base (Fig 6–19). Distal to the pseudoaneurysm, the carotid artery was patent, and there was good cross circulation via the circle of Willis. A CT scan showed that the pseudoaneurysm was very close to the left tonsil (Fig 6–20). Because of the danger of further bleeding, the left internal carotid artery was ligated. The patient recovered with no further bleeding and without neurologic deficit. The pseudoaneurysm was considerably reduced on follow-up CT scan 5 weeks later.

Discussion.—Pseudoaneurysms of the cervical internal carotid artery are rare, but they have been found after gunshot or stab wounds, blunt head injury, needle puncture, arterial grafting, tonsillectomy, and before the advent of antibiotics, as a sequel to parapharyngeal or retropharyngeal sepsis. Ligation of the internal carotid artery in the neck is standard treatment, but if cross circulation cannot be demonstrated by carotid angiography, gradual clamping of the carotid or carotid ligation plus intracranial and extracranial bypass may be a safer procedure.

▶ The complications of tonsillitis—so prevalent in yesteryear—must not be forgotten. Even in this antibiotic era, they are still around. Tonsillitis complications are a special challenge to primary care physicians and otolaryngologists who treat children. The authors show that current imaging methods of CT and angiography are excellent in demonstrating the complication of pseudoaneurysm of the internal carotid artery. Other recent articles of related interest concerning aneurysms and infections are listed (1–5).—L.W. Young, M.D.

References

1. Mootz W, et al: *HNO* 28:197, 1980.
2. Stevens HE: *J Otolaryngol* 19:206, 1990.
3. Stromquist C, et al: *J Perinatol* 12:81, 1992.
4. Gurin MA: *Vestn Otorhinolaryngol* 1:79, 1990.
5. Wells RG, et al: *Pediatr Radiol* 21:402, 1991.

MR of Intracranial Neuroblastoma With Dural Sinus Invasion and Distant Metastases

Wiegel B, Harris TM, Edwards MK, Smith RR, Azzarelli B (Indiana Univ, Indianapolis)
AJNR 12:1198–1200, 1991   6–20

Background.—Primary cerebral neuroblastoma is a rare condition that has been classified as a form of primitive neuroectodermal tumor. A patient with primary cerebral neuroblastoma that had invaded the dural sinuses and metastasized to the lungs at the time of diagnosis was evaluated.

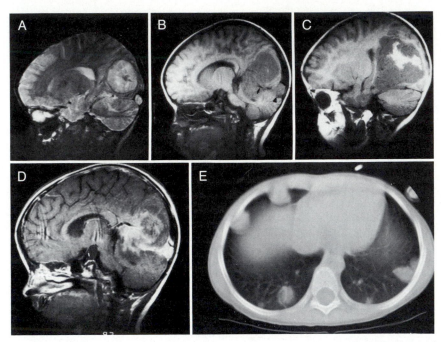

Fig 6–21.—A girl, 3 years, with a 2-month history of rapidly progressive loss of vision and crossed eyes. **A,** left parasagittal T1-weighted (700/20/1) MR image shows an irregular area of high signal intensity consistent with hemorrhage within the occipital tumor. **B,** sagittal T1-weighted (700/20/1) MR image shows occipital tumor traversing the tentorium with encasement of the straight sinus (*arrow*). Note that the soft tissue mass is isointense with tumor in the torcula (*arrowhead*). **C,** right parasagittal T2-weighted (2,500/80/1) MR image shows invasion of the tumor into the right occipital lobe. Note that the abnormal signal is isointense with tumor in right transverse sinus. **D,** axial T2-weighted (2,500/80/1) MR image shows tumor invading the falx, spreading from left to right occipital lobe. The tumor is flanked by high-signal cystic or necrotic areas. **E,** left parasagittal T1-weighted (700/20/1) postcontrast MR image. The parenchymal and dural sinus components of the tumor show marked contrast enhancement. **F,** axial CT scan through lower chest reveals multiple pulmonary metastatic lesions. (Courtesy of Wiegel B, Harris TM, Edwards MK, et al: *AJNR* 12:1198–1200, 1991.)

Case Report.—Girl, 3 years, had a 2-month history of rapidly progressing loss of vision and crossed eyes. She had a lack of coordination but no history of seizures, nausea, or emesis. Physical examination revealed mild developmental delay, marked irritability, bilateral papilledema, and a right esotropia. Pupils were bilaterally reactive but sluggish. Other neurologic findings were normal. Magnetic resonance imaging revealed a left parietooccipital mass measuring 8.5 cm. Unenhanced T_1- and T_2-weighted images showed a predominantly isointense mass with gray matter with large irregular areas of high signal consistent with hemorrhage (Fig 6–21). Abnormal soft tissue was identified in the torcula and both proximal transverse sinuses. The straight sinus was encased, and the tumor had invaded through the tentorium into the superior vermis. There was also invasion through the falx. High signal areas flanking the main tumor represented tumor necrosis or cyst formation. Contrast-enhanced T_1-weighted sagittal images showed marked irregular enhancement of the tumor and intrasinus mass. Preoperative differential diagnoses included primitive neuroectodermal tumor and cerebral or meningeal sarcoma. A chest CT scan after subtotal resection of the left occipital lobe mass revealed a right upper-lobe parenchymal mass and numerous other pulmonary mass lesions. There was no paraspinal mass. Other imaging procedures found no additional metastases. During 6 months, the child underwent 6 courses of systemic chemotherapy, followed by external beam radiation therapy to the occipital mass. Serial MR studies showed enlargement of the occipital mass and decreased contrast enhancement. Chest CT showed resolution of the pulmonary masses.

Discussion.—Neuroblastoma may occur in any region of the CNS. Tumors may be large, and they often contain calcification, hemorrhage, or both, and have cystic areas. A magnetic resonance examination shows marked enhancement and mass inhomogeneous lesions that have low signal intensity on short repetition time images and mixed low and high signal intensity on long repetition time images. If, as in this study patient, there is dural sinus invasion, distant metastases should be suspected.

▶ Recognition of primary cerebral neuroblastoma as distinct from primary extracranial neuroblastoma with CNS metastases gets into the realm of the neuropathologists and their ultrastructural and immunohistochemical analyses (1, 2). Imaging findings may be similar to those of other primary CNS tumors, such as astrocytomas, ependymomas, and meningomas, as well as other primitive neuroectodermal tumors. Davis et al. (3) have indicated that CT may be preferable to noncontrast medium MR for baseline initial examinations and for follow-up to identify calcification, recurrent tumor and leptomeningeal disease. Another recent article of related interest is listed (4).—L.W. Young, M.D.

References

1. Burger PC, et al: *Neurol Clin* 9:249, 1991.
2. Dehner LP, et al: *Ultrastruct Pathol* 12:479, 1988.
3. Davis PC, et al: *AJR* 154:831, 1990.
4. Kellie SJ, et al: *Cancer* 68:1999, 1991.

Primary Extracranial Neuroblastoma With Central Nervous System Metastases Characterization by Clinicopathologic Findings and Neuroimaging
Kellie SJ, Hayes FA, Bowman L, Kovnar EH, Langston J, Jenkins JJ III, Pao WJ, Ducos R, Green AA (St Jude Children's Research Hosp, Memphis; Univ of Tennessee; Children's Hosp of New Orleans, New Orleans)
Cancer 68:1999–2006, 1991   6–21

Background and Methods.—Direct involvement of the brain and spinal cord parenchyma and of the pia-arachnoid and subarachnoid membranes after relapse of classic childhood neuroblastoma must be recognized and treated early. This is a serious complication that is usually attributed to direct extension from metastatic deposits in adjacent structures. The clinicopathologic and neuroimaging findings were documented in 10 children with primary abdominal or thoracic neuroblastoma who relapsed in the CNS. No patient had neuroimaging or pathologic evidence of concurrent intracranial extension from adjacent bone, dura, or dural sinus metastases. At diagnosis, patients ranged in age from .3 to 4.5 years. From diagnosis, the times to CNS relapse ranged from 2 to 34 months. Seven patients relapsed 1 to 14 months after electively discontinuing treatment. In 4 patients, CNS relapse was the primary isolated adverse event. Four patients, who could not be treated at relapse, died of progressive CNS disease within 7 days. The remaining 6 patients underwent craniospinal irradiation.

Results.—Four of the 6 treated patients had complete remissions of from 4 to more than 62 months after treatment with a platinum compound, an epipodophyllotoxin, and craniospinal irradiation. Two patients had progressive disease despite combined chemotherapy and craniospinal irradiation. Neuroimaging and autopsy findings showed that CSF was the major pathway for neuraxis dissemination by neuroblastoma cells.

Conclusions.—Neurologic deterioration may signal relapse in the neuraxis in patients with neuroblastoma. A combination of craniospinal irradiation and administration of a platinum compound and an epipodophyllotoxin can induce complete responses in some patients. However, the risk of relapse outside the CNS also remains high. Children with CNS relapse should be retreated with systemic chemotherapy independent of evidence of extracranial disease.

▶ What is the mechanism of spread of neuroblastoma to the CNS without evidence of concurrent intracranial extension from adjacent bone, dura, or dural sinus metastases? Computed tomography, MRI, and autopsy findings implicate CSF as the major pathway for neuroaxis dissemination of neuroblastoma. One recent article on neuroblastoma determines the GD-DTPA–enhanced MR has promise in demonstrating residual neuroblastoma even when CT and 1-metaiodobenzylguanidine scintigraphy have been negative for residual disease (1). Another recent article of related interest on neuroblastoma and CNS involvement is listed (2).—L.W. Young, M.D.

References

1. Kornreich L, et al: *Pediatr Radiol* 21:566, 1991.
2. Munro FD, et al: *Arch Dis Child* 66:1246, 1991.

Early Detection of Heterotopic Ossification in Young Patients With Traumatic Brain Injury

Citta-Pietrolungo TJ, Alexander MA, Steg NL (Alfred I DuPont Inst, Wilmington, Del)
Arch Phys Med Rehabil 73:258–262, 1992   6–22

Introduction.—Severe head injury often is complicated by heterotopic ossification (HO), which frequently goes undetected until clinical manifestations appear. Most reports of HO have addressed adults only. The frequency and incidence of HO in children and adolescents with traumatic brain injury (TBI) were studied.

Methods.—The 3-year prospective study was conducted at a pediatric brain injury rehabilitation unit. One hundred eleven patients aged 6 to 21 years were admitted with the primary diagnosis of TBI. Each patient underwent triple-phase bone scans within 3 weeks of admission, followed by early intervention with intensive physical therapy and indomethacin.

Findings.—Twenty-five cases of HO were detected, for an incidence of 22.5%. There were 55 separate sites of HO; about half were in the hip, followed by the elbow, knee, shoulder, and other sites. Seventy-two percent of the sites had true neurogenic HO. The lesions were clinically significant, that is, they impeded the rehabilitation process, in 5 patients, although none of these needed operative intervention. Fifteen asymptomatic sites were detected by bone scanning. In symptomatic patients, bone scans often showed HO in unsuspected sites (table).

Sites of Suspected HO vs. Sites Confirmed by Bone Scan

Patient	Site Suspected (Based on Clinical Signs)	Site Detected (Based on Bone Scan)
1	Right hip	Right hip
4	Bilateral hips	Bilateral hips
5	Bilateral hips	Bilateral hips, bilateral elbows, left shoulder
6	Right knee	Right knee, bilateral hips
7	Right elbow	Right elbow, bilateral shoulders
9	Bilateral elbows	Bilateral elbows, bilateral hips, bilateral knees
10	Right elbow	Right elbow
11	Left knee	Left knee, left shoulder
15	Left knee	Left knee
16	Left hip	Left hip
18	Right knee	Right knee, bilateral hips
19	Bilateral hips	Bilateral hips
20	Right hip, right knee	Right hip, right knee, left hip
22	Left elbow	Left elbow
24	Left shoulder, left elbow	Left shoulder, left elbow, left hip

(Courtesy of Citta-Pietrolungo TJ, Alexander MA, Steg NL: *Arch Phys Med Rehabil* 73:258–262, 1992.)

Conclusions.—In young patients with TBI, HO may be more common than has been previously thought. Bone scans to screen for HO may be performed in high-risk patients, though the benefits of early intervention need to be specifically evaluated. Few patients were left with decreased range of motion in the affected joint, and none needed surgical intervention.

▶ Symptomatic HO after severe head injury is the motivation for finding the ossification before pain and decreased range of motion occur. Triple-phase radionuclide scintigraphy seems to be an effective method for trying to accomplish this. Another recent article on this subject uses cineradiography to assess joint motion (1). Among the recent articles of related interest (2–4) are 2 about myositis ossificans (2, 3).—L.W. Young, M.D.

References

1. Subbarao JV: *Am J Phys Med Rehabil* 69:88, 1990.
2. Heifetz SA, et al: *Pediatr Pathol* 12:223, 1992.
3. Nuovo MA, et al: *Skeletal Radiol* 21:87, 1992.
4. Garland DE: *Clin Orthop* 263:13, 1991.

Neurodevelopmental Outcome in Neonates After Extracorporeal Membrane Oxygenation: Cranial Magnetic Resonance Imaging and Ultrasonography Correlation
Griffin MP, Minifee PK, Landry SH, Allison PL, Swischuk LE, Zwischenberger JB (Univ of Texas, Galveston, Tex)
J Pediatr Surg 27:33–35, 1992   6–23

Purpose.—In neonates with severe respiratory failure, irreversible ligation of the right common carotid artery and right internal jugular vein is common with initiation of venoarterial extracorporeal membrane oxygenation (ECMO). This may increase the risks of cerebral hemorrhage or infarction and jeopardize neurodevelopmental outcome. Magnetic resonance imaging was used to detect abnormalities of the CNS after ECMO and the findings were correlated with the outcome.

Methods.—The study sample comprised 22 consecutive neonatal ECMO survivors treated over a 27-month period. Two patients who received ECMO died during this period. Cranial ultrasound findings, MRI scans, and neurodevelopmental outcome for each infant were reviewed. Neurologic examination included use of the Bayley Scales of Infant Development, at 3, 6, 12, and 24 months of follow-up. All patients had cranial ultrasound studies, 19 had MRI, and 20 had the Bayley tests.

Results.—None of the imaging studies showed focal abnormal findings attributable to ECMO, and there was no evidence of cerebral hemorrhage or infarction. There were 2 cases of generalized cerebral atrophy detected by MRI, and the Bayley developmental tests were abnormal in

1 of these infants. One infant had a right focal seizure 4 days after ECMO; findings at MRI were normal in this case. There were only 3 abnormal Bayley test results; mental indices ranged from 72 to 135 and motor indices from 71 to 150.

Conclusions.—The occurrence of cerebral hemorrhage or infarction after ECMO appears to be less common than has been generally reported. When ultrasound or MRI studies show no intracranial hemorrhage, cerebral infarct, or cerebral atrophy, short-term neurodevelopmental outcome is usually normal.

▶ Extracorporeal membrane oxygenation has increasing applicability in neonates treated for hypoxemia, acidosis, and cerebral ischemia. Focus on neurodevelopmental outcome of ECMO deserves attention because the technique can cause cerebral hemorrhage, infarction, or atrophy. Ultrasonography and MRI are used by these authors to exclude these findings and assure normal short-term neurodevelopmental outcome. Computed tomography (1), color Doppler imaging (2), and 3-dimensional (volume) MR angiography (3) also may be helpful. Other recent reports about intracranial imaging findings or outcome from ECMO are listed (4, 5).—L.W. Young, M.D.

References

1. Mendoza JC, et al: *Pediatrics* 88:1004, 1991.
2. DeAngelis GA, et al: *Radiology* 182:521, 1992.
3. Wiznitzer M, et al: *Am J Dis Child* 144:1323, 1990.
4. von Allmen D, et al: *J Pediatr Surg* 27:36, 1992.
5. Alexander AA, et al: *Radiology* 182:527, 1992.

Maternal Cocaine Abuse: The Spectrum of Radiologic Abnormalities in the Neonatal CNS

Heier LA, Carpanzano CR, Mast J, Brill PW, Winchester P, Deck MDF (New York Hosp-Cornell Univ Med Ctr, New York)
AJR 157:1105–1110, 1991   6–24

Background.—An unusual constellation of midline CNS malformations noted in neonates in 1 institution had a common denominator of maternal cocaine abuse. The pattern and frequency of CNS abnormalities in infants born to cocaine-abusing mothers were examined.

Methods.—A retrospective review was conducted of 43 neonates who met the criteria for use of maternal cocaine. A control group of 62 infants was matched for gestational age and race. Because the groups were matched for gestational age, it was possible to screen for intracranial abnormalities other than those seen with prematurity. Radiologic studies were analyzed by 2 independent reviewers and CNS abnormalities were assessed by sonography, CT, or MRI.

Radiologic Abnormalities

Abnormality	Study Group (n = 43)	Control Group (n = 62)	p Value
Subependymal hemorrhage	35% (15)	34% (21)	NS
Intraventricular hemorrhage	22% (10)	21% (13)	NS
Intraparenchymal hemorrhage	12% (5)	3% (2)	NS
Ventricular dilatation	14% (6)	16% (10)	NS
Periventricular leukomalacia	14% (6)	6% (4)	NS
Porencephaly	19% (8)	8% (5)	NS
Infarction	17% (7)	2% (1)	$p < .05$ ($p = .02$)
Congenital abnormalities	12% (5)	0% (0)	$p < .05$ ($p = .01$)

Abbreviation: NS, not significant.
(Courtesy of Heier LA, Carpanzano CR, Mast J, et al: AJR 157:1105–1110, 1991.)

Findings.—The frequency of the various forms of intracranial hemorrhage, porencephaly, periventricular leukomalacia (PVL), and ventricular enlargement was not significantly different in the study and control groups although the frequency of intraparenchymal hemorrhage, PVL, and porencephaly was higher in the study group (table). The higher frequency of infarctions and congenital abnormalities in the study group was statistically significant. The frequency of cortical infarction and major congenital malformations was 17% and 12%, respectively, in the study group and 12% and 0% in the control group. All 5 congenital malformations were midline CNS abnormalities, particularly neural tube defects.

Conclusions.—The higher statistically significant frequency of congenital malformations and stroke in the infants of maternal cocaine abusers appears to be related to vasospasm caused by cocaine when used in the first and third trimesters. Cocaine has a teratogenic potential and a tendency to cause cerebral vascular events in the neonate. An investigation of neonatal stroke and neural tube defects should include a history of drug use and urine screening.

▶ This is a nicely designed retrospective study that compares cocaine-abused neonates with age-related controls. It establishes, with the help of sonographic, CT, and MRI findings, the validity of the association of neonatal CNS malformation and stroke to maternal cocaine abuse. Another study indicates that some of the anomalies may be incidental rather than cause and effect (1). Two additional recent articles of related interest are listed (2, 3).—L.W. Young, M.D.

References

1. Link EA, et al: *Clin Pediatr* 30:506, 1991.
2. Neuspiel DR: *Am J Dis Child* 146:278, 1992.
3. Dominguez R, et al: *Am J Dis Child* 145:688, 1991.

Musculoskeletal

Characterization and Intraoperative Localization of a Soft Tissue Arteriovenous Malformation Via Ultrasound

Bober SE, Asnis S, Goldman MA, Gould ES, Russo B (North Shore Univ Hosp/Cornell Univ Med College, Manhasset, NY)
Orthopedics 14:1007–1010, 1991   6–25

Background.—Ultrasound provides less anatomical detail than CT, but it can play a significant role in the diagnosis of soft tissue masses of the extremities. Magnetic resonance imaging can differentiate between proton relaxation characteristics in normal muscle and pathologic tissue.

Case Report.—Girl, 14 years, had plain radiography and CT that revealed no abnormalities. She had pain in the medial left thigh of 1½-year's duration. However, MRI revealed a subtle asymmetric area of increased signal in the area of the intermuscular septum in the left lower medial thigh between the sartorius and vastus medialis muscles. Ultrasound revealed an echogenic region corresponding to MRI findings. Real-time sonography was used at surgery to confirm the site of the lesion, which proved to be a soft tissue arteriovenous malformation. The pain disappeared after excision of the lesion.

Discussion.—Because CT must detect the difference in x-ray attenuation between mass and surrounding normal tissue, a soft tissue tumor with the same density as surrounding muscle will go undetected. In contrast, MRI demonstrates superb contrast difference between hemangiomas and surrounding muscle tissue on T_2-weighted images. Therefore, MRI is effective in diagnosing soft tissue arteriovenous malformations. Arteriovenous malformations usually have relatively low signal intensity—similar to muscle—on T_1-weighted images but a relatively high signal intensity on T_2-weighted images relative to surrounding muscle. The low on T_1, high on T_2 characteristics are caused by the predominance of cystic spaces in the architecture of the masses. However, lesions with very rapid blood flow may display low signal intensities on both T_1- and T_2-weighted images. Intraoperative ultrasound can be used to guide neurosurgical procedures, detect pathologic processes of the biliary tree, detect neoplastic and inflammatory processes of the pancreas, intraoperatively visualize the kidneys, and detect intra-abdominal abscesses not apparent on abdominal exploration. Ultrasound can also be used during vascular procedures and to localize thyroid and parathyroid adenomas. Real-time intraoperative ultrasound imaging of the extremities has not been previously reported, but Doppler ultrasound has been used intraoperatively for localizing vascular lesions.

Conclusions.—This case study illustrates the capability of ultrasound to characterize soft tissue lesions of the extremities. It also demonstrates the intraoperative value of ultrasound to guide surgical excision.

▶ Abnormal findings of an arteriovenous malformation in the soft tissue of this girl's thigh were clearly shown by MRI and were refined by intraoperative ultrasonography for more precise localization and management. Intraoperative ultrasonography also is complementary during surgery on spinal cord lesions (1). One recent article of related interest includes a biologic classification of soft tissue vascular anomalies as demonstrated by MRI (2). Another technique that can be used for distinguishing vascular malformations from soft tissue hemangiomas is technetium-labeled red blood cell scintigraphy (3).—L.W. Young, M.D.

References

1. Brunberg JA, et al: *Radiology* 181:573, 1991.
2. Meyer JS, et al: *AJR* 157:559, 1991.
3. Barton DJ, et al: *Plast Reconstr Surg* 89:46, 1992.

Use of Ultrasonography in Dysplasia of the Immature Hip
Millis MB, Share JC (Children's Hosp, Boston)
Clin Orthop 274:160–171, 1992   6–26

Background.—Real-time ultrasonography has dramatically affected the diagnosis and treatment of patients with hip dysplasia. The use of this new imaging technique in dysplasia of the immature hip was reviewed.

Ultrasonographic Anatomy of the Hip.—Most of an infant's hip is cartilaginous, which allows clear ultrasonic visualization of most joint components. The standard plane of imaging includes a coronal section through the acetabular fossa containing the lower iliac margin, the superior bony acetabular rim, and the acetabular labrum. This standard image should include a contour of the iliac wall that is straight. The landmarks seen in a satisfactory coronal ultrasonogram are the vertical iliac line

---

Sonographic Anatomical Classification of Infant Hip Dysplasia (Modified From Graf)

Classification	α-Angle	Superior Bony Rim	% Coverage
Type I (mature)	>60°	Sharp	>50%
Type IIA (immature) (<3 months old)	50°–59°	Rounded	40–50%
Type II (mild–moderate) (>3 months old)	50°–59°	Rounded	40–50%
Type IIC (critical zone dysplasia)	43°–49°	Rounded	40–50%
Type III (severe dysplasia; subluxation)	<43°	Rounded	<40%
Type IV (dislocation)	<43°	Rounded	0%

(Courtesy of Millis MB, Share JC: *Clin Orthop* 274:160–171, 1992.)

ending inferiorly in the superior bony rim of acetabulum, the cartilaginous acetabular roof ending in the labrum, the lower iliac margin, the joint capsule, and the hypoechoic femoral head. The transverse view may also be useful.

Sonographic Anatomical Classification.—Graf has classified infant hips into 4 basic anatomical types, based on the standard plane coronal sonogram (table). This classification scheme is widely used, although some believe that the dynamic assessment is at least as important as the static one.

Conclusions.—Ultrasonography is almost ideal for assessing the presence and character of hip dysplasia and for monitoring the progress of the treatment program during most of the first year of life. In the second 6 months of life and thereafter, ultrasound and conventional radiography are complementary. As the hip becomes more ossified, conventional radiography becomes more accurate, and ultrasound images progressively deteriorate in quality.

▶ The application of ultrasound to demonstrate the status of the immature hip continues to gain in popularity and usage. In real time, it dynamically assesses the soft tissue, cartilaginous, and bony structures about the hip. It has a major advantage of no ionizing radiation to the infant. Gross instability can be observed with application of appropriate maneuvers. Ultrasound's affordability also contributes to its usage in preference to CT or MRI. Terjesen and co-workers recommend ultrasound as a primary imaging technique to evaluate hip joints throughout childhood and as a guide to closed reduction of dislocated hips in children less than 2 years of age (1–3). Sonography of the infant hip is a popular topic, and additional recent articles are recommended (4, 5).—L.W. Young, M.D.

References

1. Terjesen T, et al: *Clin Orthop* 262:159, 1991.
2. Terjesen T, et al: *J Pediatr Orthop* 12:54, 1992.
3. Terjesen T, et al: *J Pediatr Orthop* 11:608, 1991.
4. Walter RS, et al: *Am J Dis Child* 146:230, 1992.
5. Rungee JL, et al: *J Pediatr Orthop* 12:61, 1992.

The Spondylometaphyseal Dysplasias: A Tentative Classification
Maroteaux P, Spranger J (Hôpital des Enfants-Malades, Paris; Johannes Gutenberg University, Mainz, Germany)
Pediatr Radiol 21:293–297, 1991   6–27

Background.—Spondylometaphyseal dysplasias are a complex group of constitutional bone diseases. A preliminary classification of these disorders, in addition to the previously described Kozlowski type, have

Classification of Spondylometaphyseal Dysplasias

Severe coxa vara	Mild vertebral abnormalities { discrete metaphyseal changes	: type A1 (Sutcliffe)
	mores severe metaphyseal changes	: type A2 (Schmidt, Langer)
	Round vertebral bodies	: type A3
	Flattened vertebral bodies with tongue like deformity	: type A4
Moderate changes of the femoral neck	– Slight irregularity of the vertebral bodies Short tubular bones of the hand with irregular metaphyses	: type B1
	– Generalized platyspondyly (close to brachyolmy)	: type B2
Discrete metaphyseal changes of the femoral neck	– Squared form of the vertebral bodies with irregular contour	: type C1
	– Moderately flattened and long vertebral bodies in the lateral view	: type C2
	– Trapezoidal aspect of the vertebral bodies	: type C3

(Courtesy of Maroteaux P, Spranger J: *Pediatr Radiol* 21:293–297, 1991.)

been proposed; 3 subgroups are distinguished by the appearance of the femoral neck (table).

The First Major Group.—The type A forms show severe changes of the femoral neck. Four subtypes have been observed. In A1, mild vertebral and metaphyseal abnormalities are manifested in early childhood with gait abnormalities. The children have a relatively short trunk and a moderately protuberant sternum. Radiologic studies show a severe coxa vara, short iliac wings, and slightly flattened vertebral bodies. In A2, the metaphyseal changes of the long bones are more severe with irregular, fragmented, and cupped metaphyseal margins. The A3 type is characterized by round vertebral bodies, and A4 is characterized by severe platyspondyly and anterior tonguing of vertebral bodies.

The Second Major Group.—Type B forms show moderate changes of the femoral neck. B1 is characterized by marked involvement of the hand bones and B2 by platyspondyly. Both result in short stature and short limbs.

The Third Major Group.—Type C forms have minor spinal changes and become apparent at varying ages. Patients may show mild leg deformities, hip pain, or prepubertal scoliosis. In contrast with types A and B, the femoral neck is well developed without varus deformity.

Conclusions.—This system of classification brings some order to a confusing group of bone diseases. The fact that all but 1 of the cases were sporadic suggests dominant mutations. Additional, very rare forms of spondylometaphyseal dysplasia exist and do not fit entirely into this classification.

▶ This classification is an attempt to bring order to spondylometaphyseal dysplasias. As Hall (1) has aptly indicated, the mystique of skeletal dysplasias is gradually vanishing largely because of advances: bone marrow transplants, bone lengthening and growth hormone therapy successes. Rybak et al. (2) have described yet another spondylometaphyseal dysplasia. Recent articles of related interest on skeletal dysplasias and their classification are listed (3–7).—L.W. Young, M.D.

References

1. Hall BD: *Pediatr Clin North Am* 39:279, 1992.
2. Rybak M, et al: *Am J Med Genet* 40:304, 1991.
3. Goldblatt J, et al: *Am J Med Genet* 39:170, 1991.
4. Meinecke P, et al: *Am J Med Genet* 39:232, 1991.
5. Hanscom DA, et al: *J Bone Joint Surg* 74-A:598, 1992.
6. Shebib SM, et al: *Pediatr Radiol* 21:298, 1991.
7. Greenspan A: *Skeletal Radiol* 20:561, 1991.

Microcephalic Osteodysplastic Primordial Dwarfism Type I/III in Sibs

Meinecke P, Passarge E (Altonaer Kinderkrankenhaus, Hamburg, Germany; Universitätsklinikum, Essen, Germany)
J Med Genet 28:795–800, 1991   6–28

Background.—There is growing evidence that types I and III microcephalic osteodysplastic primordial dwarfism (MOPD) are identical. A pair of siblings with this condition shared characteristics of both types I and III. The proband was first seen in 1968 at the age of 16 months because of severe developmental retardation with dwarfism and microcephaly. In 1974, the younger sister was seen at 1 month of age, with striking similarities to the proband. The parents were young, healthy, and nonconsanguineous.

Case 1.—Male infant, born with microcephaly, dwarfism, hypotrichosis, large eyes, deep-set and small ears, and tapered fingers. He had poor growth and severely retarded psychomotor development. His electroencephalogram showed generalized dysrhythmia and signs of convulsive potential. Radiologic findings included a small skull with particularly small and sloping frontal bones, only 11 pairs of ribs, mild platyspondyly of the spine, rounded iliac wings with nearly horizontal, irregular acetabular roofs. Both femora had mildly bowed shafts; ossification of the epiphyses in the knee region was absent. Joint spaces were narrow, hands and feet were small, the first metacarpals were short, and the proximal phalanges of the big toes were short and rounded. The boy apparently remained dwarfed and microcephalic with severely retarded psychomotor development, and died at 5½ years of an acute aphthous stomatitis with complications.

Case 2.—A female infant was born at term after an uneventful pregnancy, with craniofacial anomalies, short limbs, short neck, generalized hypotrichosis, and a dry, hyperkeratotic, and scaling skin. Laboratory tests and G-banded chromosomes were normal. Radiologic findings included a small skull with a steep and sclerotic cranial base, small and sloping frontal bone, and well-ossified occipital bone with bathrocephaly. Long clavicles, poor ossification of the sternum, and only 11 pairs of ribs, which were dorsally narrow, were noted. The spine was abnormal with platyspondyly and coronal clefts of lumbar vertebral bodies. Psychomotor development was severly retarded. She died unexpectedly at 6 months of unexplained causes.

Conclusions.—Both patients had primordial dwarfism, severe microcephaly, and various external abnormalities, including large and protruding eyes; deep-set, small, poorly differentiated ears; micrognathia; short neck; short limbs; tapering fingers; and dry, scaling skin. Both also had severely retarded psychomotor development. Radiologically, both patients showed small neurocranium, long clavicles, 11 pairs of ribs, rounded iliac wings with horizontal acetabular roofs, short tubular bones, narrow joint spaces, and retarded epiphyseal maturation. The survival of the 2 patients differed, illustrating the intrafamilial variable prognosis of this disorder. The patients shared characteristics of both types I and III of MOPD, providing evidence that the 2 types are identical. These cases also provide further evidence that this condition is transmitted by autosomal recessive inheritance.

▶ Microcephalic dwarfs with severe intrauterine and postnatal growth retardation were divided into at least 4 varieties by Majewski et al. (1) in 1982. This article suggests that the division might be too broad and that the type I/III includes Taybi-Linder syndrome. I heartily support this kind of attention to detail that helps in refining concepts and advancing understanding. Recent articles of related interest are listed (2–6).—L.W. Young, M.D.

References

1. Majewski F, et al: *Am J Med Genet* 12:37, 1982.
2. Taybi H: *Am J Med Genet* 43:628, 1992.
3. Shebib S, et al: *Am J Med Genet* 40:146, 1991.
4. Meinecke P, et al: *Am J Med Genet* 39:232, 1991.
5. Haan EA, et al: *Am J Med Genet* 39:232, 1991.
6. Herman TE, et al: *Pediatr Radiol* 21:602, 1991.

Hypoplastic Posterior Arch of C-1 in Children With Down Syndrome: A Double Jeopardy

Martich V, Ben-Ami T, Yousefzadeh DK, Roizen NJ (Univ of Chicago Hosps, Wyler Children's Hosp, Chicago)
Radiology 183:125–128, 1992   6–29

Introduction.—Children with Down syndrome have an increased prevalence of cervical spine abnormalities. An anomaly not previously documented in Down syndrome, hypoplasia of the posterior arch of C1, was reported.

Methods.—At age 2 to 3 years, 38 neurologically asymptomatic children with Down syndrome had undergone routine screening for cervical spine abnormalities. The radiographs were reviewed to determine the incidence of hypoplasia of the posterior arch of the C1 vertebra. Relevant measurements were compared with those of age- and sex-matched controls. Similarly evaluated were the posterior arches of C2 to C5.

Results.—In 6 of the 23 boys and 4 of the 15 girls with Down syndrome hypoplasia of the posterior arch of C1 was diagnosed; none had abnormal C2 to C5 posterior arch measurements. Children with abnormalities had C1 measurements and C1 to C2 ratios that were more than 2 SDs less than the mean in the controls.

Conclusions.—A hypoplastic posterior arch of C1 in children with Down syndrome may increase the risk of spinal cord damage after atlantoaxial subluxation (Fig 6–22). Thus, C1 vertebral abnormalities carry a potential for "double jeopardy" and serious neurologic impairment. Cer-

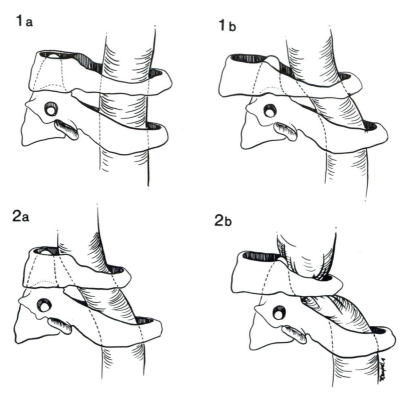

Fig 6–22.—Diagram of a normal C-1 vertebra (*1a*), a normal C-1 vertebra with concurrent atlantoaxial subluxation (*1b*), a hypoplastic posterior arch of C-1 with persistent posterior impingement on the cervical vertebral canal (*2a*), and a hypoplastic posterior arch of C-1 with concurrent atlantoaxial subluxation (*2b*). Note extensive narrowing of the vertebral canal with concomitant extrinsic compression of the spinal cord. (Courtesy of Martich V, Ben-Ami T, Yousefzadeh DK, et al: *Radiology* 183:125–128, 1992).

vical spine radiographic evaluations are essential for documenting the presence of a hypoplastic posterior arch of C1 and any associated vertebral canal impingement.

▶ In addition to atlantoaxial instability, patients with Down syndrome may have hypoplasia of the posterior arch of C1—"double jeopardy." This is a noteworthy observation because at least a quarter of patients with Down syndrome have this finding. The authors refer also to a clivo-odontoid alignment abnormality, presumably laxity, which renders "triple jeopardy" for the upper cervical spine in children with Down syndrome. Recent articles of related interest that concern trauma to the upper cervical spine are listed (1, 2).—L.W. Young, M.D.

References

1. Maves CK, et al: *Pediatr Radiol* 21:504, 1991.
2. Parisi M, et al: *Pediatr Radiol* 21:367, 1991.

Cranial Imaging in Autosomal Recessive Osteopetrosis: I. Facial Bones and Calvarium

Elster AD, Theros EG, Key LL, Chen MYM (Bowman Gray School of Medicine, Winston-Salem, NC)
Radiology 183:129–135, 1992   6–30

Introduction.—Osteopetrosis, a bone disorder caused by defective osteoclast function, is characterized by a "marble-bone" appearance. The most severe form of this rare disorder is transmitted as an autosomal recessive trait and is typically fatal in childhood. There is little in the radiology literature concerning cranial findings. Cranial images in 13 affected infants and children were reviewed to characterize patterns of facial and calvarial involvement at initial diagnosis and with disease progression.

Methods.—Seven girls and 6 boys ranging in age at initial diagnosis from 3 weeks to 9.8 years were seen over a 6-year period. All were undergoing an extensive metabolic, clinical, and radiologic work-up. Studies included radiographs, CT scans, MR images, and bone marrow scintigrams. The images were evaluated by an experienced neuroradiologist and a skeletal radiologist.

Results.—All patients had defective dentition; all 6 patients older than 1 year had dental caries and generalized mild sclerosis of the mandible. In 10 cases, the mandible showed a characteristic triangular opacity on each side (Fig 6–23). The bones of the middle of the face revealed disease involvement in all cases, with at least mild distortion of the general

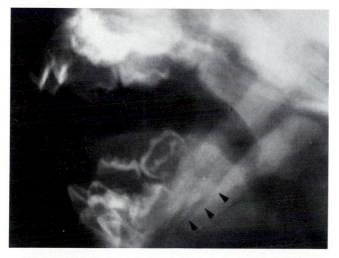

Fig 6–23.—Oblique radiograph of the mandible shows characteristic triangular opacity (the "endobone") extending from the condyle to the midbody (*arrowheads*). This was seen in 10 of the 13 patients. (Courtesy of Elster AD, Theros EG, Key LL, et al: *Radiology* 183:129–135, 1992.)

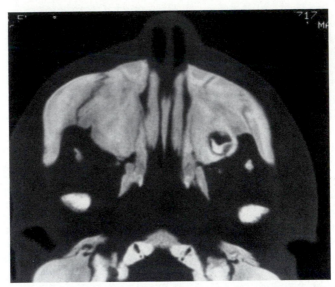

Fig 6–24.—Maxillary sinuses are unformed and filled with osteopetrotic bone (seen in 12 of 13 patients) on CT scan. (Courtesy of Elster AD, Theros EG, Key LL, et al: *Radiology* 183:129–135, 1992.)

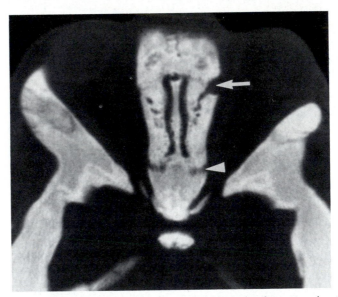

Fig 6–25.—Prominent channels for the anterior ethmoidal (*arrow*) and posterior ethmoidal (*arrowhead*) arteries were routinely visualized on CT scans in 8 patients. (Courtesy of Elster AD, Theros EG, Key LL, et al: *Radiology* 183:129–135, 1992)

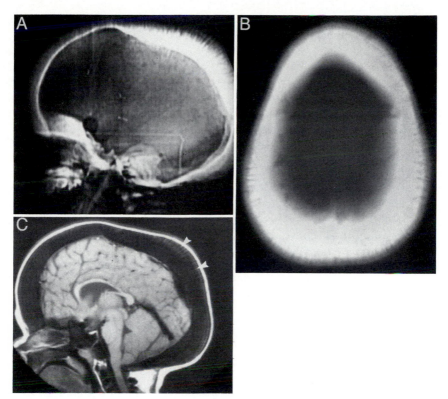

Fig 6–26.—**A,** radiograph obtained at age 5 years demonstrates progressive calvarial thickening. There is partial healing of the craniotomy site. **B,** sagittal T1-weighted MR image (repetition time, 500 ms; echo time, 20 ms) shows striations of low-to-intermediate signal intensity (*arrows*) corresponding to regions of active marrow. (Courtesy of Elster AD, Theros EG, Key LL, et al: *Radiology* 183:129–135, 1992.)

shape and proportions of the facial skeleton. A common complaint of nasal stuffiness was linked to narrowing of the nasal cavities. In 12 patients, the maxillary sinuses remained completely unpneumatized (Fig 6–24). Dense sclerosis was seen in the ethmoid sinuses in 8 patients (Fig 6–25). Calvarium involvement was present in all cases, and its pattern was related to patient age. Macrocephaly became universal with disease progression (Fig 6–26).

Conclusions.—Many new radiologic features of osteopetrosis have been identified and related to pathophysiologic characteristics. Abnormalities in the face involve the teeth, mandible, and middle of the face and sinuses. Abnormalities of the calvarium result in an increased head circumference and a "hair-on-end" appearance. Two children in this study appeared to have an intermediate recessive form of osteopetrosis with a milder clinical course.

▶ Characteristic imaging findings of osteopetrosis in the face and the calvaria are the mandibular finding of "endobone," as well as the "hair-on-end" appearance in the calvaria, on radiography. Osteopetrotic change in maxillary sinuses and ethmoid sinuses on CT and intermediate signal intensity striations representing active calvarial marrow on MRI are also reported. Certainly this is the most extensive imaging demonstration of facial bone, calvarial, skull base, and brain findings in osteopetrosis. Recent related articles of interest concerning osteopetrosis are listed after part II (Abstract 6–31).—L.W. Young, M.D.

Cranial Imaging in Autosomal Recessive Osteopetrosis: II. Skull Base and Brain

Elster AD, Theros EG, Key LL, Chen MYM (Bowman Gray School of Medicine, Winston-Salem, NC)

Radiology 183:137–144, 1992   6–31

Introduction.—Osteopetrosis is a rare disease characterized by an increase in the density of the skeleton. In the conclusion of a 2-part study, the radiologic abnormalities of those parts of the skull derived principally from cartilage were reviewed in 13 infants and children seen over a 6-year period.

Methods.—The patients had the severe, autosomal recessive form of osteopetrosis. All had undergone extensive clinical evaluation of the head and nervous system. Cranial imaging studies included radiographs, CT scans, and MR images.

Results.—A relatively large number of new findings concerning involvement of the skull base by osteopetrosis were observed. There was marked sclerosis and deposition of osteopetrotic bone along the anterior occipitomastoid suture in 8 cases, along the spheno-occipital synchondrosis in 8 cases, and at the basioccipital-exoccipital synchondrosis in 9 cases. Eleven patients showed endobones in the sphenoidal body and basioccipital bone. Three demonstrated marked cupping at the basioccipital-exoccipital synchondrosis. Metaphyseal lucencies and cupping are commonly found in the peripheral skeleton of patients with osteopetrosis (Fig 6–27). Neurologic deficits were common in these children; 11 were blind, 11 had conductive hearing loss, and 4 had facial nerve palsies. Magnetic resonance imaging revealed delayed myelination in 2 of 5 retarded infants. Five of the 8 developmentally normal children had prominent extracerebral CSF spaces over the frontal lobes.

Conclusions.—Involvement of the skull base is a prominent and universal feature of osteopetrosis. Abnormalities are seen in the occipital bone, sphenoid bone, temporal bones, and brain. Improved CT scan-

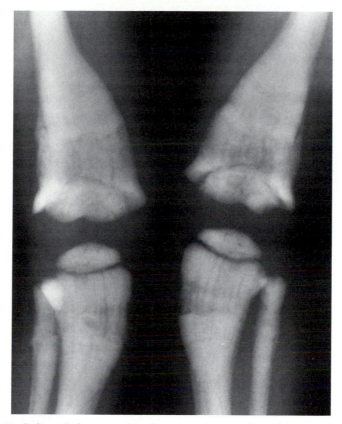

Fig 6–27.—Radiograph shows metaphyseal cupping, sclerosis, and remodeling errors—typical features of osteoporosis in the peripheral skeleton—in the knees. (Courtesy of Elster AD, Theros EG, Key LL, et al: *Radiology* 183:137-144, 1992.)

ning techniques and a larger patient population have extended many of the observations previously reported in the literature and should lead to a better understanding of this rare disease.

▶ Although the focus of the lesions shown by imaging in this article is on the cranial region, skull base, and brain, Figure 6–27 shows typical and familiar major limb bone findings of osteopetrosis. Noteworthy are MRI findings of delayed myelination and parenchymal calcifications. Elster et al. (1) and Ostuka et al. (2) in more recent articles correlate the bone marrow MRI findings in osteopetrosis with technetium 99m sulfur colloid or indium 111 chloride scintigraphy findings of hematopoeisis. This report opens a "new atlas" on osteopetrosis. A recent article of related interest is listed (3).—L.W. Young, M.D.

References

1. Elster AD, et al: *Radiology* 183:129, 1992.
2. Otsuka N, et al: *Clin Nucl Med* 16(6):443, 1991.
3. Demirici A, et al: *AJNR* 12(4):781, 1991.

Schimke Immuno-osseous Dysplasia: A Newly Recognized Multisystem Disease

Spranger J, Hinkel GK, Stöss H, Thoenes W, Wargowski D, Zepp F (University of Mainz, Mainz, Germany; Children's Hospital, Dresden, Germany; University of Erlangen, Erlangen, Germany; Clinical Genetics Ctr, Madison, Wis)
J Pediatr 119:64–72, 1991   6–32

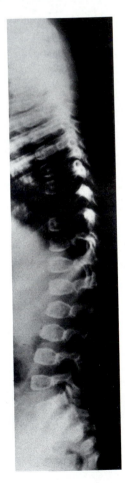

Fig 6–28.—Radiograph taken when patient was 2 years of age. (Courtesy of Spranger J, Hinkel GK, Stöss H, et al: *J Pediatr* 119:64–72, 1991.)

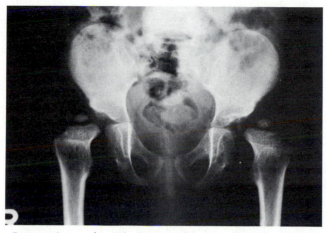

Fig 6–29.—Patient at 3 years of age. The ilia are small because of hypoplasia of the lower portions. The acetabular roofs are slanted with wide iliac angles. The femoral heads are laterally displaced with small epiphyses and dislocated. Coxa valga is present. (Courtesy of Spranger J, Hinkel GK, Stöss H, et al: *J Pediatr* 119:64–72, 1991.)

Background.—A new, hereditary multisystem disorder affecting chondrocytes, lymphocytes, and possibly melanocytes has been identified in 5 children. Because the 5 cases reported are similar to a single case described by Schimke et al. in 1974, the disease has been called Schimke immunoosseous dysplasia.

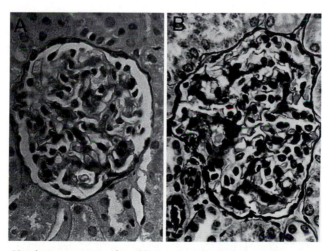

Fig 6–30.—Histologic appearance of renal biopsy tissue obtained when patient was 4 years of age. **A,** slight mesangial thickening is accentuated in the perihilar region. (Periodic acid-Schiff-hemalum stain; original magnification, x1,000.) **B,** red-staining deposits are seen in some mesangial regions. (Chromotrope 2R stain; original magnification, x1,000). (Courtesy of Spranger J, Hinkel GK, Stöss H, et al: *J Pediatr* 119:64–72, 1991.)

Case Report.—Girl, 5 years, was evaluated for short stature and proteinuria. Her early development was normal, but delayed growth was noted at 18 months. A diagnosis of nephrosis was made when the child was scheduled to undergo operative correction of bilaterally dislocated hips at age 3½ years. At age 5, she showed a short-trunk type of dwarfism, a peculiar face, thin hair, a high-pitched voice, and numerous pigmented spots on the abdomen. Radiographs revealed findings of spondyloepiphyseal dysplasia (Figs 6–28 and 6–29). Progressive signs of renal insufficiency developed during the next 3 years. The child died of renal failure at 8 years of age. An autopsy showed small kidneys and marked arteriosclerotic changes in the aorta, carotid, and coronary arteries. Renal biopsy tissue obtained when the girl was 4 years old showed focal changes characterized by perihilar mesangial deposition of proteinaceous material, a process spreading to all glomeruli (Fig 6–30).

Conclusions.—All 5 patients had small stature and an appearance like that described in the first case. Immunologic studies revealed defective T-cell function. Renal disease progressed rapidly and was resistant to corticosteroid and immunosuppressive treatment. Other hereditary diseases associated with skeletal and immunologic defects do not have the renal and pigmentary skin changes found in Schimke immunoosseous dysplasia. The pathogenesis remains unknown, but the presence of the disease in a brother and sister suggests that it is genetically determined.

▶ Schimke immuno-osseous dysplasia, a new multisystem disease with renal and pigmentary skin changes, is distinguished from the other hereditary diseases associated with skeletal and immunologic defects. This is another important contribution from this productive author in the field of skeletal dysplasias. Other recent articles of related interest in the immuno-osseus dysplasia group are listed (1, 2).—L.W. Young, M.D.

References

1. MacDermot KD, et al: *J Med Genet* 28:10, 1991.
2. Chakravarti VS, et al: *Pediatr Radiol* 21:447, 1991.

Transoral Decompression and Posterior Stabilisation in Morquio's Disease
Ashraf J, Crockard HA, Ransford AO, Stevens JM (Natl Hospitals for Neurology and Neurosurgery, University College, London, England)
Arch Dis Child 66:1318–1321, 1991   6–33

Background.—Morquio's disease is an inherited connective tissue disorder caused by absence or reduced activity of either N-acetylgalactosamine 6-sulphatase or β-galactosidase. Clinical signs include disproportionate dwarfing dysplasia with joint hypermobility caused by lax restraining ligaments. Spinal cord compression in the thoracolumbar and

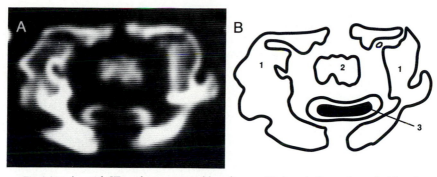

Fig 6–31.—An axial CT myelogram **(A)** and line diagram **(B)** through the craniovertebral junction, showing compression of the spinal cord in flexion by the soft tissue surrounding a malformed odontoid process and anterior arch of atlas. *1* = lateral mass of C1; *2* = odontoid base; *3* = spinal cord. (Courtesy of Ashraf J, Crockard HA, Ransford AO, et al: *Arch Dis Child* 66:1318–1321, 1991.)

sometimes in the cervicothoracic regions is caused by kyphosis and narrowing of the spinal canal. At the craniovertebral junction, localized soft tissue thickening is the dominant compressing agent. Computed tomography and MRI show that, in some patients, the spinal cord has so little available space that posterior fusion could be hazardous. Prior anterior decompression is desirable in these patients. Immediate decompression can also aid in neurologic recovery.

Case Report.—Boy, 3½ years, who had Morquio's disease, was seen with a persisting left hemiparesis 4 months after a fall. History included a pigeon chest deformity at birth and short stature and physical weakness during early development; however, he had no ocular or cardiac manifestations of Morquio's disease. Computed tomographic myelography demonstrated craniocervical junction compression caused by atlantoaxial subluxation (Fig 6–31) and significant anterior soft tissue compression. Spinal cord compression was reduced in extension but

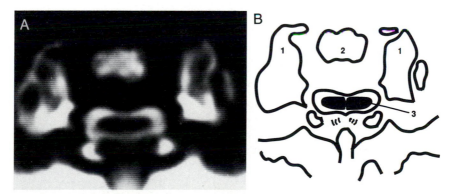

Fig 6–32.—An axial scan **(A)** and a line diagram **(B)** of the same area in extension, showing that the compression is reduced. *1* = lateral mass of C1; *2* = odontoid base; *3* = spinal cord. (Courtesy of Ashraf J, Crockard HA, Ransford AO, et al: *Arch Dis Child* 66:1318–1321, 1991.)

was not completely relieved (Fig 6–32). Transient unconsciousness at the time of the fall was probably caused by medullary concussion resulting from hyperextension rather than a head injury. Because of the significant anterior compression, early occipitocervical fusion was considered unwise. Instead, the patient was treated with skull halo traction to provide preliminary reduction after which he underwent transoral excision of the odontoid, the body of C2, and adjacent soft tissue compressing the spinal cord. This was followed by a posterior occipitocervical fusion. Recovery was uneventful. After removal of the halo body jacket at 6 weeks, the left hemiparesis was considerably improved.

Conclusions.—Spinal cord compression resulting from atlantoaxial subluxation of the craniovertebral junction is a major cause of disability and death in patients with Morquio's disease. If spinal cord compression is mild, patients are best treated with posterior occipitocervical fusion. Patients with more severe compression may require anterior decompression before surgery. This approach also offers a greater likelihood of reversing the neurologic deficit.

▶ Computed tomography shows anterior and posterior spinal cord compression in this patient. The combined effect of atlantoaxial subluxation and anterior soft tissue compression can be shown well by CT myelography. Lack of complete relief of spinal cord compression on cervical extension can lead to transoral removal of the odontoid. Other conditions that cause cervical vertebral canal narrowing are spondyloepiphyseal dysplasia congenita (1) and diatrophic dysplasia (2). Other recent articles of related interest are listed (3, 4).—L.W. Young, M.D.

References

1. Takeda E, et al: *Acta Paediatr Jpn* 33:633, 1991.
2. Richards BS: *J Bone Joint Surg* 73-A:614, 1991.
3. Stevens JM, et al: *J Bone Joint Surg* 73-B:851, 1991.
4. Wang H, et al: *Radiology* 164:515, 1987.

Occult Spinal Dysraphism in Patients With Anal Agenesis
Davidoff AM, Thompson CV, Grimm JK, Shorter NA, Filston HC, Oakes WJ
(Duke University Med Ctr, Durham, NC)
J Pediatr Surg 26:1001–1005, 1991   6–34

Background and Methods.—Congenital anorectal anomalies may be associated with dysraphic lesions of the spinal cord. During a 14-year period, 87 patients underwent treatment for anorectal anomalies. One patient had a myelomeningocele, and another had a tethered spinal cord that were recognized at birth. Two others had progressive neurologic deficits in early childhood; both proved to have tethered spinal cords. To further investigate this association, investigators performed MRI of the spine on 44 patients. Twenty-three patients had routine MRI before

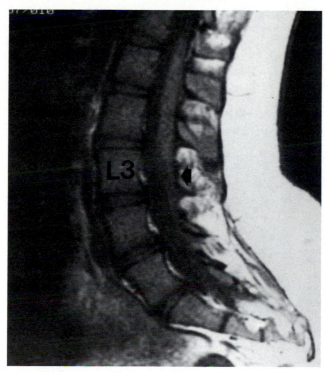

Fig 6–33.—An MRI demonstrating the presence of a tethered spinal cord. Note the position of the tip of the conus at the top of the L3 vertebral body (*arrow*). (Courtesy of Davidoff AM, Thompson CV, Grimm JK, et al: *J Pediatr Surg* 26:1001–1005, 1991.)

the age of 2 years, whereas 21 were asymptomatic former patients recalled for MRI screening.

Results.—The spinal cord anomalies most commonly detected by MRI were tethering of the cord (Fig 6–33) and fatty infiltration of the filum terminale (Fig 6–34). Four of 44 patients had significant occult dysraphism. In each case, the child had undergone neurosurgery without morbidity. Magnetic resonance imaging showed that each child had a tethered spinal cord. Two patients had only tethered spinal cords, 1 had an associated syrinx, and another had a lipomyelomeningocele. One patient had a neurologic deficit detected on preoperative evaluation, whereas 3 had no detectable deficits. Neither the extent of anorectal malformation, the absence of associated congenital abnormalities, nor the demonstration of normal vertebral anatomy on plain films of the spine precluded the presence of occult spinal dysraphism.

Conclusions.—All patients with anorectal abnormalities should undergo spinal MRI during initial evaluation to screen for occult spinal

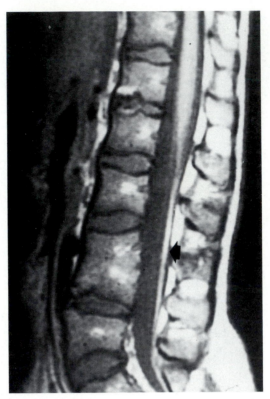

Fig 6–34.—A MR image demonstrating significant fat in the filum terminale (*arrow*). Note the similar intensity of the image of the filum with that of the subcutaneous fat. (Courtesy of Davidoff AM, Thompson CV, Grimm JK, et al: *J Pediatr Surg* 26:1001–1005, 1991.)

dysraphism. It might also be prudent to recall older patients for MRI evaluation.

▶ Occult spinal dysraphism in patients with anal agenesis should be suspected. The recommendation for MRI of patients with anorectal abnormalities for spinal dysraphism is worthwhile. Magnetic resonance imaging is the gold standard, but ultrasonography is just as effective with its ease of use, no need for sedation, and lesser cost. Other recent articles of related interest are listed (1–3), including, at the overt end of the spectrum, Wulfsberg et al.'s (1) reference to the caudal "dysplastic" sequence of lumbosacral vertebral defects, genitourinary anomalies, and imperforate anus, plus its overlap with the VATER association; and O'Riordain et al's. (2) discussion of the Currarino triad of hereditary sacral agenesis with presacral teratoma and anorectal stenosis.—L.W. Young, M.D.

References

1. Wulfsberg EA, et al: *Am J Med Genet* 42:766, 1992.
2. O'Riordain DS, et al: *Br J Surg* 78:536, 1991.
3. Taccone A, et al: *Radiol Med* 82:638, 1991.

Arteriographic Findings in Radial and Ulnar Deficiencies
Inoue G, Miura T (Nagoya University, Nagoya, Japan)
J Hand Surg 16B:409–412, 1991   6–35

Background.—Radial and ulnar deficiencies may range from hypoplasia of the thumb or ulnar digits to deficiencies of the radius and ulna themselves. Patients with these deficiencies frequently have other anomalies of the musculoskeletal, cardiac, or gastrointestinal systems, but there have been few reports of concomitant vascular malformations. The arteriographic findings were examined in a series of children with radial or ulnar deficiency.

Methods.—The arteriographic studies were performed over a 10-year period in 13 children with radial deficiency and 6 with ulnar deficiency. Average age of the 9 boys and 10 girls at time of arteriogram was 2.25 years. Three children had radial dysplasia with hypoplastic thumb and 10 had thumb hypoplasia only; 3 patients had ulnar dysplasia with ulnar digit hypoplasia and 3 had ulnar digit hypoplasia only.

Findings.—An absent or small radial artery was noted in 84.6% of children with radial deficiency and 50% of those with ulnar deficiency. A median artery, which entered into the formation of the superficial palmar arch, was present in 76.9% of cases of radial deficiency and 16.7% of ulnar deficiency. In 1 case of radial deficiency the radial artery divided into 2 branches (table). Twelve patients showed an absent or small deep palmar arch, proportional to the radial artery dysplasia. In some cases, the digital artery to the affected digit was absent.

Abnormal Arterial Patterns in the Forearm

	Number	Radial artery	Median artery	Unusual division of the artery
Radial deficiency	13			
Radial dysplasia	3	● ● ○	+ + −	
Hypoplastic thumb only	10	● ● ● ● ⊕	+ + + + +	+(U) +(R)
		⊕ ⊕ ⊕ ⊕ ○	+ + + − −	
Ulnar deficiency	6			
Ulnar dysplasia	3	● ● ⊕	+ − −	
Ulnar digit hypoplasia only	3	○ ○ ○	− − −	+(U)

Abbreviations: +, present; −, absent; +U, ulnar artery; +R, radial artery.
Note: Filled circles, absent; sectioned circles, small; open circles, normal.
(Courtesy of Inoue G, Miura T: *J Hand Surg* 16B:409–412, 1991.)

Conclusions.—Arteriographic findings in children with radial deficiency and ulnar deficiency with dysplasia of the ulna show an arterial pattern that is strikingly similar to that noted in stages III and IV of embryonic arterial development. Thus, these deficiencies appear to result from a teratogenic insult to the limb bud at stage IV or earlier. The teratogenic injury may be different in ulnar deficiency without dysplasia of the ulna, because these patients do not show arteriographic abnormalities.

▶ Knowledge of the arteriographic patterns associated with radial and ulnar deficiency broadens understanding of the genesis of these deficiencies. The authors do not include associated anomalies of musculoskeletal, cardiac, or gastrointestinal systems in this evaluation, but Singer's (1) 5 stages of arterial development are reviewed and related to these anomalies. I wonder how the arterial deficiencies fit into North and McCredie's (2, 3) embryonic neural crest injury schematic as analyzed on a neurotone/sclerotone/viscerotone basis. Perhaps some correlations might be made. Recent articles of related interest (4–6) include prenatal ultrasonographic demonstration of radial-ray reduction malformations (4, 5) and limb reduction defects in humans associated with prenatal isotretinoin exposure (6).—L.W. Young, M.D.

References

1. Singer E: *Anat Rec* 55:403, 1933.
2. North K, et al: *Am J Med Genet* 3, 29, 1987.
3. Osborne J, et al: *Pediatr Radiol* 19:425, 1989.
4. Brons JT, et al: *Prenat Diagn* 10:279, 1990.
5. Donnenfeld AE, et al: *Prenat Diagn* 10:29, 1990.
6. Rizzo R, et al: *Teratology* 44:599, 1991.

Familial Caffey's Disease and Late Recurrence in a Child
Borochowitz Z, Gozal D, Misselevitch I, Aunallah J, Boss JH (Bnai-Zion Med Ctr, Haifa, Israel)
Clin Genet 40:329–335, 1991
6–36

Background.—Cortical infantile hyperostosis, or Caffey's disease, is benign and self-limited. Later recurrence or persistence of symptoms appears to be extremely rare. Two different forms—a sporadic and a familial—are recognized. In the familial form, the tibia is the main bone affected; the mandible is mostly affected in the sporadic form. In a family with 2 affected siblings, 1 child had recurrent Caffey's disease at 11 years of age.

Case Report.—Girl, 12 years, the proband, was hospitalized for assessment of intermittent pain in the right lower leg. Her parents were healthy and nonconsanguineous, of Lebanese origin and Arabic-Christian ancestry. At the age of 5 months, the girl was noted to avoid moving her left leg. Radiographs showed

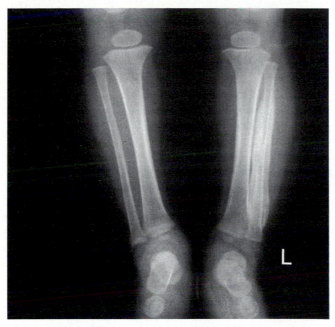

Fig 6–35.—Roentgenogram of the lower limbs of propositus at 5 years of age. The anteroposterior view shows cortical hyperostosis of the left fibula. (Courtesy of Borochowitz Z, Gozal D, Misselevitch I, et al: *Clin Genet* 40:329–335, 1991.)

cortical hyperostosis of the left fibula (Fig 6–35) without evidence of mandibular or other bony involvement. Caffey's disease was diagnosed at that time, and the girl was asymptomatic until the age of 11 years, when the pain in her right leg started. The pain gradually became continuous. The girl limped and had swelling over the midtibial region. Radiographs revealed cortical thickening in the right midtibial shaft, and technetium 99m bone scans showed increased uptake in the area affected (Fig 6–36). However, MRI showed no pathologic features in the cortex or marrow. A punch biopsy revealed several irregular, hard fragments. Histologically, only 1 fragment consisted of cortical bone. The periosteal aspect showed a multiplicity of parallel cement lines. The other fragments consisted of slender bony trabeculae set in a densely packed and cellular collagenous connective tissue. In places, they were separated from each other by spacious sinusoidal blood vessels.

Clinical assessment of the proband's parents, 2 sisters, and 1 brother showed no abnormal findings. However, another brother had been hospitalized at 4 months of age for swelling of the face, fever, and restlessness. Caffey's disease was diagnosed clinically and radiographically.

Conclusions.—This is the third family to be reported from Israel with familial infantile cortical hyperostosis. A thorough investigation indicated

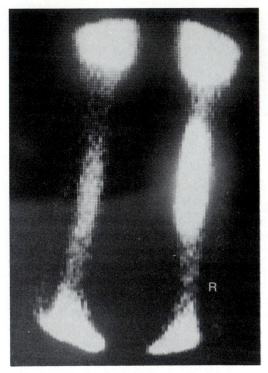

Fig 6–36.—Technetium 99m bone scan of the propositus at age 11 years shows increased uptake in the affected right midtibial shaft area and normal uptake of the left tibia. (Courtesy of Borochowitz Z, Gozal D, Misselevitch I, et al: *Clin Genet* 40:329-335, 1991.)

that the 3 families were not related. The mode of inheritance appears to be autosomal dominant with incomplete penetrance.

▶ When a new case of Caffey's disease (infantile cortical hyperostosis) comes along, it always raises the questions: What is it, and what causes it? Yet Caffey's disease has been linked to a single gene defect with an autosomal dominant mode of inheritance. It seems that not as many cases are occurring, but perhaps that's true only of the sporadic type. This report concerns 2 interesting issues about enigmatic and heterogeneous Caffey's disease, that is, its rare recurrence and its familial occurrence, the familial form. Most recurrences have been noted to be of the familial type, but it has been suggested that the recurrent cortical hyperostosis is a distinct homogeneous syndrome (1). There are several recent reports of Caffey's disease from around the world: from Greece, a lone scapula lesion (the kind that might be mistaken for a neoplasm) (2); affected twins in India (3); 6 cases in 5 years in 1 clinic in Prague (4); in utero diagnosis in France (5); effects of corticosteroid therapy in Scotland (6); and a familial form in rhesus monkeys (7). Concerning imaging, periostitis is still best demonstrated by radiography and corroborated by radionuclide scintigraphy. Curiously, MRI on the lower limbs in the subject of this report did not show abnormal cortical or marrow MR findings. Perhaps no more should be expected from a process that histologically is a typical ossifying periostitis (8). Histologic, ultrastructural, and immunohistochemical studies that might help in unraveling this disease or at least its histiogenesis are the focus of 2 recent reports (8, 9).—L.W. Young, M.D.

References

1. de Boissieu D, et al: *Arch Fr Pediatr* 46:439, 1989.
2. Papavasiliou VA, et al: *Rev Chir Orthop* 77:57, 1991.
3. Datta T, et al: *Indian Pediatr* 28:1346, 1991.
4. Ciharova K, et al: *Cesk Pediatr* 46:94, 1991.
5. Bercau G, et al: *Ann Pediatr [Paris]* 38:15, 1991.
6. Barr DG, et al: *Arch Dis Child* 66:140, 1991.
7. Snook SS, et al: *Vet Pathol* 26:274, 1989.
8. Stiller D: *Zentralbl Allg Pathol* 136:151, 1990.
9. Quacci D, et al: *Histol Histopathol* 5:187, 1990.

Multifocal Osteomyelitis in Childhood: Review by Radionuclide Bone Scan

Howman-Giles R, Uren R (Childrens Hospital; Missenden Med Centre, Camperdown, Sydney, NSW, Australia)
Clin Nucl Med 17:274–278, 1992   6–37

Introduction.—Multifocal osteomyelitis is an uncommon but well-described complication of acute osteomyelitis in neonates. The diagnosis of osteomyelitis is typically confirmed by radionuclide bone scan. Twenty-seven infants and children with multifocal osteomyelitis with no predisposing conditions were studied with radionuclide bone scanning.

Patients.—Of 139 patients with acute osteomyelitis who underwent radionuclide bone scanning over a 3-year period, 136 were younger than 16 years. Mean age was 5.3 years, with 46% being from 6 weeks to 3 years old. Twenty-seven patients had multifocal osteomyelitis, a rate of 19%. This included 31% of the patients in the neonatal groups and 44% the of older patients. Focal areas of increased uptake were present in all patients, including 3 who also had absent or reduced uptake. The older patients had 3 distinct clinical manifestations: acute illness with shock and septicemia, nonspecific bone and joint pain, and typical clinical osteomyelitis with bone pain and focal point tenderness. Several of the nonspecific group had been studied for several months before the final diagnosis was made after bone scanning. The most common sites of involvement were the femur and tibia. An organism was isolated, most commonly *Staphylococcus aureus,* in 56% of patients.

Conclusions.—Although multifocal osteomyelitis is best recognized in neonates, it may be more common than previously thought in older patients. Increased use of radionuclide bone scanning early in the condition and its high sensitivity in detecting osteomyelitis probably account for this higher incidence. All patients investigated for osteomyelitis should undergo a total-body bone scan.

▶ The authors indicate that multifocal osteomyelitis as a complication of acute osteomyelitis is more frequent in the older patient than previously described. Radionuclide scintigraphy has been effective in clarifying this increased incidence. This important observation should be recognized and applied in appropriate clinical settings. Recent articles of related interest on osteomyelitis are listed (1–6), including multifocal chronic osteomyelitis with exuberant periosteal new bone (1), multifocal skeletal tuberculosis (2), the role of Gd-enhanced MRI in childhood osteomyelitis (3), and the value of technetium 99m HMPAO–labeled leukocytes in the detection of osteomyelitis in children (4).—L.W. Young, M.D.

References

1. Starinsky R: *Pediatr Radiol* 21:455, 1991.
2. Lackenauer CS, et al: *Pediatr Infect Dis J* 10:940, 1991.
3. Dangman BC, et al: *Radiology* 182:743, 1992.
4. Lantto T, et al: *Clin Nucl Med* 17:7, 1992.
5. Beauchamp RD, et al: *Can J Surg* 34:618, 1991.
6. Yeo EE, et al: *Clin Nucl Med* 16:686, 1991.

Primary Pyogenic Abscess of the Psoas Muscle
Malhotra R, Singh KD, Bhan S, Dave PK (All India Institute of Medical Sciences, Ansari Nagar, New Delhi, India)
J Bone Joint Surg 74A:278–284, 1992   6–38

Introduction.—Most abscesses of the psoas muscles occur secondary to spinal tuberculosis. A primary abscess of the psoas muscle can be difficult to diagnose because of its rarity, its deep location, and its mimickry of septic arthritis of the hip.

Patients and Methods.—Data were reviewed on 9 children treated for primary pyogenic abscesses in 1986 to 1990. The patients ranged in age from 8 months to younger than 9 years. In only 3 patients was the correct diagnosis made at the time of admission to the hospital. In the remaining 6 patients, septic arthritis of the hip or spasm of the psoas muscle secondary to irritation from iliac lymphadenitis was suspected. All patients had fevers for 2 to 5 days before admission, and none had a history of an infective focus. The most common symptoms were fever, limp, irritability, anorexia, weight loss, and emaciation. Pain was located in the groin, the front of the thigh and knee, the iliac fossa, back, or abdomen; 2 patients were unable to walk. All patients had a flexion deformity and a lack of extension of the hip. None had palpable masses in the abdomen nor a tender spine. All patients had significantly increased

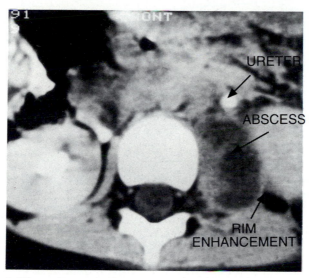

Fig 6–37.—A CT scan showing the abscess and its relationship to the kidney. Contrast medium is seen in the kidney and also enhances the rim of the margin of the abscess. (Courtesy of Malhotra R, Singh KD, Bhan S, et al: *J Bone Joint Surg* 74A:278–284, 1992.)

erythrocyte sedimentation rates, often with anemia and leukocytosis. Radiographs of the pelvis, hips, and chest were normal for all patients. In 1 patient there was a loss of definition of the margin of the affected psoas muscle, and 6 had mild scoliosis. The psoas muscle often appeared bulky or hypoechoic or both on ultrasonography; abscesses were sometimes seen. The presence of an abscess was usually confirmed by CT (Fig 6–37). When contrast medium was injected, the rim of the abscess was enhanced.

Results.—Drainage of the abscesses resulted in evacuation of foul-smelling, yellowish, purulent material that most often yielded *Staphylococcus aureus*. Antibiotic treatment continued for 3 weeks after patients became afebrile. All patients recovered.

Conclusions.—Ultrasonography was the least expensive and easiest method for detection of an abscess of the psoas muscle. It can be used to help differentiate between septic arthritis of the hip and abscess of the psoas muscle. In CT scanning enlargement, a rounded contour, a low-density center of the muscle, or gas within the muscle may be visualized. Gallium scanning can be useful for the localization, diagnosis, and follow-up of these abscesses.

▶ Pyogenic abscess of the psoas muscle can be a diagnostic dilemma because the symptoms and signs may point to the hip. Pyogenic abscess of the psoas muscle may be shown by CT, as well as by ultrasonography. In this report ultrasonography was reliable in demonstrating the lesion and was easily performed. In a related article, plasma cell granuloma in the iliopsoas region is demonstrated by CT and has morphologic similarities to psoas abscess (1). It also should be remembered that psoas abscess can be a complication of Crohn's disease (2, 3). Another recent article is listed (4).—L.W. Young, M.D.

References

1. Shedden AI, et al: *Pediatr Radiol* 21:444, 1991.
2. Cellier C, et al: *Gastroenterol Clin Biol* 16:235, 1992.
3. Procaccino JA, et al: *Dis Colon Rectum* 34:784, 1991.
4. Hresko MT, et al: *Spine* 17:590, 1992.

The Contribution of Magnetic Resonance Imaging in a Rare Ischiatic Localization of Osteoid Osteoma
Magnan B, Caudana R, Morelli N, Pregarz M, Regis D (University of Verona, Verona, Italy)
Ital J Orthop Traumatol 17:407–411, 1991   6–39

Background.—Most cases of osteoid osteoma are characterized symptomatically by night pain responsive to aspirin and radiographically by the presence of a radiolucent area surrounded by large regions of reactive host bone sclerosis. The lesion is usually of intracortical origin and most commonly localized in the long bones (71%) and the hands and feet (20%). An osteoid osteoma was localized in the ischiatic ramus, a rare finding, in a 10-year-old boy. Magnetic resonance imaging was particularly valuable in identifying the "nidus" of the osteoid osteoma.

Case Report.—Boy, 10 years, had a 6-month history of pain in the right hip. Symptoms appeared mainly at night and were responsive to aspirin. Conventional radiography and tomography revealed a lytic lesion surrounded by reactive sclerosis, which was localized in the right ischiatic ramus and had a dense nidus. The exact location of the lesion was demonstrated by CT. Magnetic resonance imaging revealed a hypointense halo and a change in the signal of the cancellous bone surrounding the lesion. A posterior approach was used for en bloc excision of the tumor.

Conclusions.—Conventional radiography is usually sufficient for diagnosing osteoid osteoma, although CT may be required when the lesion is small or has an uncommon localization. Magnetic resonance imaging allows detection of the nidus of the osteoid osteoma, which usually emits an intermediate signal on T_1-weighted images. The intense sclerotic reaction may make some tumors difficult to diagnose with conventional radiography and CT.

▶ This article beautifully demonstrates the value of MRI in the diagnosis of ischial osteoid osteoma. Computed tomography and conventional radiography are excellent in showing osteoid osteoma in most locations except when there is an excessive sclerotic reaction around the nidus. Other recent articles of related interest, including an unusual epiphyseal osteoid osteoma (Brody et al. [1]), are listed (1–4).—L.W. Young, M.D.

References

1. Brody JM, et al: *AJR* 158:609, 1992.
2. Bell RS, et al: *Can J Surg* 4:276, 1989.
3. Bettelli G, et al: *Clin Orthop* 247:261, 1989.
4. Moser RP, et al: *Skeletal Radiol* 19:181, 1990.

Melanotic Neuroectodermal Tumor of Infancy: Clinical, Radiologic, and Pathologic Findings in Five Cases

Mirich DR, Blaser SI, Harwood-Nash DC, Armstrong DC, Becker LE, Posnick JC (Hospital for Sick Children, Toronto, Ont, Canada)
AJNR 12:689–697, 1991   6–40

Background.—Melanotic neuroectodermal tumor (MNT) of infancy is a rare tumor, usually characterized by a firm mass near the midline adherent to bone, most frequently the maxilla. This aggressive neoplasm causes facial disfigurement, with blue-black discoloration from melanin pigment. Five MNTs of infancy and 1 similar melanotic neoplasm of the face were treated at 1 institution.

Methods.—Six patients were identified by a retrospective review of infantile melanotic neoplasms undertaken to correlate their clinical, radiologic, and pathologic features. Five were infants with rapidly growing facial or calvarial masses; the other had ataxia, and an MNT was discovered in the cerebellar vermis. In 5 patients, axial and coronal CT images were obtained before and after contrast administration; in 2 patients, MRI at 1.5 tesla was performed. All 6 tumors were resected, and pathologic examination was performed on fixed, embedded samples.

Results.—In 5 of the 6 cases, the clinical histories were similar, consisting of a rapidly enlarging maxillary or calvarial mass, usually in the first 6 months of life. One child had ataxia. Unenhanced and enhanced CT identified 4 homogeneous enhancing maxillary neoplasms and 1 cerebellar vermian neoplasm. One maxillary neoplasm, initially diagnosed as a schwannoma, was a large, lobular, disfiguring mass that eroded and expanded the left maxilla and orbit. Enhanced CT showed that the tumor filled the infratemporal fossa, bulged medially into the pharynx, laterally into the temporal fossa, and superiorly into the orbit and globe. Examination with MR showed a mass with isointense T_1-weighted signal compared with that of muscle. The T_1-weighted images showed the margins clearly. The left external carotid artery was the primary supplier to the maxillary neoplasm. In this case, the neoplasm was pathologically diagnosed as a congenital melanoma. Five tumors were completely resected. The calvarial tumor, which was incompletely resected, recurred and invaded the brain. In the 5 cases of complete resection, the children remained well and free from disease after 1 month to 7 years of follow-up.

Conclusions.—This rare neoplasm of infancy occurs most often in the maxilla, followed by the calvaria and mandible, but also has been seen in the shoulder, mediastinum, epididymis, and uterus. These locally aggressive tumors usually occur in infants less than 6 months of age, and are reported to have a malignant potential of 1.9% to 3.2%. In the cases described, CT scans showed predominantly lytic and expansile bone changes; 3-dimensional scans were useful for surgical planning and reconstruction. Imaging by MR showed the soft tissue component and extent of the neoplasm better than CT did, with isointense T_1-weighted and slightly hyperintense T_2-weighted signals. These findings are in contrast with those of most melanin-containing tumors, which show enhanced T_1 and T_2 relaxation.

▶ As with other lesions that affect bone, CT more clearly shows bony change of the melanotic neuroectodermal tumor, whereas MRI better demonstrates its full extent and soft tissue component. The isointense T_1-weighted and slightly hyperintense T_2-weighted signals differ from most melanin-containing tumors that have shortened T_1 and T_2. Apparently, variables other than the absolute amount of melanin may determine the MR signal. In a related article, melanotic neuroectodermal tumor of the epididymis is reported by Diamond et al. (1). Other recent articles of related interest are listed (2–5).—L.W. Young, M.D.

References

1. Diamond DA, et al: *J Urol* 147:673, 1992.
2. Pettinato G, et al: *Am J Surg Pathol* 15:233, 1991.
3. Siracusano S, et al: *Eur Urol* 20:49, 1991.
4. Atkinson GO Jr, et al: *Pediatr Radiol* 20:20, 1989.
5. Jones HH, et al: *Skeletal Radiol* 19:527, 1990.

Primary Spinal Epidural Extraosseous Ewing's Sarcoma

Kaspers G-J JL, Kamphorst W, van de Graaff M, van Alphen AM, Veerman AJP (Free University Hospital, Amsterdam, The Netherlands)
Cancer 68:648–654, 1991   6–41

Introduction.—There are striking morphological and ultrastructural similarities between extraosseous Ewing's sarcoma (EES) and Ewing's sarcoma of bone (ESB), and the same translocations involving band g12 of chromosome 22 found in both diseases suggest that ESB and EES are identical tumor types. Extraosseous Ewing's sarcoma has been reported to originate in different locations, and in 15 patients it originated in the epidural space of the spine.

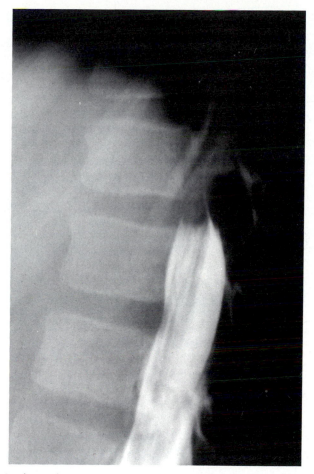

Fig 6–38.—Lumbar myelogram showing a complete obstruction at the level of L1-2 with displacement of the conus anteriorly. (Courtesy of Kaspers G-J JL, Kamphorst W, van de Graaff M, et al: *Cancer* 68:648–654, 1991.)

Case Report.—Boy, 7 years, had low back pain, weakness of the legs, neck pain, urinary retention, and loss of anal sphincter control. Neurologic examination showed a flaccid paresis of the legs, absent patellar and Achilles tendon reflexes, and a left extensor plantar reflex. Examination of the spine showed slight pain on axial compression. General examination was grossly normal, and blood and urine analyses, including catecholamine excretion, were normal. The CSF protein level was increased. Myelography (Fig 6–38) and CT (Fig 6–39) showed an extradural tumor at the level of L1-L2 that displaced the spinal cord ventrally. An epidural tumor without bone involvement was subtotally resected, with rapid and complete recovery of bladder and bowel function postoperatively. No other tumor sites were identified. The diagnosis was EES of the spinal epidural space.

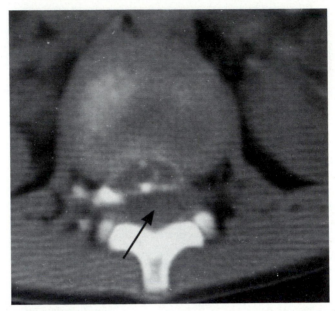

Fig 6–39.—Postmyelogram CT scan at the level of the disk L1–2, showing the extradural tumor and the anterior displacement of the tip of the conus and cauda. The *arrow* points toward the middle of the tumor. (Courtesy of Kaspers G-J JL, Kamphorst W, van de Graaff M, et al: *Cancer* 68:648–654, 1991.)

After combination chemotherapy but without radiation treatment, the patient was in clinical remission without neurologic deficit.

Comment.—Most reported patients were predominantly male, age 4 to 47 years. All had back pain or radicular pain, or both; also common were paresis of one or both legs, sensory disturbances, and bladder and bowel dysfunction. Signs and symptoms were similar to those in other spinal epidural disorders. Differential diagnosis required imaging studies; MRI was superior to myelography based both on complications and tumor delineation. Ultimate diagnosis often required histopathologic examination. Resection and adjuvant therapy usually gave good neurologic results, but 62.5% of patients died an average of 16 months after diagnosis. The 5-year survival appears to be lower than that of ESB. When young patients complain of back pain or radicular pain or both, and especially when neurologic signs are noted, a spinal epidural tumor should be considered. The preferred method for detecting such a tumor is MRI.

▶ Extraosseous Ewing's sarcoma is a rare malignant neoplasm that should be included in the differential diagnosis when the clinical context suggests an epidural tumor or even disk herniation. Although MRI should be used as the imaging examination of choice, myelography with CT demonstrated the lesion in this patient. Relatively recent articles on EES are by Ushigome et al.

(1) and Shimada et al. (2). Other recent articles of related interest on Ewing's sarcoma include multifocal simultaneous or synchronous occurrence of Ewing's sarcoma (3), Ewing's sarcoma of the temporal bone (4), and flare response (delayed increased tracer uptake after initial chemotherapy) in Ewing's sarcoma (5). The latter article emphasizes the importance of correlative clinical and radiographic assessment for interpretation of radionuclide scintigrams in oncologic patients with bony involvement to help to clarify lack of tumor spread. Another article by Ehara et al. (6) on the radiographic pattern of healing and bony complication in patients with long-term survival is quite useful and is highly recommended.—L.W. Young, M.D.

References

1. Ushigome S, et al: *Cancer* 64:52, 1989.
2. Shimada H, et al: *Hum Pathol* 19:442, 1988.
3. Beluffi G, et al: *Pediatr Radiol* 21:452, 1991.
4. Davidson MJ: *Oral Surg Oral Med Oral Pathol* 72:534, 1991.
5. Meyer JR, et al: *Clin Nucl Med* 16:807, 1991.
6. Ehara S, et al: *Cancer* 68:1531, 1991.

Calcific Cervical Intervertebral Disc Herniation in Children
Heinrich SD, Zembo MM, King AG, Zerkle AJ, MacEwen GD (Louisiana State Univ, Tulane Univ, New Orleans)
Spine 16:228–231, 1991

6–42

Background.—Only about 130 cases of calcification of an intervertebral disk in a child have been reported since 1924. In 12 symptomatic cases calcified intervertebral disk protrusions resolved after nonoperative therapy.

Case Report 1.—Boy, 4 years and 1 month, had a 4-day history of neck pain without radiation and limitation of neck motion at initial diagnosis. Radiographs of the cervical spine showed calcification of the C3–C4 intervertebral disk (Fig 6–40), and CT revealed protrusion of the calcified C3–C4 nucleus pulposus into the right anterolateral aspect of the bony neural canal with encroachment of the intervertebral neural foramina (Fig 6–41). Magnetic resonance imaging suggested disk degeneration (Fig 6–42). The pain and torticollis were resolved after 9 days in head halter-traction. A follow-up CT scan 6 months later showed a small residual nidus of calcification in the middle of the C3–C4 intervertebral disk.

Case Report 2.—Boy, 7 years and 9 months, had intermittent neck and midback pain of 2 months' duration. His medical history included a C7–T1 intervertebral disk calcification (IDC) 3 years earlier. Plain radiographs showed an IDC at C7–T1 and T5–T6, and CT scanning showed a small protrusion of the nucleus pulposus at the C7–T1 interspace. He was treated with nonsteroidal anti-inflammatory agents but returned 1 month later with new radicular symptoms. Computed tomography scanning demonstrated an IDC at C7–T1 with progression of the posterior disk protrusion superiorly along the posterior aspect of the verte-

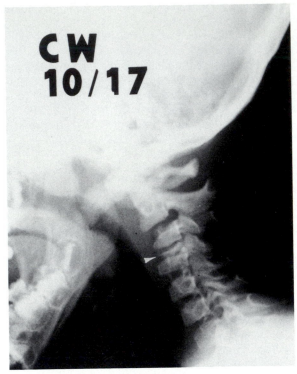

Fig 6–40.—Lateral radiograph of the cervical spine in a boy, 4 years, showing abnormal opacification of the C3–C4 interspace consistent with calcification of the invertebral disk. (Courtesy of Heinrich SD, Zembo MM, King AG, et al: *Spine* 16:228–231, 1991.)

bral body of C-7 almost to the C6–C7 disk space. No protrusion was noted at T5–T6. The patient's pain resolved after 7 days in head halter-traction. At 8 months after traction treatment there was complete resolution of the C7–T1 disk protrusion and calcification.

Conclusions.—Pediatric cervical IDC is rare. The symptoms of pain and decreased range of motion may be accompanied by fever, leukocytosis, and an elevated erythrocyte sedimentation rate. These symptoms are secondary to a protrusion of the disk complex into the neural canal.

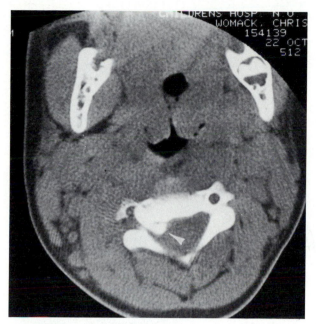

Fig 6–41.—A CT scan demonstrating abnormal calcification of posterolateral aspect of C3–C4 disk space with displacement of calcified nucleus pulposus into the right lateral aspect of the bony neural canal, with encroachment of intervertebral foramina of C3–C4. Same child as in Figure 6–40. (Courtesy of Heinrich SD, Zembo MM, King AG, et al: *Spine* 16:228-231, 1991.)

▶ Calcific intervertebral disk herniation is a relatively well-recognized, but unusual, childhood finding. The exact cause of this intervertebral disk calcification is not clear, although traumatic injury and presumably infectious inflammation have been implicated. Computed tomography and MRI contribute to the morphologic demonstration of the process that includes protrusion of the nucleus pulposus into the bony neural canal. That this is the cause of the symptomatic cervical protrusion seems quite reasonable. Recent articles of related interest, including 1 on Schmorl's nodes (Walters et al. [1]), that intraspongious herniation of the disk into the vertebral endplate, are listed (1–4). Schmorl's nodes are well shown on MRI, the modality more sensitive to showing the lesion than radiography and scintigraphy.—L.W. Young, M.D.

References

1. Walters G, et al: *Pediatr Emerg Care* 7:294, 1991.
2. Hoeffel JC, et al: *Eur J Pediatr* 149:695, 1990.
3. Dias MS, et al: *Neurosurgery* 28:130, 1991.
4. Wong CC, et al: *Spine* 17:139, 1992.

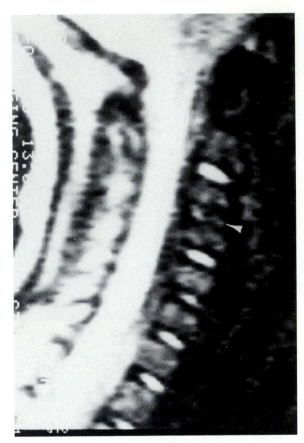

Fig 6–42.—An abnormal MR image of disk space signal intensity at C3–C4 consistent with intervertebral disk calcification. These changes suggest a degenerated disk. There is no evidence of inflammation. Same child as in Figure 6-40. (Courtesy of Heinrich SD, Zembo MM, King AG, et al: *Spine* 16:228-231, 1991.)

Bone Scintigraphy in Preschool Children With Lower Extremity Pain of Unknown Origin

Englaro EE, Gelfand MJ, Paltiel HJ (Children's Hosp Med Ctr, Cincinnati; Univ of Cincinnati; Istituto di Medicina Nucleare, Udine, Italy)
J Nucl Med 33:351–354, 1992   6–43

Background.—Preschool children who limp often are unable to describe the site or nature of their pain. If the abnormal gait is a result of trauma, the injury causing it may not have been witnessed by an adult.

Patients and Methods.—Bone scans were reviewed in 56 preschool children who were seen with a limp or refusal to walk, or who indicated the presence of lower extremity pain. The patients, all less than 5 years of age, included 41 boys and 15 girls. In only 2 instances had a fall been witnessed. An injection of .185 mCi/kg of technetium 99m–medronate was given, and blood-pool and delayed whole-body bone images were acquired, as well as delayed pinhole images of the hips when indicated.

Findings.—Thirty of the children had bone scan abnormalities, 16 of them in about the same site as the signs or symptoms suggested. Abnormalities of the tarsal bones were relatively frequent and included abnormal uptake in or near the cuboid bone and in the calcaneus. Other findings included changes of hip synovitis, avascularity of the femoral head, synovitis of the knee, and various abnormalities of the proximal femur, tibia, or fibula. Correlative imaging studies demonstrated focal bone abnormalities at only 5 of 26 sites.

Conclusions.—Preschool children who have an abnormal gait and pain in the lower extremity frequently have abnormal bone scan findings. Abnormalities are frequent in the feet and often reflect injury of the calcaneus or cuboid.

▶ The common problem of the cause of limping in the toddler (the preschool child) is well recognized. Bone radionuclide scintigraphy and skeletal survey from pelvis to feet are essential examinations to confirm or to rule out occult "toddler" fractures. Recent and pertinent articles of related interest are listed (1–5).—L.W. Young, M.D.

References

1. Aronson J, et al: *J Pediatr Orthop* 12:38, 1992.
2. Oudjhane K, et al: *J Trauma* 28:858, 1988.
3. Blatt SD, et al: *Pediatrics* 87:138, 1991.
4. Blumberg K, et al: *Radiology* 179:93, 1991.
5. Moss EH, et al: *Skeletal Radiol* 19:575, 1990.

The Lateral Pillar Classification of Legg-Calvé-Perthes Disease
Herring JA, Neustadt JB, Williams JJ, Early JS, Browne RH (Texas Scottish Rite Hosp for Children, Dallas; Georgetown Univ Hosp, Washington, DC; Norfolk and Norwich Hospital, Norwich, England)
J Pediatr Orthop 12:143–150, 1992   6–44

Introduction.—A number of different radiographic classification systems have been used for Legg-Perthes disease based on type of femoral head, the amount of head involved, or the extent of the subchondral fracture line. The system of Catterall, based on the amount of head involved, has been widely used, but a recent study reported an interobserver agreement of only 0.42 for Catterall groupings. It is known that age at onset is a prognostic feature in Legg-Perthes disease, with poorer outcomes occurring in children who are older at onset. The relationship of age at onset and a new lateral pillar classification grouping to the ra-

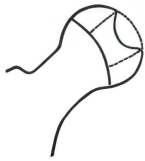

Fig 6–43.—Femoral head pillars. The pillars were derived by noting the lines of demarcation between the central sequestrum and the remainder of the epiphysis on the anteroposterior radiograph. (Courtesy of Herring JA, Neustadt JB, Williams JJ, et al: *J Pediatr Orthop* 12:143–150, 1992.)

diographic outcome at skeletal maturity was investigated, and its intraobserver and interobserver reproducibility was also studied.

Methods.—Data on 93 hips in 86 patients with Legg-Perthes who were treated with the Craig or the Atlanta Scottish Rite brace were reviewed. Radiographs taken during and before the fragmentation phase were classified using the lateral pillar classification system. Radiographs obtained at skeletal maturity were separately reviewed and the results were classified by the Stulberg method. To determine interobserver reproducibility, 16 trained observers independently classified 32 hips by the lateral pillar method; intraobserver reproducibility was assessed by the duplication of 7 patients within the interobserver reproducibility classification test.

Classification.—The system is based on the observation that fragmentation in Legg-Perthes occurs in distinct sectors of the femoral head. This method divides the femoral head as seen on anteroposterior radiograph into lateral, central, and medial pillars (Fig 6–43). Group A is identified with a radiographically normal lateral pillar. In group B, greater than 50% of the normal lateral pillar height is maintained. In group C, less than 50% of the lateral pillar height is maintained, and there is more lucency than in group B. Group A corresponds to Catterall's groups I

Classification system	Interobserver reliability
Lateral pillar	.78
Catterall classification*	.42
Head at Risk signs*	.35

Fig 6–44.—Interobserver reliability of lateral pillar classification, Catterall classification, and risk factors (*asterisk* refers the reader to Uhthoff HK, et al: *Behavior of the Growth Plate.* New York, Raven Press, 1988, pp 393–400. Courtesy of Herring JA, Neustadt JB, Williams JJ, et al: *J Pediatr Orthop* 12:143–150, 1992.)

and II, group B includes those in Caterall II or III, and group C includes Catterall groups III and IV.

Results.—Both the lateral pillar classification and the age at onset were significantly correlated with the final Stulberg result, but the classification group was the stronger determinant in predicting outcome. The interobserver agreement was .78 for 16 investigators (Fig 6–44), and the intraobserver agreement was .79.

Conclusions.—The lateral pillar classification appears to have satisfactory reproducibility and a good capability to predict the amount of flattening of the femoral head at skeletal maturity. Together with the age at onset, this system can provide meaningful comparisons for evaluating treatment.

▶ Healing prognosis in Legg-Perthes disease is a subject of ongoing evaluation for improving the outcome from treatment. The lateral pillar classification shows excellent promise for this purpose as being more consistently reproducible than the Catterall method. This needs to be proved with the test of time. These methods use "old-fashioned" radiography alone for their evaluation. Others have found the Catterall classification an important prognostic index with acceptable interobserver agreement (1, 2). Two articles that relate to possible early development of Legg-Perthes discuss the use of ultrasonography in transient synovitis of the hip (3, 4).—L.W. Young, M.D.

References

1. Simmons ED, et al: *J Bone Joint Surg* 72-B:202, 1990.
2. Mukherjee A, et al: *J Pediatr Orthop* 10:153, 1990.
3. Futami T, et al: *J Bone Joint Surg* 73-B:635, 1991.
4. Terjesen T, et al: *J Pediatr Orthop* 11:608, 1991.

Ultrasonography in the Study of Prevalence and Clinical Evolution of Popliteal Cysts in Children With Knee Effusions
Szer IS, Klein-Gitelman M, DeNardo BA, McCauley RGK (Tufts Univ, Boston)
J Rheumatol 19:458–462, 1992   6–45

Introduction.—The prevalence and clinical evolution of popliteal cysts in children has not been studied. High-resolution ultrasonography was used to establish the prevalence and clinical evolution of popliteal cysts in 44 children with clinically detectable knee effusions, including 35 with juvenile arthritis, 3 with spondyloarthritis, 2 with psoriasis associated knee effusion, 2 with sepsis-associated knee effusion, and 2 with lupus-associated knee effusion.

Methods.—All children, as well as 10 control children, were examined clinically and by real-time ultrasonography using either a 5- or 7.5-MHz linear array transducer to produce sagittal and transverse views of the knee. Popliteal cysts were defined as hypoechoic masses in the popliteal

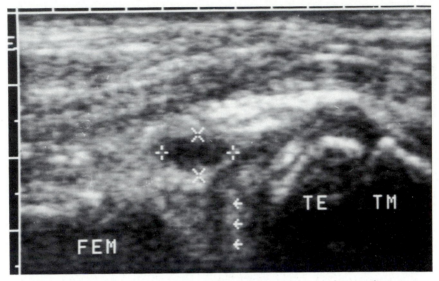

Fig 6–45.—Sagittal view posterior knee. An oval hypoechoic cyst (*c*) is seen between the *stars* posterior to the joint space. *Abbreviations:* FEM indicates distal posterior femur; TE, tibial epiphysis; TM, tibial metaphysis. The *arrows* point to the straplike hypoechoic posterior cruciate liagment curving posteriorly to attach to the posterior tibial epiphysis. (Courtesy of Szer IS, Klein-Gitelman M, DeNardo BA, et al: *J Rheumatol* 19:458–462, 1992.)

space of at least 1 × 1 cm. The posterior cruciate ligament was identified if possible to distinguish it from small hypoechoic cysts in the notch adjacent to the medial femoral condyle (Fig 6–45).

Results.—Popliteal cysts were found in 61% of the children, which were often small and asymptomatic. In 37% of children with bilateral arthritis there were bilateral cysts. The cysts measured 1 to 40 cm³ (median, 2 cm³). The presence of cysts did not correlate significantly with the patient's age or the duration, treatment, or cause of arthritis. The size of the cysts correlated significantly with the size of the suprapatellar effusion. All 10 children with posterior knee pain had cysts. Large cysts were generally Baker's cysts associated with the gastrocnemiosemimembranous bursa, but others were located in the region of the popliteal bursa, deep to the popliteal artery in the intercondylar notch. These were usually adjacent to the medial femoral condyle. Although most cysts were partly or completely hypoechoic, small, and of a flattened ovoid shape, some were anechoic and some formed infiltrating multilobular extensions as they enlarged. Plain radiographs did not show these popliteal cysts. When used, MRI and CT confirmed their presence. Prospective follow-up ultrasonography in 25 children with cysts showed that, in half, the suprapatellar effusion improved over 18 to 24 months, with only conventional arthritis treatment. The size of the popliteal cysts also improved but lagged behind the changes in the effusions. In all pa-

tients in whom the effusions improved, the cysts became smaller or resolved. In 2 children with very large cysts, clinical rupture occurred.

Conclusions. —Ultrasonographic evidence suggests that children with
knee arthritis have a high frequency of popliteal cysts, the size of which
correlates with that of the suprapatellar effusion. These cysts are often
painless and usually improve or resolve.

▶ These authors contribute useful ultrasound findings for bursae and tendons. Ultrasonography, sensitive and noninvasive, is particularly suited to examine popliteal cysts of rheumatoid arthritis. This is another good application
of ultrasound. Recent or pertinent articles on other interesting applications of
ultrasonography and MRI to bursal and tendon sheath cysts are listed
(1–5).—L.W. Young, M.D.

References

1. Toolanen G, et al: *Acta Orthop Scand* 59:294, 1988.
2. Lieberman JM: *Can Assoc Radiol j* 39:295, 1988.
3. Massari L, et al: *Chir Organi Mov* 75:245, 1990.
4. Vaughan BF: *Clin Radiol* 41:24, 1990.
5. Baldrati L, et al: *Radiol Med* 81:234, 1991.

Ifosfamide: A New Cause of Rickets
Silberzweig JE, Haller JO, Miller S (State Univ of New York, Brooklyn, NY)
AJR 158:823–824, 1992   6–46

Introduction. —Ifosfamide is a synthetic analogue of cyclophosphamide that is part of the first-line management of several recurrent tumors, including Ewing's sarcoma, rhabdomyosarcoma, soft tissue sarcomas, and Wilms' tumor. This chemotherapeutic agent has numerous
adverse effects, including nephrotoxicity. Recently hypophosphatemic
rickets was recognized as an additional complication. A child developed
hypophosphatemic rickets after ifosfamide treatment.

Case Report. —Girl, 2 years, with normal renal function and normal serum levels of calcium, phosphate, and alkaline phosphate, underwent surgery, radiation,
and chemotherapeutic therapy for stage III abdominal rhabdomyosarcoma. Chemotherapy consisted of ifosfamide (total cumulative dose, 175 g/m^2) vincristine,
and actinomycin D over an 18-month period, after which she had normal renal
function and no evidence of tumor recurrence. However, 1 year after the end of
chemotherapy, a rachitic rosary was noted on physical examination, and laboratory tests showed an increased serum alkaline phosphatase level, a low serum
phosphate level, and a normal serum calcium level. The diagnosis of rickets was
confirmed by chest and wrist radiographs (Fig 6–46).

Conclusions. —Ifosfamide can induce a nephrotoxicity that includes
low serum bicarbonate and phosphate concentrations with glucosuria,

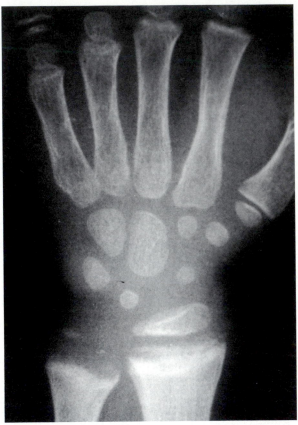

Fig 6–46.—A girl, 5 years, with stage III abdomnial rhabomyosarcoma 3 years after intitation of ifosfamide chemotherapy. A radiograph of the wrist shows growth-plate widening with metaphyseal fraying and cupping typical of rickets. (Courtesy of Silberzweig JE, Haller JO, Miller S: AJR 158:823-824, 1992.)

aminoaciduria, and hypochloremic metabolic acidosis. In this patient, this resulted in rachitic changes. In another patient, a girl aged 7 years with stage II Wilms' tumor, hypophosphatemic rickets developed 20 months after initiation of ifosfamide chemotherapy for tumor recurrence. Although no other chemotherapeutic agent has been reported to be associated with rickets, the radiologist should be aware of this possibility when examining radiographs obtained for tumor surveillance.

▶ Ifosfamide therapy is an important new cause of rickets. Ifosfamide is a chemotherapeutic agent that causes hepatic reduction in synthesis of 1,25-dihydroxyvitamin D_3. This is apparently a similar mechanism to the 1 involved in anticonvulsant therapy rickets. Other recent related reports are listed (1–6). Although Pratt et al. (1) indicate that the ifosfamide rickets may be irreversible, van Gool et al. (2) and DeSchepper et al. (3) report spontaneous resolution after ifosfamide was discontinued.—L.W. Young, M.D.

References

1. Pratt CB, et al: *J Clin Oncol* 9:1495, 1991.
2. Van Gool S, et al: *Med Pediatr Oncol* 20:254, 1992.
3. DeSchepper J, et al: *Am J Pediatr Hematol Oncol* 13:39, 1991.
4. Skinner R, et al: *Arch Dis Child* 65:732, 1990.
5. Burk CD, et al: *J Pediatr* 117:331, 1990.
6. Devalck C, et al: *J Pediatr* 118:325, 1991.

Cardiopulmonary

Digital Imaging With a Photostimulable Phosphor in the Chest of Newborns

Cohen MD, Katz BP, Kalasinski LA, White SJ, Smith JA, Long B (Riley Hosp for Children; Regenstreif Inst; Indiana Univ, Indianapolis)
Radiology 181:829–832, 1991   6–47

Introduction.—The photostimulable phosphor imaging technique makes it possible to acquire digital images of the chest with a lower radiation dose than that used for conventional screen-film images. The use of a digital photostimulable phosphor imaging system in the neonatal nursery was evaluated.

Chest Radiographs in Newborns

Structure or Film Density	Mean Score			Significant Difference	P Value
	SFR	CR	0.5 CR		
Mediastinum	3.36	3.43	3.06	CR and 0.5 CR	.017
	(0.623)	(0.707)	(0.718)		
Lung	3.32	3.43	2.97	CR and 0.5 CR	<.001
	(0.611)	(0.486)	(0.460)	SFR and .5 CR	
Bone	3.62	3.57	3.32	CR and 0.5 CR	<.001
	(0.451)	(0.356)	(0.362)	SFR and 0.5 CR	
Soft tissue	3.75	3.64	3.36	CR and 0.5 CR	<.001
	(0.353)	(0.292)	(0.335)	SFR and 0.5 CR	
Tubes	3.72	3.82	3.69	NS	.21
	(0.406)	(0.271)	(0.268)		
Film density	2.20	2.47	2.47	CR and SFR	.001
	(0.456)	(0.393)	(0.369)	0.5 CR and SFR	

Abbreviation: NS, not siginificant.
Notes: Table is a comparison of screen-film radiographs (SFRs) and computed radiographs (CRs) obtained with the same radiation dose and CRs obtained with 50% reduction in the radiation dose (.5 CRs). *The numbers in parentheses* are standard deviations.
(Courtesy of Cohen MD, Katz BP, Kalasinski LA, et al: *Radiology* 181:829–832, 1991.)

Methods.—The study group included 150 consecutive newborns who were randomly allocated into 3 groups of 50. In the first 2 groups, screen-film and computed radiographs of the chest were obtained at the usual standard radiation exposure. Infants in the third group had computed radiographs which were obtained with a 50% radiation dose reduction. Three observers blindly scored the images.

Results.—The image quality of the first 2 groups was similar with regard to visualization of the mediastinum, lungs, bones, soft tissues, and tubes. Computed radiographs, however, had more consistently uniform image density. Images obtained with a reduced dose of radiation were consistently rated of lesser quality than those acquired with the higher dose (table).

Conclusions.—Half-exposure computed radiographs yield generally poorer images than higher dose computed or screen-film radiographs. Although the result of dose reduction on diagnostic value was not examined in this study, the use of higher dose computed radiographs, with their more uniform density, may reduce the need for repeat radiographs.

▶ Most users of a computerized radiography system for imaging the newborn chest have observed that the overall image quality—even with a 50% dose reduction (half-exposure computed radiography)—is consistently higher than by analog radiography (1). The authors have one of the longer experiences with use of this technique and attest its consistency and *potential* for a lower radiation dose. Others have identified some problems (2). Recent articles of related interest are listed (3–5).—L.W. Young, M.D.

References

1. Vossenrich R, et al: ROFO 156:107, 1992.
2. Arthur RJ, et al: *Pediatr Radiol* 22:5, 1992.
3. Kiuru A, et al: *Acta Radiol* 32:114, 1991.
4. Franken EA Jr, et al: *Pediatr Radiol* 21:336, 1991.
5. Murphy MD, et al: *Invest Radiol* 26:590, 1991.

Receiver-Operating-Characteristic Study of Chest Radiographs in Children: Digital Hard-Copy Film vs 2K × 2K Soft-Copy Images

Razavi M, Sayre JW, Taira RK, Simons M, Huang HK, Chuang K-S, Rahbar G, Kangarloo H (Univ of California, Los Angeles; Univ of Utah, Salt Lake City)
AJR 158:443–448, 1992   6–48

Introduction.—Picture archiving and communication systems (PACS) may have an advantage over film-based radiology by permitting image-analysis tools to prescreen specific conditions and by improving operational efficiency. The digital data from PACS can be visualized either by laser-printed analog film or by a soft-copy display. It is unclear which of these media provides the most useful output. Observers' performances in detecting various pediatric chest abnormalities using soft-copy 2048K × 2048K byte displays were compared with those using digital laser-printed film.

Methods.—Data for images were derived from computed radiography. Five observers, including fellows and experienced pediatric radiologists screened 239 images previously judged to contain sufficient samples of each disease with the full range of its subtleties and normal findings. The observers viewed and interpreted the images using soft-copy displays in half of the patients and hard-copy images in the remainder. All images again were interpreted 2 months later with the alternative viewing technique. The findings using both viewing techniques were compared with those independently determined by senior pediatric radiologists who had access to all available images, records, and image processing tools.

Area Under Receiver-Operating-Characteristic (ROC) Curve and Level of Significance for Hard-Copy and Soft-Copy Viewing Methods

Abnormality/Observer No.	Area Under ROC Curve (SD)		Significance (p Value)	95% Confidence Intervals for Area Differences
	Hard Copy	Soft Copy		
Pneumothorax				
1	.9253 (.046)	.9469 (.044)	.62	(−.039, .088)
2	.8310 (.119)	.7840 (.114)	.63	(−.209, .115)
3	.8969 (.071)	.8818 (.087)	.88	(−.136, .106)
4	.9351 (.043)	.9243 (.090)	.89	(−.136, .114)
5	.9513 (.023)	.9071 (.041)	.18	(−.102, .014)
Average	.9079 (.060)	.8888 (.075)	–	
Interstitial disease				
1	.8952 (.031)	.8728 (.032)	.43	(−.062, .013)
2	.8858 (.022)	.8675 (.028)	.42	(−.053, .016)
3	.7956 (.036)	.8335 (.032)	.04	(.004, .071)
4	.8141 (.030)	.9392 (.020)	.001	(.086, .164)
5	.8390 (.028)	.8243 (.028)	.54	(−.051, .022)
Average	.8459 (.029)	.8675 (.028)	–	
Linear atelectasis				
1	.7841 (.125)	.8056 (.112)	.82	(−.147, .191)
2	.8762 (.050)	.8770 (.057)	.86	(−.079, .080)
3	.7487 (.112)	.9337 (.038)	.05	(.012, .357)
4	.8470 (.068)	.9616 (.018)	.04	(.003, .226)
5	.9183 (.020)	.8536 (.063)	.20	(−.162, .033)
Average	.8349 (.075)	.8863 (.058)	–	
Air bronchograms				
1	.7441 (.046)	.8203 (.060)	.08	(−.007, .159)
2	.7828 (.069)	.8263 (.080)	.46	(−.053, .140)
3	.7789 (.033)	.7592 (.056)	.62	(−.095, .056)
4	.7973 (.038)	.8305 (.044)	.32	(−.024, .089)
5	.7820 (.183)	.7522[a] (.122)	–	
Average	.7770 (.074)	.7803 (.072)	–	

Note: Significance and 95% confidence intervals were not calculated for average values.
[a] One of the data sets did not meet the convergence criterion in the CORROC2 program. In this case, the areas were obtained separately by the ROCFIT program, which does not calculate P values.
(Courtesy of Razavi M, Sayre JW, Taira RK, et al: AJR 158:443–448, 1992.)

Results.—An abnormality was found in 162 images. All radiologists performed equally using both hard and soft-copy images for the detection of pneumothoraces (table). For the detection of interstitial disease and linear atelectasis, senior pediatric radiologists performed better on the soft-copy displays, but the pediatric fellows performed equally well on both displays. For the detection of air bronchograms, 4 of the 5 observers performed equally on both the soft-copy display and the film. The overall mean times spent examining the images did not differ significantly for soft and hard copy.

Conclusions.—No significant difference exists in the detection of pneumothoraces and air bronchograms using digital hard-copy and soft-copy images. For the detection of interstitial disease and linear atelectasis, soft-copy images appear slightly better. These findings are consistent with the feasibility of PACS as an alternative to film-based radiology.

▶ My guess is that digital display stations will replace stationary and motorized viewers in our reading rooms probably sooner than is generally thought. Pediatric radiology departments may lead the way in this conversion. Several are the major current testing sites for these systems because resolution problems for smaller radiographic images are less complex. This article helps to set the stage. Anticipation is high on the road to a 21st century–envisioned all-PACS environment. Other recent articles of related interest are listed (1–4).—L.W. Young, M.D.

References

1. Manninen H, et al: *Eur J Radiol* 14:164, 1992.
2. Arthur RJ, et al: *Pediatr Radiol* 22:5, 1992.
3. Cohen MD, et al: *Radiology* 181:829, 1991.
4. Vosshenrich R, et al: ROFO 156:107, 1992.

Magnetic Resonance Imaging of the Pediatric Airway: Compared With Findings at Surgery and/or Endoscopy
Auringer ST, Bisset GS III, Myer CM III (Brenner Children's Hosp, Winston-Salem, NC; Children's Hosp Med Ctr, Cincinnati)
Pediatr Radiol 21:329–332, 1991   6–49

Background.—The complexity of the pediatric airway may require multiple imaging techniques and invasive procedures for accurate evaluation. To determine whether invasive procedures might be avoided by the use of MR imaging, MR findings were compared with those obtained by surgery and/or endoscopy.

Methods.—Thirty-four infants and children with a mean age of 2.8 years and symptoms of chronic airway obstruction underwent thoracic MRI. Oral or intravenous sedation was used as needed; 2 examinations

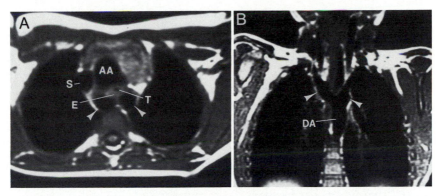

Fig 6–47.—**A,** transaxial, gated (SE 500/20) scan through the upper thorax in a patient with chronic upper-airway obstruction. The 2 limbs of a double aortic arch (*arrowheads*) encircle the trachea (*T*) and esophagus (*E*). *AA,* ascending aorta; *S,* superior vena cava. **B,** coronal scan in the same patient demonstrates the junction of the 2 limbs of the aortic arch (*arrowheads*) joining the form the descending aorta (*DA*). (Courtesy of Auringer ST, Bisset GS III, Myer CM III: *Pediatr Radiol* 21:329–332, 1991.)

required general endotracheal anesthesia. The total examination time averaged approximately 45 minutes.

Results.—Magnetic resonance imaging indicated vascular compression of the airway in 15 of the 34 patients. A double aortic arch (Fig 6–47)

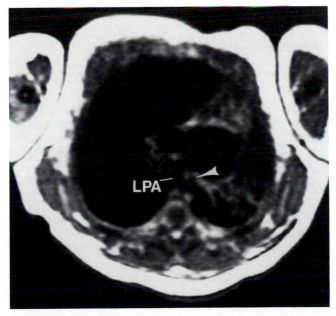

Fig 6–48.—Transaxial, gated (SE 444/20) scan through the pulmonary arteries in a 1-week-old infant with progressive hyperinflation of the right lung and respiratory distress. The left pulmonary artery (*LPA*) originates aberrantly in the right pulmonary artery and encircles the compressed trachea (*arrowhead*). (Courtesy of Auringer ST, Bisset GS III, Myer CM III: *Pediator Radiol* 21:329–332, 1991.)

was revealed in 2 patients. Other vascular causes of airway compression included pulmonary artery sling (Fig 6–48), a malpositioned aorta, dilated pulmonary arteries, and enlarged left atria. Twelve patients had primary tracheomalacic states. Magnetic resonance imaging also revealed 4 mediastinal masses, and three patients were judged to have a normal airway. The findings with MRI agreed with surgical findings in 21 of 21 cases and with endoscopic findings in 25 of 28 cases.

Conclusions.—Pulmonary artery sling usually requires angiography for confirmation; in 1 patient, MRI accurately diagnosed the condition noninvasively. In many other cases, the specific information gained through MRI can obviate the need for more invasive procedures. Following plain film and barium studies, MRI in pediatric patients with suspected chronic airway obstruction is recommended.

▶ Magnetic resonance imaging of the pediatric airway gives answers noninvasively concerning the airway and major vessels. Airway analysis is one of the difficult imaging areas of pediatric radiology. Magnetic resonance imaging findings do correlate well with surgery and endoscopy. Recent articles of related interest concerning imaging of the airways are listed (1–6).—L.W. Young, M.D.

References

1. Schuster T, et al: *Prog Pediatr Surg* 27:231, 1991.
2. Hofmann U, et al: *Prog Pediatr Surg* 27:221, 1991.
3. Vogl T, et al: *Pediatr Radiol* 21:89, 1991.
4. Jaffe RB: *Semin Ultrasound CT MR* 11:206, 1990.
5. Shepard JO, et al: *Clin Chest Med* 12:151, 1991.
6. Ryan CF, et al: *Am Rev Respir Dis* 144:939, 1991.

Countercurrent Aortography: An Alternative to Cardiac Catheterization in Infancy
Anjos R, Kakadekar A, Murdoch I, Baker E, Tynan M, Qureshi (Guy's Hospital, London, England)
Pediatr Cardiol 13:10–13, 1992   6–50

Introduction.—Cross-sectional echocardiography usually permits the diagnosis of aortic coarctation and interruption of the aortic arch, but in some patients, cardiac catheterization and angiography may be required. A previous study in a small number of patients showed that countercurrent aortography was a safe and effective alternative procedure. In a larger study, 25 infants underwent countercurrent aortography to clarify suspected anomalies of the aortic arch.

Methods.—Aortic coarctation was suspected in 21 infants, interrupted aortic arch was suspected in 2, recoarctation was suspected in 1, and vascular ring was suspected in 1. Standard biplane angiography or digital subtraction angiography was performed using Niopam 370. The mean number of angiograms per patient was 1.5.

Results.—In 96% of patients, countercurrent aortography provided adequate diagnostic information. Aortic coarctation was confirmed in 15 infants, interruption of the aortic arch was confirmed in 2, and vascular ring was confirmed in 1. Anomalies of the aortic arch were excluded in 6 infants. In 1 patient with an anomalous origin of the right subclavian artery from the descending aorta, the information was incomplete, and cardiac catheterization was required. Cannulation of 2 arteries was required for 2 neonates. There were complications except for 1 episode of transient ischemia of the arm.

Conclusions.—Countercurrent aortography is a less invasive procedure than cardiac catheterization and can usually provide excellent images of the aortic arch. Injection into the right brachial artery provides the best results. Although MRI is the method of choice for imaging the aortic arch when echocardiographic results are insufficient, countercurrent aortography provides an excellent alternative when MRI is unavailable.

▶ Countercurrent aortography via a peripheral artery is an excellent method to demonstrate arch anomalies. It's used when cross-sectional and Doppler ultrasonographic evaluation is inconclusive, when MRI is not available, or when associated lesions (e.g., large ventricular defect) mitigate against left ventriculography. This report of findings in 25 infants beautifully demonstrates the value of countercurrent aortography. Other relatively recent articles on countercurrent aortography are listed (1–3).—L.W. Young, M.D.

References

1. Patres PR, et al: *Arch Inst Cardiol Mex* 58:27, 1988.
2. Qureshi SA, et al: *Int J Cardiol* 15:333, 1987.
3. Ueda K, et al: *Pediatr Cardiol* 2:231, 1982.

Lung Perfusion Scans in Patients With Congenital Heart Defects
Tamir A, Melloul M, Berant M, Horev G, Lubin E, Blieden LC, Zeevi B (Beilinson Med Ctr, Petah Tiqva, Israel; Tel Aviv University, Tel Aviv, Israel)
J Am Coll Cardiol 19:383–388, 1992   6–51

Background.—Congenital or postoperative lung perfusion abnormalities in patients with a congenital heart defect may negatively affect outcomes. Children with reduced lung perfusion, particularly if it is unilateral, are usually asymptomatic, and these conditions are not detected easily by chest radiography or 2-dimensional echocardiography. An accurate, noninvasive way to assess the relative pulmonary blood flow quantitatively in patients with a congenital heart defect is needed. Lung perfu-

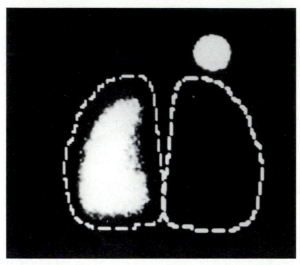

Fig 6–49.—Lung perfusion scintigram (posterior view) in a patient with multiple large apical ventricular septal defects after pulmonary artery banding, demonstrating severe underperfusion of the right lung (right lung 18%; left lung 82%). (Courtesy of Tamir A, Melloul M, Berant M, et al: *J Am Coll Cardiol* 19:383–388, 1992.)

sion scintigrams using albumin macroaggregates labeled with technetium 99m were evaluated in 63 patients with various congenital heart defects.

Patients and Findings.—Patients' ages ranged from 6 months to 40 years. In 34 cases, or 54%, right lung perfusion abnormalities were documented. There was a particularly high incidence in patients who had had a systemic to pulmonary artery shunt as the initial palliative procedure or who had had right ventricular outflow reconstruction. The incidence was also especially high in those with bilateral pulmonary artery stenosis. Serial evaluations were helpful in the assessment of functional results of different transcatheter interventions for optimizing pulmonary blood flow. The quantitative relative perfusion radionuclide technique was more sensitive than chest radiography in detecting abnormal lung perfusion (Fig 6–49).

Conclusions.—The lung perfusion scintigram is a fairly easy, reliable, noninvasive method for accurately determining relative pulmonary blood flow. The method permits the detection of changes in pulmonary flow and enables clinicians to plan more invasive studies or special transcatheter or surgical interventions.

▶ The lung perfusion scintigram is easy, reliable, relatively noninvasive, and more sensitive than chest radiography in problems of patients with congenital heart disease. Although the Sugimura et al. (1) article is written in Japanese, the table and figure English captions very nicely support the findings of the abstracted article. Other recent articles of related interest are listed (2, 3).—L.W. Young, M.D.

References

1. Sugimura H, et al: *Kaku Igaku [Jpn J Nucl Med]* 27:1337, 1990.
2. del Torso S, et al: *Int J Cardiol* 20:107, 1988.
3. Dowdle SC, et al: *J Nucl Med* 31:1276, 1990.

Sequential Transcatheter Treatment of Combined Coarctation of Aorta and Persistent Ductus Arteriosus

Pavlovic D, de Lezo JS, Medina A, Romero M, Hernández E, Pan M, Tejero J, Melian F (Hospital Reina Sofia, University of Córdoba, Córdoba, Spain; Hospital del Pino, University of Las Palmas, Las Palmas, Spain)
Am Heart J 123:249–250, 1992   6–52

Background.—In some cases of congenital heart disease, a number of percutaneous transluminal procedures may be done for palliation or definitive treatment. Sequential angioplasties have been used for combined stenotic lesions, but no previous authors have reported such treatment for stenosis associated with a shunting defect. In this study, hemodynamic findings in a patient with combined aortic coarctation and persistent ductus arteriosus (PDA) treated by coarctation angioplasty are reported.

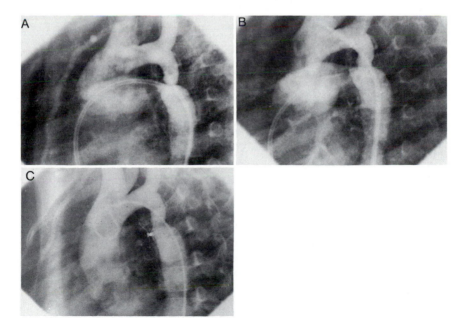

Fig 6–50.—Angiographic sequences of the aorta in our patient (60-degree left anterior oblique projection). **A,** basal angiogram; **B,** immediately after coarctation angioplasty; **C,** 7 months after percutaneous closure of ductus. (Courtesy of Pavlovic D, de Lezo JS, Medina A, et al: *Am Heart J* 123:249–250, 1992.)

Case Report.—Boy, 23 months, was slightly underweight, with no palpable femoral pulses and a maximum instantaneous Doppler gradient of 50 mm Hg between the upper and lower extremities. Systolic and continuous murmurs were auscultated at the left parasternal borders, and the diagnosis of coarctation of the aorta and PDA was made. On left- and right-sided heart catheterization, PDA and percutaneously dilated aortic coarctation were observed. A 9-mm diameter balloon was used. Transcoarctation gradient decreased from 46 to 25 mm Hg; left to right shunt increased from 21% to 59%. There were no complications, and the patient had palpable femoral pulses at discharge. He was followed up every 6 months, with echo-Doppler studies done annually. When the patient was 5 years of age, hemodynamic reevaluation showed that the pressure relief at the coarctation persisted, with a 27% left-to-right shunt across the ductus. When the patient was aged 5.5 years, percutaneous closure of the PDA was done with a 17-mm Rashkind umbrella. The ductus was immediately occluded with no complications, and the patient was discharged within 48 hours. Repeat coarctation 7 months postoperatively showed a 13 mm Hg gradient and no left-to-right shunt.

Discussion.—In some patients, coarctation of the aorta associated with PDA can be treated by sequential transcatheter treatment. This may be done if the transcoarctation gradient can be sufficiently relieved and if the ductus is of suitable size for percutaneous closure; the 2 procedures should not be done at the same time. The resulting blood flow through the aorta may affect beneficial remodeling of the arch (Fig 6–50).

▶ This sequential transcatheter treatment of a combined coarctation of the aorta and persistent ductus arteriosus is noteworthy. Although these procedures are now done by pediatric cardiologists, radiologists' knowledge of them in consultation is useful. Other recent articles on intervention in coarctation and other major congenital heart lesions, mostly in infants, are listed (1–7). Each shows informative illustrations of such imaging procedures as angiography, cardiac ultrasonography with Doppler, and MRI.—L.W. Young, M.D.

References

1. Jain A, et al: *Am Heart J* 123:514, 1992.
2. Allada V, et al: *Am Heart J* 122:1464, 1992.
3. Anjos R, et al: *Am J Cardiol* 69:655, 1992.
4. Cambier PA, et al: *Am J Cardiol* 69:815, 1992.
5. Baylen BG, et al: *J Am Coll Cardiol* 19:1025, 1992.
6. DaCosta AG, et al: *Pediatr Cardiol* 13:104, 1992.
7. Marin-Garcia J, et al: *Pediatr Cardiol* 13:41, 1992.

Life-Threatening Fluid Extravasation of Central Venous Catheters
Krasna IH, Krause T (UMDNJ-Robert Wood Johnson Med School, New

Brunswick, NJ)
J Pediatr Surg 26:1346–1348, 1991

Introduction.—Even apparently successful placement of central venous catheters may result in migration outside the vein with subsequent extravasation of fluid. Four infants aged 2½–14 months showed no external evidence of extravasation prior to rapid deterioration of their condition.

Case Report 1.—Infant girl, 6 months, had chronic diarrhea and reflux esophagitis at initial diagnosis. Three days after placement of a catheter in the superior vena cava she had acute respiratory distress. A chest film showed the catheter to be in the mediastinum. A contrast study revealed extravasation into the mediastinum, confirming the diagnosis of catheter perforation (Fig 6–51). The infant rapidly improved after bilateral chest tubes were placed, hyperalimentation fluid was removed from both pleural spaces, and the line was replaced by a new central line in the groin.

Case Report 2.—Infant girl, 9 months, had a fever, a distended abdomen, and a white blood cell count of 35,000 at 8 days after closure of a colostomy and placement of a central line. The catheter tip was found to have migrated slightly to the left and perforated into the retroperitoneum (Fig 6–52). After removal of the catheter and antibiotic treatment, the child improved and was able to be sent home.

Conclusions.—In each of the 4 cases, blood could no longer be withdrawn from the catheters when the infants became symptomatic. Occlu-

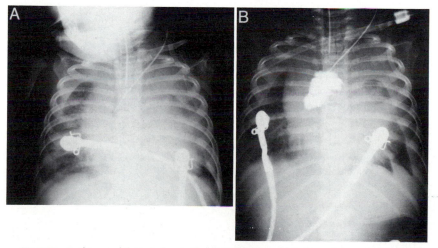

Fig 6–51.—**A,** there are bilateral pleural effusions and an unusual position of the central line in the mediastinal location. **B,** contrast injected through the catheter shows dye in the mediastinum, and the catheter is not located in subclavian vein or the superior vena cava. (Courtesy of Krasna IH, Krause T: *J Pediatr Surg* 26:1346–1348, 1991.)

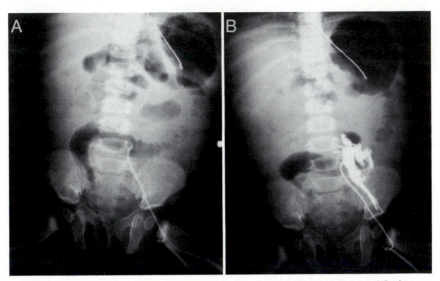

Fig 6–52.—A, at the time of laparotomy, the catheter tip is angulated at L-5. Peritoneal fluid is present, separating the bowel loops. **B,** contrast injected into the left catheter shows extravasation into the retroperitoneum. (Courtesty of Krasna IH, Krause T: *J Pediatr Surg* 26:1346–1348, 1991.)

sion was not registered when the catheters migrated from the vein and pressure from the intravenous infusion pumps forced large quantities of fluid into the thoracic and abdominal cavities. Newer model pumps, however, may be more sensitive to pressure. A patient with a central line who has acute respiratory or abdominal symptoms should be examined for proper function and location of the line.

▶ Central venous catheter lines play an important role in the neonate, as well as in the child who has need for long-term chemotherapy. Complications can be extravasation (in the mediastinum in this patient), thrombosis, and infection. We use the Broviac cathetergram as an examination to demonstrate extravasation, thrombosis, or obstruction. Other recent articles of related interest on this subject are listed (1–5).—L.W. Young, M.D.

References

1. Seguin JH: *Am J Perinatol* 9(3):154, 1992.
2. Casado-Flores J, et al: *Intensive Care Med* 17:350, 1991.
3. Giacoia GP: *JPEN J Parenter Enteral Nutr* 15:110, 1991.
4. Carey BE: *Neonatal Netw* 7:17, 1989.
5. Russell L, et al: *Scott Med J* 35:11, 1990.

Cystic Fibrosis: Scoring System With Thin-Section CT
Bhalla M, Turcios N, Aponte V, Jenkins M, Leitman BS, McCauley DI, Naidich DP (Med Univ of South Carolina, SC; Univ of Medicine and Dentistry of

New Jersey, Newark, NJ; New York Univ Med Ctr, New York)
Radiology 179:783–788, 1991

Summary of CT Scoring System

Category	0	Scores 1	Scores 2	Scores 3
Severity of bronchiectasis	Absent	Mild (luminal diameter slightly greater than diameter of adjacent blood vessel)	Moderate (lumen 2–3 times the diameter of vessel)	Severe (lumen >3 times diameter of vessel)
Peribronchial thickening	Absent	Mild (wall thickness equal to diameter of adjacent vessel)	Moderate (wall thickness greater than and up to twice the diameter of adjacent vessel)	Severe (wall thickness >2 times the diameter of adjacent vessel)
Extent of bronchiectasis (no. of BP segments)	Absent	1–5	6–9	>9
Extent of mucus plugging (no. of BP segments)	Absent	1–5	6–9	>9
Sacculations or abscesses (no. of BP segments)	Absent	1–5	6–9	>9
Generations of bronchial divisions involved (bronchiectasis/plugging)	Absent	Up to 4th generation	Up to 5th generation	Up to 6th generation and distal
No. of bullae	Absent	Unilateral (not >4)	Bilateral (not >4)	>4
Emphysema (no. of BP segments)	Absent	1–5	>5	...
Collapse/consolidation	Absent	Subsegmental	Segmental/lobar	...

Note: The CT score is calculated from this table. Add the letter *P* for plugging and *T* for peribronchial thickening when present. Subtract the CT score from 25 to determine the patient's score. The latter can be used with the Doershuk modification of the Shwachman-Kulczycki clinical scoring system.

Abbreviation: BP, bronchopulmonary.

(Courtesy of Bhalla M, Turcios N, Aponte V, et al: *Radiology* 179:783–788, 1991.)

Background.—Chest radiography is used to evaluate the progression of lung disease and the efficacy of therapeutic regimens in patients with cystic fibrosis (CF). Two scoring systems, the Chrispin and Birmingham methods, use imprecise and subjective terms. Thin-section CT allows a more accurate definition of the extent and severity of disease, but heretofore no scoring system had been developed for use with CT. Such a system was designed based on a retrospective study of patients with CF.

Methods.—The 14 patients ranged in age from 5 to 42 years. All had undergone chest CT. Three radiologists independently reviewed and scored the scans on the basis of the severity and/or extent of 9 morphologic changes (table). Each category was scored as 0 (absent), 1 (mild), 2 (moderate), or 3 (severe). Chest radiographs obtained in 9 cases were used for a comparative analysis of the 2 modalities.

Results.—The CT scores ranged between 8 and 17. The scoring method had excellent interobserver reliability. Computed tomography was superior to chest radiography in detecting bronchiectasis and mucus plugging. Mucous plugs, which play a crucial role in the pathogenesis of airway disease in CF, were detected in 38 bronchopulmonary segments with CT, but in only 4 segments with chest radiography.

Conclusions.—Thin-section CT has proved superior to chest radiography in evaluating lung disease in patients with CF. The scoring system presented here incorporates all of the lung changes seen in CF and may help in making treatment decisions and evaluating outcome.

▶ Cystic fibrosis is an important disease in pediatrics and in all of medicine. Thin-section CT is very useful for defining extent and progression of pulmonary disease in these patients. Advances in the genetics of CF are being correlated with imaging findings and help to identify patients afflicted with the disease. Scoring of findings of bronchiectasis and mucoid impaction by ultrafast CT allows comparison with findings from conventional chest radiography (1). The value of CT over conventional radiography is paramount, especially in the older CF patient who has mild pulmonary disease (2, 3). Evaluation of paranasal sinusoses with CT and MRI relative to therapy should become increasingly important. Other recent articles of related interest on varying aspects of CF are listed (4, 5).—L.W. Young, M.D.

References

1. Nathanson I, et al: *Pediatr Pulmonol* 11:81, 1991.
2. Taccone A, et al: *Radiol Med* 82:79, 1991.
3. Santis G, et al: *Clin Radiol* 44:20, 1991.
4. Wine JJ, et al: *Am J Physiol* 261:L218, 1991.
5. Lynch DA, et al: *Radiology* 176:243, 1990.

Antral Choanal Polyp Presenting as Obstructive Sleep Apnea Syndrome

Rodgers GK, Chan KH, Dahl RE (Univ of Pittsburgh, Pittsburgh)
Arch Otolaryngol Head Neck Surg 117:914–916, 1991   6–55

Background.—Obstructive sleep apnea syndrome (OSAS) in children may manifest as chronic mouth breathing, snoring, disrupted sleep patterns, and behavioral disturbances consistent with disrupted sleep. The diagnosis of sleep apnea in children is not as well delineated as in adults. In children apneic periods may be less than the 10-second hallmark in adult sleep apnea. Although OSAS is commonly caused by adenotonsillar hypertrophy, 1 case was caused by an antral choanal polyp.

Case Report.—Boy, 10 years, was referred to the psychiatry service for evaluation of behavior disturbances, snoring with restless sleep, daytime hypersomnolence, and enuresis. His medical history included a seizure disorder treated with carbamazepine, attention deficit disorder, and a diagnosis of multiple inhalant allergies. Roentgenography revealed bilateral maxillary sinusitis (Fig 6–53) and adenoidal enlargement (Fig 6–54). An overnight electroencephalogram sleep study revealed frequent obstructive apneic episodes, which usually occurred during rapid eye movement sleep. Rapid eye movement sleep was approximately 7% compared with normal for age 20%, and the proportion of delta sleep was markedly increased. The patient was scheduled for adenoidectomy when antibiotics failed to improve his obstructive symptoms. A large polyp, which filled the entire nasopharynx, was avulsed during surgery, and a nasal antral window was created.

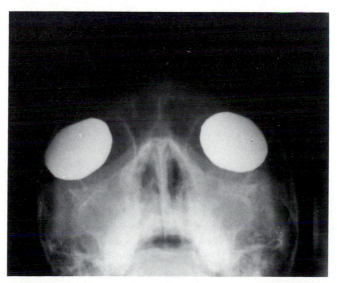

Fig 6–53.—Water's view revealing bilateral maxillary sinusitis. (Courtesy of Rodgers GK, Chan KH, Dahl RE: *Arch Otolarnygol Head Neck Surg* 117:914-916, 1991.)

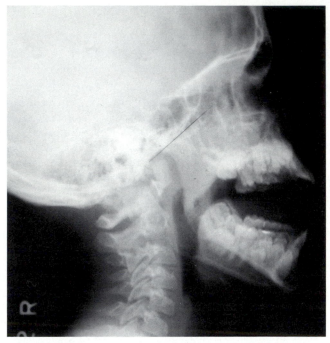

Fig 6–54.—Lateral soft tissue radiograph showing adenoid hypertrophy with an adenoid-nasopharynx ratio of .8 (97th percentile for a child aged 10 years). (Courtesy of Rodgers GK, Chan KH, Dahl RE: *Arch Otolaryngol Head Neck Surg:* 117:914-916, 1991.)

Polypoid nasal mucosa recurred in 2 months, and a Caldwell-Luc procedure was performed. The signs and symptoms of disturbed sleep resolved completely after surgery.

Conclusions.—Certain mass lesions of the nasopharynx have been reported to cause sleep apnea, but this is the first documented case in which an antral choanal polyp produced OSAS. The antral choanal polyp should be added to the differential diagnosis of nasopharyngeal obstructions that produce OSAS.

▶ The authors use the adenoidal/pharyngeal ratio radiographic assessment method for measuring a pharyngeal mass simulating enlargement of the adenoids (1). Antral choanal polyp is an additional lesion in the list of causes of OSAS. Cineradiography and cine CT (ultrafast CT) are being used to improve assessment of the airway in the surgical management of OSAS (2, 3). In another article on OSAS, MRI findings suggest compression of the respiratory center by an aberrant vertebral artery as a central cause of sleep apnea (4). Another recent article of related interest is listed (5).—L.W. Young, M.D.

References

1. Fujioka M, et al: *AJR* 133:401, 1979.
2. Koopmann CF Jr, et al: *Otolaryngol Clin North Am* 23:787, 1990.
3. Galvin JR, et al: *Radiology* 171:775, 1989.
4. Miyazaki M, et al: *Ann Neurol* 29:564, 1991.
5. Gaultier C, et al: *Arch Fr Pediatr* 48:429, 1991.

Anterior Mediastinal Masses With Calcifications on CT in Children With Histiocytosis-X (Langerhans Cell Histiocytosis): Report of Two Cases

Odagiri K, Nishihira K, Hatekeyama S, Kobayashi K (Kanagawa Cancer Ctr; Kanagawa Children's Medical Center; Gumma Children's Hospitals, Yokohama City, Japan)
Pediatr Radiol 21:550–551, 1991   6–56

Purpose.—Some patients with histiocytosis X have masses in the anterior mediastinum at the time of diagnosis. Two infants with histiocytosis X had anterior mediastinal masses with punctate calcifications.

Case Report.—Girl, 3 months, and boy, 7 months, had a rash, fever, and hepatosplenomegaly. The girl also had tachypnea and tachycardia. On chest radiography, she had a mediastinal mass with diffuse reticular shadows in both lung fields. On CT, the mass contained multiple punctate foci of calcification. Skin biopsy revealed the diagnosis of histiocytosis-X. Additional findings in the boy included lymphadenopathy, anemia, and increased erythrocyte sedimentation rate. He also had an anterior mediastinal mass on plain radiographs. The mass was solid with small strong echoes on ultrasound examination and showed scattered, fine calcifications and a lytic change of the left scapula on CT (Fig 6–55). Both patients responded well to chemotherapy.

Discussion.—Generalized histiocytosis-X can show anterior mediastinal masses on diagnostic imaging. The fine calcifications described may

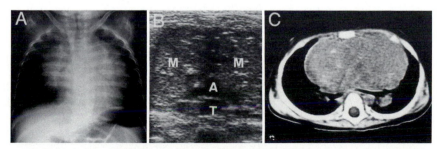

Fig 6–55.—A, radiograph of the chest showing a mediastinal mass. **B,** ultrasonogram revealing multiple strong echoes in the solid mass (T, trachea; A, aorta; M, mass). **C,** CT showing punctate calcifications in the mass in the anterior mediastinum. (Courtesy of Odagiri K, Nishihara K, Hatekeyama S, et al: *Pediatr Radiol* 21:550–551, 1991.)

be seen more often because CT is used more extensively in investigation of mediastinal masses and may help to make the differential diagnosis.

▶ Diffuse reticular calcifications in an anterior mediastinal mass of histiocytosis-X as shown by CT is an interesting observation. A previous report of calcification in thymus histiocytosis was associated with cytomegalic inclusion disease (1). Calcifications also have been reported in a soft tissue mass of histiocytosis-X adjacent to a lytic mandibular osseous lesion (2).—L.W. Young, M.D.

References

1. Tirnoveanu G, et al: *Monatsschr Kinderheilkd* 119:144, 1971.
2. Shenouda NF, et al: *Skeletal Radiol* 20:620, 1991.

Radiation Recall Supraglottitis in a Child
Wiatrak BJ, Myer CM III (Univ of Michigan, Ann Arbor, Mich)
Am J Otolaryngol 12:227–229, 1991   6–57

Purpose.—There have been many reports of recrudescence and modification of radiation effects precipitated by use of chemotherapy. There has been a report of radiation recall supraglottitis in an adult patient with diffuse histiocytic lymphoma. A case of radiation recall supraglottitis involving dactinomycin therapy in a child is reported.

Case Report.—Girl, 4 years, was seen at 2 years of age with a rapidly enlarging mass in the right neck, which proved to be pleomorphic rhabdomyosarcoma. There were no signs of metastasis or CNS involvement. The patient was started on dactinomycin, ifosfamide, and vincristine therapy, but the tumor did not resolve completely and resection was done. After surgery the patient received 60 Gy of hyperfractionated radiation and a second 2-week course of ifosfamide and vincristine. On microlaryngoscopy and bronchoscopy 3 months postoperatively, the larynx and subglottis were normal, though the posterior glottis was slightly inflamed. Chemotherapy continued after decannulation. At 4 months, after a course of dactinomycin, vincristine, and ifosfamide, the patient developed increased airway obstruction with intermittent stridor. She was monitored closely at home, with a pulse oximeter applied during sleep. An MRI scan, done for routine tumor surveillance, showed a marked decrease in the supraglottic airway (Fig 6–56). These structures showed increased signal intensity on T2-weighted images, suggesting edema rather than tumor involvement, and the supraglottic larynx was noted to be within the previous radiation port. The patient was readmitted to the hospital. Microlaryngoscopy and bronchoscopy showed marked edema of the epiglottis and supraglottis. The glottis could be seen only after tracheotomy and was normal. Inflammation was noted on biopsy of the epiglottis. The supraglottic edema was decreased but persistent 1 month later. The swelling decreased sufficiently over the following year to allow decannulation. The pa-

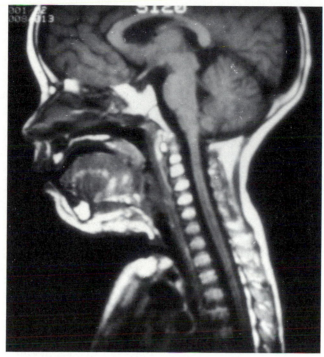

Fig 6–56.—An MRI scan of the neck after the administration of dactinomycin. Notice the fatty infiltration of cervical vertebrae 1-4 on the T1-weighted image, consistent with postradiation changes. The significant edema noted in the supraglottic airway lies within the previous radiation ports. (Courtesy of Wiatrak BJ, Myer CM III: *Am J Otolaryngol* 12:227-229, 1992.)

tient required stoma closure, but she remains decannulated with normal exercise tolerance and minimal residual edema.

Conclusions.—This is first known case of radiation recall supraglottitis in a child, which is believed to have resulted from dactinomycin treatment for rhabdomyosarcoma. With many new chemotherapeutic agents being used in conjunction with radiation therapy, the possibility of augmentation or recurrence of radiation toxicity should be borne in mind.

▶ Radiation recall supraglottitis is a confusing phenomenon at any age and is especially unusual in childhood (1). The recognition and demonstration of this phenomenon is made easier with MRI and should expedite early diagnosis and subsequent appropriate life-saving management. A similar massive production of granulation tissue reported in the larynx and facial sinuses of the elderly may occur after radiation therapy for carcinoma even without chemotherapeutic stimulation (2).—L.W. Young, M.D.

References

1. Wallenborn PA III, et al: *Arch Otolaryngol* 110:614, 1984.
2. Weidner N, et al: *Cancer* 59:1509, 1987.

Chest Radiograph Scoring System for Use in Pre-Term Infants

Yuksel B, Greenough A, Karani J, Page A (King's College Hospital, London, England)
Br J Radiol 64:1015–1018, 1991   6–58

Background.—Chest radiographs can assess the progression of respiratory distress syndrome (RDS) in neonates but are not reliable predictors of survival or of the development of bronchopulmonary dysplasia. The predictive value of a scoring systems designed to identify infants at risk for lung function abnormalities was evaluated.

Methods.—Chest radiographs taken at age 1 months in 20 very low birth weight infants with RDS were scored according to abnormalities of lung volume, presence of opacification, interstitial changes, and cystic elements (table). The possible range of scores was 0 to 17, with 17 indicating the most abnormal appearance.

Results.—The median chest radiograph score in these infants was 4. Five scores above the median ranged from 5 to 14. All 20 infants showed opacification-haziness of the lungs, and 15 had abnormalities of lung volume. The scoring system documented accurately the severity of neonatal RDS. Infants who required the most prolonged respiratory support also had the highest scores. The system had a sensitivity of 88% in identifying infants with the most severe lung function abnormalities at age 6 months.

Conclusions.—This scoring system has a high reproducibility and compared favorably with previous systems. In addition to documenting the severity of neonatal respiratory distress, the method is a useful predictor of chronic respiratory problems.

▶ Preterm infant chest radiographic pulmonary findings can be so similar that any effort to establish a method for determining severity is worth knowing and using. Radiologists experienced in neonatal chest interpretation recognize that no longer do we see the findings initially described for the stages of bronchopulmonary dysplasia (1). Another article reports a case of air embolism and pulmonary interstitial emphysema in a preterm infant with hyaline membrane disease and also reminds us of the Macklin and Macklin pathogenesis (2, 3). Other related articles concerning neonatal chest that are worthy of attention are included (4–6).—L.W. Young, M.D.

References

1. Northway WH, et al: *N Engl J Med* 276:357, 1967.
2. Richter A, et al: *Pediatr Radiol* 21:521, 1991.

Chest Radiograph Scoring System

	Score				
	0	1	2	3	4
Volume of thorax	Normal	Decreased	Increased		
Degree of inflation of lung fields	Normal	Underinflated	Overinflated		
Opacification	Absent	Perihilar *or* regional	Perihilar *and* regional	Complete opacification	
Air bronchogram	Absent	Present			
Pulmonary interstitial emphysema	Absent	Present			
Interstitial changes (coarse shadowing)	Absent	Present in one zone	Two zones	Three zones	Four zones
Cystic element	None	Single	Multiple		
Size of largest cyst	(not applicable)	Up to one-third of ipsilateral lung field	Larger than one-third of ipsilateral lung field		

(Courtesy of Yuksel B, Greenough A, Karani J, et al: *Br J Radiol* 64:1015–1018, 1991.)

3. Macklin MT, et al: *Medicine (Baltimore)* 23:281, 1944.
4. Bucky B, et al: *Acta Paediatr Hung* 30:351, 1990.
5. Levine D, et al: *AJR* 157:371, 1991.
6. Yip YY, et al: *J Paediatr Child Health* 27:34, 1991.

Imaging of Neonatal Arterial Thrombosis

Gudinchet F, Dreyer J-L, Payot M, Duvoisin B, Laurini R (University Hospital, Lausanne, Switzerland)
Arch Dis Child 66:1158–1159, 1991   6–59

Background.—Thrombosis of the aorta, great vessels, and veins is rare in the neonatal period when not related to umbilical catheterization. In 1 infant, thrombi associated with antenatal stroke were demonstrated by color Doppler sonography (CDS) and digital subtracted angiography (DSA).

Case Report.—Infant boy, 2 days, was referred because of the absence of spontaneous movement and cyanosis of the right arm. The pregnancy had been uneventful, but shoulder dystocia resulted in a prolonged delivery. Color Doppler sonography and DSA of the aorta were carried out, revealing reversed flow through the right carotid and vertebral arteries consistent with an obstructing thrombus in the brachiocephalic trunk (Fig 6–57). Further thrombi were visible at the emergence of the left common carotid artery (Fig 6–58). The findings of contrast enhanced CT were suggestive of a prenatal thromboembolic event (Fig 6–59). Therapy consisted of heparin and aspirin for 10 days and nicoumalone for 3 months. The left carotid artery thrombus had resolved after the first CDS. A left hemiparesis became apparent at 3 months; at 23 months, the child has a complete left hemiplegia.

Conclusions.—Only 2 similar cases of primary arterial and venous thromboses associated with antenatal stroke have been reported. Other

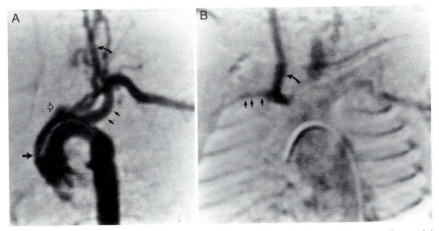

Fig 6–57.—A, aortic DSA. The tip of the catheter has been placed in the ascendant aorta (*large solid arrow*). Opacification of the left subclavian (*small arrows*) and left carotid (*curved arrow*) arteries. Absent opacification of the brachiocephalic trunk (*open arrow*). **B,** a late image showing opacification of the right subclavian artery (*small arrows*) via retrograde flow through the right carotid artery (*curved arrow*). (Courtesy of Gudinchet F, Dreyer J-L, Payot M, et al: *Arch Dis Child* 66:1158–1159, 1991.)

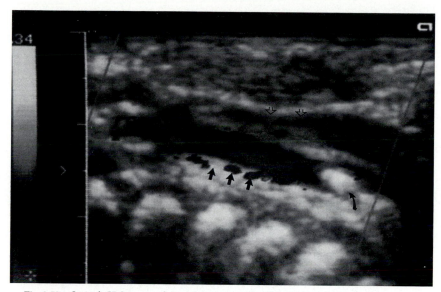

Fig 6–58.—Sagittal CDS image of the left common carotid (*solid straight arrows*) with proximal partially obstructing mural thrombus (*curved arrow*). The arterial flow is blue, and the venous jugular flow is red (*open arrows*). (Courtesy of Gudinchet F, Dreyer J-L, Payot M, et al: *Arch Dis Child* 66:1158–1159, 1991.)

causes for such thromboses are sepsis, birth trauma, and asphyxia. Color Doppler sonography displayed the thrombi and DSA confirmed the findings without femoral puncture. Because obstructive lesions in relation to the great vessels may be associated with cerebral infarction, brain imaging should also be carried out.

▶ Primary arterial thrombosis in the neonate is unusual. It was demonstrated by CDS and DSA in this neonate boy who had suffered antenatal stroke. One recent article reports thrombosis of the abdominal aorta demonstrated by sonography after catheterization of the umbilical artery (1), the usual cause of thrombosis in this age group. On the related subject of abdominal aortic aneurysm, both aortography and CT demonstrated the lesions (2, 3). Other recent articles of related interest are included (4, 5).—L.W. Young, M.D.

References

1. Teissier JM, et al: *Ann Radiol* 34:256, 1991.
2. Saad SA, et al: *J Pediatr Surg* 26:1423, 1991.
3. van Reedt Dortland RWH, et al: *J Pediatr Surg* 26:1420, 1991.
4. Pavlakis SG, et al: *Adv Pediatr* 38:151, 1991.
5. Singer R, et al: *J Pediatr Orthop* 11:588, 1991.

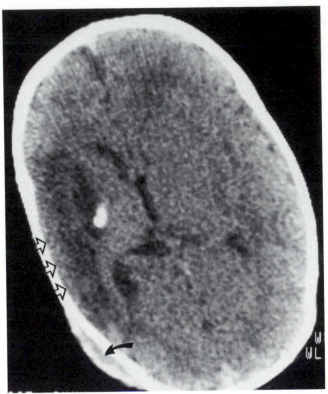

Fig 6–59.—Contrast-enhanced cerebral CT scan demonstrating a superficial infarct in the territory of the middle carotid artery (*open arrows*). The atrophic aspect and the deep focal calcification suggest a prenatal ischemic event. Cephalhematoma (*curved arrow*). (Courtesy of Gudinchet F, Dreyer J-L, Payot M, et al: *Arch Dis Child* 66:1158–1159, 1991.)

Pulmonary Hemorrhage Complicating Systemic Lupus Erythematosus: Role of MR Imaging in Diagnosis

Hsu BY, Edwards DK III, Trambert MA (Univ of California, San Diego)
AJR 158:519–520, 1992   6–60

Introduction.—Although pleuropulmonary involvement in systemic lupus erythematosus (SLE) is common, it is rarely symptomatic. Pulmonary hemorrhage is a rare and possibly fatal complication, which has nonspecific radiographic features. A case of this complication in a child with SLE, emphasizing the usefulness of MRI in making the diagnosis is reported.

Case Report.—Girl, 12 years, with a 1-month history of fever, lethargy, and intermittent joint pain, was serologically diagnosed as having SLE. Her chest radiographic findings were normal at admission. She had pleuritic chest pain,

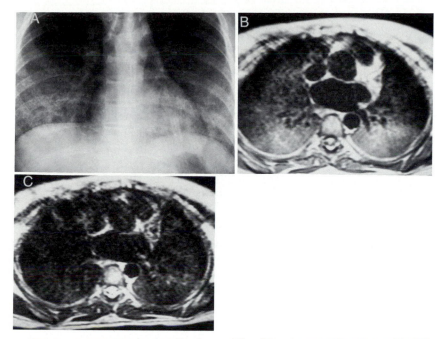

Fig 6–60.—A, anteroposterior chest film shows a diffuse, bilateral, nonspecific, reticulonodular infiltrate. **B,** and **C,** axial dydrogen-density MR images show a diffuse signal isointence with muscle in the midlung regions, with a decrease of signal intensity from first echo (2,169/20) (**B**) to second echo (2,169/70) (**C**). (Courtesy of Hus By, Edwards DK III, Trambert MA: AJR 158:519-520, 1992.)

cough, and tachypnea 7 days later, with no hemoptysis or sputum production. Chest radiographs showed a diffuse reticulonodular pattern. Her condition worsened, and the next day she was moved to the intensive care unit. Bronchoscopy showed bloody mucus, and bronchoalveolar lavage yielded bloody return. The patient was treated with high-dose corticosteroids and cyclophosphamide and was able to leave the intensive care unit on day 20. On day 24, however, her chest pain returned, with hypoxemia, falling hematocrit, and worsening alveolar opacities. Transaxial MRI through the lungs suggested recurrent hemorrhage (Fig 6-60). Corticosteroids were resumed, with no need for repeat bronchoscopy.

Conclusions.—Magnetic resonance imaging may be useful in diagnosing pulmonary hemorrhage as a complication of SLE. Preferential T_2 shortening is seen as a result of the paramagnetic effects of ferric iron in the blood. In this way, more invasive procedures can be avoided.

▶ Magnetic resonance imaging of the lung to show hemorrhage as a complication of SLE is a unique but practical use of the modality. It is always worthwhile to avoid invasive procedures. There appears to be much promise for MRI to be used to show pulmonary hemorrhage. The authors interestingly speculate that the signal changes of T_2-weighted images in the pulmonary hemorrhage might vary with time in a similar manner as blood in the brain. Two other articles refer to hemorrhage in the lung and MRI: 1 in a case of pulmonary sequestration (1) and the other in invasive pulmonary aspergillosis (2). Most other recent articles of related interest are about MRI findings in lupus erythematosus involving the CNS (3–5). L.W. Young, M.D.

References

1. Ohtomo K, et al: *Radiat Med* 6:58, 1988.
2. Herold CJ, et al: *Radiology* 173:717, 1989.
3. Sibbitt WL Jr, et al: *Ann Rheum Dis* 48:1014, 1989.
4. Boumpas DT, et al: *J Rheumatol* 17:89, 1990.
5. McAbee GN, et al: *Pediatr Neurol* 6:186, 1990.

Wegener's Granulomatosis in Childhood
McHugh K, Manson D, Eberhard BA, Shore A, Laxer RM (Hospital for Sick Children, Toronto, Ont, Canada)
Pediatr Radiol 21:552–555, 1991   6–61

Introduction.—Wegener's granulomatosis (WG), a disease characterized by vasculitis involving the upper and lower respiratory tracts and kidney, may be more common in children than previously thought.

Methods.—In 1984 to 1990, WG was diagnosed in 5 girls aged 11 to 16 years. The disease was histologically confirmed and involved both upper and lower respiratory tracts. Renal disease was proved in the 4 who underwent renal biopsies. Prednisone treatment was successful in 3 patients; the 2 remaining patients had multiple relapses during the mean follow-up period of 28 months.

Results.—Initial chest radiographs were abnormal in all patients. In 3 patients there was pulmonary hemorrhage and 1 required a tracheotomy because of subglottic stenosis. Thoracic CT examinations showed a highly variable expression of the disease, but the most common manifestations were multifocal parenchymal infiltrates with or without small peripheral nodules. In 2 patients, classic cavitary lung nodules were seen, 1 at initial diagnosis and another at relapse. There were 2 examples of extensive sinus mucosal disease (Fig 6–61).

Conclusions.—Corticosteroids and cyclophosphamide have improved prognosis for patients with WG. Examination with CT is valuable in localizing the site of lung parenchymal involvement, assessing the extent of respiratory tract involvement, and monitoring the results of therapy.

▶ Cross-sectional CT imaging for lung lesions is proving to be increasingly valuable for chronic lung disease, as in this article about Wegener's granulomatosis. Application of CT to systemic lupus erythematosus and cystic fibrosis also has been fruitful. Computed tomography imaging of the paranasal

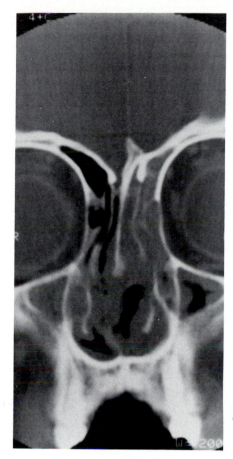

Fig 6–61.—Coronal CT showing mucosal thickening of the maxillary and ethmoid sinuses also at presentation. There is no air-fluid level or evidence of bone destruction (W = 4,000; L = 500). (Courtesy of McHugh K, Manson D, Eberhard BA, et al: *Pediatr Radiol* 21:552–555, 1991.)

sinuses may show soft tissue swelling but no osseous disturbance (1–3). Recent or pertinent related articles of interest are listed (4–7).—L.W. Young, M.D.

References

1. Singer J, et al: *Clin Radiol* 42:50, 1990.
2. Teng MM, et al: *Neuroradiology* 31:498, 1990.
3. Milford CA, et al: *Clin Otolaryngol* 11:199, 1986.
4. Guhl L, et al: *Bildgebung* 585:33, 1991.
5. Weir IH, et al: *Can Assoc Radiol J* 43:31, 1992.
6. Satorre J, et al: *Can J Ophthalmol* 26:174, 1991.
7. Leavitt JA, et al: *Cornea* 10:542, 1991.

Splenic Necrosis in Wegener's Granulomatosis

McHugh K, Manson D, Eberhard BA, Laxer RM, Shore A (Hospital for Sick Children, Toronto, Ont, Canada)
Pediatr Radiol 21:588–589, 1991   6–62

Background.—Although multiorgan involvement can occur in Wegener's granulomatosis, there are few reports of the disorder affecting the spleen. Splenic necrosis secondary to Wegener's granulomatosis appeared in a pediatric patient.

Case Report.—Girl, 11 years, was seen for treatment with a 2-month history of arthralgia, headaches, and episodes of epistaxis. A week before admission, a rash, sore eyes, and increasing dyspnea on exertion had developed. Examination revealed a palpable spleen and a decreased range of movement in the knees and ankles. Renal biopsy showed a focal segmental necrotizing glomerulonephritis with crescent formation. A plain chest radiograph on the fourth day after admission was suggestive of pulmonary hemorrhage. With a working diagnosis of Wegener's granulomatosis, pulse corticosteroids and cyclophosphamide therapy was started. The patient's symptomatic response was good. Computed tomography a week later demonstrated marked low attenuation within the spleen (Fig 6–62). No focal splenic lesion could be identified on sonography, and the girl had no abdominal symptoms.

Conclusions.—Despite patency of the splenic vessels, the splenic lesion was determined to be the result of necrosis secondary to Wegener's granulomatosis. Normal attenuation of the girl's spleen is seen on CT, although follow-up has revealed relapses of the disease in the lower respiratory tract. Splenic involvement may go unnoticed in some patients with Wegener's granulomatosis.

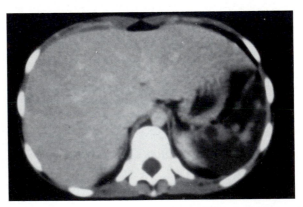

Fig 6–62.—Contrast-enhanced CT scan demonstrating marked low attenuation within the spleen. Subsequent CT examinations showed return to a normal attenuation with lobulation and shrinkage of the spleen (W = 300, L = 114). (Courtesy of McHugh K, Manson D, Eberhard BA, et al: *Pediatr Radiol* 21:588–589, 1991.)

▶ Wegener's granulomatosis is a disease of multiorgan involvement with the respiratory tract and kidney most commonly affected. Observation of splenic involvement in a child has not been previously reported. Both CT and ultrasound showed changes—decreased attenuation on CT and inhomogeneous echotexture with ultrasound. Recent articles of involvement of Wegener's granulomatosis in unusual organs—heart (1), lacrimal gland (2), ear (3), and orbit (4)—are listed.—L.W. Young, M.D.

References

1. Kosovsky PA, et al: *J Comput Assist Tomogr* 15:1028, 1991.
2. Leavitt JA, et al: *Cornea* 10:542, 1991.
3. Ito Y, et al: *Auris Nasus Larynx* 18:281, 1991.
4. Satorre J, et al: *Can J Ophthalmol* 26:174, 1991.

Gastrointestinal

Contribution of Ultrasonography in the Diagnosis of Achalasia

Bergami GL, Fruhwirth R, Di Mario M, Fasanelli S (Bambino Gesù Pediatric Hospital, Rome)
J Pediatr Gastroenterol Nutr 14:92–96, 1992   6–63

Introduction.—Ultrasonography can be used to study the abdominal esophagus and cardia. There are 2 sonographic views: along the main axis of the distal esophagus and along its transverse plane. Gastroesophageal reflux, hiatal hernia, neoplastic diseases, local vascular anomalies, and postoperative aspects are well demonstrated. In addition to clinical manometric and endoscopic examination ultrasonography was used to diagnose achalasia in a young child.

Case Report.—Girl, 3 years, with Down syndrome, had intermittent vomiting and frequent regurgitation. A metallic foreign body in the esophagus was identified on a chest roentgenogram and confirmed by a barium meal study. The latter also showed a marked narrowing of the distal tract and cardia of the esophagus, whereas the esophagus above was dilated, atonic, and hypoperistaltic. Ultrasonography showed symmetric thickening of the muscular wall of the distal tract of the esophagus (Fig 6–63) and a dilated distal esophagus after ingestion of water. Manometry showed a failure of relaxation of the lower esophageal sphincter and an absence of primary or secondary peristalsis. Endoscopy showed an undamaged mucosa of the prestenotic esophagus, which permitted the extraction of a toy coin of lightweight metal. Extramucosa cardiomyotomy and Nissen fundoplication were performed. The patient was discharged from the hospital on day 14 of remission.

Conclusions.—In patients with achalasia, the narrowing of the distal esophagus is radiologically evident, and ultrasonography permits the visualization of the muscular wall and the evaluation of the degree of

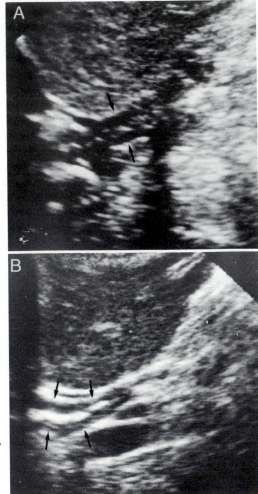

Fig 6-63.—Ultrasonography. **A,** longitudial view of a normal esophagus (*arrows*), which shows regular aspect of the walls. **B,** a longitudinal view of an achalasial esophagus with moderate thickening of the muscular walls (*arrows*), restricted lumen, and abnormally oriented longitudinal axis (visibility of the abdominal aorta). (Courtesy of Bergami GL, Fruhwirth R, Di Mario M, et al: *J Pediatr Gastroenterol Nutr* 14:92-96, 1992.)

thickening and the extension of the stenotic tract. Ultrasonography shows that the major axis of the distal esophagus becomes almost parallel to the aorta in achalasia. Preoperative demonstration of a symmetric thickening of the muscular layer of the esophagus by ultrasonography helps exclude other diseases of the gastroesophageal junction.

▶ Ultrasound is valuable in corroborating the diagnosis of achalasia. There are some conditions that simulate achalasia on plain and contrast medium radiography. In a recent article on leiomyomatosis of the esophagus in a 5-year-old girl, the diagnosis might not have been made without the use of MRI and CT (1). Another article on ultrasonography in achalasia is useful, although not specific to childhood (2). Two recent articles on esophageal stricture obstructions of another type are listed; 1 is one Stevens-Johnson syndrome involving esophageal stricture and chronic lung disease (3), and the other is on balloon dilatation of esophageal strictures in children (4).—L.W. Young, M.D.

References

1. Lerone M, et al: *Pediatr Radiol* 21:578, 1991.
2. Zhou FX, et al: *Clin Med J* 103:50, 1990.
3. Edell DS, et al: *Pediatrics* 89:429, 1992.
4. Meyer CM III, et al: *Arch Otolaryngol Head Neck Surg* 117:529, 1991.

Pyloric Stenosis Associated With Malrotation
Croitoru D, Neilson I, Guttman FM (Montreal Children's Hospital; McGill University, Montreal)
J Pediatr Surg 26:1276–1278, 1991   6–64

Introduction.—Pyloric stenosis associated with malrotation is thought to be genetically transmitted. All reported familial patients have had congenitally a shortened bowel and a poor prognosis. However, 3 infants were encountered who did not have a short bowel and recovered after surgery.

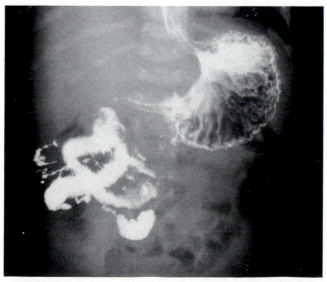

Fig 6–64.—Upper gastrointestinal tract series showing pyloric stenosis and malrotation in patient 1. (Courtesy of Croitoru D, Neilson I, Guttman FM: *J Pediatr Surg* 26:1276–1278, 1991.)

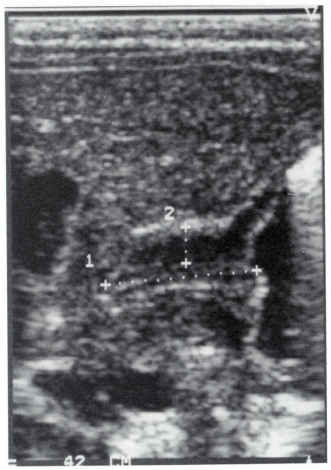

Fig 6-65.—Ultrasonogram of pylorus in patient 1. (Courtesy of Croitoru D, Neilson I, Guttman FM: *J Pediatr Surg* 26:1276-1278, 1991.)

Case Report.—Boy, 5 weeks, had projectile nonbilious vomiting. He was dehydrated, and the upper half of his abdomen was distended. Ultrasonography confirmed a pyloric tumor. When the nasogastric drainage became bilious, an upper gastrointestinal tract series was performed. Pyloric stenosis and malrotation were confirmed (Fig 6-64). Repeated ultrasonographic measurements met the standard for pyloric stenosis (Fig 6-65). After a pyloromyotomy and Ladd's procedure, the vomiting ceased and the infant began to gain weight.

Conclusions.—In the 2 other patients, Ladd's procedure was performed after malrotation was diagnosed. Vomiting continued and pyloric stenosis was diagnosed. The finding of malrotation and pyloric stenosis occurring together and without a familial inheritance association is unusual. Discordant findings in patients with intestinal obstruction manifested as pyloric stenosis or malrotation should prompt further investigation.

▶ Association of pyloric stenosis and malrotation is unusual and probably coincidental. Good morphologic demonstration by gastrointestinal and contrast medium and ultrasound examinations is possible, but the contrast medium exam is distinctly better for malrotation. Other recent reports are similar to the abstracted article (1, 2). One of them reports the combination of hypertropic pyloric stenosis, intestinal malrotation, and gastric antral diaphragm (2). Other recent articles of related interest are listed (3–5).—L.W. Young, M.D.

References

1. Baumgartner F, et al: *Eur J Pediatr Surg* 2:42, 1992.
2. Dassonville M, et al: *Z Kinderchir* 41:112, 1986.
3. Ford EG, et al: *Ann Surg* 215:172, 1992.
4. Courtney SP, et al: *Br J Clin Pract* 44:370, 1990.
5. Rollins MD, et al: *Gut* 32:612, 1991.

Congenital Choledochal Dilatation With Emphasis on Pathophysiology of the Biliary Tract

Iwai N, Yanagihara J, Tokiwa K, Shimotake T, Nakamura K (Children's Research Hosp, Kyoto, Japan)
Ann Surg 215:27–30, 1992   6–65

Background.—Although the relationship between congenital choledochal dilatation and abnormalities of the choledochopancreaticoductal junction has been well studied, little is known about the pathophysiology of the biliary tract in patients with congenital choledochal dilatation. Morphologic abnormalities and the pathophysiology of the biliary tracts were analyzed in 26 patients with congenital choledochal dilatation.

Patients and Methods.—Thirty-seven patients were treated between 1978 and 1990 at 1 center. There were 28 girls aged 1 month to 12 years and 9 boys aged 8 days to 5 years. All had undergone excision of the choledochal cyst with Roux-en-Y hepaticojejunostomy. Twenty-six patients could be analyzed for morphologic abnormalities and pathophysiology of the biliary tract.

Findings.—Ninety-six percent of the patients analyzed had an abnormal choledochopancreaticoductal junction. Ten of the 12 patients with cystic-type choledochal dilatation had the C-P type of abnormal choledochopancreaticoductal junction. Of the 13 children with fusiform-type choledochal dilatation, 9 had the P-C type. Amylase levels in the choledochal cyst and gallbladder were increased, regardless of the form of choledochal dilatation. One child had an adenocarcinoma in a cystic choledochal dilatation.

Conclusions.—Long-standing inflammation of the biliary tract caused by the reflux of pancreatic juice may be 1 factor in carcinogenesis of the biliary tract. Free reflux of pancreatic juice was shown both by amylase levels in the biliary tract and by intraoperative biliary manometry. The lack of sphincter function at the junction of the common bile and pancreatic ducts may explain this reflux.

▶ Findings on endoscopic retrograde cholangiopancreatography as used in this report, were classified into 3 defined types: (1) the C-P type, the pancreatic duct is the major duct and the bile duct joins it; (2) the P-C type, the bile duct is the major duct and the pancreatic duct joins it; and (3) the miscellaneous type, the complexity of the ductal connection defies categorization. This study provides additional information and gives added support to the Babbitt proposal (1) that the abnormal choledochopancreatoductal junction is a cause for congenital choledochal dilatation. Recent articles of related interest are listed (2, 3).—L.W. Young, M.D.

References

1. Babbitt DP: *Ann Radiol* 12:231, 1969.
2. Young WT, et al: *Br J Radiol* 65:33, 1992.
3. Okada A, et al: *Surg Gynecol Obstet* 171:291, 1990.

Radionuclide Blood Pool Scintigraphy in a Child With Intestinal Arteriovenous Malformation (Juvenile Angiodysplasia): A Case Report and Review of the Literature
Garty I, Siplovich L, Horowitz J, Miron D, Verstandig A, Dharan M (Central Emek Hospital, Afula; Hadassah Medical Organization, Jerusalem, Israel)
Eur J Nucl Med 18:992–995, 1991   6–66

Introduction.—Gastrointestinal arteriovenous (AV) malformation or angiodysplasia very rarely causes bleeding in children; only 15 such cases have been reported. A child had a type II AV malformation of the distal ileum that was diagnosed by radionuclide blood pool scanning and angiography and treated by local resection.

Case Report.—Boy, 4 years, was admitted with severe anemia. He was pale and tachycardic and had frank melena. Hemoglobin was 4.5 g%, hematocrit 22, reticulocytes 6%, platelets 250,000, prothrombin time 60%, and partial thromboplastin time 20 seconds. Two units of blood were given immediately to stabilize the patient's condition. No pathologic changes were found on gastroscopy, colonoscopy, barium studies, or technetium 99m–sodium pertechnetate abdominal scan. However, delayed ^{99m}Tc red blood cell scan showed an area of abnormal concentration in the right lower quadrant (Fig 6–66). Selective superior mesenteric angiography showed a vascular malformation in the distal small bowel. Exploratory laparotomy revealed a submucosal vascular lesion in the distal ileum,

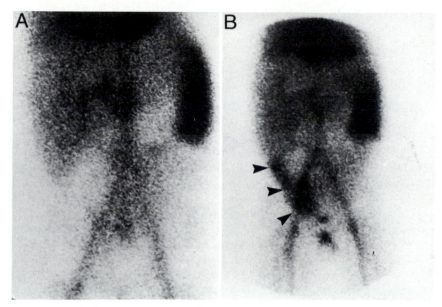

Fig 6–66.—Blood pool scintigraphy using ^{99m}Tc red blood cells. No pathologic concentrations were demonstrated by this early (1.5-hour) blood pool scan. A region of pathologic concentration consistent with a large blood pool in the lower right abdomen is shown by the delayed (2.5-hour study) (**B**) and is marked by *arrows*. No movement of blood down the gastrointestinal tract was demonstrated by sequential images. The study was interpreted as abdominal AV malformation with no evidence of active bleeding. (Courtesy of Garty I, Siplovich L, Horowitz J, et al: *Eur J Nucl Med* 18:992–995, 1991.)

which was resected using end-to-end anastomosis. After an uneventful postoperative course, the child's hemoglobin was 11.7 g% at 4 months.

Discussion.—Intestinal AV malformations are very rare congenital anomalies, thought to be of hamartomatous origin. The patient described appears to be the youngest yet reported. Radionuclide blood pool scintigraphy appears to be an accurate, simple, and noninvasive diagnostic procedure. If the diagnosis is made early enough, prompt surgical intervention with complete cure can be achieved.

▶ Radionuclide blood pool scintigraphy is valuable in diagnosing juvenile angiodysplasia. This case of congenital hamartomatous vascular anomaly beautifully shows how scintigraphy correlates with angiography. Relatively recent and pertinent articles of related interest are listed (1, 2).—L.W. Young, M.D.

References

1. Heyman S, et al: *Clin Nucl Med* 15:119, 1990.
2. Wesselhoeft CW Jr, et al: *J Pediatr Surg* 21:71, 1986.

Air Enema for Diagnosis and Reduction of Intussusception: Clinical Experience and Pressure Correlates
Shiels WE II, Maves CK, Hedlund GL, Kirks DR (Children's Hosp Med Ctr, Univ of Cincinnati, Cincinnati)
Radiology 181:169–172, 1991   6–67

Background and Methods.—Air enema has become increasingly popular for evaluation and treatment of intussusception in children. Air enema was used for exclusion, diagnosis, initial movement, and complete reduction of intussusception in 186 patients. Fluoroscopic times, findings, and the success rate were also evaluated.

Results.—Seventy-five patients were diagnosed as having intussception; intussception was successfully reduced in 65. In comparison, reduction was successful in only 55 of 100 patients who underwent hydrostatic reduction. The average pressure required for initial movement of intussusception with air enema was 56.5 mm Hg. An increase to an average maximum pressure of 97.8 Hg was necessary for complete reduction, which required from 1 to 3 attempts. The average fluoroscopy time for reduction was 94.8 seconds, while for exclusion of intussusception, it was 41.8 seconds.

Discussion.—The number or air enemas required to find intussusception depends on the experience of the examining physician and that of the radiologist interpreting the abdominal plain films. An experienced radiologist can exclude the diagnosis of intussusception in 5–10 seconds of fluoroscopy time and reduce an uncomplicated intussusception in 14–30 seconds. Because air insufflation is quick and easy, surgeons have a lower threshold for obtaining the examination in suspected cases of intussusception. With air insufflation, short fluoroscopy time and lower required kilovolt peak and milliamperes result in a lower radiation dose to the patient compared with barium or water-soluble contrast enemas.

Conclusions.—Air enema is a safe and effective method of diagnosing and treating intussusception in infants and children. Complete intussusception reduction requires copious reflux of air into the small bowel and disappearance of the soft tissue mass. In experienced hands, air insufflation is the method of choice for radiologic treatment of intussusception.

▶ This is another informative article—there have been several over the last 2 years (1)—on air enema for pneumatic reduction of ileocolic intussusception. One of the realistic aspects about enema reduction is that radiologist, experienced with hydrostatic reduction without complication using barium or other liquid positive contrast media, feel no urgency to change to the air enema for pneumatic reduction. Yet those gaining experience with pneumatic reduction find it to be relatively innocuous. Theoretically, it should require less radiation. I suspect that the air enema, or a modification of it, eventually will become the method of choice even in this country for this diagnosis and treatment. However, I am not convinced that, in the everyday careful practice of radiology, there is a significant morbidity associated with use of barium for hydrostatic reduction of ileocolic intussusception. Recent articles of related interest either on diagnosis of ileocolic intussusception, reduction, or both, or on isolated small bowel intussusceptions (2, 3) are listed (1–7).—L.W. Young, M.D.

References

1. 1992 YEAR BOOK OF DIAGNOSTIC RADIOLOGY, p 448.
2. Ratcliffe JF, et al: *AJR* 158:619, 1992.
3. Hu SC, et al: *Arch Dis Child* 66:1065, 1991.
4. McGrath FP, et al: *Pediatr Radiol* 21:590, 1991.
5. Sargent MA, et al: *Pediatr Radiol* 21:346, 1991.
6. Schmitz-Rode T, et al: *Pediatr Radiol* 21:341, 1991.
7. Woo SK, et al: *Radiology* 182:77, 1992.

Differences in the Clinical and Radiologic Patterns of Rotavirus and Non-rotavirus Necrotizing Enterocolitis

Keller KM, Schmidt H, Wirth S, Queisser-Luft A, Schumacher R (Johannes Gutenberg University, Mainz, Germany)
Pediatr Infect Dis J 10:734–738, 1991   6–68

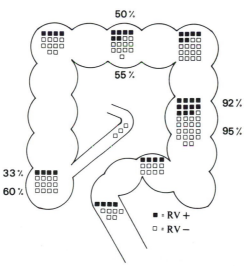

Fig 6–67.—Distribution of pneumatosis intestinalis in RV + NEC and RV − NEC infants. *Filled box* indicates localization of pneumatosis intestinalis in the 13 infants with RV + NEC; *open box*, positive findings of pneumatosis in the 19 infants with RV − NEC. The percentages refer to the relative distribution of pneumatosis in RV + infants (*figures at top*) and in RV − patients (*figures below*) over the different intestinal segments: ascending, transverse, and descending colon, respectively. (Courtesy of Keller KM, Schmidt H, Wirth S, et al: *Pediatr Infect Dis J* 10:734–738, 1991.)

Background and Methods.—Necrotizing enterocolitis (NEC) is the principal gastrointestinal emergency in neonates. To improve the understanding of a subgroup of patients with NEC associated with rotavirus (RV) infection, investigators retrospectively analyzed 13 infants with NEC and RV and compared the findings with those from 19 infants with NEC alone.

Results.—All cases had moderate to severe radiologic grades. All had at least pneumatosis intestinalis, and all but 1 had risk factors for perinatal asphyxia. There was a significant difference between infants with NEC who were RV positive and those who were RV negative. Infants who were positive for RV had higher birth weights and were born at later gestational ages. They had begun oral feeding earlier, but symptoms had developed later and more insidiously than in infants who were RV negative. Radiologic studies showed that RV positive infants had less severe and more distal colon involvement than did those who were RV negative, but radiologic changes of pneumatosis coli of RV-positive and RV-negative patients were equally distributed in the transverse and descending colon (Fig 6–67). The NEC patients without RV had predominantly small intestinal or ileocecal changes and more frequent complications of pneumoportogram and intestinal perforations. Patients with these complications often had rapid clinical deterioration, and 84% required surgery.

Conclusions.—Significant differences were found between NEC patients who were RV positive and those who were RV negative. Although infants with NEC are predominantly affected in the ileocecal region, this part of the intestine was not generally involved in RV-positive patients. The reasons for this are not clear. However, this distinction is 1 method of differentiating RV-positive patients from RV-negative patients.

▶ The differences in RV NEC vs. non–RV NEC are interesting, but whether they will stand the test of time for application in the everyday clinical problem of the neonate with possible NEC is uncertain. The relatively common RV-positive gastroenteritis has less severe necrotizing enterocolitis findings than RV-negative NEC. Perhaps more significant is what causative organisms, if any, might be causing the RV-negative NEC. What must be kept in mind is that whichever is the causative organism, late complications can occur that may require surgery. Another recent article is about the finding of an empty rectum on the plain radiograph of the infant abdomen and its relation to NEC, generalized sepsis, or Hirschsprung's disease (1). Recent articles of additional related interest are listed (2–4).—L.W. Young, M.D.

References

1. Bradley MJ, et al: *Clin Radiol* 43:265, 1991.
2. Nigro G: *J Pediatr Gastroenterol Nutr* 12:280, 1991.
3. Uauy RD, et al: *J Pediatr* 119:630, 1991.
4. Avni EF, et al: *Pediatr Radiol* 21:179, 1991.

Hepatic Abscess Caused by a Ventriculoperitoneal Shunt

Paone RF, Mercer LC (Texas Tech Univ, El Paso, Tex)
Pediatr Infect Dis J 10:338–339, 1991

6–69

Background.—Although the ventriculoperitoneal (VP) shunt is the preferred method of diverting CSF in patients with hydrocephalus, this technique has resulted in numerous intra-abdominal complications. In 1 case the catheter portion of a VP shunt was embedded in the liver and caused a hepatic abscess.

Case Report.—Girl, 2 years and 2 months, had been born with a meningomyelocele, clubbed feet, and hydrocephalus. A Pudenz-type VP shunt was inserted at age 3 weeks. She had a 2-day history of abdominal pain, emesis, and subjective fever 2 weeks after treatment for a urinary tract infection. The child was then treated for a presumptive diagnosis of sepsis, secondary to a urinary tract infection or to a VP shunt infection. *Enterococcus faecalis* was cultured in fluid from the VP shunt reservoir. Ultrasonography revealed a large cystic structure deep within the left lobe of the liver. She underwent exploratory laparotomy, which confirmed the VP shunt catheter had entered the left lobe. After antibiotic treatment and removal of the shunt the child became afebrile and was discharged within 1 week.

Conclusions.—Abdominal complications are common in patients with VP shunt systems. The present case, however, involving penetration of the liver and formation of a hepatic abscess, is 1 of only a few reported complications of this type. The abscess may have formed as the result of either translocation of gut flora or intra-abdominal sepsis with seeding of the liver through the portal vein. A hepatic abscess should be considered as a possibility in patients with VP shunts and abdominal symptoms.

▶ The child with a VP shunt, abdominal pain, and fever needs a diagnostic workup, including imaging for an intra-abdominal complication. The imaging workup includes a radiographic shunt series, abdominal sonography, or abdominal CT. In this patient, the imaging findings led to the unusual diagnosis of hepatic abscess around the caudal tip of the shunt tube. A shunt-related hepatic abscess in an adult also was recently reported (1). In another unusual complication, a ventriculoatrial shunt fragment lodged in the right atrium and became the source for recurrent *Staphylococcus aureus* bacteremia (2). Standard imaging techniques did not detect an intravascular foreign body, but ultrafast CT of the heart showed the catheter fragment, which was successfully excised (2). A shunt-related brain abscess in an infant also was recently reported (3). Other recent articles of related interest are listed (3–5).—L.W. Young, M.D.

References

1. Peterfy CG, et al: *AJR* 155:894, 1990.

2. McKinsey DS, et al: *Rev Infect Dis* 13:893, 1991.
3. Gower DJ, et al: *J Child Neurol* 5:318, 1990.
4. Ashpole RD, et al: *Br J Neurosurg* 5:515, 1991.
5. Chow CC, et al: *Pediatr Radiol* 21:305, 1991.

Granulomatous Hepatitis in Cat-Scratch Disease: Ultrasound and CT Observations

Port J, Leonidas JC (Long Island Jewish Med Ctr)
Pediatr Radiol 21:598–599, 1991   6–70

Introduction.—Cat-scratch disease (CSD) is a self-limited disease resulting from a pleomorphic gram-negative bacillus. In a patient with rare granulomatous involvement of the liver and spleen, imaging of the liver suggested a neoplastic process, but clinical manifestation and a liver biopsy confirmed CSD.

Case Report.—Boy, 2 years, from Honduras, was admitted with a 1-month history of persistent fever. He was treated orally for a suspected viral infection with cefaclor, followed by erythromycin, 2 weeks before admission. Except for a temperature of 40.5°C, the physical examination was unremarkable. Abdominal ultrasonography and CT revealed lesions in the liver at first thought to be metastatic (Figs 6–68 and 6–69). Tissue specimens obtained at biopsy showed delicate pleomorphic gram-negative bacilli, which are characteristic of CSD. Contact with

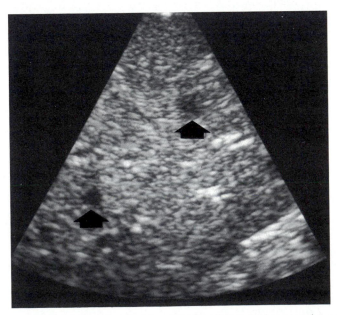

Fig 6–68.—Magnified view of the right lobe of the liver (longitudinal sonogram) reveals multiple small hypoechoic lesions (*arrows*). (Courtesy of Port J, Leonidas JC: *Pediatr Radiol* 21:598–599, 1991.)

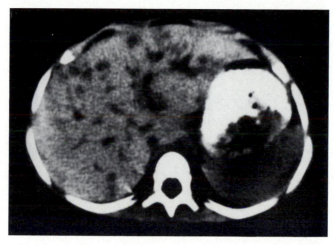

Fig 6–69.—A CT scan of the liver without intravenous contrast shows multiple low-density lesions throughout the substance of the liver. Although initially thought to represent metastatic lesions from an unknown primary tumor, biopsy proved them to be granulomas associated with cat-scratch disease. (Courtesy of Port J, Leonidas JC: *Pediatr Radiol* 21:598–599, 1991.)

a cat was confirmed, and gentamycin sulfate was administered intravenously. Improvement was rapid.

Conclusions.—Symptoms of CSD may take months to resolve. The most common manifestations are fever and malaise, headache, and peripheral adenopathy. Hepatic and splenic involvement have rarely been reported but may be more prevalent than previously suspected. Such findings lead to fear of more ominous diseases in young children, but a simple skin test can usually confirm or exclude CSD without the need for biopsy or further diagnostic work-up.

▶ It is important to know about the graphic imaging findings of ultrasound and CT in granulomatous hepatitis of CSD. The involvement of liver and spleen may be more prevalent than previously suspected (1). Recent articles of related interest are listed (2, 3).—L.W. Young, M.D.

References

1. Rappaport DC, et al: *AJR* 156:1227, 1991.
2. Delahoussaye PM, et al: *J Infect Dis* 1611:71, 1990.
3. Weintrub P: *Pediatr Infect Dis J* 101:80, 1991.

Pediatric Abdominal Lymphangiomas: A Plea for Early Recognition

Kosir MA, Sonnino RE, Gauderer MWL (Rainbow Babies and Childrens Hosps of Cleveland, Cleveland)
J Pediatr Surg 26:1309–1313, 1991
6–71

Background.—Although abdominal lymphangiomas are typically grouped with mesenteric cysts, they are considerably different in histologic features, location, and clinical behavior.

Case Report.—Boy, 9 years, had had increasing abdominal distention, mild pain, anorexia, and decreased bowel movements for 3 days. In retrospect, his appetite and energy had been decreased for about 6 months. Examination revealed a distended abdomen with a firm, slightly tender central mass. Ultrasound and CT showed a large septated cystic mass that was separate from the liver, gallbladder, kidneys, and spleen (Fig 6–70). At laparotomy the mass was adherent to the transverse colon, extending to the base of the small bowel mesentery and involved the superior mesenteric artery and vein, duodenum, and pancreatic surface. Most of the lesion was removed without damage to those structures, although part of the posterior wall had to be left behind. The diagnosis of lymphangioma was confirmed; the child showed no signs of recurrence at 19 months' follow-up.

Review.—Thirteen children, mean age 5.8 years, with abdominal lymphangiomas were seen over a 15-year period. Twelve had symptoms, including 11 with abdominal pain, 8 with vomiting, 8 with increased abdominal girth, and 6 with nausea. Average duration of symptoms was 2 months, although it was less than 1 week in 7 cases. Ten had a palpable mass. Diagnostic yield was best with ultrasound and CT. Surgical find-

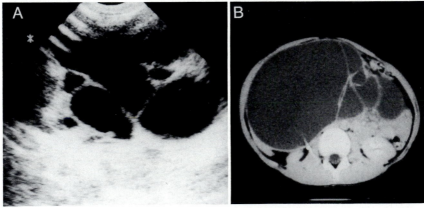

Fig 6–70.—A, preoperative ultrasound of lymphangioma. A large multiloculated cystic lesion measured 12 × 16 × 18 cm in maximum dimensions. **B,** a preoperative CT scan of the same patient. A cystic mass with septations is well visualized. (Courtesy of Kosir MA, Sonnino RE, Gauderer MWL: *J Pediatr Surg* 26:1309–1313, 1991.)

ings included bowel obstruction in 5 patients, volvulus in 4, and gangrenous bowel in 2. Eight required bowel resection, and 2 of the tumors could not be resected completely. Tumors ranged in size from 5 to 27.5 cm in their maximal dimensions. One child had a recurrence at 4 months. At an average of 8 years of follow-up, none of the children had died.

Discussion.—In a series of 13 children with abdominal lymphangioma, the lesions were frequently symptomatic, commonly causing pain and a mass in the abdomen. Earlier diagnosis can avoid catastrophic complications. These lesions are accurately diagnosed by ultrasound and CT; the former should be used promptly in children with intermittent or ill-defined abdominal pain.

▶ Early recognition of lymphangioma by ultrasound or CT is important because morbidity increases with age. For example, 38% of this series had volvulus and gangrene, and 61% needed bowel resection. Another recent article in this general category is about infantile hemangioma and its diagnosis with Doppler ultrasound (1). Recent articles of related interest are listed (2–5).—L.W. Young, M.D.

References

1. Paltiel HJ, et al: *Radiology* 182:735, 1992.
2. Caro PA, et al: *Clin Imaging* 15:41, 1991.
3. Patel RV, et al: *Indian Pediatr* 28:814, 1991.
4. Buonomo C, et al: *Radiographics* 11:1146, 1991.
5. Davidson AJ, et al: *Radiology* 175:507, 1990.

Safety-Belt Injuries in Children With Lap-Belt Ecchymosis: CT Findings in 61 Patients
Sivit CJ, Taylor GA, Newman KD, Bulas DI, Gotschall CS, Wright CJ, Eichelberger MR (Children's Natl Med Ctr, George Washington Univ, Washington, DC)
AJR 157:111–114, 1991   6–72

Background.—Children involved in vehicular crashes are at risk for incurring linear abdominal or flank ecchymosis if they are wearing lap safety belts. These injuries, which often involved the lumbar spine and hollow viscera, are difficult to identify on CT scan.

Methods.—Between 1983 and 1990, 61 children involved in vehicular crashes incurred "lap-belt ecchymosis." Demographic data, indications for CT, clinical records, radiologic findings, and clinical outcome were reviewed.

Results.—Thirteen children (21%) had lumbar spine injuries; 14 (23%) had hollow viscus injuries. Of these 14, 12 had bowel injuries and 2 had bladder injuries. Five children (8%) had both spine and hollow viscus in-

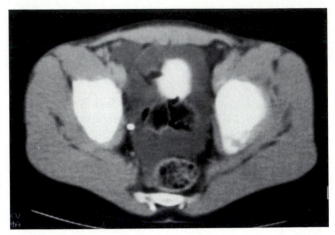

Fig 6–71.—Partial jejunal tear with unexplained peritoneal fluid. A CT scan through the pelvis shows a moderate amount of fluid. (Courtesy of Sivit CJ, Taylor GA, Newman KD, et al: AJR 157:111–114, 1991.)

juries. Retrospectively, abdominal CT showed abnormal findings in only 3 of 13 children with lumbar spine injuries, but lateral radiographs of the spine showed the injuries in all cases. Computed tomography noted free intraperitoneal air in 3 of 12 children with bowel injury, an incidence of 25%. However, CT showed large unexplained collections of peritoneal fluid in 8 of these children (Fig 6–71). Two children with intraperitoneal bladder ruptures were identified by the first CT scan. In both cases, ex-

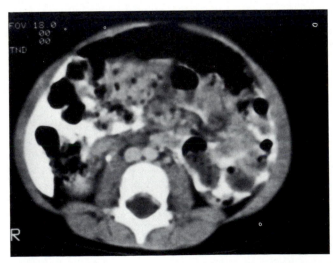

Fig 6–72.—Intraperitoneal bladder rupture. A CT scan shows intraperitoneal contrast material. Bladder perforation was noted during surgery. (Courtesy of Sivit CJ, Taylor GA, Newman KD, et al: AJR 157:111–114, 1991.)

travasation of intravenous contrast material was present throughout the peritoneal cavity (Fig 6–72).

Conclusions.—The presence of lap-belt ecchymosis should alert the clinician to search for spine, bowel, and bladder injury. However, CT has limited capability to diagnose these injuries. Findings of intestinal trauma may be nonspecific and subtle on CT. The presence of pneumo-peritoneum is neither specific nor sensitive for the diagnosis of bowel injury. Observers have rarely noted peritoneal fluid or blood as an iso-lated finding after blunt trauma. In the absence of a solid viscus injury, pelvic fracture, or hypoperfusion complex, peritoneal fluid was identi-fied in only 17 of 965 children studied by CT after blunt trauma. Ten of these patients had bowel injuries.

▶ The use of lap belts—designed for adults—in small children can cause such children substantial intra-abdominal injury. Abdominal CT as the imag-ing method of choice for such injury is well demonstrated by this report. An-other fascinating trauma consequence in a small child is the entrapment of bowel within a spinal fracture shown by combined imaging of plain radiogra-phy, upper gastrointestinal contrast fluororadiography, and CT (1). Other re-cent articles of related interest that are listed (2–7) include splenic injuries (2) and liver injuries in nonaccidental trauma (3).—L.W. Young, M.D.

References

1. Rodger RM, et al: *J Pediatr Orthop* 11:783, 1991.
2. Bethel CAI, et al: *Am J Dis Child* 146:198, 1992.
3. Coant PN, et al: *Pediatrics* 89:274, 1992.
4. Hara H, et al: *J Comput Assist Tomogr* 16:94, 1992.
5. Anderson PA, et al: *J Orthop Trauma* 5:153, 1991.
6. Ebraheim NA, et al: *Orthopedics* 14:1010, 1991.
7. Hayes CW, et al: *Radiographics* 11:23, 1991.

Vascular Compromise Prior to Intestinal Manifestations of Crohn's Disease in a 14-Year-Old Girl

Van Elburg RM, Henar EL, Bijleveld CMA, Prins TR, Heymans HSA (University Hospital of Groningen, Groningen, The Netherlands)
J Pediatr Gastroenterol Nutr 14:97–100, 1992   6–73

Background.—Vascular manifestations as extraintestinal symptoms of Crohn's disease are rare. Only occasionally are they reported in children. A patient with a long history of arthropathy and severe systemic signs had symptoms from severe vascular involvement 6 weeks before gastro-intestinal complaints.

Case Report.—Girl, 14 years, was referred for assessment of severe rectal blood loss. She was seen initially 6 years earlier with general malaise, recurrent fever, weight loss, and painful swelling in 1 knee. Rheumatoid arthritis was sus-

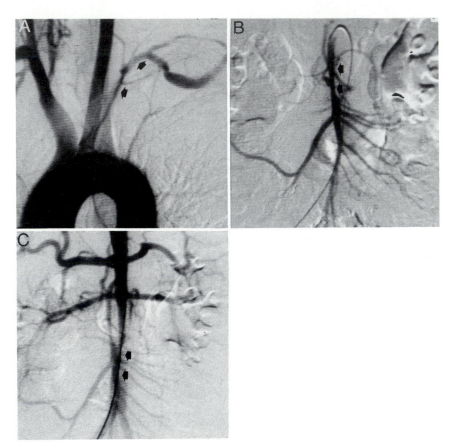

Fig 6–73.—Angiography of the patient showing: **(A)** moderate stenosis of the left subclavian artery; **(B)** segmental stenosis of the superior mesenteric artery; and **(C)** segmental stenosis of the abdominal aorta below the level of the renal arteries. (Courtesy of Van Elburg RM, Henar EL, Bijleveld CMA, et al: *J Pediatr Gastroenterol Nutr* 14:97–100, 1992.)

pected, and she was treated with nonsteroid anti-inflammatory drugs (NSAIDs). She improved steadily, but her symptoms recurred over the following years, all treated with a variety of NSAIDs. Three months before the current referral, she suffered an episode particularly resistant to treatment. She was eventually hospitalized with acute lower abdominal pain. She began to produce mucoidy bloody stools and complained of pain in her jaw and ankle. Several days later severe rectal bleeding suddenly developed with circulatory collapse. Sigmoidoscopy showed skip lesions of many large and deep ulcers in the sigmoid between areas with a normal mucosa. The lesions abated distally, and only a few superficial, aphthous lesions were found in the rectum. On referral, repeat sigmoidoscopy showed the same abnormalities as the initial test. Histologic assessment of the sigmoidal and rectal biopsies showed chronic inflammatory changes with a few giant cells, consistent with Crohn's disease. Angiography revealed segmental stenosis to the left subclavian artery, superior mesenteric artery, and abdominal aorta below the level of the renal arteries (Fig 6–73). These findings resembled those in Takayasu's disease. Iridocyclitis developed during the patient's hospitalization but responded well to treatment. High-dose corticosteroids were given, and she was started on an exercise program to enhance the development of collateral circulation. The patient was doing well 6 months later, but she still had severe active chronic inflammation with erosive mucosa on sigmoidoscopy.

Conclusions.—This case demonstrates an uncommon manifestation of large vessel involvement before the onset of recognizable enteric signs in a girl with Crohn's disease. The kind of vascular involvement seen in this patient is different from that seen in Crohn's disease. It is more like Takayasu's disease. Until the pathogenetic mechanisms of Crohn's disease and Takayasu's disease are established, the relationship between them is open to speculation.

▶ Vascular involvement before enteric signs in Crohn's disease is an unusual but recognized phenomenon. The angiographic imaging findings in this case were segmental areas of stenosis in multiple vessels similar to lesions of Takayasu's disease, but biopsy specimens of the sigmoid and rectal segments of the colon showed Crohn's disease. This relationship is fascinating regarding vagaries of pathogenesis. The case is similar to the report by Yassinger et al. (1). Other relatively recent articles of related interest are listed (2–4).—L.W. Young, M.D.

References

1. Yassinger S, et al: *Gastroenterology* 71:844, 1976.
2. Friedman CJ, et al: *Dig Dis Sci* 24:954, 1979.
3. Buckley A, et al: *J Rheumatol* 18:1073, 1991.
4. Lenhoff SJ, et al: *Postgrad Med J* 58:386, 1982.

Genitourinary

Results of a Survey of Doses to Paediatric Patients Undergoing Common Radiological Examinations

Chapple C-L, Faulkner K, Lee REJ, Hunter EW (Newcastle Gen Hospital; Royal Victoria Infirmary, Newcastle-Upon-Tyne, England)
Br J Radiol 65:225–231, 1992
6–74

Introduction.—There are few data on the radiation doses to children during diagnostic radiologic procedures. Typical radiation dose values were obtained for children of different ages from a number of common radiologic examinations.

Methods.—Patients were divided into age groups of infants younger than 1 year, those aged 1 to 5 years, and those aged 6 to 18 years. In each group, 10 to 20 children were monitored during 8 procedures with a Diamentor ionization chamber to measure dose-area product and ther-

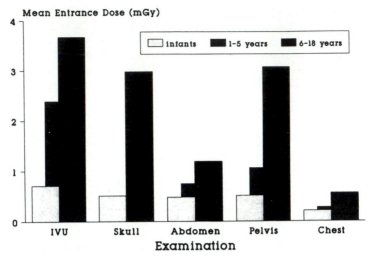

Fig 6–74.—Variation in entrance dose: radiographic examinations. (Courtesy of Chapple C-L, Faulkner K, Lee REJ, et al: *Br J Radiol* 65:225–231, 1992.)

moluminescent dosimeters to determine entrance and organ doses. The 5 radiographic procedures studied were chest, abdomen, pelvis, skull, and intravenous urography. The 3 fluorographic procedures studied were barium meal, barium enema, and micturating cystourethography (MCUG). Data were collected in a dedicated pediatric x-ray room and were automated with a personal computer.

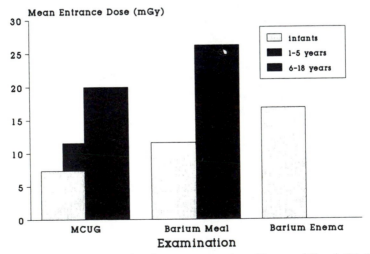

Fig 6–75.—Variation in entrance dose: fluoroscopic procedures. (Courtesy of Chapple C-L, Faulkner K, Lee REJ, et al: *Br J Radiol* 65:225–231, 1992.)

Results.—Measured entrance doses included radiation from all radiographs taken and any fluoroscopic time. For radiographic examinations, up to 100-fold differences were found among dose-area products, and fourfold differences in entrance doses were found in different age groups (Fig 6–74). For fluoroscopic investigations, ten fold differences in dose-area products were seen, as were fourfold differences in entrance doses (Fig 6–75). For radiographic examinations, entrance doses were .3 to 5.7 mGy, and those for fluoroscopic examinations were 7.4 to 26.2 mGy. Screening times did not generally differ between age groups.

Conclusions.—These findings provide typical values of radiation doses to children of different age groups from 3 fluorographic and 5 simple radiographic procedures. These dosages varied widely in children of different ages because of their different sizes and builds. These values can be used as baselines for comparisons by other hospitals.

▶ Awareness of radiation dose from radiologic imaging examinations is essential in the pediatric patient. Infants and children have a longer time to live and greater risk of developing radiation injury. Doses from the common radiographic and fluoroscopic exams and CT exams should be obtained from all radiofluorographic and CT units. Comparisons should be made with the results contained in this article or with other documented standards. Not enough attention of practicing radiologists is given to the issue of diagnostic radiologic radiation doses. Recent articles of related interest are listed (1–4).—L.W. Young, M.D.

References

1. Arroe M: *Acta Paediatr Scand* 80:489, 1991.
2. Faulkner K, et al: *Br J Radiol* 62:230, 1989.
3. Nakano Y, et al: *Pediatr Radiol* 19:167, 1989.
4. Kling TF Jr, et al: *Spine* 15:880, 1990.

Voiding Cystourethrography in Children: Value of Digital Fluoroscopy in Reducing Radiation Dose
Cleveland RH, Constantinou C, Blickman JG, Jaramillo D, Webster E (Massachusetts Gen Hosp, Boston; Brockton Hosp, Brockton, Mass)
AJR 152:137–142, 1992   6–75

Introduction.—The diagnosis and treatment of urologic diseases accounts for up to 25% of genetically significant radiation in infants and children. To reduce the radiation dose during voiding cystourethrography (VCUG), a digital fluoroscope has been adapted for pediatric use. This device was evaluated for its ability to reduce the dose of radiation during VCUG.

Methods.—Using the digital fluoroscope, digital spot films, and 105-mm spot films, entrance and midplane doses were calculated on child-

Comparative Clinical Doses From Voiding Cystourethrography

Dose in mGy (1 SD)

Age Group (yr)	Digital Spot Film			105-mm Spot Film			Radionuclide	
	Fluoroscopy	Spot	Total	Fluoroscopy	Spot[a]	Total[a]	Bladder	Ovary
Neonate to 1								
Skin	1.738 (0.519)	0.455 (0.155)	2.193 (0.537)	1.738 (0.519)	3.003	4.741	0.3	0.04–0.05
Midplane	0.510 (0.273)	0.118 (0.041)	0.628 (0.276)	0.510 (0.273)	0.719	1.228		
1–5								
Skin	1.829 (1.019)	0.537 (0.346)	2.367 (1.074)	1.829 (1.019)	3.494	5.323	0.3	0.04–0.05
Midplane	0.528 (0.291)	0.136 (0.091)	0.664 (0.309)	0.528 (0.291)	0.837	1.365		
5–7								
Skin	4.477 (6.206)	0.919 (0.955)	5.396 (6.279)	4.477 (6.206)	6.024	10.501	0.3	0.04–0.05
Midplane	1.301 (1.802)	0.227 (0.237)	1.589 (1.820)	1.301 (1.802)	1.447	3.294		

[a] Values are estimates.
(Courtesy of Cleveland RH, Constantinou C, Blickman JG, et al: AJR 152:137–142, 1992.)

size phantoms. Data were collected on 47 children ranging in age from neonates to 7 years. The VCUG was performed in the children using the same exposure factors as those for the phantoms. Average skin and ovarian doses were calculated for the children and compared with previously reported doses for fluoroscopic and radionuclide VCUG. Three experienced pediatric radiologists independently assessed the quality of images obtained with digital fluoroscopy.

Results.—Average midplane and skin doses with digital spot films for children younger than 5 years were equal to or less than .66 and 2.37 mGy, respectively, compared with 1.37 and 5.32 mGy with the 105-mm spot films. In previous reports, ovarian doses ranged from 2.52 to 10 mGy for fluoroscopic VCUG and from .04 to .05 mGy for radionuclide VCUG. Digital spot films reduced the radiation dose approximately 50% compared with 105-mm spot films, whereas the ovarian dose was .62 mGy greater than for radionuclide VCUG (table).

Conclusions.—Image quality must not be compromised in the search for lower radiation doses. Images from the digital device and 105-mm images obtained on a conventional fluoroscope both were considered by the pediatric radiologists to have the degree of resolution needed for clinical interpretation. The increase in ovarian dose to children younger than 5 years needs to be weighed against the gain in anatomical resolution.

▶ The gonads can't be avoided by the primary x-ray beam in VCUG; therefore, the lowest possible radiation dose for diagnostic information should be consciously and conscientiously pursued. The value of the digital technique in reducing dose is unrefutable even though with most fluororadiographic equipment it is still slightly greater than the dose of radionuclide VCUG. I have used digital fluororadiographic equipment with similar reduced radiation dose (1) to that of the authors and concur with their observations and methods. Recent articles of related interest are listed (1–4).—L.W. Young, M.D.

References

1. Young LW, et al: *Pediatr Radiol* 20:418, 1990.
2. Kiuru A, et al: *Acta Radiol* 32:114, 1991.
3. Tarver RD, et al: *J Thorac Imaging* 5:31, 1990.
4. Salvini E, et al: *Radiol Med* 77:44, 1989.

Doppler Waveforms in the Renal Arteries of Normal Children
Friedman DM, Schacht RG (New York Univ Med Ctr, New York)
J Clin Ultrasound 19:387–392, 1991   6–76

Introduction.—Until the advent of Doppler ultrasonography, renal vascular resistance could be measured only with intravascular catheters and infused indicators. There is considerable variation in the blood ve-

Relationships Between Various Parameters in Normal Children

Linear Correlations[b]

Variable[a]	Mean ± SD	1	2	3	4	5	6	7	8	9	10	11	12	13
1. L renal A/B	2.9 ± .74	—	-.22	-.54	-.58	-.59	-.10	-.11	-.25	-.23	-.55	-.49	+.23	+.10
2. L renal HR (bpm)	85 ± 13	—	—	-.19	-.21	-.36	.72	-.02	-.07	-.07	-.01	-.01	+.05	+.21
3. Weight (kg)	37.6 ± 15	—	—	—	+.98	+.80	-.27	+.48	+.56	+.61	+.72	+.66	-.29	-.22
4. BSA (m²)	1.2 ± .32	—	—	—	—	+.85	-.32	+.40	+.52	+.55	+.69	+.68	-.37	-.26
5. Age (months)	119 ± 37	—	—	—	—	—	-.44	+.25	+.29	+.32	+.58	+.60	-.37	-.32
6. HR (bpm)	80 ± 13	—	—	—	—	—	—	+.11	-.15	-.09	-.07	-.21	+.37	+.53
7. Systolic BP (mm Hg)	106 ± 7.4	—	—	—	—	—	—	—	+.46	+.71	+.41	+.24	+.16	+.01
8. Diastolic BP (mm Hg)	68 ± 7.7	—	—	—	—	—	—	—	—	+.95	+.38	-.46	-.37	-.10
9. BP (mm Hg)	81 ± 6.7	—	—	—	—	—	—	—	—	—	+.44	+.44	-.23	-.07
10. LVED (cm)	3.7 ± .51	—	—	—	—	—	—	—	—	—	—	+.88	-.18	+.13
11. LVES (cm)	2.4 ± .37	—	—	—	—	—	—	—	—	—	—	—	+.63	-.07
12. EF (%)	74.7 ± 6.2	—	—	—	—	—	—	—	—	—	—	—	—	+.25
13. CI (L/min/M²)	6.21 ± 1.58	—	—	—	—	—	—	—	—	—	—	—	—	—
14. SVR (µ-M²)	14.0 ± 4	—	—	—	—	—	—	—	—	—	—	—	—	—
15. R/L A/B	1.01 ± .23	—	—	—	—	—	—	—	—	—	—	—	—	—

[a]*Abbreviations:* BP, blood pressure; bpm, beats per minute; BSA, body surface area; CI, cardiac index; EF, ejection fraction; HR, heart rate; LVED, left ventricular end diastolic dimension; LVES, left ventricular end systolic dimension; R, right; L, left; SVR, systemic vascular resitance.

[b]$p \le .05$ if $r \ge .43$.

(Courtesy of Friedman DM, Schacht RG: J Clin Ultrasound 19:387–392, 1991.)

locity waveforms of the peripheral arteries; as vascular resistance decreases, diastolic velocity at steady state increases. The feasibility of Doppler evaluation of renal and central hemodynamic status in children was assessed, both to establish the range of normal values and to investigate the relationships between systemic and renal circulatory variables within this range.

Methods.—The subjects were 20 normal children, mean age 119 months, studied during echocardiographic evaluation of insignificant murmurs. Image-directed Doppler echocardiography was used to record M-mode measurements and cardiac index. For Doppler sampling, the renal hila were visualized by way of the flank. Peak systolic and minimal diastolic velocities were also measured.

Findings.—In each subject, Doppler waveforms were easily recorded from the renal artery. The waveforms showed a characteristic bilateral continuous forward diastolic flow. Ratio of peak systolic to minimal diastolic velocity in the renal artery was 2.9, with no differences bilaterally (table). Within the resting normal range, this ratio was independent of the subjects' central hemodynamic findings, although it was inversely associated with age and size. Doppler waveforms from the hilar vessels were easily obtained within 10 minutes.

Discussion.—Normal renal Doppler waveform values were obtained noninvasively from a small group of children. In patients with acute renal function disturbances, this technique may become a useful index of renal vascular resistance. Both central and renal hemodynamic variables can be assessed noninvasively in older children.

▶ Normal values for Doppler waveforms of the renal artery establish a baseline for the noninvasive evaluation of acute disturbances in renal function. The authors were encouraged to obtain the renal artery waveforms based on reliable quantitation of cardiac output by Doppler measurements. Recent articles of related interest are listed (1–8). The large number of recent articles on this subject reflects the high level of interest in Doppler sonography for functional renal vascular evaluation in children.—L.W. Young, M.D.

References

1. Lamont AC, et al: *Br J Radiol* 64:413, 1991.
2. Mari G, et al: *J Clin Ultrasound* 19:15, 1991.
3. van Bel F, et al: *J Pediatr* 118:621, 1991.
4. Buckley A, et al: *J Rheumatol* 18:1073, 1991.
5. Palmer JM, et al: *J Urol* 146:605, 1991.
6. Arduini D, et al: *Obstet Gynecol* 77:370, 1991.
7. Bunchman TE, et al: *Pediatr Radiol* 21:312, 1991.
8. Visser MO, et al: *Radiology* 183:441, 1992.

Renal Obstructive Dysplasia: Ultrasound Diagnosis and Therapeutic Implications

Blane CE, Barr M, DiPietro MA, Sedman AB, Bloom DA (Univ of Michigan, Ann Arbor, Mich)
Pediatr Radiol 21:274–277, 1991   6–77

Background.—Renal obstructive dysplasia is a nonhereditary developmental renal abnormality of nephronic and ductal structures. It can be cortical, medullary, total, or partial and is thought to be the result of early obstruction of the urinary tract. Ultrasound diagnosis and therapeutic implications were studied in 57 children with renal obstructive dysplasia.

TABLE 1.—Associations Found in 42 Patients

Involvement	Status	Other kidney	Other problems
Bilateral ODK (14)	Dead (12)	12 ODK	1 cloacal plate malformation 1 imperforate anus, VACTERL assoc. 1 malrotation of bowel 1 hypothyroid 2 CHD 1 chromosome translocation 5 none
	Alive (2)	2 ODK CRF	1 ambiguous genitalia, no bladder 1 developmentally delayed, cardiac arrest
Unilateral ODK (28)	Dead (4)	Solitary kidney	none
		3 normal	2 VACTERL assoc, congenital hydrocephalus, CHD 1 conotruncal defect, velopalatine incompetence assoc
	Alive (24)	2 CRF 1 UPJ	none
		1 PUV	
		+ reflux	none
		5 reflux	1 tracheoesophageal atresia & fistula, coloboma 1 VACTERL assoc, imperforate anus, tethered cord, CHD 3 none
		2 UPJ 1 PUV	none
		15 normal	13 none 1 vertebral anomalies & scoliosis 1 meatal stenosis

Abbreviations: ODK, obstructuve dysplastic kidney; CFR, chronic renal failure; UPJ, ureteropelvic junction obstruction; PUV, posterior urethral valves; CHD, congenital heart disease; *assoc.*, association.
(Courtesy of Blane CE, Barr M, DiPietro MA, et al: *Pediatr Radiol* 21:274–277, 1991.)

TABLE 2.—Associations Found in 15 Stillborns

Involvement	Other kidney	Other problems
Bilateral ODK (10)	10 ODK	1 Melnick-Needles syndrome 3 cloacal plate malformation 1 omphalocele; anal atresia, CHD 1 omphalocele, hydrocephalus 1 anal artresia, single orbit, alobar holoprosencephaly 3 none
Unilateral ODK (5)	2 solitary kidney	1 CHD 1 alobar holoprosencephaly
	3 normal	1 omphalocele 1 anencephaly, CHD 1 Trisomy 18, CHD

Abbreviations: ODK, obstructive dysplastic kidney; CHD, congenital heart disease.
(Courtesy of Blane CE, Barr M, DiPietro MA, et al: *Pediatr Radiol* 21:274–277, 1991.)

Methods.—Sonographic findings, renal and other associated anomalies, and current status of the children were documented.

Findings.—More than one third had bilateral disease. Although not uniformly fatal, bilateral involvement was associated with significant mortality and morbidity. In 12 of the 33 patients with unilateral dysplasia, the condition was associated with contralateral renal problems, such as obstruction of the ureteropelvic junction, vesicoureteral reflux, and aplasia. Almost 50% of the children had congenital anomalies, including vertebral abnormalities, anal atresia, cardiac abnormalities, tracheo-esophageal fistula and/or esophageal atresia, renal agenesis and dysplasia, and limb defects association; congenital heart disease; cranial abnormalities; and gastrointestinal malformations. Fifteen babies were stillborn. In addition, 12 children with bilateral involvement and 4 with unilateral involvement have died. Four others require dialysis. Only one fourth are otherwise healthy (Tables 1 and 2).

Conclusions.—In this mixed-age population with obstructive renal dysplasia, more serious problems occurred than have been reported in previous studies. This new age-expanded population must be considered in future management decisions.

▶ This report shows that ultrasound and radionuclide scintigraphy help to define the variable morphology of renal obstructive dysplasia. The retrospective review also is valuable for collating the associated multisystem anomalies and in defining therapeutic implications. Prenatal ultrasound examinations now allow for imaging observations of the urinary tract of the fetus and the early recognition of some of these renal anomalies. In another recent article, isotretinoin exposure is reported to cause multicystic dysplastic kidney (1). Recent articles of related interest are listed (2–5).—L.W. Young, M.D.

References

1. Rizzo R, et al: *Teratology* 44:599, 1991.
2. Hammond DI: *Can Assoc Radiol J* 43:179, 1992.
3. Paduano L, et al: *J Urol* 146:1094, 1991.
4. Daneman A, et al: *Radiol Clin North Am* 29:351, 1991.
5. Estroff JA, et al: *Radiology* 181:135, 1991.

MRI in Distal Vaginal Atresia
Hugosson C, Jorulf H, Bakri Y (King Faisal Specialist Hospital and Research Centre, Riyadh, Saudi Arabia)
Pediatr Radiol 21:281–283, 1991   6–78

Background.—Increasingly, MRI is being used for preoperative assessment of vaginal-uterine malformations.

Case Report.—Girl, 14 years, had a 6-month history of lower abdominal pain. The referring hospital attempted "hymenotomy," which failed to provide a functioning vaginal canal for menstrual outflow. The patient had an abdominal pelvic mass extending up to the xiphoid process and atresia of the distal vagina. Rectal examination showed that the vaginal lumen was 5 cm from the external genitalia. She also had polydactyly of both feet and of the left hand. On ultrasound, an elongated, homogeneous, echo-free mass was seen extending nearly to the xiphoid process, above which was an elongated structure interpreted as being the uterus. On MRI, a sagittally oriented pelvic-abdominal mass with high but homogeneous signal intensity was seen, suggestive of blood or fat. There was a distance of 5 cm from the perineum to this fluid-filled cavity. The high-signal inten-

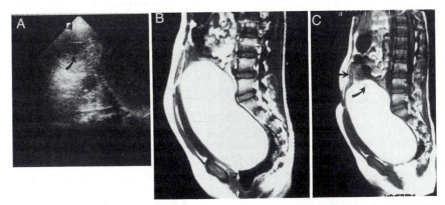

Fig 6–76.—**A,** ultrasound midline longitudinal scan. Fluid-filled mass extends from pelvis. Possible uterus (*curved arrow*) is seen at the top of the mass. **B,** MRI SE 600/20. Sagittal midline image shows a blood-filled distended vagina. The atretic segment measured to 5 cm (< >). **C,** MRI SE 600/20. Sagittal, off midline, again shows blood-filled distended vagina. Uterus with endometric canal (*straight arrow*) and uterine vaginal flow (*curved arrow*). (Courtesy of Hugosson C, Jorulf H, Bakri Y: *Pediatr Radiol* 21:281–283, 1991.)

sity structure above the mass was interpreted as being the uterus, with functional endometrium and uterine-vaginal flow (Fig 6–76). Vaginal atresia with massive hematocolpos but normal cervix and uterine body was diagnosed. At surgery, the hymen ring was found in conjunction with the atretic vagina, which was 5 cm long. The patient underwent carbon dioxide laser canalization, and surgical findings agreed with the MRI measurements.

Discussion.—Two girls with vaginal atresia were evaluated by MRI. This technique is superior to ultrasound for presurgical examination, including measurement of the obstructed segment.

▶ As with anorectal abnormalities, the high-resolution multiplanarity and exquisite tissue differentiation of MRI makes it an excellent modality for evaluating genital tract abnormalities. It is superior to CT and ultrasound for that purpose. It is less invasive and expensive than laparoscopy. Ultrasound, however, is less expensive than all the others and may be a screening tool before MRI. Recent articles of related interest are listed (1–3).—L.W. Young, M.D.

References

1. Kelley JL III, et al: *Obstet Gynecol* 75:521, 1990.
2. Fedele L, et al: *Obstet Gynecol* 76:593, 1990.
3. Rosenblatt M, et al: *Pediatr Radiol* 21:536, 1991.

RARE-MR-Urography in the Diagnosis of Upper Urinary Tract Abnormalities in Children

Sigmund G, Stoever B, Zimmerhackl LB, Frankenschmidt A, Nitzsche E, Leititis JU, Struwe FE, Hennig J (Univ of Freiburg, Freiberg, West Germany)
Pediatr Radiol 21:416–420, 1991   6–79

Background.—Urography using the rapid acquisition with relaxation enhancement technique (RARE) is a rapid MRI technique that selectively shows fluid by heavy T2 weighting. The method uses no ionizing radiation, and it does not require contrast medium.

Methods.—To diagnose upper urinary tract anomalies in 55 children, RARE-MR urograms were obtained and evaluated. Images were obtained in several planes and combined with a coronal T_1-weighted spin-echo sequence. All children also underwent ultrasound; 27 underwent excretory urography (EU); 39 underwent voiding cystourethrography (VCUG); and 41 underwent renal scintigraphy. Two observers subjectively classified the quality of images based on absence of motion artifacts and good signal-to-noise ratios.

Results.—Fifty-nine RARE-MR urograms and 51 T_1-weighted sequences were either satisfactory or excellent. In each case, at least 1 of the 2 techniques provided evaluable diagnostic images. The RARE-MR urography successfully identified all 19 pelviureteric obstructions (Fig 6–77)

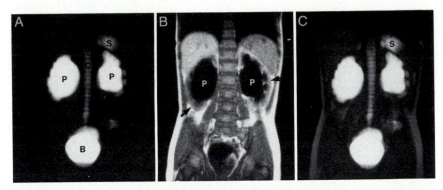

Fig 6–77.—Boy, 2.5 years, with mild urinary tract infection. **A,** coronal RARE-MR urography: massive dilation of renal pelvis (P) and calices on both sides. Note the fluid-filled stomach (S), cerebrospinal fluid (C), and urinary bladder (B). Ureters are not delineated, i.e., not dilated. **B,** representative T1-weighted slice shows thin parenchyma (*arrows*), but no severe atrophy. Urine is depicted dark (long T1 = low signal). **C,** algebraic addition of figures A and B. Image postprocessing allows for better anatomical-topographic orientation, for example, to locate the fluid in the stomach (S). (Courtesy of Sigmund G, Stoever B, Zimmerhackl LB, et al: *Pediatr Radiol* 21-416–420, 1991.)

and all 8 renal duplications with dilated segments. The technique clearly depicted the urinary tract even when the kidneys were nonfunctioning. However, RARE-UR urography was unable to differentiate between vesicoureteral reflux and nonrefluxing dilatation of the ureter or renal pelvis. There were no false positive MRI findings.

Conclusions.—As a new diagnostic tool, RARE-MR urography can be used for examining urinary tract abnormalities in children, including neonates. It is independent of excretory function, requires no contrast medium, uses no ionizing radiation, and has a scan time of only 23 seconds per slice. One slice images the entire urinary tract without interference from bowel motion or gas. These qualities make it superior to ultrasound or EU. When combined with T_1-weighted images, RARE-MR urography provides additional information on nondilated segments of renal parenchyma. Because RARE-MR urography cannot presently identify vesicoureteric reflux, VCUG is still mandatory for differential diagnosis.

▶ The use of RARE MR is perhaps a rare breakthrough for urography without contrast medium or ionizing radiation. The role of RARE at this time is mainly corroborative with ultrasonography and renal scintigraphy in the imaging of upper urinary tract abnormalities. It may have an increasingly significant use in the future, because the "habit" of excretory urography fades even more. A recent article of related interest to the application of MR to the urinary tract is listed (1).—L.W. Young, M.D.

Reference

1. Feinberg DA, et al: *Radiology* 181:597, 1991.

The Normal and Abnormal Scrotum in Children: Evaluation With Color Doppler Sonography

Atkinson GO Jr, Patrick LE, Ball TI Jr, Stephenson CA, Broecker BH, Woodard JR (Egleston Children's Hosp; Emory Univ, Atlanta, Ga)
AJR 158:613–617, 1992   6–80

Background.—Testicular perfusion must be studied when testicular torsion cannot be distinguished clinically from nonoperative causes of scrotal pain. Color Doppler sonography is a useful initial imaging procedure in adults, but in children, smaller arteries and slow testicular blood flow may make this an unreliable means of diagnosing testicular torsion.

Study Design.—A fourth-generation color unit having a 7-MHz linear transducer was used to study prospectively 32 patients, aged 1 day to 18 years (mean age, 8.6 years) who were seen because of scrotal pain or swelling. The findings were correlated with the scintigraphic appearances in 23 patients examined using pertechnetate, and with the operative findings in 12 patients.

Findings.—Acute torsion was diagnosed by color Doppler sonography in 2 of 8 surgically confirmed cases. In 1 of those patients scintigraphy showed reduced activity in the affected hemiscrotum. The other 6 patients had late torsion and exhibited absent flow within central arteries, sometimes associated with increased peritesticular flow. Doppler study correctly demonstrated perfusion of the testis in the other patients, most of whom had torsion of the appendix testis or epididymitis.

Conclusions.—Color Doppler sonography provides an accurate assessment of the presence or absence of perfusion in the symptomatic hemiscrotum. It may, however, be difficult to detect blood flow in the prepubertal testis, making the addition of scintigraphy reasonable.

▶ Color Doppler sonography and radionuclide scintigraphy is the right combination for examining the child's scrotum for torsion and for showing perfusion. Small prepubertal testes may not be flow detectable, but can be shown with scintigraphy. Recent articles of related interest are listed (1–6). Splenogonadal fusion, the focus of another recent report, is a fascinating diagnosis that should be considered in the differential diagnosis of scrotal swellings (1). In another article MRI is reported to be excellent for localizing the nonpalpable undescended testis (2).—L.W. Young, M.D.

References

1. Henderson RG, et al: *Clin Radiol* 44:117, 1991.
2. Miyano T, et al: *J Pediatr Surg* 26:607, 1991.
3. Middelton WD, et al: *Radiology* 177:177, 1990.
4. Lerner RM, et al: *Radiology* 176:355, 1990.
5. Tumeh SS, et al: *Semin Ultrasound CT MR* 12:115, 1991.
6. Fenner MN, et al: *Urology* 38:237, 1991.

Posterior Urethral Valves Presenting as Venous Obstruction

Bauchner H, Cranley W, Vinci R (Boston City Hosp, Boston)
Urology 38:57–59, 1991   6–81

Background.—Posterior urethral valves (PUVs) are congenital abnormalities whose signs and symptoms include abdominal mass, urinary tract infection, failure to thrive, incontinence, sepsis, anemia, and renal failure. A neonate with unilateral right leg swelling as a result of PUV complicated by venous obstruction was described.

Case Report.—Male infant, 15 days, previously well, was seen with a swollen right leg. The bladder was easily palpated, and both kidneys appeared to be significantly enlarged. Abdominal radiography revealed bilateral retroperitoneal masses; renal ultrasound demonstrated bilateral moderate to marked hydronephrosis and a mildly distended bladder. A voiding cystourethrogram showed PUVs with grade V reflux on the right but no reflux on the left. Plethysmography revealed diminished respiratory variation of the right femoral venous flow consistent with iliac or femoral vein obstruction. A Foley catheter—placed during the voiding cystourethrogram—was maintained for drainage. After stabilization, the patient underwent fulguration of the PUV and dilatation of the urethra. At discharge, the child appeared healthy and had a normal right leg.

Discussion.—Overdistention of the bladder causes increased venous pressure and lower-leg edema secondary to urinary retention in adults with bladder-outlet obstruction from hypertrophied prostates and in those with atonic bladders and massive urinary retention. Since PUV was originally described in 1919, considerable variation has been noted in the age at presentation and in the manner of presentation. However, there has been only 1 other case in which venous obstruction was the presenting sign of PUVs. Although distended bladder is frequently associated, vascular obstruction is a rare manifestation of PUV. Nevertheless, the anatomical relationship of the distended bladder and iliac veins makes such obstruction possible. In infants who have evidence of venous obstruction in the leg, PUV should be considered in the differential diagnosis.

▶ Venous obstruction is a rare association with PUVs (1). Plain radiographs showed that the infant's leg swelling was not from an osseous cause. Cystourethrography showed the posterior urethral valve and hydronephrosis. Why this manifestation is not more commonly seen is not understood. Recent articles of related interest are listed (2–4).—L.W. Young, M.D.

References

1. Carlsson E, et al: *Acta Radiol* 53:449, 1960.
2. Connor JP, et al: *J Urol* 144:1209, 1990.
3. Silver RK, et al: *Obstet Gynecol* 76:951, 1990.
4. Fernbach SK, et al: *Pediatr Radiol* 20:543, 1990.

Salt Losing Nephropathy Simulating Congenital Adrenal Hyperplasia in Infants With Obstructive Uropathy and/or Vesicoureteral Reflux: Value of Ultrasonography in Diagnosis

Levin TL, Abramson SJ, Burbige KA, Connor JP, Ruzal-Shapiro C, Berdon WE (Columbia Presbyterian Med Ctr, Babies Hosp; Mem Sloan-Kettering Cancer Ctr, New York)

Pediatr Radiol 21:413–415, 1991   6–82

Background.—Salt-losing nephropathy, occurring mainly in infant boys, has been associated with a variety of urologic diseases, including obstructive uropathy and massive, infected vesicoureteral reflux. Ultrasonography is a useful tool in diagnosis.

Case Report.—Male infant, 1 month, was previously healthy before the onset of vomiting and dehydration. He was admitted to a different center to exclude hypertrophic pyloric stenosis. A left upper quadrant abdominal mass was palpated, and ultrasonography showed a cystic structure in the left upper quadrant. Laboratory results indicated hyponatremia, hyperkalemia, and metabolic acidosis, which prompted the diagnosis of salt-losing congenital adrenal hyperplasia (CAH). The infant was transferred to the Babies Hospital, and a repeat ultrasonogram was obtained. It showed a thick-walled bladder, dilated posterior urethera, bilateral hydronephrosis, and a left perinephric fluid collection consistent with urinoma. Voiding cystourethrography confirmed posterior urethral valve and showed bilateral vesicoureteral reflux and filling of a left urinoma. The infant underwent drainage of the kidney and left urinoma. Transurethral resection of the posterior urethral valve was done. The patient's electrolyte levels eventually normalized, and he has done well.

Conclusions.—In this case, the signs and symptoms of vomiting, dehydration, hyponatremia, and hyperkalemia suggested the diagnosis of CAH. Ultrasonography showed the mass to be a urinoma in an infant with posterior urethral valve and obstructive hydronephrosis.

▶ Ultrasonography showed posterior urethral valves with bilateral vesicoureteral reflux and a variety of other lesions. These boy infants had salt-losing nephropathy that simulated CAH. The infant had normal adrenal function and normal renal morphology. This article nicely documents how these findings were sorted out with the imaging help of ultrasonography. A relatively recent article of related interest is listed (1).—L.W. Young, M.D.

Reference

1. Rodriquez-Soriano J, et al: *J Pediatr* 103:375, 1983.

Diagnosis of Acute Pyelonephritis in Children: Comparison of Sonography and ^{99m}Tc-DMSA Scintigraphy

Björgvinsson E, Majd M, Eggli KD (Children's Natl Med Ctr, Washington, DC)
AJR 157:539–543, 1991   6–83

Background.—Animal studies suggest that renal cortical scintigraphy with dimercaptosuccinic acid (DMSA), labeled with technetium 99m is sensitive and reliable in detecting and localizing acute pyelonephritis. With that as the standard of reference, the use of sonography in the diagnosis of acute pyelonephritis was studied in 91 children from 2 centers.

Methods.—All of the children were aged 1 week to 10 years and had culture-documented febrile urinary tract infection. Renal sonograms and DMSA scans were done within 72 hours of the child's admission to the hospital. Sonographic criteria for pyelonephritis were one or more areas of increased or decreased cortical echogenicity and/or loss of corticomedullary differentiation, with or without renal enlargement. Eighty-seven children also underwent voiding cystography.

Results.—According to DMSA scan, 63% of the children had acute pyelonephritis. Sonographic signs of the disease were seen in only 24% of the whole group and 39% of those with positive DMSA scans. Fourteen patients showed increased cortical echogenicity, and 8 showed decreased echogenicity; 3 of the latter had renal abscesses. Nine patients had dilatation of the collecting system, and all had evidence of acute pyelonephritis on DSMA scans.

Conclusions.—Renal sonography is not an appropriate primary technique for diagnosing acute pyelonephritis because it is relatively insensitive for detection of acute inflammatory changes of the renal cortex. Defects seen on DMSA scan can be evaluated sonographically, however, as can obstructive uropathies associated with urinary tract infection.

▶ This excellent article shows that ^{99m}Tc-DMSA scintigraphy is clearly superior to sonography in the diagnosis of acute pyelonephritis in children. Findings from scintigraphy can help to guide the sonographic examination for correlation and follow-up. Many recent articles of related interest are listed (1–7).—L.W. Young, M.D.

References

1. Rickwood AMK, et al: *BMJ* 304:663, 1992.
2. Rushton HG, et al: *J Urol* 147:1327, 1992.
3. Farnsworth RH, et al: *J Urol* 145:542, 1991.
4. Jacobson SH, et al: *Pediatr Nephrol* 6:19, 1992.
5. Smellie JM, et al: *Pediatr Nephrol* 6:223, 1992.
6. Wikstad I, et al: *Pediatr Nephrol* 4:331, 1990.
7. Verboven M, et al: *Pediatr Radiol* 20:540, 1990.

Vesical Manifestations of Chronic Granulomatous Disease in Children: Its Relation to Eosinophilic Cystitis

Bauer SB, Kogan SJ (Children's Hosp, Harvard Med School, Boston; Weiler Hosp of the Albert Einstein College of Medicine and Montefiore Med Ctr, Bronx, NY)

Urology 37:463–466, 1991   6–84

Background.—Chronic granulomatous disease (CGD), a congenital disorder, is characterized by the failure of granulocytes to destroy bacteria intracellularly after they are phagocytized. Two boys with CGD involving the bladder were seen.

Case Report. Boy, 3 years, was initially brought for medical attention because of severe pain in his penis, dysuria, and infrequent urination. A cystogram and cystoscopy showed an edematous inflammatory area on the left posterior bladder wall. Treatment with nitrofurantoin relieved his symptoms, but he continued to have exacerbations and remissions of pain over the next 3 months. Two years later, he began to complain again of dysuria. A sonogram showed thickening of the left bladder wall and some irregularity of the dome of the bladder was seen on excretory urography. A bladder CT scan showed a small endophytic mass intrinsic to the bladder and separate from the bowel. Cystoscopy showed a pale, scarred lesion on the left posterior wall of the bladder, with the trigone pulled and rotated toward the lesion. A deep resectoscopic biopsy revealed acute and chronic inflammation with multinucleate giant cells, necrosis, and a predominance of eosinophils. His symptoms again abated over the next 3 months, but recurred episodically. Spiking fevers developed. A chest radiograph showed right upper lobe consolidation. Eventually, a thoracotomy was done, exposing a mass lesion in the upper right lobe. The lesion was unresectable. Biopsy specimens showed a granulomatous infiltration and necrosis. Immunohematologic study indicated impaired phagocytosis and ability to generate free radicals by ingestion of opsonized zymosin. He had no further bladder disease, despite other organ system involvement.

Conclusions.—The manifestation and radiologic, cystoscopic, and histologic appearances of CGD and eosinophilic cystitis are similar. For children with eosinophilic cystitis or CGD and lower urinary tract symptoms, excretory urography and cystoscopy, granulocyte nitroblue tetrazolium testing, and biopsy and culture of all lesions in the bladder or retroperitoneum are recommended.

▶ Correlative imaging by sonography and CT helped to identify this vesical CGD. Clinical suspicion and appropriate laboratory testing and histologic findings from biopsy yield the diagnosis. A recent article of related interest is listed (1).—L.W. Young, M.D.

Reference

1. Speirs RT, et al: *Urol Radiol* 12:106, 1990.

Can MR Contribute to the Diagnosis of Nephroblastomatosis?: A Report of One Case

Hausegger KA, Fotter R, Flückiger F, Sorantin E (University Hospital Graz, Austria)
Pediatr Radiol 21:533–535, 1991   6–85

Introduction.—Different imaging modalities usually result in detection of Wilms' tumors and its variants, although the detection of foci of nephroblastomatosis (NB), potential precursors of Wilms' tumor, can be difficult.

Case Report.—Female infant, 10 months, had blood in her diapers. Physical examination was normal, but an ultrasound study of the abdomen showed a solid tumor in the right kidney, with bright echoes in the margins that indicated calcium deposits. The left kidney showed subtle increases in echogenicity with an enlargement of a column of Bertini. Contrast-enhanced abdominal CT showed some calcifications in the right kidney. The left kidney had 1 nonenhancing, partially calcified cortical lesion and 2 additional slightly calcified lesions. Examinations with MRI using T_1- and T_2-weighted spin-echo sequences showed no pathologic foci in the left kidney and a homogeneous mass lesion in the right kidney. Wilms' tumor with accompanying NB was diagnosed based on the CT findings. A right nephrectomy was performed along with simultaneous biopsies of the left kidney. Their histologic features were consistent with metanephric hamartoma, considered to be an involuted form of NB. Postoperative follow-up included ultrasonography and contrast medium–enhanced MRI. At 6 months postoperatively, the latter clearly showed 3 nonenhancing cortical lesions in the left kidney. These findings were identical to the lesions previously seen by contrast-enhanced CT but were more clearly shown with contrast medium–enhanced MRI.

Conclusions.—It appears that contrast medium–enhanced MRI can contribute to the diagnosis of DB, although contrast medium–enhanced CT studies are still essential in the investigation of Wilms' tumors or NB in children. Because ultrasonography may not detect foci of NB, it is not the preferred modality when Wilms' tumors or NB is suspected.

▶ Contrast medium–enhanced MRI can contribute to the diagnosis of NB. In this article contrast medium–enhanced MRI in 1 case showed a focus of NB more clearly than did contrast-enhanced CT. Ultrasound did not show the lesion. The MRI capability to show NB has been observed by others (1, 2). Other recent articles of related interest are listed (3, 4).—L.W. Young, M.D.

References

1. Horak J, et al: *Cesk Radiol* 44:1, 1990.
2. Baskin LS, et al: *J Urol* 146:1591, 1991.
3. Weese DL, et al: *J Pediatr Surg* 26:64, 1991.
4. Gigli F, et al: *Radiol Med* 82:415, 1991.

Abdominal Neuroblastoma With Inferior Vena Caval Tumor Thrombus: Report of Three Cases (One With Right Atrial Extension)

Day DL, Johnson R, Cohen MD (Univ of Minnesota Hosp, Minneapolis; Riley Hosp for Children, Indianapolis)
Pediatr Radiol 21:205–207, 1991   6–86

Background.—Primary adrenal neuroblastoma, often large, can compress or invade adjacent organs and encase retroperitoneal vessels. Intravascular tumor thrombus is rarely associated with neuroblastoma. Three patients with large abdominal neuroblastomas and inferior vena cava tumor thrombi were seen.

Case Report.—Boy, 3 years, underwent an exploratory laparotomy for suspected splenic rupture after he had suffered abdominal trauma. A large adrenal mass was discovered. The patient was further assessed and given a diagnosis of stage III left adrenal neuroblastoma. Imaging studies performed at initial diagnosis demonstrated a large left suprarenal mass and an intracaval mass (Fig 6–78). Chemotherapy significantly reduced the size of the adrenal tumor, which was resected 4 months after diagnosis. The intracaval tumor was also removed and proved to be neuroblastoma on histologic examination.

Conclusions.—The 3 cases presented demonstrate that a large abdominal neuroblastoma can be associated with inferior vena caval tumor thrombus. In an infant or young child, the main diagnostic considerations of a large solid upper abdominal mass include neuroblastoma, Wilms' tumor, and hepatoblastoma. Certain features of the mass, such as calcification, necrosis, homogeneity, margins, encasement of vessels, and deformity of the renal collecting system, may make 1 of these lesions most likely on the basis of radiographic results.

▶ Inferior vena cava tumor thrombus occurs in the pediatric patient most frequently in Wilms' tumor or hepatoblastoma. Tumor thrombosis in neuroblastoma is rare, but has been previously reported (1). Other recent articles of related interest are listed (2–6).—L.W. Young, M.D.

References

1. Paneul M, et al: *Eur J Radiol* 14:201, 1992.
2. Shamberger RC, et al: *J Pediatr Surg* 26:1113, 1991.
3. Ritchey ML, et al: *J Urol* 140:1113, 1988.
4. Colletti PM, et al: *Magn Reson Imaging* 10:177, 1992.
5. Gigli F, et al: *Radiol Med Torino* 82:415, 1991.
6. Hoffman JC, et al: *Radiology* 149:793, 1983.

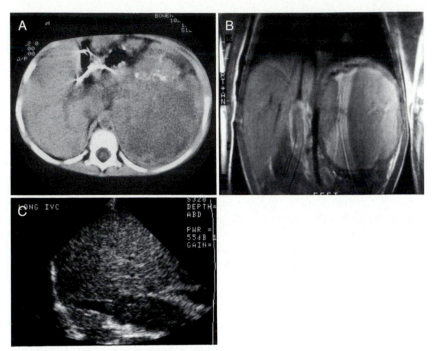

Fig 6–78.—A, CT scan at presentation demonstrated a large left adrenal mass. Calcifications and low density areas consistent with hemorrhage and necrosis are seen within the mass. **B,** coronal T1-weighted (833-20) MRI demonstrated a large left adrenal mass and a sausage-shaped mass within the inferior vena cava. **C,** a longitudinal sonogram confirms the presence of a mass within the inferior vena cava. (Courtesy of Day DL, Johnson R, Cohen MD: *Pediatr Radiol* 21:205–207, 1991.)

Renal Atrophy or Infarction in Children With Neuroblastoma

Day DL, Johnson RT, Odrezin GT, Woods WG, Alford BA (Univ of Minnesota, Minneapolis; Univ of Alabama at Birmingham, Children's Hosp of Birmingham, Birmingham, Ala; Univ of Virginia, Charlottesville, Va)
Radiology 180:493–495, 1991   6–87

Background.—The 5-year survival rate in children treated for neuroblastoma is only about 55%. The poor prognosis is at least partially related to adverse effects of aggressive treatment. Ipsilateral renal damage through infarction or atrophy is 1 such complication that has not been specifically addressed in the radiologic literature.

Methods.—Twelve children with adrenal or upper abdominal para-aortic neuroblastoma developed unilateral or bilateral renal atrophy or infarction after treatment with surgery, chemotherapy, localized abdominal irradiation, and/or bone marrow transplantation. Patients ranged in

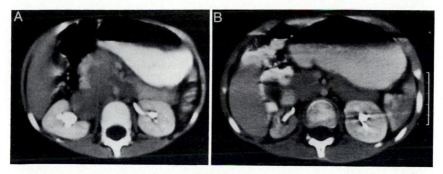

Fig 6–79.—Computed tomography scans obtained in a boy, 5 years, with right adrenal stage IV neuroblastoma. **A,** at the time of diagnosis, tumor growth across the midline and into the right renal hilum was evident. The right kidney is displaced slightly laterally and is mildly obstructed. **B,** 6 months later, marked reduction in tumor size and atrophy of the right kidney are evident. (Courtesy of Day DL, Johnson RT, Odrezin GT, et al: *Radiology* 180:493–495, 1991.)

age from 2 weeks to 9.7 years. Seven children had stage IV neuroblastomas; 2 each had stages III and IV-S; and 1 had stage II. Medical records and radiologic findings were reviewed, and children were studied by CT at initial diagnosis and/or periodically during treatment.

Results.—Acute perioperative ipsilateral or bilateral renal infarction developed in 5 children, and ipsilateral renal atrophy developed in 6 (Fig 6–79). One patient experienced contralateral renal infarction unrelated to surgery. Two patients who required hemodialysis during treatment subsequently died. In 8 patients, creatinine concentrations have remained within the normal range, whereas 2 have had mild, but persistently elevated, creatinine levels.

Conclusions.—Children with upper abdominal or adrenal neuroblastoma can develop renal damage from the primary effects of the tumor. Aggressive treatment, particularly surgical resection of the primary tumor, irradiation, and chemotherapy, can add further damage.

▶ Distinguishing primary effects of neuroblastoma as a cause of renal atrophy or infarction vs. results of associated injury from therapy may not be possible. The authors used CT to determine renal size. Ultrasound might be the better modality to measure renal size, although not as good as CT to assess morphologic damage. Recent articles of related interest are listed (1, 2).—L.W. Young, M.D.

References

1. Sagerman RH, et al: *Ann Radiol (Paris)* 12:278, 1969.
2. Schullinger JN, et al: *J Pediatr Surg* 13:429, 1978.

Stenosing Hemorrhagic Ureteritis in a Child With Henoch-Schönlein Purpura: CT Appearance

Smet M-H, Marchal G, Oyen R, Breysem L (Univ Hosps KU Leuven, Belgium)
J Comput Assist Tomogr 15:326–328, 1991   6–88

Introduction.—Ureteral obstruction in children may rarely result from anaphylactoid purpura in children with Henoch-Schönlein purpura (HSP). Hydroureteronephrosis may be seen on renal ultrasound and intravenous urography, but no specific diagnosis can be made. Computed tomography was used to differentiate between 2 rare complications of HSP in 1 child.

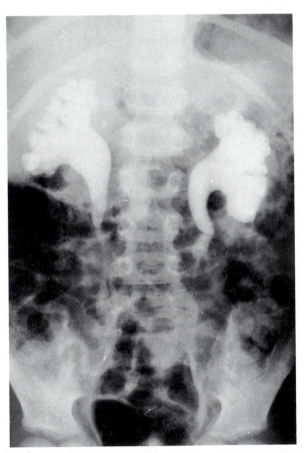

Fig 6–80.—Intravenous urogram reveals bilateral hydroureteronephrosis as a result of incomplete stenosis of both midlumber ureters. (Courtesy of Smet M-H, Marchal G, Oyen R, et al: *J Comput Assist Tomogr* 15:326–328, 1991.)

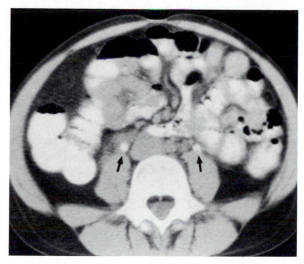

Fig 6–81.—Precontrast CT scan depicts in each midlumbar ureter a small nodular hyperdensity (*arrows*), which proved to be ureteral wall calcifications on histology. (Courtesy of Smet M-H, Marchal G, Oyen R, et al: *J Comput Assist Tomogr* 15:326–328, 1991.)

Case Report.—Girl, 6 years, had a purpuric rash of the extremities, abdominal pain, arthritis, and microscopic hematuria, the characteristic symptoms of HSP. Ultrasound showed bilateral hydroureteronephrosis, and excretory urography showed incomplete stenosis of both midlumbar ureters (Fig 6–80). Precontrast CT also showed bilateral hydroureteronephrosis, along with bilateral calcifi-

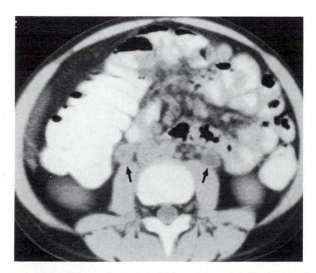

Fig 6–82.—Postcontrast CT scan demonstrated bilateral ureteral wall contrast enhancement (*arrows*) and considerable ureteral wall thickening, predominantly on the right side. (Courtesy of Smet M-H, Marchal G, Oyen R, et al: *J Comput Assist Tomogr* 15:326–328, 1991.)

cations of the ureteral wall at the midlumbar level (Fig 6–81). After administration of contrast medium, the ureteral wall was enhanced both proximal and distal to the calcifications (Fig 6–82). Despite long-term corticosteroid treatment, both midlumbar ureters became completely occluded 6 months after the onset of the disease. Rigid calcified stricutres of both ureters were surgically excised in 2 operations, performed 1 week apart. Histologic examination revealed hemorrhagic ureteritis with calcifications. Three months postoperatively, the child had mild functional impairment of the right kidney.

Discussion.—In a child with HSP CT was able to distinguish between intrinsic and extrinsic ureteral stenosis—hemorrhagic ureteritis and retroperitoneal fibrosis, respectively.

▶ Computed tomography may differentiate the nonspecific findings of excretory urography and renal sonography. According to the authors, intrinsic hemorrhagic ureteritis of HSP can be grossly distinguished morphologically from extrinsic retroperitoneal fibrosis of HSP. Relatively recent articles of related interest are listed (1, 2).—L.W. Young, M.D.

References

1. Garcia-Merida M, et al: *Actas Urol Esp* 13:118, 1989.
2. Grasso E, et al: *Pediatr Med Chir* 10:319, 1988.

Hyperechoic Renal Medullary Pyramids in Infants and Children
Shultz PK, Strife JL, Strife CF, McDaniel JD (Children's Hosp Med Ctr, Univ of Cincinnati, Cincinnati)
Radiology 181:163–167, 1991   6–89

Background.—Normally medullary pyramids in infants and children are hypoechoic compared with the renal cortex. Sonographic findings of increased echogenicity stem from a number of conditions. Common clinical conditions associated with hyperechoic renal medullary pyramids were reviewed.

Methods.—Fifty-five children—34 boys and 21 girls—whose ultrasonic scans demonstrated hyperechoic renal medullary pyramids were retrospectively identified. Patients ranged in age from 1 day to 18 years; approximately half the children were less than 6 months old. Serum and urine calcium concentrations were correlated with results of renal function tests to determine a specific cause for the increased echogenicity. Clinical diagnoses were divided into 2 groups based on whether the patient did or did not have hypercalciuria.

Results.—The pattern of increased medullary echogenicity was not specific for any diagnosis. Ten infants had drug-induced hypercalciuria after treatment with furosemide. Two with hypercalciuria were treated with long-term corticosteroid therapy, and 1 was treated with excessive

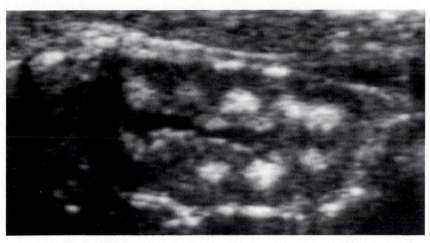

Fig 6–83.—Longitudinal ultrasound scan reveals strikingly increased echogenicity of the medullary pyramids in a 2-year-old child with Bartter syndrome. (Courtesy of Shultz PK, Strife JL, Strife CF, et al: *Radiology* 181:163–167, 1991.)

amounts of vitamin D. Other clinical conditions associated with hypercalciuria included renal tubular acidosis in 10 cases, Bartter syndrome in 5 (Fig 6–83), hyperparathyroidism in 3, Williams syndrome in 2, and medullary sponge kidney in 2. There were 10 children with transient renal insufficiency and 3 with sickle cell disease who had normal urine cal-

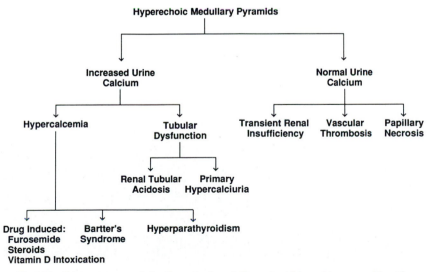

Fig 6–84.—Schematic approach for diagnosis of renal disease in children with sonographic evidence of hyperechoic medually pyramids. (Courtesy of Shultz PK, Strife JL, Strife CF, et al: *Radiology* 181:163–167, 1991.)

cium concentrations. The remaining patients without hypercalciuria had a variety of conditions.

Conclusions.—The clinician can usually make a specific diagnosis in children with hyperechoic renal medullary pyramids based on careful clinical evaluation that includes consideration of the patient's age, serum and urine calcium concentrations, and renal function (Fig 6–84).

▶ The ultrasonographic finding of hyperechoic renal medullary pyramids in infants and children is nonspecific. Several conditions associated with hyper-calciuria give this finding. Furosemide therapy is another cause. The causes of hyperechoic renal medullary pyramids are compiled by the authors along multipe pathophysiologic pathways. This is a useful contribution concerning a finding that has generated substantial interest over the years. Recent articles of related interest are listed (1–4).—L.W. Young, M.D.

References

1. Jequier S, et al: *J Clin Ultrasound* 19:85, 1991.
2. Herman TE, et al: *Pediatr Radiol* 21:270, 1991.
3. Downing GJ, et al: *Pediatr Radiol* 21:563, 1991.
4. Hernanz-Schulman M: *Radiology* 181:9, 1991.

Furosemide-Related Renal Calcifications in the Premature Infant: A Longitudinal Ultrasonographic Study
Downing GJ, Egelhoff JC, Daily DK, Alon U (Children's Mercy Hosp, Univ of Missouri, Kansas City, Mo)
Pediatr Radiol 21:563–565, 1991   6–90

Background.—Intrarenal calcifications can develop in premature infants who receive chronic furosemide therapy. Ultrasound has improved diagnosis of these calcifications over plain radiography. In a prospective,

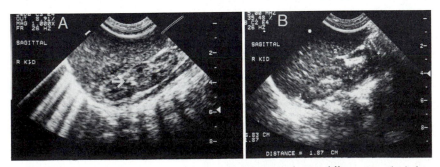

Fig 6–85.—A, renal ultrasound of an infant, 26 weeks' gestation, showing diffuse intrarenal calcifications (*arrow*); **B,** repeat ultrasound peformed 7 months later, demonstrating resolution of the intrarenal calcification. (Courtesy of Downing GJ, Egelhoff JC, Daily DK, et al: *Pediatr Radiol* 21:563–565, 1991.)

longitudinal study the associations among furosemide use, clinical course, and serial ultrasound findings were studied in low birth weight infants with furosemide-related internal calcifications.

Methods.—Over a 30-month period, 117 infants with birth weights less than 1,750 g, respiratory distress syndrome, and chronic lung disease were treated with furosemide. Before discharge, each infant underwent ultrasound imaging of the urinary tract. If renal calcifications were found, sonographic imaging was repeated every 3–6 months.

Findings.—Intrarenal calcifications were found in 20 patients, an incidence of 17%. Twelve patients were boys, and 15 had bilateral calcifications. At age 16.3 months, 6.6 months after cessation of furosemide therapy, 8 patients had sonographic resolution of calcifications (Fig 6–85). Four of the remaining 12 children died of severe pulmonary disease, and autopsy confirmed the presence of calcifications in 3 of those patients. Ten of the children continued to receive furosemide; the association between chronic use of loop diuretics and persistent calcifications was significant. Nephrolithotomy was required in 2 patients, and recurrent urinary tract infections developed in 4. Five kidneys in 4 patients were noted to be small in size, and 2 patients had bilateral dilatation of the collecting system.

Conclusions.—In premature infants with furosemide-related renal calcifications, cessation of therapy is associated with resolution of the calcifications as assessed by ultrasound. Patients in whom furosemide is continued have high renal morbidity and need careful clinical and ultrasonographic follow-up.

▶ Infants who are on furosemide therapy need ultrasonic monitoring of their kidneys for associated calcifications. Furosemide-induced calcifications do regress after the therapy is stopped. This report shows that ultrasound is preferable to radiography for this assessment. There also has been an association of the furosemide therapy with cololithiasis in premature infants (1). Furosemide decreases bile salt formation. Another recent article of related interest is listed (2).—L.W. Young, M.D.

References

1. Blickman JG, et al: *Pediatr Radiol* 21:363, 1991.
2. Shultz PK, et al: *Radiology* 181:163, 1991.

7 Technical Developments, Economics, Education, and Quality Assurance

Introduction

Selections for this section are made from hundreds of articles that do not fit clearly into 1 of the major organ system groups. The wide variety of topics makes it an interesting and enjoyable task to pick appropriate articles for inclusion in the 1993 YEAR BOOK. The subjects range from economics to ethics, from training to computer applications. Because an attempt is made to include issues that are most important to the field of radiology at a particular time, topics vary considerably from year to year. This chapter emphasizes several general areas of interest: (1) the emergence of the relative value system for reimbursement; (2) the challenges associated with the introduction of new, expensive high technology; (3) the emergence of computed radiography; (4) the special aspects of digital imaging; (5) challenges to training programs; (6) MRI; (7) quality assurance and effectiveness studies; (8) computer-assisted diagnosis; and (9) radiology and risks.

The relative value scale (RVS) system of the American College of Radiology and Hsiao's resource-based RVS system have gained considerable attention from radiologists during the past 3 years. Comparable value between studies is 1 of the goals of these systems. Also, the RVS system attempts to standardize reimbursement among radiologists across the country. Why should 1 study cost $2\frac{1}{2}$ times more in southern Illinois than in St. Joseph, Missouri? The need for reimbursement standards has been recognized for some time; however, radiologists have not accepted implementation of this RVS system without comment. Some believe the system is inequitable among subspecialty groups. With some refinements, however, it will make reimbursement more uniform and may provide a means for comparing the productivity between radiologists and practice groups. Dr. Hsiao's system would also decrease payments to "procedural" physicians (radiologists, surgeons) and increase pay to "cognitive" ones (family practitioners, internists).

The introduction of new high technology has changed the practice of radiology over the past 25 years, but similar progress may not be as easy to accomplish in the future. Government, through regulations imposed by its various agencies such as the Food and Drug Administration, the Office of Technology Assessment, and the Health Care Financing Agency may attempt to slow down the infusion of new technology and the payment for new high-cost procedures. The impact of these regulations on such technology as PET and high-speed MRI could be significant.

Digital radiology is making an impact on radiology; it is already used extensively in ultrasound, nuclear medicine, CT, and MRI. Its popularity is no surprise, because resolution is adequate and much is gained by processing these images. Computed radiography, however, for plain film has been limited primarily to chest applications (1), particularly to portable examinations done in intensive care units. Studies are under way, however, to determine the physical, as well as the clinical, requirements for the successful application of digital radiology to what has been traditionally the exclusive domain of film. In time, the advantages of processing, storage, display, and transmission of digitized images will lead radiology to become primarily electronics based instead of film based. It is now only a matter of time before the implementation of a practical, comprehensive picture archiving and communication system (PACS); mini-PACS already exist.

The need will continue for developing more academic radiologists, particularly those with an interest in research careers. It will be extremely important that we become involved in the areas of outcome research and cost-effectiveness studies. Currently, we do not have adequate numbers of radiologists who are trained in these techniques. How to get substantial numbers of our current, bright residents to consider such careers is a common topic of discussion among members of the Society of Chairmen of Academic Radiology Departments. Courses such as the Introduction to Research program given at the annual meetings of the American Roentgen Ray Society and the Radiological Society of North America are not enough. We need to expand the Intramural Diagnostic Radiology Research Program at the National Institutes of Health and to develop genuine research fellowships in many of our medical center training programs.

The training of radiologists becomes increasingly challenging each year. The number of subspecialty areas to be covered grows steadily, and the complexity of the procedures makes it difficult for residents to become across the board experts. With the recent approval by the American Council on Graduate Medical Education of fellowship programs in neuroradiology, pediatric radiology, and cardiovascular interventional radiology, it is clear that subspecialization is here.

Significant advances continue in the field of MRI. Again, Dr. Kerry M. Link, a member of the Department of Radiology at the Bowman Gray School of Medicine of Wake Forest University, was asked to assist in selecting appropriate technical articles in this area for inclusion in the 1993 YEAR BOOK. His comments are affixed to these selections. Improved resolution, output, speed, MR angiography, and specialized image processing are topics of major importance.

Quality control, quality assurance, total quality management, effectiveness studies, outcome studies—all of these terms are becoming familiar to radiologists. What they really mean is that radiologists must make certain that a procedure is appropriate for the condition under investigation, the study is technically correct, the interpretation is proper, and the exam result is important to the outcome for the patient. We will see more and more quality assurance and outcome studies in the radiology literature in the future on topics ranging from quality control of equipment to comparisons of the accuracy of interpretations by radiologists and nonradiologists.

Applications of expert systems and neural networks to the interpretation of imaging studies will increase during the next 5 years. Many young radiologists trained extensively in computer science will lead the way in these research areas. Computer-assisted diagnosis actually has considerable promise. Replacing radiologists by machines, however, is a long way off!

Controversy over the use of low-osmolarity contrast media continues. Whether adverse reactions justify the universal use of low-osmolarity contrast agent or whether some selection criteria should be employed is an issue that has yet been resolved satisfactorily by the health care industry. Increased cost of nonionic contrast material is still the primary focus of the debate.

Because increasing numbers of HIV-positive patients are being seen in radiology departments, more attention must be directed toward implementing adequate safeguards to protect radiology staff. The Occupational Safety and Health Administration has published extensive regulations to provide protection from blood-borne pathogens.

Radiologists seem to face more and more issues that fall outside of the realm of their clinical training as radiology residents, such as economics, ethics, and administration. Perhaps we need to take a second look at our training programs. These issues are not going away.

C. Douglas Maynard, M.D.

Reference

1. Jost RG: *Digital Imaging* 5: 67, 1992.

Relative Value Scale (RVS) System

The Impact of New Payment Systems on the Specialty of Radiology
Evens RG (Washington Univ, St Louis)
Radiology 182:613–620, 1992   7–1

Introduction.—In the past 25 years, diagnostic radiologic procedures have been revolutionized and patients have reaped marked benefits as a result. Radiology initially was placed near the top of the list of "rich" specialities. Estimated overevaluation for radiologic examinations was about 26%, but later estimates were closer to 21%.

Current Payment System.—An American College of Radiology (ACR) relative value scale (RVS) system is used by the Health Care Financing Administration for payment for radiologic services throughout the United States. This approach made radiologists aware of components of the Medicare payment system that had existed for years. Since the original regional conversion factors were announted, there has been considerable effort to develop a "fairer," or at least a more standard, geographic distribution of conversion factors.

Impact on Subspecialties.—Under the ACRRVS system, Medicare would pay more for general radiologic, angiographic, and interventional procedures and for radiation therapy. Fewer units were assigned to CT and MRI and to nuclear radiology. The differences relate to local patterns of subspecialty payment existing before the impact of the ACRRVS system.

Likely Consequences.—Overall there is expected to be an average 3% reduction in Medicare reimbursement with the ACRRVS system operating. An impact on patient care is inevitable. Resources will be used more efficiently, or referring physicians and consumers will be displeased. Radiologists and facilities will be consolidated and concentrated. Groups of radiologists will have to decide whether to continue practicing with their incomes at the 1990 level; time and money will be trade-offs.

▶ If you want to understand the evolution of the RVS system and the current and future impact of the Hsiao proposal on radiology practice, this is your article. Facts and philosophy are intertwined in an easy to read and understand discussion of the reimbursement issues surrounding radiology practice today. Mandatory reading for every radiologist!—C.D. Maynard, M.D.

Analysis of the Resource-Based Relative Value Scale for Medicare Reimbursements to Academic and Community Hospital Radiology Departments
Liang BA, Austin JHM, Alderson PO (Columbia Univ College of Physicians

and Surgeons, Columbia-Presbyterian Med Ctr, New York)
Radiology 179:751–758, 1991   7–2

Introduction.—Dissatisfaction with the customary, prevailing, and reasonable (CPR) charge system based on original Medicare legislation resulted in the development of a resource-based relative value scale (RBRVS). A sample of 40 radiologists from 4 academic centers and 4 community hospitals was surveyed to assess this reform of Medicare.

Methods.—The survey instrument was a personal interview covering the radiologists' knowledge of RBRVS. Radiologic vignettes were presented to the radiologists so that they might estimate the relative intraservice work values of 12 radiologic services.

Results.—Only 2 radiologists had no knowledge of the RBRVS. The primary source of information on RBRVS was the *ACR Bulletin.* The radiologists' knowledge of RBRVS was relatively accurate, but only 3 knew of the involvement of the American Medical Association in the scale. Most (73%) supported the concept of Medicare reform, particularly fee reallocation. Academic and community hospital radiologists appeared to differ qualitatively in their perceptions of intraservice work.

Conclusions.—Although scales of relative values such as the RBRVS are an important step in the direction of equitable payment for Medicare services, the relative value concept needs additional study and modification before the goal of appropriate pricing for services is achieved. The RBRVS may not now accurately represent the spread of perceived relative work values among radiologists.

▶ Any relative value system will have imperfections. Practice patterns, perception, and prejudice all contribute to these imperfections. The RVS system is a start, but it will need to be refined and changed frequently to adapt to the dynamic field of radiology.—C.D. Maynard, M.D.

Productivity of Radiologists: Estimates Based on Analysis of Relative Value Units

Conoley PM, Vernon SW (Kelsey-Seybold Clinic; Univ of Texas Health Science Ctr, Houston)
AJR 157:1337–1340, 1991   7–3

Background.—Radiology services have been quantified for purposes of reimbursement by means of relative value units (RVUs). Interpretation of a posteroanterior chest radiograph was assigned the value of 1 RVU; all other procedures received a value in relation to this service, taking into account the technical and professional components of each procedure. The list of these values is the relative value scale. Using this scale, the productivity of radiologists in multispecialty group practices was quantified.

Methods.—Data were sought from 22 large clinics throughout the United States. Clinics were asked to provide a comprehensive list of the volume of procedures performed during a recent 12-month period for each of the codes in the diagnostic radiology section of the relative value scale.

Results.—Nineteen practices responded with comprehensive lists, reporting 3,234,451 examinations corresponding to 7,356,462 RVUs. Five productivity indexes were calculated. The overall physician index, the ratio of the total number of physicians in the clinic to the total number of radiologists, was 20:1. The availability index, the fraction of radiologists available to perform clinical work after deductions are made for time away from clinical work, was .77. The difficulty index, which measures (in RVUs per examination) the level of complexity of the overall examination mix, was 2.27. The examination index—examinations per year per available radiologists—was 14,098. Finally, the RVU index, which measures RVUs per available radiologist, was 32,065. The RVU index was higher for single-site practices, high-prepaid practices, outpatient-only practices, and practices without radiology training programs.

Conclusions.—The RVU method, developed for comparing radiology practices within multispecialty groups, can also serve as a model for making workload comparisons among specialties. These workloads are likely to be related by third-party payers to compensation.

▶ If the relative value scale established for reimbursement for radiologic service is at all valid, it should make it possible to compare productivity between individual radiologists and individual radiology practices. Efficiency increases in importance as payment decreases for each study we perform. A management tool to look at productivity will be useful. Although individual practices vary considerably, this approach may be a reasonable place to start.—C.D. Maynard, M.D.

Introduction of High Technology

Analysis of Economics and Use of MR Imaging Units in the United States in 1990
Evens RG, Evens RG Jr (Washington Univ, St Louis; Iowa Methodist Med Ctr, Des Moines, Iowa)
AJR 157:603–607, 1991   7–4

Background.—Magnetic resonance imaging is widely available in the United States, and the number of MR units continues to grow. The economic impact of MR units is considerable because of their significant capital and operating costs and the billings generated each year. Three surveys of data related to the economics and use of MRI facilities were conducted, the latest in 1990.

Methods.—The 72 facilities surveyed were those in operation before October 1984. Those imaging installations were sent a 2-page question-

TABLE 1.—Comparison of MRI Data From 1985, 1987, and 1990

Variable	Mean Value		
	1985	1987	1990
No. of respondents	47	52	45
No. of imaging units	47	74	93
Operation days/week	5.2	5.4	5.6
Scheduled hours/week	55	68	66
Procedures/week	35	58	68
Schedule delay (days)			
Inpatient	1.0	1.6	0.9
Outpatient	5.3	11.4	6.9
Procedure mix (%)			
Head	66	49	40
Spine	11	33	33
Bone and joint	4	6	17
Body (other)	19	12	10
Global charge ($)			
Head	652	713	945
Spine	NA	735	955
Bone and joint	NA	NA	932
Body (other)	702	753	959
Revenue reduction (%)	40	15	21

Note: The "global" charge is the terminology used by many third-party payers for total charge in outpatient procedure.
Abbreviation: NA, not available.
(Courtesy of Evens RG, Evens RG Jr: AJR 157:603–607, 1991.)

naire requesting economic and use data for April or May 1990. Of the 45 facilities responding, 30 were installations in hospitals and 15 were in outpatient locations. The installations had a total of 93 imaging units. Data from 1990 were compared with results from the 2 earlier (1985 and 1987) studies.

Results.—A typical unit operated about 66 hours per week, imaging 68 patients. The mean number of patients per year increased dramatically from 1,200 per MR unit in 1985 to 3,400 in 1990. Most examinations were of the head and spine (73%). Delays in scheduling MR studies decreased for both inpatients and outpatients since 1987 (Table 1). Technical and professional charges were approximately $950 per examination; intravenous contrast material, used in 40% of head and 20% of spine studies, was an additional $200. Net revenues in 1990 were almost $1.9 million and annual operating costs about $1.3 million, yielding an annual net profit of approximately $500,000. In contrast, each unit was losing almost $400,000 annually in 1985 (Table 2).

Conclusions.—Since 1985, the 72 oldest MRI installations have experienced marked changes in number of patients examined, mix of patients, revenues, and expenses. Demand appears to be met by available MR services, and the financial position of the units is highly favorable.

TABLE 2.—Financial Performance of a Typical MR Unit in
1985, 1987, and 1990

Variable	Mean Value		
	1985	1987	1990
No. of respondents	47	52	45
No. of patients billed/year	1260	2024	3140
Typical technical charge ($)	500	589	754
Gross billings* †	630	1193	2372
Net revenues *†	378	1014	1873
Estimated costs *†	820	968	1338
Net profit (loss)*	(440)	46	535

* In thousands of dollars.
† Excluding cost or charge for contrast material.
(Courtesy of Evens RG, Evens RG Jr: AJR 157:603–607, 19991.)

The pattern seen here is typical of that for many new medical technologies.

▶ Ron Evens is the "guru" of radiology economics. Again, he has teamed up with his son, who holds an MBA degree, this time to study the financial history of MRI units in the United States. It is an excellent example of the successful introduction of a new medical technology into the health care system. The question is, will current reimbursement schemes allow this pattern in the future?—C.D. Maynard, M.D.

Hurdles to Technology Diffusion: What Are Expectations for PET?
McGivney WT (American Med Assoc, Chicago)
J Nucl Med 32:660–664, 1991   7–5

Introduction.—New and expensive medical technologies face a number of regulatory and economic hurdles before approval by the Food and Drug Administration (FDA) and coverage under private insurance and Medicare. The mechanics of these hurdles and their impact on the availability of PET were examined.

FDA Approval.—The Medical Device Amendments of 1976 charged the FDA with ensuring the safety and effectiveness of any health care devices introduced into interstate commerce. Congress established 3 classes of devices, each to have different standards of control. Class III devices are those that may be used to support human life, may prevent impairment of human health, or present an unreasonable risk of injury. Most devices, those judged to be substantially equivalent to ones marketed in the United States before May 28, 1976, have been approved under the premarket notification ("510K") provision of the Medical Device

Amendments. Other devices require the more rigorous premarket approval application (PMAA).

PET Regulation.—At first, marketing of PET instrumentation did not fall under requirements of either a 510K or PMAA process, but the FDA reclassified PET on November 20, 1990, thereby making positron cameras subject to the 510K provision. Because the FDA classifies imaging agents used in PET as pharmaceuticals, PET technology is controlled under both the drug and device provisions of the Food, Drug and Cosmetic Act.

Coverage.—Major payers have stringent requirements for "big-ticket" devices and procedures. Payers may ask for more data even after FDA approval, yet without some form of payment it is difficult to generate supporting data for the devices. Some, but not all, private payers cover certain PET cardiologic applications. The utilization of PET is also restricted by the fact that requisite imaging agents are classified as investigational by the FDA.

Conclusions.—Positron emission tomography and other new, expensive technologies can continue to be developed only through compromise between advocates of the technology and those who demand a careful evaluation of this technology. Adequate coverage for limited use could provide outcome data and lead to a mutual decision on the future use and payment for new devices such as PET.

▶ The success of PET will depend to some extent on reimbursement. The hurdles to overcome before FDA approval can be obtained are not inconsequential. Still undecided is the question of who, if anyone, has jurisdiction over cyclotron-produced pharmaceuticals. Should it be the FDA, or is it within the jurisdiction of state pharmacy regulations? If national road blocks are placed before each and every new radiopharmaceutical to be used in PET studies, general clinical applications of this technology could be derailed before they get started.—C.D. Maynard, M.D.

The Diffusion of Medical Technology: Free Enterprise and Regulatory Models in the USA
James AE, Perry S, Warner SE, Chapman JE, Zaner RM (Vanderbilt Univ, Nashville, Tenn; Georgetown Univ, Washington, DC)
J Med Ethics 17:150–155, 1991   7–6

Introduction.—The diffusion of costly medical technologies poses formidable problems for those whose task it is to formulate health care policy. Attempts to limit health care costs often are directed at areas with high unit costs, among which are instruments used for diagnostic medical imaging such as CT scanners, MRI devices, and PET machines.

Problems.—Certificates of need (CON) legislation requires those who are considering acquiring medical technology or facilities above a certain value to demonstrate both qualifications and clinical need. Hospitals have incurred substantial debts for equipment whose efficacy was not yet fully established. Groups of physicians have formed to allow the purchase of CT and MR devices, and the members have a vested financial interest in the economic viability of these enterprises. Problems exist despite efforts by the doctors not to refer their patients to facilities they own. Some physicians may forego procedures if they will deplete institutional resources or their personal income.

Implications.—Understanding the relationship between a free enterprise or marketplace model and governmental regulation will allow more rational policies to be developed for diffusing medical technology. If a regulatory model is adopted, the entire health care system should be regulated. Penalties will be necessary but must be imposed so as not to compromise patient welfare.

▶ I am always amazed at Everett James's breadth of interest and knowledge. This article should be read by all radiologists. It clearly presents the ethical dilemma associated with radiology's high-cost technology and the government action to regulate it. The government has pushed for competition in the health care market but at the same time restricts competition by regulation. This "schizophrenia" does not help radiologists cope with the system.—C.D. Maynard, M.D.

The Volume and Cost of Radiologic Services in the United States in 1990
Sunshine JH, Mabry MR, Bansal S (American College of Radiology, Reston, Va)
AJR 157:609–613, 1991   7–7

Introduction.—Data on the number and cost of radiologic procedures performed in the United States each year are of interest to radiologists, equipment manufacturers, and health care administrators. Yet neither the total number of procedures nor their cost is known. Estimates for all radiologic services, including radiation oncology, nuclear medicine, and radiologic services performed by nonradiologists, were developed.

Methods.—Two largely independent estimates of each total were developed, 1 based principally on surveys of radiologists and the other on Medicare data. The 2 estimates served purposes of cross-validation. An important assumption used in the Medicare-based estimate is that Medicare pays for one third of radiologic services. Another important assumption was that, in the hospital setting, the total of payments for professional services plus technical services equals 2.5 times the payments for professional services alone.

Results.—It was estimated that 260 million to 330 million radiologic procedures were performed in the United States in 1990. Payments for those services, including payments for technical components in the hospital setting, were estimated to be $19 billion to $22 billion. That total represents approximately 3.5% of national spending on personal health care. High-technology radiology accounted for less than half the total. The annual number of procedures per capita—1 to 1.3—represents an increase of 10% to 40% since 1980. Approximately half of the total cost was paid to physician practices, with a substantial part of this amount going to office practice expenses.

Conclusions.—Some observers of health care costs in the United States believe that high-technology radiology is responsible for much of the increased spending. The findings of this study suggest that high-technology radiology accounts for only approximately 1.5% of personal health care expenditures.

▶ Because radiology has many high-cost procedures (CT, MRI, PET), it is often selected as an example of the high cost of medicine. This study by the American College of Radiology shows that we really are only a small part of the total "problem." Here is one time when high visibility is not helpful!—C.D. Maynard, M.D.

Digital Radiology

Single-Exposure Conventional and Computed Radiography Image Acquisition

Chotas HG, Dobbins JT III, Floyd CE Jr, Ravin CE (Duke Univ Med Ctr, Duke Univ, Durham, NC)
Invest Radiol 26:438–445, 1991   7–8

Background.—Computed radiography (CR) systems based on photostimulable phosphor image detectors have been in use for about 8 years. Many reports have been favorable, and the CR system has gained wide clinical acceptance. To compare CR performance with conventional film-screen imaging techniques, researchers developed a hybrid cassette containing both film and a CR imaging plate.

Methods.—Five detector configurations were evaluated: standard film (conventional film-screen cassette), standard CR (CR plate in standard CR cassette), CR reversed (CR plate, backward in CR cassette), hybrid A (first screen replaced with CR plate), and hybrid B (second screen replaced with CR plate) (Fig 7–1). Areas examined included gray-scale (optical density) measurements, spatial resolution, and signal-noise ratio (SNR).

Results.—Gray-scale values in both the hybrid A and hybrid B images were well matched with the standard film densities (Fig 7–2). Spatial resolution was slightly degraded in all nonstandard detector configurations, but there seemed to be no perceptible decrease in image detail. There were no significant differences in SNR values derived from the CR images. Hybrid A was selected as the preferred detector configuration for

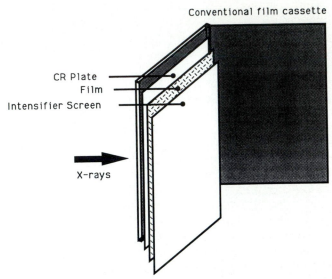

Fig 7–1.—Hybrid film-CR imaging plate detector. One intensifier screen in conventional film cassette is removed and replaced with a CR imaging plate, phosphor side facing film. Hybrid A is illustrated here. Hybrid B is similar, but the order is reversed. (Courtesy of Chotas HG, Dobbins JT III, Floyd CE Jr, et al: *Invest Radiol* 26:438–445, 1991.)

acquiring 2 radiographic images with a single x-ray exposure. The resultant image pair was judged to be most like the 2 standard images in overall image quality.

Conclusions.—Quantitative investigations of CR performance relative to conventional film-screen imaging have been difficult to perform. Duplicate exposures of the same patient doubles the radiation burden, whereas single exposures of 2 matched patient groups will have many variables. In addition to clinical applications, the technique described here will facilitate such comparative studies.

▶ Studies comparing conventional film and CR are still needed. These researchers have developed a unique method of obtaining both simultaneously. Widespread use of a method such as this could assist in this comparison.—C.D. Maynard, M.D.

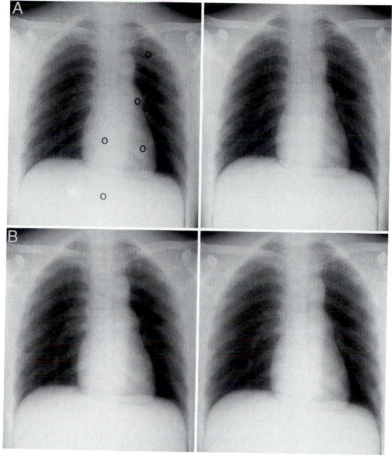

Fig 7–2.—Image pairs illustrate the absence of significant changes in image grayscale in a hybrid (nonstandard) cassette relative to the standard images. **A,** standard and hybrid A CR images (with optical density measurement points indicated). **B,** standard and hybrid A analog film images. (Courtesy of Chotas HG, Dobbins JT III, Floyd CE Jr, et al: *Invest Radiol* 26:438–445, 1991.)

Comparison of Imaging Properties of a Computed Radiography System and Screen-Film Systems

Sanada S, Doi K, Xu X-W, Yin F-F, Giger ML, MacMahon H (Univ of Chicago, Chicago)
Med Phys 18:414–420, 1991

7–9

Introduction.—Though computed radiography (CR) based on photostimulable phosphor technology has been in clinical use for some time, the diagnostic value of this modality has not been clearly defined. To compare CR and conventional screen-film systems, researchers devised a dual system recording system.

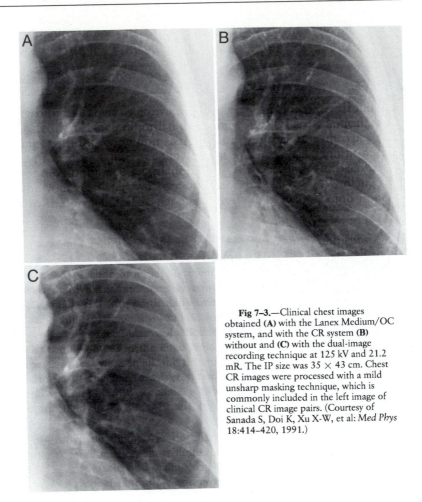

Fig 7–3.—Clinical chest images obtained (**A**) with the Lanex Medium/OC system, and with the CR system (**B**) without and (**C**) with the dual-image recording technique at 125 kV and 21.2 mR. The IP size was 35 × 43 cm. Chest CR images were processed with a mild unsharp masking technique, which is commonly included in the left image of clinical CR image pairs. (Courtesy of Sanada S, Doi K, Xu X-W, et al: *Med Phys* 18:414–420, 1991.)

Methods.—The dual system makes it possible to obtain 2 images at once, 1 from each system, in a clinical examination with the same patient positioning, the same degree of patient motion, the same geometric unsharpness, and no additional exposure. Images of various test objects were also compared, and measurements of Hunter and Driffield (H & D) curves, modulation transfer functions (MTFs), and Wiener spectra were obtained.

Results.—Compared with the MTFs of the screen-film systems, the MTFs of the CR system, with and without the dual imaging recording techniques, were greater at lower frequencies and lower at high frequencies. The noise Wiener spectra of the CR images at the plane of the imaging plate were greater than those of the screen-film systems. Because of reduction in image size, however, the noise Wiener spectra of CR were comparable to those of screen-film systems at the plane of the printed film. Clinical chest images appeared comparable when obtained with the dual image recording technique. This may result from image size reduction and the use of mild unsharp mask processing (Fig 7–3).

Conclusions.—Computed radiography images appear to be unfavorable for the detection of high-frequency anatomical structures or lesions, such as pneumothorax and breast microcalcifications. Because the noise level of the CR images was significantly greater than that of the screen-film images examined here, it is important to objectively examine the physical and diagnostic quality of these images. Dual-image recording should be a useful tool for this purpose.

▶ Like the authors of the previous article, these researchers are attempting to define the advantages and limitations of CR by measuring and comparing certain physical characteristics. As important as this type of study is to the understanding of this new technology, its ultimate acceptance will undoubtedly rest on more radiologists applying the systems to clinical practice.—C.D. Maynard, M.D.

Clinical Experience in the Use of Photostimulable Phosphor Radiographic Systems

Murphey MD, Huang HKB, Siegel EL, Hillman BJ, Bramble JM (Univ of Kansas Med Ctr, Kansas City, Kan; UCLA School of Medicine, Los Angeles; Univ of Arizona College of Medicine, Tucson)
Invest Radiol 26:590–597, 1991   7–10

Background.—Computed radiography (CR), a digital radiographic imaging system that uses a photostimulable phosphor imaging plate, has been evaluated at a number of clinical sites. Most reports have been favorable (Fig 7–4), although results of 1 study suggested poorer detectability of pneumothoraces with CR than with conventional radiography. The experience with CR at 3 institutions was reviewed.

University of California–Los Angeles.—The first CR was installed in October 1985 in the pediatric radiology section. Between October 1986 and December 1988, there were 40,717 CR images performed (70% were of the chest). Daily reviews made it clear that positioning and collimation were critical to obtaining adequate studies. The plates were found to be more prone to damage than their conventional counterparts and to require weekly cleaning to avoid artifacts. The small size of the images may be a problem in some cases.

University of Arizona.—The first study cohort included 100 symptomatic patients undergoing excretory urography. Experienced staff radiologists evaluated matched CR and screen-film exposures. No significant differences were found in the evaluation of these studies. The accuracy of radiologists making etiologic diagnoses was similar for CR and con-

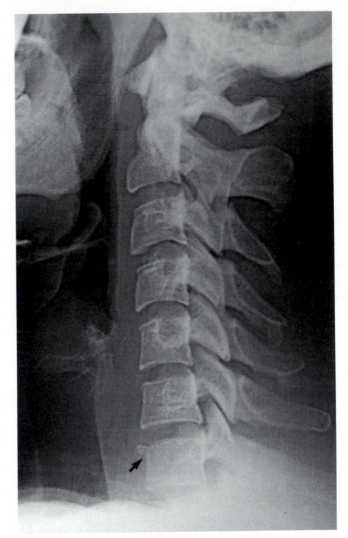

Fig 7–4.—Phosphor plate image of the lateral cervical spine shows an acute flexion compression fracture of the superior end plate of the seventh cervical vertebra (*arrow*). The cervicothoracic junction could not be evaluated on the conventional radiograph (not shown). (Courtesy of Murphey MD, Huang HKB, Siegel EL, et al: *Invest Radiol* 26:590–597, 1991.)

ventional radiographs. The CR urograms allowed a 47% reduction in radiation exposure.

University of Kansas.—More than 10,000 CR examinations were completed since 1989. This center reported problems in establishing proper enhancement parameters for pediatric and extremity studies, as well as examinations requiring contrast media. Chest images can be obtained with a 30% exposure reduction and mammograms with a 50% reduction.

Conclusions.—Some advantages of CR are the reduction in radiation exposure, a decrease in the number of repeat examinations required, the capability to archive electronically all images by means of a digital optical storage system, and the ability to adjust the display parameters. Disadvantages of CR include its current high costs, edge enhancement (which may obscure pathology), a graininess of the image with excessive exposure reduction, and the lack of available interfaces inhibiting use of local and wide-area networks.

▶ Researchers from the University of Kansas, the UCLA School of Medicine, and the University of Arizona College of Medicine jointly reported their experiences with photostimulable phosphor radiographic systems. They outlined clearly the technical advantages and disadvantages of these systems as applied to many organ systems. Further comparative clinical studies are needed.—C.D. Maynard, M.D.

Diagnostic Efficacy of Digitized Images vs Plain Films: A Study of the Joints of the Fingers

Richmond BJ, Powers C, Piraino DW, Freed H, Meziane MA, Hale JC, Schluchter MD, Schils J, Gragg LA (Cleveland Clinic Found, Cleveland)
AJR 158:437–441, 1992   7–11

Objective.—The ability to transmit digital radiographic images between locations has many advantages, as in emergency departments and rural areas. Whether digital images are equal in quality to plain films was studied by comparing high- and low-resolution digital images with plain radiographs.

Methods.—A total of 415 finger joints of 30 patients were examined for joint space erosion, narrowing, and degenerative spurring. Five experienced radiologists examined plain films; low-resolution digitized images (1024 × 840 bytes × 12 bit matrix); and high-resolution digitized images (2048 × 1680 bytes × 12 bit matrix). The digital images were displayed on a 1K × 1K monitor. It was possible to alter level, window, orientation, and brightness. Two skeletal radiologists not participating in the study provided a consensus view of whether or not abnormality was present. Receiver operating characteristic (ROC) curves were recorded for each of the interpreters.

Results.—There were no significant differences in areas under the ROC curves for the 2 imaging methods. Except in detecting erosions, there were no significant differences in predicted true positive rates.

Conclusions.—In this study of the digital joints, digitized imaging in both high- and low-resolution modes performed similarly to plain radiography.

▶ Many of us have been concerned that the spatial resolution afforded by computed radiography (CR) will limit its usefulness in skeletal radiography, particularly of the small bones such as those in the hands. This report, however, is very encouraging. If, in fact, CR technology could be satisfactorily applied to the extremities, many emergency rooms in various geographic locations could be staffed by 1 radiologist using teleradiography. Could this be the future (1)?—C.D. Maynard, M.D.

Reference

1. Brogdon BG, et al: *Computer Applications to Assist Radiology* (SCAR 92), Symposia Foundation, Carlsbad, Calif, 1992, p 505.

Photostimulable Phosphor Digital Radiography of the Extremities: Diagnostic Accuracy Compared With Conventional Radiography
Wilson AJ, Mann FA, Murphy WA Jr, Monsees BS, Linn MR (Washington Univ, St Louis)
AJR 157:533–538, 1991   7–12

Background.—Reports on photostimulable phosphor digital radiography (PPDR) have indicated a much greater dynamic range compared with conventional radiography but lower spatial resolution. The system has been used to a limited extent in such settings as the emergency department.

Objective.—A direct comparison of the PPDR system with a conventional screen/film combination was carried out in patients requiring extremity imaging in an emergency department after minor trauma.

Methods.—Matched sets of images were acquired, using the same exposure factors, from 103 patients having injuries of the hand, wrist, foot, or ankle. One set was obtained using a conventional screen/film system and the other with photostimulable phosphor digital cassettes (Fig 7–5). The image sets were independently interpreted by 3 radiologists in a blinded manner and the findings compared with the consensus opinion of 2 other radiologists. Receiver operating characteristic (ROC) curves were plotted for each of the 3 primary readers.

Results.—There were no significant differences in areas under the ROC curves for the 2 imaging systems, but conventional radiography was slightly better. When true positive fractures for detecting fractures were compared at false positive fractions of 0.1, conventional screen/film radiography was significantly more sensitive than the PPDR system.

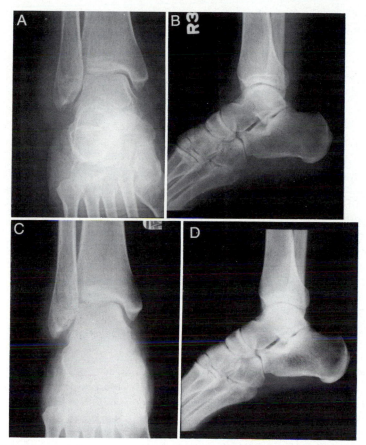

Fig 7–5.—Computed (**A, B**) tomography and conventional (**C, D**) radiographs of an ankle showing lateral and posterior malleolar fractures with soft-tissue swelling laterally. Although fractures are readily visible on both sets of radiographs, increased dynamic range of computed images make both soft tissues and densest bony areas easier to see. (Courtesy of Wilson AJ, Mann FA, Murphy WA Jr, et al: *AJR* 157:533–538, 1991.)

Conclusions.—Photostimulable phosphor digital radiography was less accurate than conventional screen/film radiography in assessing acute minor extremity trauma. The spatial resolution of current photostimulable phosphor systems may not be adequate for clinical use.

▶ This group found computed radiology (CR) to be slightly less accurate than conventional radiography in detecting acute trauma, but, like the previous authors considered, believe CR to be acceptable. Differences in results by groups comparing this technology is common. Perhaps some of the discrepancies are related to variability between radiologists and the population studied. It should be noted that 1 advantage of CR for musculoskeletal work is that 2 views, 1 to demonstrate bony abnormalities and another to see soft tissue injury, can be accomplished with 1 exposure, because computer processing is available with CR.—C.D. Maynard, M.D.

Comparison of a PACS Workstation With Conventional Film for Interpretation of Neonatal Examinations: A Paired Comparison Study

Franken EA Jr, Smith WL, Berbaum KS, Kao SCS, Sato Y (Univ of Iowa College of Medicine, Iowa City, Iowa)
Pediatr Radiol 21:336–340, 1991   7–13

Objective.—Picture archiving and communication systems (PACS) are increasingly used to display imaging studies. In this study the diagnostic value of the PACS in pediatric radiology was compared with that of plain film interpretation in 202 consecutive abdominal and chest examinations on 72 patients.

Methods.—The PACS work station used was a Siemens Diagnostic Reporting Console having 8 monitors, which allows test images to be altered in various ways by computerized processing. A rigorously paired comparison was carried out to review plain films and PACS images alternately in an unbiased manner.

Results.—There was a slight overall preference for the PACS method. A change in diagnosis or in the degree of diagnostic confidence was more than twice as likely to occur with the PACSs after hard copy than on assessment of conventional radiographs after the PACS. When new findings were recognized by the PACS, the ability to alter contrast replaced a loss of resolution (Figs 7–6 and 7–7).

Conclusions.—It appears that the PACS and conventional radiographic interpretation hold similar diagnostic value for assessing studies of the neonatal chest and abdomen.

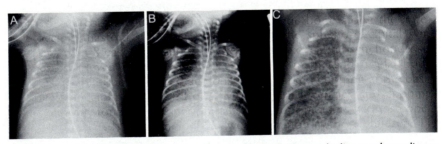

Fig 7–6.—A–C, pulmonary interstitial emphysemia (PIE) complicating hyaline membrane disease (HMD) in a 3-day-old girl. **A,** the plain film image was interpreted as HMD, although there is retrospective evidence of an abnormal right upper lobe. **B,** the PACS image shows to much better advantage the cystic lucencies in the right upper lobe. **C,** examination several hours later shows diffuse PIE of the right lung. (Courtesy of Franken EA Jr, Smith WL, Berbaum KS, et al: *Pediatr Radiol* 21:336–340, 1991.)

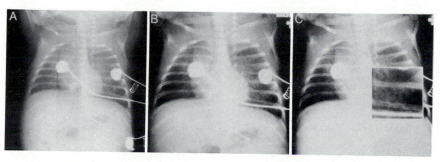

Fig 7–7.—A–C, bronchopulmonary dysplasia (BPD) in a 33-day-old boy. **A,** the plain film was interpreted as normal. **B,** the PACS image clearly shows interstitial lung disease, particularly in the right upper lobe and left lower lung field. **C,** the changes of BPD are even more evident using the "magic glass." (Courtesy of Franken EA Jr, Smith WL, Berbaum KS, et al: *Pediatr Radiol* 21:336–340, 1991.)

▶ As we gain more experience in interpreting conventional studies directly on diagnostic work stations, film will decrease in importance. What is needed is a user-friendly, high-resolution work station that radiologists are comfortable with. Even if the diagnostic accuracy is equivalent to that of plain films, for soft copy to gain widespread use, it needs to provide the radiologist with an advantage over film. The edge may be found in increased efficiency, improved diagnostic capabilities, or fewer administrative headaches.—C.D. Maynard, M.D.

MR Examination of the Knee: Interpretation With Multiscreen Digital Workstation vs Hardcopy Format
Brown JJ, Malchow SC, Totty WG, Wilson AJ, Lee JKT, Vannier MW, Jost RG (Washington Univ, St Louis)
AJR 157:81–85, 1991   7–14

Objective.—Interpreting MR studies requires the simultaneous display of multiple cross-sectional images so that the viewer may make spatial associations and rapidly scan thorough the image set. The authors developed an 8-screen imaging work station with the video display arranged like a standard film panel alternator.

Study Design.—The quality of interpretation of MR studies of the knee using the multiscreen picture archiving and communication system (PACS) was determined using studies of 30 patients who also had arthroscopy. Sixty menisci, half of them abnormal, were assessed along with 30 anterior cruciate ligaments, 5 of which were abnormal. The imaging protocol utilized a coronal T1-weighted spin-echo pulse sequence and a double-echo sagittal sequence.

Results.—Areas under the receiver operating characteristic (ROC) curves were slightly greater for PACS than for film (Fig 7–8). For neither observer was the difference significant. Both observers, however, required significantly more time for image analysis with PACS than using film; the average time per case differed about 2.7-fold.

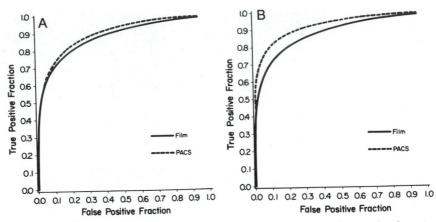

Fig 7-8.—A, receiver-operating-characteristic (ROC) curves for diagnosis of meniscal and anterior cruciate ligament tears, film vs. picture archiving and communication system (PACS), for observer 1. The areas under the curves are not significantly different (P = .47). **B,** ROC curves, observer 2. Areas under curves are not significantly different (P = .08). (Courtesy of Brown JJ, Malchow SC, Totty WG, et al: AJR 157:81-85, 1991.)

Conclusions.—These findings do not warrant replacing film with PACS when MR studies are interpreted. The accuracy of PACS, however, suggests that it may find use in some areas of clinical imaging.

▶ For digital work stations to replace radiographic film and a film alternator, they must be made much easier to use. A busy radiologist cannot afford to change to a system that requires *more* time to arrive at the same diagnosis.—C.D. Maynard, M.D.

Preliminary Assessment of Computed Tomography and Satellite Teleradiology From Operation Desert Storm
Cawthon MA, Goeringer F, Telepak RJ, Burton BS, Pupa SH, Willis CE, Hansen MF (Brooke Army Med Ctr, San Antonio, Tex; Office of the Surgeon Gen, Dept of the Army, Falls Church, Va; Fitzsimons Army Med Ctr, Aurora, Colo; Tripler Army Med Ctr, Honolulu)
Invest Radiol 26:854–857, 1991

7-15

Background.—Operation Desert Storm provided the first opportunity for the United States to use CT at military transportable hospitals. Two CT scanners were installed in standard transportable military hospital hard-wall shelters (ISO-shelters) (Fig 7-9) at the start of a full-scale test program undertaken in the fall of 1990. The outbreak of hostilities cut short the test period, and the scanners were transported to Saudi Arabia on January 16, 1991. The CT scanners became operational 1 week later.

Results.—Both scanners provided excellent clinical images and facilitated diagnoses that previously could not have been made under battle-

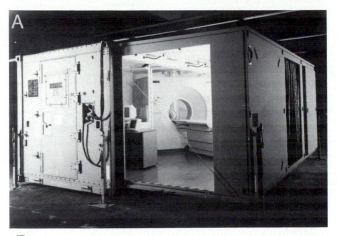

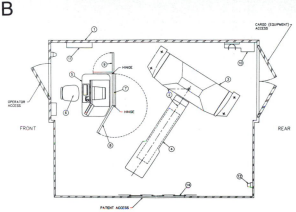

PICKER IQ SCANNER DEPMEDS INSTALLATION — OPERATIONAL CONFIGURATION

Fig 7–9.—A, picker CT scanner installed in ISO-shelter. The side panel was temporarily removed to permit photography of the scanner. A tent passageway and ramp is connected to the draped opening on the right side of the shelter when the ISO-shelter is attached to the combat hospital. **B,** an overhead drawing of the ISO-shelter configured with the CT scanner with the operator console *(5),* lead acrylic operator protection *(7–9),* gantry *(3),* table *(4),* and passageway *(14)* to the hospital. (Courtesy of Cawthon MA, Goeringer F, Telepak RJ, et al: *Invest Radiol* 26:854–857, 1991.)

field conditions. As expected from previous wartime experiences, disease and nonbattle injuries were common. One of the CT scanners was equipped with a commercially available teleradiology system that acquired video frame images from the scanner display and prepared them for transmission by an L-band portable radio to satellite. The images were then down-linked to stations in Australia and Japan and proceeded via commercial phone links to Brooke Army Medical Center in San Antonio. The scans of 41 different patients were judged to be of high quality for consultation purposes.

Conclusions.—The CT scanners operated efficiently from standard diesel generator power and produced images equal to those obtained in the United States during the abbreviated test period. The technology is anticipated to aid in decisions regarding allocation of resources, both in battlefield situations and in civilian peacetime natural disasters.

▶ Teleradiography was performed successfully during Operation Desert Storm. It is an excellent example of the future of radiology practice and what "electronic radiology" will offer. The military is clearly leading the way in the development of a practical picture archiving and communication system (PACS). The project Medical Diagnostic Imaging Support System currently being implemented at Madigan Army Hospital in Tacoma, Washington, could lead the way toward the future development of widespread PACSs.—C.D. Maynard, M.D.

Challenges to Training Programs

Academic Radiologists: Aging and Renewal
Friedman PJ (Univ of California San Diego, La Jolla, Calif)
Invest Radiol 26:858–865, 1991   7–16

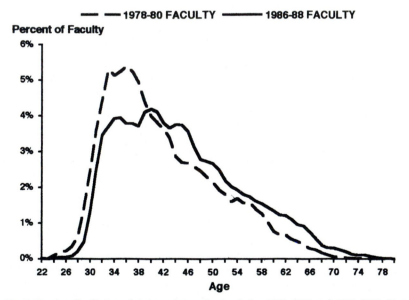

Fig 7–10.—Age distribution of active radiology faculty during 1978–1980 and 1986–1988. Notice the broadening of the peak of the curve, reflecting the aging of the larger group of new faculty recruited before growth reached its current low level. Also, there are relatively more senior faculty in the recent period. The later beginning of the curve probably reflects a longer training period in 1986–1988. (Courtesy of Friedman PJ: *Invest Radiol* 26:858–865, 1991.)

Background.—As part of a larger examination of the demographics of full-time medical school faculty, changes in the age and retirement patterns of radiology faculty since 1970 were assessed. Other trends examined include the proportions of women and PhD scientists in academic radiology and the effects of possible growth rates and resignation patterns.

Methods.—Data were obtained from the Faculty Roster, a database maintained by the Association of American Medical Colleges. Retirement was defined as a final separation from the medical school after age 60 years. The starting point for projections of the future was the 1986 distribution of faculty.

Results.—The number of full-time faculty in radiology more than doubled from 1970 to 1988, paralleling the increase in all medical school faculty. The number of women in academic radiology grew from 9% in 1970 to 16% in 1988, a proportion that still lags behind female faculty in general. Whereas the general faculty consists of 29% PhDs and 6% MD-PhDs, radiology departments contain 2% PhDs and 8% MD-PhDs. Recent trends are to more middle-aged and older faculty (Fig 7–10). The mean age of faculty radiologists has increased 5 years in the last 20 years. Radiologists have a higher turnover rate than does the general faculty, and women have a higher turnover rate than men. Women are also not promoted to full professor as quickly as men (Fig 7–11). Overall, the proportion of radiologists leaving academia has been about the same as for the general faculty. The majority of job changes for radiologists (total or final) are occurring before age 50 years. Radiologists also tend to have a lower mean retirement age than general faculty.

Conclusions.—Projections suggest that increased recruitment or an increase in the retention rate of junior faculty will be required to sustain the current 1.5% growth level. The end of mandatory requirement is not likely to affect radiologists who seem to prefer to hang up their lead aprons in their early to mid-60s.

▶ We need to attract more of our radiology residents and fellows into academic positions. The aging of our current faculty and the apparent trend toward early retirement will create a shortage. This shortage will be particularly acute in specialty areas that have not been popular in recent years, such as gastrointestinal and genitourinary radiology, chest and bone radiology, pediatric radiology, and nuclear medicine. Academic departments need to address this problem actively now.—C.D. Maynard, M.D.

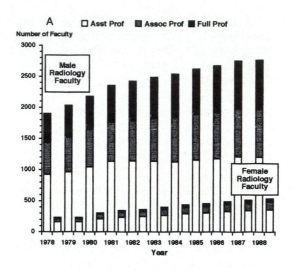

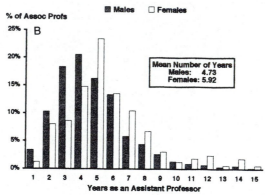

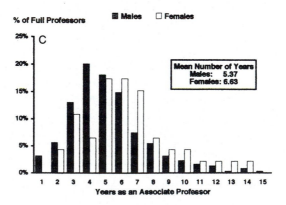

Fig 7–11 (cont).

Early Predictors of Career Achievement in Academic Medicine

Brancati FL, Mead LA, Levine DM, Martin D, Margolis S, Klag MJ (Johns Hopkins Univ School of Medicine and School of Hygiene and Public Health, Baltimore; Univ of Florida, Gainesville, Fla)

JAMA 267:1372–1376, 1992   7–17

Objective.—There has been considerable work in identifying predictors of success in medical school but relatively little in relating medical school performance to future career achievement. This study attempted to find those personal and scholastic features that predict the choice of an academic career and achievement in that career.

Methods.—A longitudinal cohort study was carried out on 944 males graduating from the Johns Hopkins University School of Medicine from 1948 to 1964. Achievement of faculty rank in 1990 was ascertained, as well as the number of citations to published work. Research-intensive institutions were those among the top 30 in total grant dollars from the NIH, those among the top 10 in number of citations, and the National Institutes of Health themselves.

Findings.—Forty-five percent of the physicians had chosen academic careers. Both scholastic performance and research experience in medical school correlated with the choice of an academic career. Nearly half the academicians, or about one fifth of all graduates, held appointments at research-intensive institutions. Scholastic performance influenced the likelihood of becoming a chairman, chief, or dean (Fig 7–12). High rank also correlated with graduation from a private college. Membership in Alpha Omega Alpha was associated independently with higher achieved rank.

Implications.—The use of a range of career achievement measures helps validate these findings. These measures account for excellence in teaching or patient care only to the extent that such excellence contributes to promotion. Both scholastic performance and research experience in medical school help predict career achievement in academic medicine.

▶ If we want to increase the number of radiology residents entering academic careers, we clearly need to attract medical students who have special

Fig 7–11.—**A,** academic ranks of radiology faculty in the past decade, excluding faculty not listed as a professor of any level. Overall, the distribution has remained fairly stable, despite faculty aging, with only a modest increase in the relative number of the higher ranks. The distribution of ranks among women differs from that of men, with continuing preponderance of assistant professors and, clearly, a much smaller proportion of full professors. **B,** the duration of appointment as assistant professor before promotion. Among all associate professors, this is the number of years since appointment as an assistant professor, by sex. There are clear differences in the distribution and the averages. Faculty who were never promoted were excluded. **C,** duration of appointment as associate professor of radiology before promotion. This is a similar distribution for all full professors in the database. Whether the difference has changed over the years was not examined. (Courtesy of Friedman PJ: *Invest Radiol* 26:858–865, 1991.)

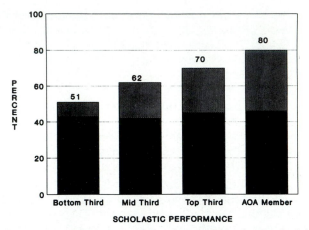

Fig 7–12.—Percentage attaining the rank of full professor (*solid bars*) and rank of chairman, chief, or dean (*shaded bars*) by scholastic performance in medical school (defined by class standing at graduation and membership in Alpha Omega Alpha (AOA) among 424 male academic physicians (test for trend, P < .001). (Courtesy of Brancati FL, Mead LA, Levine DM, et al: JAMA 267:1372–1376, 1992.)

characteristics and backgrounds. Attempts to influence them during their residency and fellowship training come too late in the educational cycle. I used to believe medical school background didn't matter; I've changed my mind.—C.D. Maynard, M.D.

The RSNA-AUR-ARRS Introduction to Research Program: The Development, First Year's Experience, and Promise of a Program to Encourage Radiology Research Careers
Hillman BJ, Maynard CD, Stanley RJ, Witzke DB, Fulginiti JV (Univ of Arizona, Tucson; Bowman Gray School of Medicine, Winston-Salem, NC; Univ of Alabama, Birmingham, Ala)
Invest Radiol 27:192–197, 1992   7–18

Background.—The number of productive clinician researchers in radiology is inadequate, prompting major efforts to obtain more of them and to improve the quality of their work. The Conjoint Committee on Diagnostic Radiology has coordinated efforts by the American College of Radiology, the Association of University Radiologists (AUR), and the Society of Chairmen of Academic Radiology Departments. In addition, the Research and Education Fund of the Radiological Society of North America (RSNA) has sponsored several programs supporting young investigators and has funded pilot research. The America Roentgen Ray Society (ARRS) now is following the lead of the RSNA.

Objectives.—The goals of these programs are to provide selected residents with a primer in research at an early stage of their residencies, to raise awareness of the importance of research in diagnostic radiology programs, and to expose residents to successful researchers.

Aspects of Programs.—Nominations of second-year residents are considered for participation. Typically a 12-hour course is offered in 90-minute sessions, ensuring 1-on-1 contact with established academicians whose research might be known to the residents. In sharing rooms it is easy for the participants to become acquainted with one another.

Effects.—Residents appeared to be significantly more interested in pursuing an academic career than persons not selected or randomly surveyed residents. Once entering practice, participants expected to spend more of their time doing research. Some participants, however, who initially rated themselves as most likely to enter academic careers, were less academically oriented after participating in the program.

▶ This effort truly represents the cooperative nature of the 3 major radiologic organizations: the ARRS, the AUR, and the RSNA. Although very few residents (80) can participate in this program annually, it is a good beginning. The field of radiology must take advantage of the current excellent resident pool to develop researchers. Radiology does not have a strong history of high-quality basic research. Our opportunity to correct that problem exists today with these young people. Let's not blow our chance.—C.D. Maynard, M.D.

Radiologic Physics Instruction for Diagnostic Radiologists: A Survey of Residency Programs
Committee on Training of Radiologists (American Assoc of Physicists in Medicine, New York)
AJR 157:409–410, 1991   7–19

Introduction.—The Committee on Training of Radiologists of the American Association of Physicists in Medicine conducted a survey designed to compare residents' impressions of their physics instruction (the subject of a previous survey) with the curricula of existing programs. Persons in 99 of 250 programs receiving the questionnaire responded.

Methods.—The survey consisted of 20 questions related to general program information, curriculum, instructors' background, and use of instructional materials. Written comments and suggestions were also invited.

Results.—Fifty-three percent of the programs were university based, 44% were hospital based, and 3% were clinic based. The mean number of residents in each year of residency was 4. Diagnostic radiology was the specialty in 73% of the physics instruction programs. Classroom hours varied and dropped to a mean of 18 during the fifth postgraduate year. Most programs (66%) offered a special in-house physics review course before the American Board of Radiology examinations. The primary physics instructor was board certified in either diagnostic or radiologic physics. Handouts were the most frequently used instructional materials. Suggestions from respondents included the need for high-quality, standardized teaching materials and the need for regular attendance.

Conclusions.—Physics instruction encompasses a significant time commitment during radiology residency programs. There appears to be a need for the development of new teaching materials or the promotion of existing materials. The lack of audiovisual materials suggests a need for correlating physics principles with images.

▶ More attention should be given to the basic science education of our residents. Physics and radiobiology have been part of our program for years, but now we need to add computer science and electrical engineering. Because of the wide variability among programs in the quality of the faculty in these areas, other methods of education, such as interactive video, might be considered.—C.D. Maynard, M.D.

Resident Interpretation of Emergency Computed Tomographic Scans
Roszler MH, McCarroll KA, Rashid T, Donovan KR, Kling GA (Wayne State Univ, Detroit)
Invest Radiol 26:374–376, 1991   7–20

Introduction.—Previous reports on the error rates of residents in interpreting emergency radiology examinations have considered only plain film (PF) studies. As part of a hospital quality assurance study, residents' preliminary reports for head CT scans were examined.

Methods.—Second- through fourth-year radiology residents give preliminary interpretations on all PF and CT studies performed after working hours and on weekends at the study institution. These reports are subsequently evaluated by a staff radiologist and significant errors are noted. During a 2-month period, 289 emergency cranial CT examinations were studied. Errors were classified as false negative, false positive, or as a misinterpretation of the pathology seen.

Results.—Significant acute pathology was found in 22% of the examinations. There were 6 minor errors in the residents' reports, 4 cases of moderate errors, and 2 cases of major errors. Three of the major and moderate errors were false negatives, 2 were false positives, and 1 was a misinterpretation. Five of these errors were made by second-year residents.

Conclusions.—The error rate here, 2%, is significantly lower than that found in previous studies of PF examinations. One possible explanation is that the limited pathology range of emergency cranial CT may be easier to evaluate. In addition, most of these CT studies (78%) were negative. As a result of the findings, the study institution gives at least 5 hours of special head trauma conferences before second-year residents begin emergency room (ER) call.

▶ This article points out the need to make certain that radiology residents are prepared in CT interpretation before taking ER call. This is certainly true for other procedures as well. The resident in the ER often covers specialized services such as nuclear medicine and ultrasound. Although manpower needs cannot be ignored, training should be a major consideration in the timing of ER call.—C.D. Maynard, M.D.

Radiotracers and the Heart: State of the Turf
Holman BL (Brigham and Women's Hosp, Harvard Med School, Boston)
Invest Radiol 26:1009–1012, 1991   7–21

Objective.—A questionnaire was sent to directors of nuclear medicine training programs to gain some understanding of how cardiac nuclear medicine is practiced in academic institutions. Sixty-four of 98 centers with approved training programs in nuclear medicine, nuclear radiology, or both responded, and data on the 55 that bill third-party payers were analyzed.

Findings.—Myocardial scintigraphy with thallium 201 accounted for 57% of all procedures. The next most common were exercise stress testing and pharmacologic stress studies. There was, however, substantial variation in the degree to which different centers rely on myocardial scintigraphy and wall motion studies (Fig 7–13). All but 13% of physicians who interpreted the studies were certified by the American Board of Nuclear Medicine.

Discussion.—It is expected that methods of measuring flow, diffusion, biochemical properties, and receptor function will proliferate in the coming years. At present, relatively few institutions rely heavily on stress

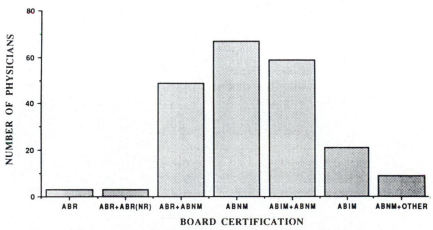

Fig 7–13.—The board certification of physicians involved in the interpretation of cardiac nuclear medicine studies. (Courtesy of Holman BL: *Invest Radiol* 26:1009–1012, 1991.)

wall motion studies to assess coronary artery reserve. Pharmacologic stress testing likely will be used more often when dipyridamole is approved for routine clinical use.

▶ Radiology is losing cardiac diagnostic studies to nonradiologists, primarily cardiologists. "Turf battles" are often won or lost in the academic centers. It is clear that radiologists in this setting are not actively pursuing nuclear cardiology. It also appears that these procedures will follow coronary angiography into the domain of cardiology. Will MR cardiac angiography be next?—C.D. Maynard, M.D.

Magnetic Resonance Imaging

Three-Dimensional MR Microscopy With Large Arrays
Suddarth SA, Johnson GA (Duke Univ Med Ctr, Durham, NC)
Magn Reson Med 18:132–141, 1991   7–22

Objective.—The development of MR microscopy has prompted interest in 3-dimensional Fourier imaging because the small signal from microscopic pixels poses a significant limit to this technique. Previously 3-dimensional Fourier transform imaging has been limited to data arrays of 16 × 256 × 256. Arrays of 256 × 256 × 256 were attempted.

Methods.—Imaging was carried out using a 300-MHz MR micro-

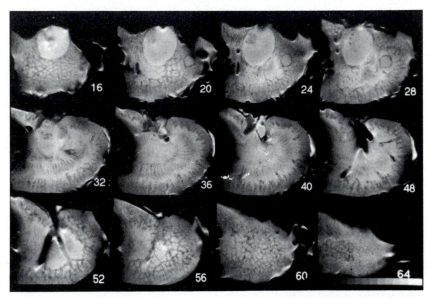

Fig 7–14.—Selected levels from a 64 × 256 × 256 array of a formalin-fixed perfused rat kidney. The animal had been treated with a compound thought to create renal tumors. A large cystic mass was removed from the lower pole (at the left side) of each image to permit higher resolution of the remaining pole. TR = 500 ms; TE = 20 ms; 70 × 70 × 190 μm voxels. (Courtesy of Suddarth SA, Johnson GA: *Magn Reson Med* 18:132–141, 1991.)

scope. Images were acquired at 7.0 T with voxels as small as $70 \times 70 \times 70$ μm (3.4×10^{-4} mm^3). The large data sets are most easily handled by separating acquisition, reconstruction, archiving, and analysis onto networked work stations. Isotropic data may be interactively displayed through any plane with no loss of in-plane resolution.

Results.—Images from a formalin-fixed rat kidney of an animal treated with ferric nitrilotriacetic acid, which may cause renal cancer, are shown in Fig 7–14. They were acquired from a $64 \times 256 \times 256$ array covering a $12 \times 18 \times 18$ mm field of view. Subtle neuroanatomical structures were clearly defined using a 256^3 array of a formalin-fixed rat brain.

Implications.—The 3-dimensional nature of the acquisitions is a definite advantage in studies where it is necessary to obtain accurate morphometric data. Problems of tissue shrinkage are eliminated. Larger arrays will be possible with higher-speed digitizers and new ways of presorting and routine data. Acquisition times can readily be shortened by applying high-speed pulse sequences, with no loss of signal/noise ratio.

▶ Dr. K.M. Link, Associate Professor of Radiology, Bowman Gray School of Medicine, Wake Forest University, Winston-Salem, North Carolina, comments:

▶ With the achievement of 70-mm^3 spatial resolution, this pioneering group continues to improve the capabilities of MR microscopy. This cutting-edge work may revolutionize the study and understanding of microanatomy.—K.M. Link, M.D.

Real-Time Flow Measurements Using Echo-Planar Imaging
Guilfoyle DN, Gibbs P, Ordidge RJ, Mansfield P (Univ of Nottingham, Nottingham, England)
Magn Reson Med 18:1–8, 1991   7–23

Objective.—The high-speed capability of echo-planar imaging (EPI) makes it well suited to flow measurements. Echo-planar imaging may be used to measure both quantitative and qualitative information in real time, as well as for real-time angiography.

Methods.—A flow-encoding gradient is used first to overcome magnetic-field inhomogeneities. After a second flow-encoding gradient pulse, the spin magnetization is tipped back along the main field axis. A spin phase scrambling gradient is then applied to eliminate any remaining signal. A normal EPI experiment follows to image the residual longitudinal magnetization.

Application.—Echo-planar imaging flow studies were done on both phantoms and human subjects. Cardiac images made using the flow-encoding method showed the sinusoidal and cosinusoidal dependence of signal intensity on flow rate. The sinusoidal variation in signal intensity results from suppression of the static spin signal.

Utility.—This way of directly exciting flowing spins may serve to perform real-time nuclear MR angiography and immediately visualize vascular structures without the need for postprocessing. Flow data are assessed from a magnitude image, minimizing sensitivity to phase errors. It should be possible to assess the 3-dimensional steady-state flow patterns within an object totally in a relatively short examination time. Full 3-dimensional velocity maps might find use in cardiac imaging where flow conditions are fairly reproducible from 1 cardiac cycle to another.

▶ The authors investigated the latest ultrafast MR technique (EPI). Their results indicate that this essentially real-time technique makes possible the visualization and the quantification of blood flow. Potentially the technique will overcome the limitations of present MR angiography techniques in studying the cardiovascular system.—K.M. Link, M.D.

Combined Chemical-Shift and Phase-Selective Imaging for Fat Suppression: Theory and Initial Clinical Experience
Chan TW, Listerud J, Kressel HY (Hosp of the Univ of Pennsylvania, Philadelphia)
Radiology 181:41–47, 1991   7–24

Introduction.—Imaging methods that can suppress the detection of fat content in disease conditions with a fat component pose some difficulties because of their short-inversion time inversion-recovery. The chemical shift–selective (CHESS) or the phase-selective (Dixon) imaging methods provide incomplete fat suppression, which is related in part to the olefinic fat component. The CHESS fat saturation technique was combined with the Dixon opposed method (called the opposed-fat suppression, or OP-FS, technique) to obtain more effective fat suppression during imaging of 10 volunteers.

Methods.—Materials included a copper sulfate and water mixture and verified unsaturated vegetable cooking oil. Instead of the manufacturer's recommended sinc pulse, the CHESS technique was performed with a 1-3-3-1 pulse. Comparison of fat saturation differences was carried out on phantom images of the vegetable oil and water using spin-echo (SE) and various combinations of the CHESS and the Dixon techniques, including OP-FS. The 10 healthy volunteers between ages 23 and 42 years underwent axial imaging of the upper half of the abdomen. Two radiologists evaluated all images.

Results.—The OP-ES technique provided better fat suppression, up to 4% of the SE signal, than the other methods. Altering the flip angle changed the measured saturation of the aliphatic fat component. Clinical analysis of images from the volunteers showed that the OP-FS method

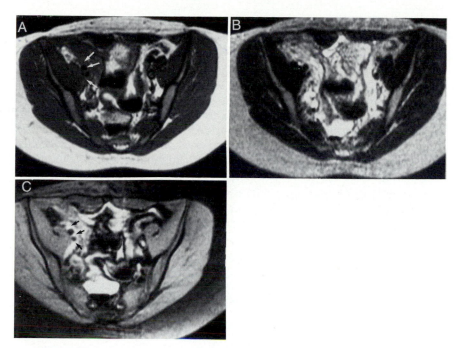

Fig 7–15.—Magnetic resonance images demonstrate aggressive fibromatosis in the right pelvis with involvement of the iliac vessels. **A,** axial T1-weighted SE image (600/20) shows soft-tissue mass (*arrows*) isointense to muscle; **B,** T2-weighted SE image (2,500/80) shows this mass to be isointense with fat, making it difficult to identify; **C,** on the OP-FS image (600/23) the mass is hyperintense and surronds the iliac vessels (*arrows*). This lesion is better visualized in **C** than in **A** or **B**. (Courtesy of Chan TW, Listerud, J, Kressel HY: *Radiology* 181:41–47, 1991.)

resulted in more complete saturation of subcutaneous and retroperitoneal fat when compared with images obtained by the CHESS technique alone. The OP-FS method gave the highest contrast/noise ratio for the pancreas to retroperitoneal fat comparison. Physician reviewers reported higher confidence in fat lesion diagnosis with the OP-FS method because of more defined lesions (Fig 7–15).

Conclusions.—The findings indicate that the OP-FS method produces better fat suppression than other compared methods. The OP-FS imaging effectiveness is related to the saturation of aliphatic fats and olefinic fat residual signal cancellation.

▶ Chemical-shift techniques for fat suppression serve an important role in MRI. However, present schemes are limited by their inability to completely suppress the signal of fatty structures. The authors present a new method, based on a combination of the chemical-shift and the opposed-Dixon methods, which more effectively suppresses fat signal.—K.M. Link, M.D.

Fast Short-Tau Inversion-Recovery MR Imaging

Fleckenstein JL, Archer BT, Barker BA, Vaughan JT, Parkey RW, Peshock RM
(Univ of Texas Southwestern Med Ctr, Dallas)
Radiology 179:499–504, 1991   7–25

Introduction.—The short-tau inversion-recovery (STIR) imaging sequence provides a high sensitivity to pathologic lesions and a high fat signal suppression, but even low-resolution images often require several minutes to achieve. Alterations of the STIR sequence were used to allow for shortened imaging times to fit in with available MR systems.

Methods.—The STIR sequence used on the .35-T MRT 35 instrument consisted of repetition time (TR) of 1,500 ms, an echo time (TE) of 30 ms, and an inversion time (TI) of 100 ms. To speed up the STIR images, lower TR, fewer excitations, and reduced phase-encoding steps were as-

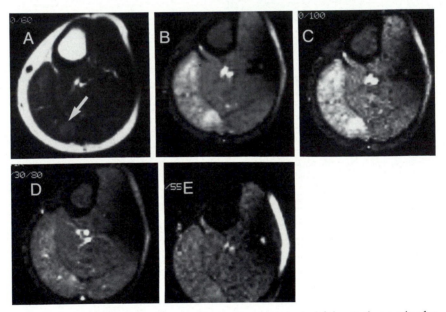

Fig 7–16.—Fast STIR images of postexercise muscle necrosis in the left leg. **A,** three weeks after injurious exercise, necrosis in the left medial gastrocnemius is barely perceptible in spin-echo image obtained with TR of 2,000 and TE of 60. **B,** abnormality is much more obvious when usual STIR sequence is used; **C,** with half-Fourier technique, a 1,500/30/100 image is obtained in 1.9 minutes and is as sensitive to the abnormality as usual STIR imaging. **D,** further threefold time savings was obtained by reducing the TR to 500 ms and the TI to 80 ms; however, the conspicuity of the lesion was decreased. **E,** an additional twofold time savings could have been obtained by reducing the TR/TI to 250/55. Four excitations were performed, which required 2.1 minutes. This procedure resulted in an overall increased signal-to-noise ratio, but the diminished conspicuity of the injured muscle was not compensated for by the greater number of excitations. High signal intensity in the lateral aspects of the image was the result of the closeness of the legs to the edge of the coil, a common pitfall in STIR imaging. (Courtesy of Fleckenstein JL, Archer BT, Barker BA, et al: *Radiology* 179:499–504, 1991.)

sessed. Each alteration of the STIR sequence underwent phantom and preliminary clinical assessments.

Results.—Results show that the use of rectangular pixels reduced image sharpness. The reduction of TR but not TI produced a suppression of the phantom samples that differed from those of the usual STIR sequence, indicating that when TR fell to less than 1,000 ms, TI had to be reduced to achieve good fat suppression. Fat suppression occurred using imaging times of 8 seconds (175/30/45). The better contrast produced by STIR sequences was achieved with one-half acquisition, leading to a threefold lowering of imaging time (Fig 7–16). Testing the fast STIR MR sequence using a gadopentetate dimeglumine infusion demonstrated that a decrease in T1 relaxation time from the Gd caused minimal change in the signal intensity at long TR, but signal intensity was greatly improved with short TRs.

Conclusions.—The STIR imaging time can be seriously reduced by using a shorter TI at a lower TR or by a shorter TR with Gd enhancement. The calculations and estimates produced by this study allow for further development of a range of TR/TI values for use at .35 T and similar techniques can be used to delineate the best field strengths for STIR imaging.

▶ Short-tau inversion-recovery is another means of suppressing fat signal. Unfortunately, this time-consuming process has limited use in day-to-day imaging, especially on low field-strength systems that are best suited to STIR sequences. By manipulating TE, and TI, the authors were able to decrease scanning time threefold. This will allow for greater versatility on lower field-strength systems, which ordinarily require longer scanning times than are necessary with field-strength MR.—K.M. Link, M.D.

Volume Rendering and Connectivity Algorithms for MR Angiography
Cline HE, Dumoulin CL, Lorensen WE, Souza SP, Adams WJ (GE Corporate Research and Development Ctr, Schenectady, NY)
Magn Reson Med 18:384–394, 1991   7–26

Problem.—The display algorithm used to render volumetric data in a 2-dimensional form can significantly limit 3-dimensional MR angiography. Volume rendering projection algorithms have been most widely used. The maximum intensity projection (MIP) method is computationally rapid and relatively insensitive to low-level background signals. An alternative approach is to extract a surface from the volume of interest, typically on the basis of pixel intensity, and display the 3-dimensional surface in 2 dimensions by simulating a light source and surface reflectivity. It frequently is necessary to enhance the surface-rendering algorithm with MR data.

Solution.—Several display algorithms for 3-dimensional angiographic data were assessed. Additive Gaussian noise was assumed to predict the background distribution function for the MIP, sum projection, and connectivity display methods. With the MIP method, the mean noise level increased with the number of voxels in the ray. With sum projection, the noise distribution width increased with the projection thickness, but the mean level remained constant. Measurements of noise distribution agreed with this analysis when the algorithms were applied to an MR angiogram of the circle of Willis. Connectivity algorithms can be combined with projection algorithms to avoid problems with surface presentation.

Conclusions.—Selecting a method for rendering vessels from 3-dimensional MR angiographic data depends on the particular medical application and on whether fine vessel resolution, flow information, or morphology is of chief importance.

▶ Manipulation of MR angiography data is a tricky and often time-consuming process. The authors, pioneers in the field of MR angiography, describe the methods currently used and how they can maximize the display of volumetric data.—K.M. Link, M.D.

T2-Weighted Spin-Echo Pulse Sequence With Variable Repetition and Echo Times for Reduction of MR Image Acquisition Time
Butts RK, Farzaneh F, Riederer SJ, Rydberg JN, Grimm RC (Mayo Clinic and Found, Rochester, Minn)
Radiology 180:551–556, 1991   7–27

Introduction.—Radiologists use the T_2-weighted spin-echo pulse sequence as the MR method of choice to assess and characterize many different kinds of lesions. Several techniques have attempted to lower the acquisition times of the T_2-weighted spin-echo (SE) pulse sequence, which can be accomplished but with reduced quality of image. The usefulness of the variable-rate spin-echo (VARSE) pulse sequence for reducing the repetition times (TRs) and echo times (TEs) was assessed.

Methods.—The usual TR for the VARSE image technique is about 8 minutes and 56 seconds, with the second image requiring an additional 2 minutes. The incorporation of VARSE into multisection imaging was measured. Both the TR and TE were reduced in various combinations to determine whether that could lower imaging times. Noise and contrast studies measured the loss of T_2-related contrast with reduction of TE. All test sequences and volunteer studies were made with a 1.5-T MRI system.

Results.—The higher frequencies became enhanced on the VARSE image on elimination of the postacquisition filter. The effects were demonstrated in studies of the volunteer, subjects knee with the superoinferior phase-encoding direction; the total acquisition time was 9 minutes 30

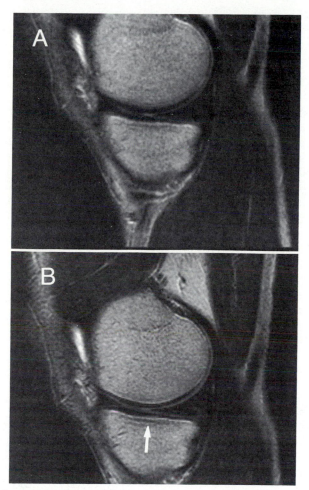

Fig 7–17.—A, standard MR image of the knee (TR/TE, 2,000/80; 256 phase encodings); **B,** VARSE image (TR$_0$/TE$_0$, 2,000/80; TR$_f$/TE$_f$, 1,000/20; n_i/n_p 20/60; 256 phase encodings) of the same volunteer as in **A.** Phase encoding is along the superior-inferior direction. Articular cartilage (*arrow*) is clearly better depicted in the VARSE image. (Courtesy of Butts RK, Farzaneh F, Riederer SJ, et al: *Radiology* 180:551–556, 1991.)

seconds using the standard SE pulse sequence (Fig 7–17). By decreasing the TR/TE, the total acquisition time was lowered to 6 minutes 21 seconds. Noise and contrast studies outlined and enhanced the smallest objects with diameters of 5 and 8 pixels, using a reconstruction filter. These studies produced an increased net contrast/noise ratio for large objects, with only objects of less than 8 pixels in diameter having lower contrast with respect to the noise decrease. Thus, filtering the data before reconstruction suppresses these outcomes and produces an overall increase in contrast/noise ratio.

Conclusions.—The T₂-weighted images with some enhancing of the contrast at the edges can reduce imaging time by changing the pulse sequence factors while acquiring the image. Altering parameters other than TR and TE, such as inversion time and bandwidth, may also reduce image acquisition time.

▶ The T₂-weighted SE pulse sequences play a major role in characterizing lesions detected with MR. Unfortunately, these sequences tend to be time consuming and therefore increase the length of the overall examination and limit the number of T₂-weighted SE sequences used during the course of a single MR examination. The authors use the VARSE pulse sequence to demonstrate that time requirements can be reduced by one third while maintaining the contrast/noise ratio. This technique should be useful in day-to-day MR scanning.—K.M. Link, M.D.

Volume Imaging With MR Phased Arrays
Hayes CE, Hattes N, Roemer PB (GE Medical Systems, Milwaukee; GE Corporate Research and Development Ctr, Schenectady, NY)
Magn Reson Med 18:309–319, 1991   7–28

Introduction.—The MR-phased array technique gathers data from a number of surface coils covering anatomy of interest. Each coil has its own data acquisition system. Individual images from the coils are com-

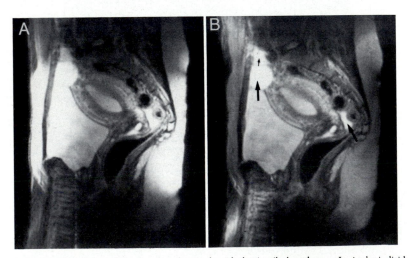

Fig 7–18.—Sagittal view of the female pelvis made with the 4-coil phased array. In **A,** the individual images were combined using the sum of squares algorithm, which gave regions of high signal intensity near the surfaces. In **B** the same individual images were combined with uniform sensitivity using an equation. The high-intensity regions marked by arrows in **B** are somewhat masked in **A** by the coil intensity effects. Imaging parameters: $T_R = 2,000$ ms; $T_E = 80$ ms, slice thickness = 5 mm; FOV = 30 cm, matrix = 256 × 256 with 1 excitation. (Courtesy of Hayes CE, Hattes N, Roemer PB: *Magn Reson Med* 18:309–319, 1991.)

bined into a composite image with the goal of obtaining an overall field of view while retaining the higher signal/noise ratio characteristic of the individual surface coils.

Objective.—A volume MR-phased array was made of 2 coils placed anteriorly and 2 posteriorly on a phantom. The combined image had a signal/noise ratio 80% better than the image from a body coil. The 4-coil phased array was compared with a 2-coil phased array and with a Helmholtz pair having the same overall dimensions. Quantitative comparisons were made by imaging a water-filled phantom.

Findings.—The composite signal/noise ratio was influenced by variations of signal amplitude and phase in the individual coils. Images of the male and female pelves (Fig 7–18) showed that the improved signal/noise ratio may be used to reduce the number of excitations, decrease the field of view, increase the echo time, or reduce the slice thickness.

Discussion.—The use of smaller surface coils in a phased array allows a better combination of individual signals. The 4-coil phased array yielded a signal/noise ratio 40% or more higher than that associated with a Helmholtz pair of coils having similar overall dimensions.

▶ The major limiting factor in MRI is the time it takes to acquire information. Attempts to examine large regions of interest in a short period of time have included the use of large fields of view, decreased matrices and number of excitations, and increased slice thickness. All of these techniques result in poorer image quality and decreased spatial resolution and signal/noise ratios. The authors describe the use of phased array coils (a series of small surface coils) to examine large fields of view. These coils provide excellent spatial resolution while improving signal/noise ratio and, just as important, decreasing overall scanning time. This new hardware device will play an important role in MR for years to come.—K.M. Link, M.D.

Quality Assurance and Effectiveness

Performance Standards in Positron Emission Tomography

Karp JS, Daube-Witherspoon ME, Hoffman EJ, Lewellen TK, Links JM, Wong W-H, Hichwa RD, Casey ME, Colsher JG, Hitchens RE, Muehllehner G, Stoub EW (Univ of Pennsylvania, Philadelphia; Natl Insts of Health, Bethesda, Md; Univ of California, Los Angeles; Univ of Washington, Seattle; Johns Hopkins Med Institutions, Baltimore; et al)
J Nucl Med 12:2342–2350, 1991   7–29

Background.—With the growing number of PET centers, the need for a standard set of performance measurements became clear. A set of measurements was developed jointly by the Computer and Instrumentation Council of the Society of Nuclear Medicine (SNM) and the National Electrical Manufacturers Association (NEMA). The individual SNM/NEMA tests are briefly studied and the rationale for each are examined. For each measurement, a comparison is made between the

SNM/NEMA protocol and that of the European Economic Community task group on PET performance standards.

Methods.—Performance tests were divided into 2 groups. The first included the basic intrinsic measurements: tests of spatial resolution, scatter fraction, true sensitivity, and count rate losses and randoms. The second group included measurements of the accuracy of corrections for physical effects, namely, uniformity correction, scatter correction, attenuation correction, and count rate linearity correction. A fillable cylinder of Lucite was designed as the PET performance phantom.

Results.—The set of measurements put forth by the NEMA and SNM committees was designed to be general enough to ensure that the tests will be valid for many years. The measurements and analysis should be able to be performed in about 2 weeks, assuming experience with the procedures and no need to repeat the experiments. Although considerable effort was made to keep the American and European measurements similar to each other, in certain cases they differ with respect to the activity distribution or the method of data analysis.

Conclusions.—The set of measurements developed by the joint committee should prove useful for evaluating and understanding the performance of PET scanners. If the proposed set of standards is adopted by many PET investigators, an expanded data base may lead to reevaluation and possible modifications.

▶ As PET technology moves from academic medical centers to widespread use in community hospital settings, performance standards must be available. This is an admirable beginning.—C.D. Maynard, M.D.

A Multicentre Audit of Hospital Referral for Radiological Investigation in England and Wales
Royal College of Radiologists Working Party (University of Wales, Cardiff, Wales)
Br Med J 303:809–812, 1991   7–30

Introduction.—A study by the Royal College of Radiologists and the National Radiological Protection Board estimated that at least 20% of x-ray examinations performed in the United Kingdom are unnecessary. A booklet distributed to physicians recommended a reduction in radiologic procedures and improvement of practice in general. A baseline audit of radiology referral practice before introduction of the booklet's guidelines was examined.

Methods.—A representative sample of centers was chosen for the audit, 4 in England and 2 in Wales. Five were district general hospitals and 1 was a district health authority. The data collection period extended from January 1987 to December 1989.

Results.—The study population consisted of 159,421 inpatient discharges, deaths, and day cases and 861,370 outpatient attendances. Patients were under the care of 722 consultants from 25 clinical specialties. There was a great variation in referral rates from 1 center to another. No consistent relation was seen between high referral for x-ray examination and teaching status of the center, specialty, or subspecialty. Referral rates for chest x-ray examinations, for example, varied fourfold for outpatients from 1 center to another. Until this survey was performed, local consultants were unaware of how their use of diagnostic radiologic services compared with that of colleagues in other institutions.

Conclusions.—Contrary to the usual assumption, teaching hospitals, which treat more complicated cases and teach medical students, did not have higher referral rates. Although British radiology practice is more selective than that of other developed countries (e.g., the United States or France). At least 20% of x-ray examinations in England and Wales may be clinically unhelpful.

▶ Although this study was done in England and Wales, it adds to the knowledge that practice patterns vary greatly between referring physicians when ordering procedures. The lack of standards of practice in the United States has been singled out as a reason for overutilization of high technology. Rationing of health care in this country is considered unnecessary by some if the money thus spent could be transferred to individuals who lack adequate care (1).—C.D. Maynard, M.D.

Reference

1. Brook RH, et al: *Issues in Science and Technology,* Fall: 68, 1986.

Efficacy of Daily Routine Chest Radiographs in Intubated, Mechanically Ventilated Patients
Hall JB, White SR, Karrison T (Univ of Chicago, Chicago)
Crit Care Med 19:689–693, 1991   7–31

Background.—There is controversy as to the efficacy of routine daily chest radiographs in critically ill patients who require intubation and mechanical ventilation. The efficacy of this approach, including its incremental benefit to more routine patient assessment; was examined prospectively.

Methods.—The study was performed in 74 patients who required 77 episodes of intubation and mechanical ventilation in a medicosurgical intensive care unit. Before the chest radiographs were reviewed every day, unit critical care physicians carefully evaluated the patients' clinical and physiologic variables. The physicians documented any new findings along with the required diagnostic and therapeutic interventions. Those findings were then compared with the radiologist's interpretation of the

---

Criteria for Major and Minor Findings

Major Finding	Minor Finding
ET tube tip at or below tracheal carina	Small change in ET tube position
ET tube tip at or above vocal cords	Interstitial emphysema
Pneumothorax	Small pleural effusion
Pneumomediastinum	Small change in chest tube position
Large pleural effusion	Atelectasis in <1 lobe
Chest tube position change out of thorax	Collapse in <1 lobe
Free air under diaphragm	Infiltrate in <1 lobe
Pulmonary edema	Small change in NG tube position
Lobar collapse or atelectasis	Small change in CV catheter position
Lobar infiltrate	Small change in PA catheter position
Pulmonary cavitary lesion	New minor abdominal finding
NG tube in airway	Small changes in vascular volume
NG tube tip in esophagus	
Evidence for pulmonary embolus	
New major abdominal finding	
CV catheter tip in RV	
CV catheter tip outside lumen	
PA catheter tip in RV	
Major new vascular redistribution in lungs	

Note: Major findings were defined as those requiring immediate diagnostic or therapeutic intervention. Minor findings were defined as those abnormalities that were present but did not require immediate intervention.

Abbreviations: ET, endotracheal; NG, nasogastric; RV, right ventricle; PA, pulmonary artery; CV, central venous.

(Courtesy of Hall JB, White SR, Karrison T: *Crit Care Med* 19:689–693, 1991.)

---

radiograph, which was done in blinded fashion. Both clinical assessment and radiographic findings were used to correlate new major and minor findings (table).

Results.—Five hundred eighty-four chest radiographs were reviewed. The most common admitting diagnoses were malignancy, aspiration pneumonia, and sepsis, followed by a variety of others. No new major or minor findings were detected on 65.8% of radiographs. Only minor new findings were detected on 30.3% of radiographs, and 40.5% of those findings were anticipated by the clinical assessment (Fig 7–19). However, chest radiography alone detected new major findings in 17.6% of patients (Fig 7–20), with tube malposition accounting for 78% of these.

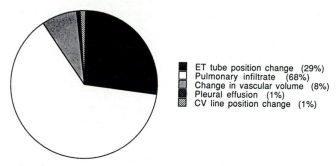

ET tube position change (29%)
Pulmonary infiltrate (68%)
Change in vascular volume (8%)
Pleural effusion (1%)
CV line position change (1%)

Fig 7–19.—Distribution of new minor findings noted by chest radiography but not by clinical assessment. A total of 97 (59.5%) of all new minor findings were not anticipated by clinical bedside assessment; these findings involved 48 (64.9%) of 74 patients. *Abbreviations:* ET, endotracheal; CV, central venous. (Courtesy of Hall JB, White SR, Karrison T: *Crit Care Med* 19:689–693, 1991.)

Conclusions.—In patients requiring intubation and mechanical ventilation, most routine chest radiographs will not disclose new findings. However, such routine daily studies have a major effect on the management of these patients in that many major findings cannot be anticipated by bedside assessment. Critically ill patients should continue to have daily chest radiographs.

▶ Portable chest radiographs in the intensive care unit are a large part of the plain-film volume of any major tertiary care medical center. Many institutions have protocols that call for routine chest films after specific surgical procedures. The usefulness of this practice is constantly under discussion between radiology faculty and intensive care physicians. This study reaffirms the value of portable chest radiographs.—C.D. Maynard, M.D.

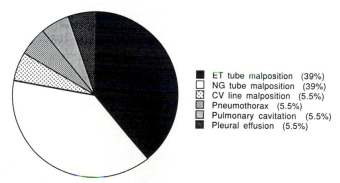

ET tube malposition (39%)
NG tube malposition (39%)
CV line malposition (5.5%)
Pneumothorax (5.5%)
Pulmonary cavitation (5.5%)
Pleural effusion (5.5%)

Fig 7–20.—Distribution of new major findings noted by chest radiography but not by clinical assessment. A total of 18 (41.9%) of all new major findings were not anticipated by clinical bedside assessment. The findings involved only 3.4% of all chest radiographs taken, but 13 (17.6%, 95% confidence interval, 9% to 26%) of 74 patients. *Abbreviations:* ET, endotracheal; NG, nasogastric; CV, central venous. (Courtesy of Hall JB, White SR, Karrison T: *Crit Care Med* 19:689–693, 1991.)

The Limited Role of Radiologic Imaging in Patients With Unknown Tumor Primary

Kagan AR, Steckel RJ (Southern California Jonsson Comprehensive Cancer Ctr, Univ of California Los Angeles School of Medicine, Los Angeles)
Semin Oncol 18:170–173, 1991   7–32

Background.—A substantial number of patients are first seen with metastatic cancer and an unknown primary tumor. Although extensive tests and procedures may be undertaken to locate the primary site, this strategy may not contribute to the patient's quality or length of life. The difficulties involved in such a search were reviewed from the radiologist's perspective.

Problems.—The physician may have little information to impart to the patient with an unknown primary tumor. The patient must be told that location of the primary tumor will probably not influence survival. A reasonable approach to help relieve the patient's frustration is the use of diagnostic imaging.

Course of Action.—Certain imaging studies are recommended for presenting sites of metastatic disease (table). Although median survival is 3–4 months for most metastatic cancers with a persistently unknown pri-

Diagnostic Imaging Recommendations for Patients With Metastatic Carcinoma and an Occult Primary

Presenting Site of Metastatic Disease	Imaging Studies to Consider Initially (chest radiographs are always indicated)
Abdominal mass	Abdominal CT scan
Hepatomegaly	Abdominal CT scan
	Consider barium enema/UGI series
Biliary tract (painless jaundice)	Percutaneous and/or endoscopic cholangio-pancreatogram
	Abdominal CT scan
Malignant ascites	Abdominal CT scan
	Consider barium enema/UGI series
Malignant pleural effusion	Mammogram in women
	Consider chest CT scan
Upper cervical lymph nodes	MRI or CT of upper airways
	Consider thyroid scan
Lower cervical lymph nodes	CT chest/abdomen
	Consider mammogram in women
Axillary lymph nodes (undifferentiated CA)	Mammography in women
	Consider chest CT scan
Brain (diagnosed on CT or MRI)	Chest/abdominal CT scans (if chest radiographs are nondiagnostic)
Spinal epidural space (on myelogram, contrast CT, or MRI)	Chest CT (if radiographs are nondiagnostic)
Bone	Radionuclide bone scan survey, with correlative radiographs
	CT of chest/abdomen (if chest radiographs are nondiagnostic)
	Consider ultrasound of prostate (men) or mammogram (women)
Lungs (multiple nodules)	CT abdomen/pelvis
	Consider BE/UGI series

Abbreviations: UGI, upper gastrointestinal; *BE*, barium enema.
(Courtesy of Kagan AR, Steckel RJ: *Semin Oncol* 18:170–173, 1991. Adapted from Kagan AR, Steckel RJ: *Invest Radiol* 23:545–547, 1988.)

mary, identification of the primary site may suggest a specific treatment and possibly result in a longer survival period.

Conclusions.—In pursuing further diagnostic testing, the physician must keep in mind the best interests of the patient. For patients with metastatic disease when first seen, vigorous treatment may not be the right choice.

▶ As we try to control the escalating costs of health care, we must attempt to identify imaging studies with low yields. This article is an excellent report of 1 such attempt. Radiologists must take a more active role in deciding the appropriateness of imaging studies. Performing diagnostic procedures only to convince the patients and their families that something is being done should be discouraged.—C.D. Maynard, M.D.

Diagnostic Radiology Peer Review: A Method Inclusive of All Interpreters of Radiographic Examinations Regardless of Specialty
Hopper KD, Rosetti GF, Edmiston RB, Madewell JE, Beam LM, Landis JR, Miller KL, Ricci JA, McCauslin MA (Pennsylvania State Univ, Hershey, Pa; Pennsylvania Blue Shield, Camp Hill, Pa)
Radiology 180:557–561, 1991   7–33

Introduction.—Peer review to measure quality assurance in health care has come to the attention of national and regional government regulatory commissions. The Joint Commission on the Accreditation of Healthcare Organizations (JCAHO) has found that 54% of hospitals do not adequately assess or observe their physician staff. The JCAHO peer review concept has influenced the practice of diagnostic radiology. A pilot program was established to evaluate peer review of physicians in the Pennsylvania Blue Shield (PBS) data files.

Methods.—The PBS and Pennsylvania State University (PSU) diagnostic radiology data files from the Harrisburg area provided frontal and lateral chest radiographs for analysis. The study monitors randomly selected 10 provider accounts, with 9 of those 10 responding promptly with 2 sets of chest radiographs (CRs). The CRs were masked and reviewed by a board-certified radiologist. At the end of the review, a written report on the professional failures was prepared and the CRs were returned to the individual provider.

Results.—Of the 10 randomly chosen providers, 7 were primary care physicians and 3 were diagnostic radiologists. Table 1 presents a summary of basic information, including PBS radiography billings, for each of the 10 providers. Of the 98 CRs reviewed, 97 had some form of patient identification; only 4 providers usually marked the CR with the patient's identification number. Table 2 summarizes the failures and errors of the providers. Two providers who infrequently assessed CRs made the 5 CR marking errors. Some 80% of the CRs appeared technically ad-

TABLE 1.—Summary of Individual Providers

Provider	Specialty	# Years Billing PBS Interpretation X-rays	# X-ray Interpretations Billed PBS 2nd Quarter 1989	# Chest X-rays Reviewed
A	Internal Medicine	12	24	10
B	Internal Medicine	23	17	9*
C	Radiology	4	218	10
D	Internal Medicine	6	101	10
E	Multi-specialty Primary Care	12	24	10
F	Radiology	19	1029	10
G	Multi-specialty Primary Care	5	62	10
H	General Practice	12	32	10
I	Radiology	16	1014	10
J	Internal Medicine	12	11	9**

*Provider miscoded porcedure on claim form.
**Provider lost 1 study plus its written interpretation.
(Courtesy of Hopper KD, Rosetti GF, Edmiston RB, et al: *Radiology* 180:557–561, 1991.)

equate. Interpretation errors occurred on 10 CRs evaluated by 5 providers, with most errors made by 3 providers assessing less than 25 CRs during a quarter.

Conclusions.—Peer review offers many advantages and allows several levels of professional analysis. If a physician fails an initial review, a more thorough peer evaluation of many more radiographs could follow to obtain a clearer picture of the practitioner's capabilities. This type of peer review suits the provider of managed care.

▶ This article presents a very interesting way to perform peer review. Grouping nonradiologists performing radiologic studies with radiologists offers a unique opportunity to determine if the push for "radiology by radiologists" is justified.—C.D. Maynard, M.D.

TABLE 2.—Summary of Results

	DISTRIBUTION OF PROVIDERS	FILM MARKINGS FAILURE	REPORT FAILURE	TECHNICAL QUALITY FAILURE	ERRORS IN INTERPRETATION	
					TOTAL	# SERIOUS MISSES
TOTAL	10	5	21	10	11	5
Radiologists	3	0	0	2	2	0
		$p=0.005$	$p<0.01$	$p=0.189$	$p=0.189$	$p=0.019$
Non-Radiologists	7	5	21	8	9	5
# Studies Billed*						
< 50	5	5	11	7	8	4
50–500	3	0	10	3	3	1
> 500	2	0	0	0	0	0

Note: NA, not applicable.
*Number of radiographic interpretations billed to PBS during the second quarter, 1989.)
(Courtesy of Hopper KD, Rosetti GF, Edmiston RB, et al: *Radiology* 180:557–561, 1991.)

Quality Assessment in an Ambulatory Care Unit: Do Training and Responsibility Conflict?
Stewart NR, Mann FA, Terrell CB, Murphy WA Jr (Washington Univ, St Louis)
Radiology 181:857–861, 1991
7–34

Background.—Until recently, primary care physicians interpreted radiographs in the ambulatory care unit (ACU) of the study institution. Discordant opinions between ACU staff and attending radiologists were audited as part of an ongoing quality assessment program. The clinical significance of such discrepancies in musculoskeletal studies was examined.

Methods.—During the 4-month study period, 521 patients underwent radiography in the ACU; 233 patients met study requirements. Emergency department physicians (EDPs) evaluated 165 patients and second-year internal medicine residents evaluated 68. A review of these studies by staff radiologists resulted in discrepancies in 55 patients.

Results.—Differences in interpretation were not significant for the study subgroups: internal medicine residents had 3 false positive errors and 17 false negative errors; EDPs had 8 false positive errors and 27 false negative errors. There were 4 errors by radiologists. Both internal medicine residents and EDPs correctly identified 95% of the normal radiographs. Internal medicine residents made more clinically significant errors than EDPs. Anatomically complex areas (e.g., the elbow, wrist, and cervical spine) contributed a higher proportion of such errors.

Conclusions.—Interpretations by nonradiologists in an ACU or emergency department should be evaluated as soon as possible by a radiologist. Double reading of all radiographs helps to ensure a high standard of patient care. Ambulatory care unit residency training programs can be improved by inclusion of selected basic radiologic principles.

▶ This study clearly demonstrates the need for radiologists to be involved in the interpretation of emergency diagnostic studies in a timely fashion. The logistics of ED coverage on a 24-hour basis, 7 days per week is not inconsequential, particularly in smaller hospitals. Coverage could some day be handled with teleradiography, which would undoubtedly improve the quality of care in the ambulatory setting.—C.D. Maynard, M.D.

Importance of Daily Rounds by the Radiologist After Interventional Procedures of the Abdomen and Chest
Goldberg MA, Mueller PR, Saini S, Lee MJ, Girard MJ, Dawson SL, Hallisey MJ, Cortell ED, Hahn PF, Brink JA (Massachusetts Gen Hosp, Boston)
Radiology 180:767–770, 1991   7–35

Introduction.—Interventional radiologic procedures have become more common, making the radiologist an active member of the patient care team. This prospective study evaluated the utility of daily rounds by the radiologist for patients who have undergone catheter-related interventional procedures.

Methods.—All inpatients with indwelling catheters in the chest and abdomen were seen daily by the interventional team or staff radiologist. During the 7-week evaluation period, the number of patients seen, the number of clinical and catheter problems observed, and the management of these problems were documented.

Results.—There were 268 visits to 37 patients during the study period. An average of 69.5 minutes per day was spent visiting an average of 7.7 patients. Catheter-related or clinical problems were identified at 57 of the visits. The most common problem involved a catheter not draining because of mechanical or structural obstructions. Most (71%) catheter problems were managed at the patient's bedside. The presence of a radiologist on rounds resulted in requests for interventional procedures on a number of new patients.

Conclusions.—Failure to recognize catheter problems could result in inadequate drainage and a prolonged hospital stay. Daily rounds are an essential component of patient care after catheter-related interventional procedures and elevate the status of the interventional radiologist to that of a valued consultant.

▶ Interventional radiology will require that radiologists function more like surgeons. Daily ward rounds will become as common in radiology as they are in other specialties of medicine. The result will be a change in the way radiologists view their specialty. Some even predict that interventional radiology will become a separate field, but I do not believe that would be good for radiology as a whole.—C.D. Maynard, M.D.

Computer-Aided Diagnosis

Computer-Assisted Fusion of Single-Photon Emission Tomographic and Computed Tomographic Images: Evaluation in Complicated Inflammatory Disease
Swayne LC (College of Physicians and Surgeons of Columbia Univ, New York)
Invest Radiol 27:78–83, 1992   7–36

Background.—Complicated inflammatory disease requires rapid diagnosis and treatment to ensure patient survival. Multiple imaging modalities may be needed to diagnose and stage the disease.

Methods.—To enhance the information obtained from SPECT and x-ray CT images, a computer-assisted fusion method was developed and used to evaluate prospectively 10 patients with suspected inflammatory disease complicated by an associated underlying condition. A software program was written to allow the CT studies to be transferred to the nuclear computer system via O.5-in, 9-track tape. Fusion of images was accomplished with standard scaling, rotation, translation, and stretching transformations, using anatomical or external landmarks.

Results.—The CT findings were nonspecific in all cases. The SPECT-CT fusion, however, correctly identified and localized the inflammatory process in all patients (Fig 7–21). In 6 cases, precise localiza-

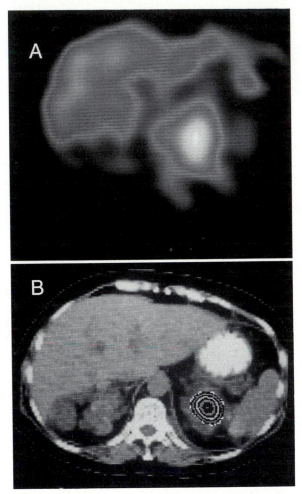

Fig 7–21.—A, woman, 52, with abdominal pain and known adult polycystic renal disease. Single-photon emission CT gallium study shows a focus of increased activity in the left upper quadrant. **B,** CT scan shows polycystic kidney disease and no evidence of an abdominal abscess. **C,** SPECT–CT fusion localized the gallium avid focus to an infected cyst in the upper pole of the left kidney. The patient's condition improved after antibiotic therapy, and results on a follow-up scan were normal. (Courtesy of Swayne LC: *Invest Radiol* 27:78–83, 1992.)

tion with SPECT-CT fusion facilitated percutaneous drainage or preoperative surgical planning.

Conclusions.—With the use of 3 different radiopharmaceuticals, the fusion technique can localize inflammatory sites accurately. Knowledge of the normal biodistribution of the radiopharmaceutical used is essential to avoid a false positive result.

▶ Superimposition of images from multiple modalities such as PET, CT, and MRI will be of diagnostic value because it affords a way to combine anatomical, physiologic, and biochemical information. Achieving adequate reregistration of the patient, however, for exact superimposition of multiple studies, will not be easy.—C.D. Maynard, M.D.

Expert Learning System Network for Diagnosis of Breast Calcifications

Patrick EA, Moskowitz M, Mansukhani VT, Gruenstein EI (Univ of Cincinnati; Heimlich Inst, Cincinnati)
Invest Radiol 26:534–539, 1991   7–37

Introduction.—Breast cancer is becoming more prevalent in the United States, although mortality remains constant. Presently about 1 in 11 women will develop breast cancer, which optimally is detected before a breast lump becomes palpable.

Objective.—The process of diagnosing breast calcification on mammograms was examined using computerized image processing in a network of trained expert learning systems (outcome advisor, or OA). The system was tested using records different from those used in training.

Methods.—Twenty difficult training and testing cases, 10 benign and 10 malignant, were randomly chosen for testing, and 108 others were used to train the network. Specialized systems in an expert learning system (ELS) network learn the manifestations of individual calcifications, clusters of calcifications, and clinical manifestations. Complex features are formed to interconnect the ELSs. There are a number of possible ways to network classification systems and complex features. For each ELS, supervised cases are stored so that the probability of a new test case being benign or malignant may be determined.

Results.—The best of 5 different ELS network configurations recognized 9 of 10 cancer clusters and 9 of 15 benign clusters, for an accuracy of 72%. The probability of this system performing at random with an accuracy of 72% or greater is 0.0216.

Implications.—This work suggests that it is feasible to develop a network of OAs that can be used to diagnose breast cancer by integrating digital mammographic image processing. Considering how many women are screened, an automated diagnostic network of ELSs that provides even a modest improvement in diagnostic accuracy or speed would have considerable value.

▶ Expert systems are not likely to replace radiologists in the near future, but perhaps they can be applied in a manner to assist radiologists with interpretations. I am sure that at 1 time cardiologists did not believe electrocardiograms could be interpreted by computers, so let's not totally disregard the possibility that expert systems will someday be valuable in screening.—C.D. Maynard, M.D.

Application of Artificial Neural Network to Computer-Aided Diagnosis of Coronary Artery Disease in Myocardial SPECT Bull's-Eye Images

Fujita H, Katafuchi T, Uehara T, Nishimura T (Gifu University, Yanagido, Gifu, Japan; National Cardiovascular Center, Osaka, Japan)
J Nucl Med 33:272–276, 1992   7–38

Objective.—Because even experienced observers interpret nuclear images variably, even using the bull's-eye technique, the authors attempted to develop a computerized system that can aid the detection and classification of coronary artery disease in thallium 201 SPECT bull's-eye images.

Methods.—The technique is based on a multilayer feed-forward neural network with a backpropagation algorithm. Thirty-six planar images of 64×64 matrix and 64 gray levels are acquired with a gamma camera, and the data are transferred to a data-processing system that produces 3 types of bull's-eye image at the same time: the original image, an image showing only the extent area of disease relative to the averaged normal case, and another showing the severity within the extent area. Image patterns are input into the network, where "synapses" connect neurons in the input layer and in a hidden layer, as well as those in the hidden and output layers. A "teacher" signal is given to the network, and the backpropagation technique modifies weight values to minimize errors in the output layer (a "training" process). The network becomes increasingly clever after repeated training procedures and begins recognizing patterns correctly, even those never used in the training process.

Results.—The neural network performs better than a radiology resident but not as well as an experienced radiologist. The results appeared to depend on the variety of training examples utilized.

Conclusions.—The neural network approach may prove useful for the computer-aided diagnosis of coronary artery disease from myocardial SPECT images.

▶ The use of artificial neural networks for image interpretation will be tested with many types of studies in the future. As the previous article concluded, computers and specialized software can't beat the radiologist yet but can help the interpreter. The amount of assistance provided by such systems depends on the expertise of the reader. In this study the system did better than the residents tested.—C.D. Maynard, M.D.

Risks in Radiology

A Survey of Risk Factors for Adverse Reactions to Intravenous Contrast Media

Sachinwalla T, Godfrey C, Palmer J (Prince Henry Hospital; Prince of Wales Hospital, Sydney, NSW, Australia)
Australas Radiol 35:106–108, 1991   7–39

Background.—Previous surveys of reactions to intervenously administered contrast media found that patients with identified risk factors and those receiving conventional ionic media were more likely to have adverse reactions than patients without risk factors and those receiving nonionic contrast media. Severe reactions were linked to the use of ionic medium, regardless of the presence of risk factors. The use of ionic vs. nonionic agents and the presence or absence of risk factors were estimated in many patients.

Methods.—Data were obtained from 13 public hospitals and 14 private practices in Australia. Returns were included from a total of 12,524 patients referred for CT or intravenous pyelography. Participants were asked to provide the patients' age, type of risk factor (if any) seen, and the type of contrast medium used.

Results.—Nonionic agents were used in 79.7%, and conventional ionic agents were used in 20.3% of the studies. Hospitals recorded the use of nonionic contrast medium in 90.6% of the patients. The presence of individual risk factors ranged from 1.4% (a previous contrast medium reaction) to 8.2% (asthma) (table).

Conclusions.—Because of the comparative high cost of nonionic contrast media, many radiologists have called for a demonstration of lower morbidity and mortality to justify this cost. Approximately 30% of patients in Australia have risk factors for adverse reactions. In addition, the risk for reactions increases with age. Patients with identified risk factors

Percentage Distribution of Individual Risk Factors

	Asthma	Hay Fever	Allergy	Previous CM Reaction	Cardiac Disease	Renal Disease	Diabetes
Hospital	7.5	3.3	6.2	1.1	6.2	2.5	3.5
Private Practice	8.6	4.2	7.8	1.6	6.0	0.9	2.3
Total	8.2	3.8	7.2	1.4	6.1	1.6	2.8

There were also 5 patients with multiple myeloma, 2 with pheochromocytoma, and 1 with sickle-cell anemia.
In 225 patients (1.8%), there was inadequate recording of risk factors.
In 2.9% of the hospital patients and .9% of the private practice patients, no history was obtainable because of coma, incapacity, language difficulties, etc.
(Courtesy of Sachinwalla T, Godfrey C, Palmer J: *Australas Radiol* 35:106–108, 1991.)

and those older than age 50 years constitute approximately 70% of the population, suggesting that the judicious course would be to use nonionic media in all patients.

▶ Palmer (from Australia) performed 1 of the first large clinical studies comparing the risks of nonionic and ionic agents (1). His group advocates the use of nonionic media for all patients. This issue is still much debated in the United States. The cost associated with 100% use of nonionics is the problem; if there were no difference in cost, universal use would occur quickly (2, 3).—C.D. Maynard, M.D.

References

1. Palmer FJ: *Australas Radiol,* 32:426, 1988.
2. Steinberg EP, et al: N Engl J Med 326:425, 1992.
3. Barrett BJ, et al: *Radiology* 183:105, 1992.

AIDS Risk and Risk Reduction in the Radiology Department
Wall SD, Olcott EW, Gerberding JL (Univ of California, San Francisco Gen Hosp, San Francisco)
AJR 157:911–917, 1991   7–40

Introduction.—With the predicted growth in the number of patients with AIDS in the United States, the risk of transmission of HIV to health care workers will increase in the coming years. The risk of occupational acquisition of HIV in the heath care setting was summarized and precautions to be taken in the radiology department were examined.

Occupational Risk.—By June 1991, 27 definite cases of occupational acquisition of HIV infection had been reported, 25 of which involved health care workers exposed to infected blood or blood-contaminated body fluids. Anecdotal case reports suggest that seroconversion usually occurs within 4 to 12 weeks after exposure and is accompanied by symptoms. Based on prospective cohort studies, the risk of infection after an accidental needle-stick injury is estimated to be 0.3% to 0.4%. The degree of risk probably depends on the volume of blood transferred and the concentration of HIV in the source fluid.

Precautions in the Radiology Department.—An infection control program is essential because HIV infection may not have been diagnosed in a patient and negative HIV test results are not 100% reliable. Most needle-stick injuries have been associated with the recapping of needles, a practice that is strongly discouraged. Needles and other sharp instruments must be disposed of immediately in a puncture-resistant container. Protective garb (e.g., gowns, gloves, and goggles), should be worn when blood or body fluids might splash. A readily available manual resuscitation bag avoids the need for mouth-to-mouth contact. Such procedures as plain film radiography, mammography, and CT and MRI when intravenously administered contrast media is not used generally require no HIV protection.

Conclusions.—Although the risk of HIV infection is low in radiologic procedures, the stakes are high. Protective procedures increase cost and time but are essential in certain settings. If exposure does occur, the exposed area should be washed immediately, and contaminated equipment should be disinfected. Azidothymidine treatment, if given after exposure, should be started within 1 hour.

▶ All radiologists should read this article. The risks associated with HIV infections in the radiology department are real, and with the increasing number of HIV-positive patients seen in radiology steadily increasing, these risks are worthy of attention.—C.D. Maynard, M.D.

Subject Index

Author Index

A Simple, Once-a-Year Dose!

Review the partial list of titles below. And then request your own FREE 30-day preview. When you subscribe to a Year Book, we'll also send you an automatic notice of future volumes about two months before they publish.

This system was designed for your convenience and to take up as little of your time as possible. If you do not want the Year Book, the advance notice makes it easy for you to let us know. And if you elect to receive the new Year Book, you need do nothing. We will send it on publication.

No worry. No wasted motion. And, of course, every Year Book is yours to examine FREE of charge for thirty days.

Year Book of **Anesthesia**® (22141)
Year Book of **Cardiology**® (22640)
Year Book of **Critical Care Medicine**® (22639)
Year Book of **Dermatology**® (22645)
Year Book of **Dermatologic Surgery**® (21171)
Year Book of **Diagnostic Radiology**® (22613)
Year Book of **Digestive Diseases**® (22625)
Year Book of **Drug Therapy**® (22630)
Year Book of **Emergency Medicine**® (22080)
Year Book of **Endocrinology**® (21174)
Year Book of **Family Practice**® (22124)
Year Book of **Geriatrics and Gerontology** (22611)
Year Book of **Hand Surgery**® (22618)
Year Book of **Hematology**® (22646)
Year Book of **Health Care Management**® (21177)
Year Book of **Infectious Diseases**® (22650)
Year Book of **Infertility** (22637)
Year Book of **Medicine**® (22638)
Year Book of **Neonatal-Perinatal Medicine** (22629)
Year Book of **Nephrology** (21175)
Year Book of **Neurology and Neurosurgery**® (22616)
Year Book of **Neuroradiology**® (21849)
Year Book of **Nuclear Medicine**® (22627)
Year Book of **Obstetrics and Gynecology**® (22636)
Year Book of **Occupational and Environmental Medicine** (22619)
Year Book of **Oncology** (22651)
Year Book of **Ophthalmology**® (22133)
Year Book of **Orthopedics**® (22644)
Year Book of **Otolaryngology – Head and Neck Surgery**® (22609)
Year Book of **Pathology and Clinical Pathology**® (21176)
Year Book of **Pediatrics**® (22130)
Year Book of **Plastic and Reconstructive Surgery**® (22635)
Year Book of **Psychiatry and Applied Mental Health**® (22649)
Year Book of **Pulmonary Disease**® (22624)
Year Book of **Sports Medicine**® (22111)
Year Book of **Surgery**® (22641)
Year Book of **Transplantation**® (21854)
Year Book of **Ultrasound** (21169)
Year Book of **Urology**® (22621)
Year Book of **Vascular Surgery**® (22612)

Mosby-Year Book, Inc. • 11830 Westline Industrial Drive • St. Louis, MO 63146